Y0-CCU-397

Basic Pediatric Nursing

Basic Pediatric Nursing

PERSIS MARY HAMILTON, R.N., P.H.N., B.S., M.S., Ph.D.

Associate Professor,
Associate Degree Nursing Program,
Napa College, Napa, California

FOURTH EDITION

*with **291** illustrations*

The C. V. Mosby Company

ST. LOUIS • TORONTO • LONDON   1982

MOSBY

A TRADITION OF PUBLISHING EXCELLENCE

Editor: Alison Miller
Assistant editor: Susan R. Epstein
Editing supervisor: Elaine Steinborn
Manuscript editor: Dale Woolery
Book design: Nancy Steinmeyer
Cover design: Diane Beasley
Production: Susan Trail

FOURTH EDITION

Copyright © 1982 by The C.V. Mosby Company

All rights reserved. No part of this book may be reproduced
in any manner without written permission of the publisher.

Previous editions copyrighted 1970, 1974, 1978

Printed in the United States of America

The C.V. Mosby Company
11830 Westline Industrial Drive, St. Louis, Missouri 63141

Library of Congress Cataloging in Publication Data

Hamilton, Persis Mary.
  Basic pediatric nursing.

  Bibliography: p.
  Includes index.
  1. Pediatric nursing. 2. Practical nursing.
I. Title. [DNLM: 1. Pediatric nursing. WY 159
H219b]
RJ245.H28 1982   610.73′62   81-18887
ISBN 0-8016-2040-6   AACR2

GC/VH/VH 9 8 7 6 5 4 3 2   03/D/357

Preface

Basic Pediatric Nursing was originally written to provide practical-vocational nurses with a comprehensive textbook in pediatric nursing suitable for their functional role on the pediatric team. Since the first edition the purpose has not changed but the practice of pediatric nursing and the health care delivery system have changed. Scientific knowledge in pathophysiology, genetics, psychology, and therapeutics has expanded. Humanistic values and social concerns have been applied to the care of children, especially in regard to family relationships. Economic necessities have shortened hospital stays and produced an expansion of outpatient services. The nursing profession has made progress in defining its roles in terms of the nursing process. A new edition of a textbook offers an opportunity to incorporate these changes in knowledge, values, and approaches into the revision and at the same time keep and refine the best of former editions. To that end, every portion of the text has been evaluated and changed to reflect current practice, while the original outline has remained the same.

The book is divided into five units: Pediatrics in Perspective; Growing, Developing Children and Their Health; Illness, Children, and Their Hospital Care; Disorders Common to Children and Their Care; and Children in Society. Each chapter includes a vocabulary list, summary outline, and study questions. Each unit is followed by a list of references, and the text is made more useful by a detailed index of its contents.

I am grateful to the many persons who have contributed their considerable knowledge and experience to the revision of this edition, to the faculty members who have reviewed it, and to the students who have made suggestions for change. Particularly, I wish to acknowledge Louise Burkett Snead, Assistant Director of Nursing, Children's Hospital Medical Center of Northern California. Her contributions and counsel have been invaluable in bringing this edition to fruition.

Persis Mary Hamilton

Contents

Pediatrics in perspective

1
Changing concepts of child care

VOCABULARY

Pediatrics
Infanticide
Quarantine
Child labor
Children's Bureau
White House conferences
UNICEF

THE SCOPE OF PEDIATRICS

Pediatrics is the study and care of children in sickness and in health. The word *pediatrics* comes from the Greek and means "child-cure." This field is one of the broadest and most fascinating of all of the medical specialties because it includes a study of the growth and development of a total person from conception through adolescence, as well as the prevention, diagnosis, and treatment of disorders affecting children during their growing years.

The medical doctor who specializes in pediatrics is called a *pediatrician.* A host of other professional persons work together with the pediatrician, including geneticists, biochemists, laboratory and prosthesis technicians, psychologists, surgeons, educators, orthodontists, physical, occupational, and inhalation therapists, dietitians, pediatric associates, and public health registered and licensed nurses and aides. These persons all form the modern pediatric team whose goal is to prevent disease and promote maximum health in every child.

HISTORICAL PERSPECTIVE

The current status of child care is part of a great historical pageant that has involved the cultures of many peoples. To appreciate more fully the present and respond to the challenge of the future, the pediatric nurse should know something of what has happened in the past. Such a historical perspective cannot fail to heighten enthusiasm and deepen respect for the study of pediatrics.

3

Ancient world
Prehistoric times (before 3000 BC)

Little is known about life in prehistoric times before written records were made, but it is believed that child care was somewhat like that still found in isolated tribes living in the world today. In these groups, the individuals of each generation follow the prescribed pattern of life taught to them by their parents in endless repetition with little variation until some catastrophe destroys or alters their lives. Because of the hostile environment in which the tribe exists, the good of the whole must come before that of the individual. As a result, babies who are undesirable in any way may be allowed to die. Such babies are those born with defects, those born under the wrong sign or at the wrong time of year, or those who are of an unwanted sex. Tribal life of the surviving children is one that modern psychologists might consider ideal. While they are infants, they are held or carried by their mothers almost continuously, fed at the breast, watched and fostered, carefully taught the customs, beliefs, skills, and history of the tribe, and protected and included as members of the whole. Children learn a strong dependency on the group and in turn gain the security of knowing they belong.

Although every tribe differs from the next, in most, childhood is a period of relative freedom and preparation for adulthood. At puberty, children take on the full responsibility of adults, sometimes by means of harrowing puberty rites. Girls marry and are expected to produce children and to feed and care for their family. Boys become hunters and warriors and father future generations, thus continually repeating the cycle.

Ancient civilizations (3000 BC to 500 AD)

In the ancient civilizations of Egypt, India, and China, children were reared in the traditions passed down from the previous generation. Their education was usually limited to the social station and vocation of their parents—girls following their mothers, boys their fathers. So, for example, a scribe's son in ancient Egypt might begin his long years of tedious copying of hieroglyphs at 5 years of age. Peasants' sons became farmers, artisans' sons become artisans, kings' sons became kings.

The practice of medicine combined both medical knowledge and magic. In such old writings as the Papyrus Ebers, written about 1500 BC, there are prescriptions for the treatment of urinary ailments in children. In China, herbalists compounded complex formulas for the treatment of childhood fevers and convulsions. Smallpox vaccination was first done in ancient China and India. Among the ancient Jews the hygienic measures prescribed by the Mosaic Law greatly influenced maternal and child care. Parenthood was honored, the individual's life was held sacred, and large families were considered a blessing of God.

Adoption of orphaned children and the continuation of the family name held an important place in the ancient cultures. The Babylonian Code of Hammurabi included a well-defined contractural relation between children and their adoptive parents. Jewish law made careful provision for orphaned or widowed family members. In the fourth century BC in Greece, funds were provided for the orphans of soldiers and for their free medical care. Japanese history records a charitable concern for its orphans, and early Christian teaching stated that "Pure religion and undefiled before God and the Father is this, To care for the fatherless and the widow . . ." (James 1:26).

Medical care for mothers and children was an early concern. Hippocrates wrote much on child care, and in the first century AD Celsus reportedly was the first to state that children require different treatment from that of adults. Soranus, an obstetrician and gynecologist of the same century, was a pioneer in the treatment of diseases of mothers and children.

Even though there was concern for the lives and well-being of children in the ancient cultures, there was also a widespread acceptance of infanticide as a means to eliminate defective children and to limit family size. Roman law gave fathers absolute authority over their children, including administration of cruel punishments, imprisonment, death, or their sale into slavery. The humane teachings of the Greek and Roman Stoics, the Hebrews, and later the Christians played an important part in the development of a new philosophy of the sanctity of human life. The child's lot was better in cultures when regarded as a valuable individual and not merely as an old-age insurance policy for the parents.

In the Western world Christianity became the official religion and the Roman Catholic Church became the repository of scholarly work and the administrator of charitable and medical care. Its teachings of care for the sick and helpless motivated continued medical progress, but advances did not go on unhampered. Wars, invasions from barbaric tribes, and the burning of great libraries destroyed valuable records, and arguments over church doctrine impeded progress. Some scholarly works were preserved by being hidden away in monasteries to be unearthed in later years.

Medieval world (450 to 1350 AD)

In Europe, wars and epidemics swept back and forth across the land, leaving great sickness, suffering, and death in their wake. Religious orders sprang up to meet the many human needs. Noble women gave their money and time to relieve the suffering. Leprosy, plague, influenza, and smallpox were the most prevalent diseases. The death rate was appallingly high among children, especially in the city slum areas. One fourth the entire population is believed to have died in the pandemic of "Black Death" in 1347. To forestall the spread of the disease, the chief maritime cities of the Mediterranean Sea adopted a 40-day detention period for all vessels entering their ports, or a *quaranta*. From this word is derived the modern term *quarantine*.

Although the religious temples of the ancient peoples had long been centers for healing, the first infant asylum or hospital was founded in Italy in 787. This one and others like it were not hospitals in the modern sense but were shelters for abandoned children. Because of a lack of understanding of sanitation and low standards of nursing care, conditions in these foundling homes were extremely poor. In fact, the general level of public health for the entire population was low, the death rate high, and misery the way of life for a vast majority of the population.

Renaissance and early modern world (1350 to 1800 AD)

During the period called the *Renaissance* many changes took place to alter the course of human life from the static medieval social patterns that had held sway for hundreds of years. A middle class gradually emerged and world commerce developed. The dissemination of knowledge was enhanced as a result of the spread to Europe of two Chinese inventions—printing and the manufacture of paper. Two medical books that greatly influenced the practice of pediatric medicine were published in the sixteenth century. Thomas Phaer, the father of English pediatrics, wrote *The Boke of Children*, and in Germany Felix Würtz wrote *The Children's Book*. Another figure who was influential in arousing public interest in the care of children was St. Vincent de Paul, who lived from 1576 to 1660. He is called the patron saint of orphans.

The latter part of the early modern period is called the *Industrial Revolution* because of the rapid expansion of industry from small home workshops to large machine-powered factories. These factories employed large numbers of people in incredibly dangerous and inhuman conditions for very low wages. As a result, people were crowded together in unsanitary rooms. To survive, every member of the family was forced to work, including children as young as 6 years of age, for 10 or more hours a day, 6 days a week. Accidents, sickness, and death were common. Not until far into the nineteenth century were laws passed that prohibited the worst evils of child labor.

Despite the deplorable conditions in the industrial cities of England and western Europe, many advances in the sciences, medicine, literature, and political thought were made. In England, Jenner developed the smallpox vaccine. Harvey discovered the circulation of blood. The microscope, obstetrical forceps, and clinical thermometer were invented. Rousseau wrote his famous book, *Emile*, which included a section on the rights of children and another on the hygiene and nutrition of infants.

Modern world (1800 AD to the present)
Scientific and social advances

The Industrial Revolution of the late eighteenth century ushered in a period of unprecedented change that has continued up to the present. During this time people made great progress in conquering disease, hunger, thirst, ignorance, superstition, isolation, and exposure to the elements. These remarkable changes are a result of the coincidence of two facts of history: the mushrooming of scientific knowledge and the flourishing of humanistic social ideals.

People have always been curious about themselves and the world around them. Ancient peoples studied the heavens and gained much knowledge about astronomy. They sailed the oceans and explored distant lands. Yet they were always hemmed in by superstitious prejudice or political control. When these hindrances were lessened by the new intellectual climate of the Renaissance, people were able to make observations, to ask questions of what, how, and why, to perform experiments, and to leave their findings for others. As a result, the modern world has seen scientific advances never before possible in human history.

The second fact of history that worked together with scientific advance to produce change in the modern world was humanitarianism—a widespread acceptance of the idea that all people are created with an inherent dignity and value. This concept revolutionized the Western world and politically blossomed into democratic and socialistic forms of government. Practically, it focused attention on the need to improve the lot of ordinary people, thus producing social advances.

From scientific advances came knowledge of the human body and the diseases that afflict it, and new medical techniques for treating those diseases. These advances alone, however, would not have benefited the general population. From the social advance of democratic societies came concern for public health. As a result, the new medical techniques have been applied to the needs of all adults and children on an ever-widening scale.

Some of the most notable applications of scientific knowledge to public health include the purification of water supplies and sanitary waste and sewage disposal; pasteurization of commercial milk supplies; testing of milk cows for tuberculosis; immunization programs against many communicable diseases; development and mass production of antibiotic and other drugs; maternal and child health programs that include free food and medical care; laws to control child labor, child abuse, and adoption and food and drug production; inspection of hospitals and child-care facilities; accident prevention programs; counseling and recreation programs; legal aid; and many more. In the world today a country is judged according to the degree to which it has "developed" these public health and welfare measures along with its industry and commerce.

Child care in the United States

When the United States was young most children lived in rural areas. The level of nutrition, health, and education was not high, but it was considerably better than that found in the crowded slums of big cities. There child mortality was high as a result of disease and malnutrition. Milk from tuberculous cows caused many cases of tuberculosis among children. The condition of neglected children aroused public sympathy, and many charitable organizations were formed to provide for their needs. A few of the most outstanding milestones in child welfare in the United States are listed in Table 1-1.

Table 1-1. Milestones in child welfare

United States

1820	First nursery school established for working mothers in Harmony, Ind.
1836	First child labor law
1855	Children's Hospital in Philadelphia, first pediatric hospital in U.S.
1870	Elementary Education Act to provide free public education for children
1881	American Red Cross established
1893	Henry Street Settlement established by Lillian Wald in New York, N.Y.
1897	First publicly supported visiting nurse in Los Angeles, Calif.
1899	First juvenile court in United States in Cook Co., Ill.
1902	First school nurses in New York, N.Y.
1904	National Tuberculosis Association founded
1908	First municipal unit for child health organized in New York, N.Y.
1912	Children's Bureau established
1917	First Federal Child Labor Law passed
1918	Children's Year
1918	United Community Funds and Councils of American formed
1919	First law for statewide care of handicapped children in Ohio
1927	First medical social worker in health department of Los Angeles Co., Calif.
1932	Premature infant care program begun under city support in Chicago, Ill.
1935	Social Security Act passed
1938	National Foundation for Infantile Paralysis founded
1950	National Association for Mental Health and National Association for Retarded Children founded
1953	Federal Department of Health, Education, and Welfare established
1966	Child Nutrition Act passed
1966	Child Protection Act passed
1968	Child Abuse Law passed
1973	Bill of Rights for Foster Children
1979	Federal Department of Health and Human Services and Department of Education established

White House conferences

1909	White House Conference on Dependent Children
1919	White House Conference on Child Welfare Standards
1930	White House Conference on Child Health and Protection, *The Children's Charter* and *Bill of Rights for Handicapped Child* adopted
1940	White House Conference on Children in a Democracy
1950	Midcentury White House Conference on Children and Youth, *Pledge to Children* adopted
1960	Golden Anniversary White House Conference on Children and Youth
1970	White House Conference on Children and Youth amid a Changing Social Scene
1980	White House Conference on Families

Worldwide

1902	Pan-American Sanitary Bureau founded
1946	United Nations organized
1946	United Nations International Children's Fund (UNICEF) created by United Nations
1948	First World Health Assembly; World Health Organization (WHO) established
1948	Founding of the World Federation for Mental Health; *Declaration of Human Rights* adopted by the U.N. General Assembly
1949	International Children's Center established in Paris, France
1959	*Declaration of the Rights of the Child* adopted by the U.N. General Assembly
1960	International Health Research Act enacted
1979	International Year of the Child

White House conferences. The need for a nationwide attack on the many problems faced by children was recognized in 1909 when President Theodore Roosevelt called the first White House Conference on Children and Youth. A similar conference has been held every 10 years since that time. At the 1930 White House Conference on Child Health and Protection, *The Children's Charter* was drawn up. It is considered to be one of the most important documents in the history of child care. (See pp. 8-10.)

Children's Bureau. As a result of the first White House conference, The Children's Bureau was founded in 1912 by an act of Congress. It was placed under the jurisdiction of the Department of Labor because at that time child labor was believed to be the greatest problem of children. With the nation's growth, the scope and responsibilities of the bureau have been greatly expanded to include youths and families. Its present functions are described in Chapter 20.

THE CHILDREN'S CHARTER OF 1930

President Hoover's White House Conference on Child Health and Protection, 1930, recognizing the rights of the child as the first rights of citizenship, pledges itself to these aims for the children of America:

I

For every child spiritual and moral training to help him to stand firm under the pressure of life

II

For every child understanding and the guarding of his personality as his most precious right

III

For every child a home and that love and security which a home provides; and for that child who must receive foster care, the nearest substitute for his own home

IV

For every child full preparation for his birth, his mother receiving prenatal, natal, and postnatal care; and the establishment of such protective measures as will make child-bearing safer

V

For every child health protection from birth through adolescence, including: periodical health examinations and, where needed, care of specialists and hospital treatment; regular dental examinations and care of the teeth; protective and preventive measures against communicable diseases; the ensuring of pure food, pure milk, and pure water

VI

For every child from birth through adolescence, promotion of health, including health instruction and health program, wholesome physical and mental recreation, with teachers and leaders adequately trained

VII

For every child a dwelling-place safe, sanitary, and wholesome, with reasonable provisions for privacy; free from conditions which tend to thwart his development; and a home environment harmonious and enriching

VIII

For every child a school which is safe from hazards, sanitary, properly equipped, lighted, and ventilated. For younger children nursery schools and kindergartens to supplement home care

IX

For every child a community which recognizes and plans for his needs; protects him against physical dangers, moral hazards, and disease; provides him with safe and wholesome places for play and recreation; and makes provision for his cultural and social needs

X

For every child an education which, through the discovery and development of his individual abilities, prepares him for life and through training and vocational guidance prepares him for a living which will yield him the maximum of satisfaction

XI

For every child such teaching and training as will prepare him for successful parenthood, homemaking, and the rights of citizenship and, for parents, supplementary training to fit them to deal wisely with the problems of parenthood

XII

For every child education for safety and protection against accidents to which modern conditions subject him—those to which he is directly exposed and those which, through loss or maiming of his parents, affect him directly

XIII

For every child who is blind, deaf, crippled, or otherwise physically handicapped and for the child who is mentally handicapped, such measures as will early discover and diagnose his handicap, provide care and treatment, and so train him that he may become an asset to society rather than a liability. Expenses of these services should be borne publicly where they cannot be privately met

XIV

For every child who is in conflict with society the right to be dealt with intelligently as society's charge, not society's outcast; with the home, the school, the church, the court, and the institution when needed, shaped to return him whenever possible to the normal stream of life

XV

For every child the right to grow up in a family with an adequate standard of living and the security of a stable income as the surest safeguard against social handicaps

Continued.

THE CHILDREN'S CHARTER OF 1930—cont'd

XVI

For every child protection against labor that stunts growth, either physical or mental, that limits education, that deprives children of the right of comradeship, of play, and of joy

XVII

For every rural child as satisfactory schooling and health services as for the city child, and an extension to rural families of social, recreational, and cultural facilities

XVIII

To supplement the home and the school in the training of youth, and to return to them those interests of which modern life tends to cheat children, every stimulation and encouragement should be given to the extension and development of the voluntary youth organizations

XIX

To make everywhere available these minimum protections of the health and welfare of children, there should be a district, county, or community organization for health, education, and welfare, with full-time officials, coordinating with a statewide program which will be responsive to a nationwide service of general information statistics, and scientific research. This should include:

(a) Trained, full-time public health officials, with public health nurses, sanitary inspection, and laboratory workers

(b) Available hospital beds

(c) Full-time public welfare service for the relief, aid, and guidance of children in special need due to poverty, misfortune, or behavior difficulties, and for the protection of children from abuse, neglect, exploitation, or moral hazard

FOR EVERY CHILD THESE RIGHTS, REGARDLESS OF RACE, OR COLOR, OR SITUATION, WHEREVER HE MAY LIVE UNDER THE PROTECTION OF THE AMERICAN FLAG.

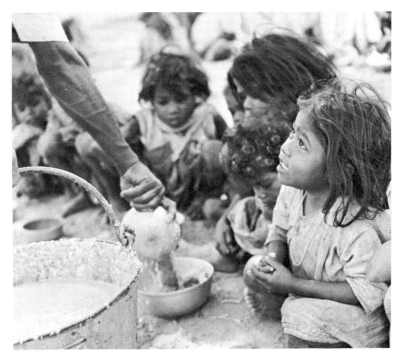

Fig. 1-1. A child waits for a bowl of corn-soy-milk powder provided by UNICEF during a famine in northern India in 1967. (Courtesy UNICEF; photograph by Mallica Vajrathon.)

Child care throughout the world

The societies of the world in the twentieth century show increasing concern for their most valuable asset—their children. In the industrialized countries of Europe, Asia, and the Americas, national programs for child health and welfare have been established to meet the unique needs of each country. In the developing countries of the world, international organizations, as well as national ones from the developed countries, have reached out to assist in raising the level of child care.

The chief international organization concerned with child welfare was established by the United Nations in 1946 as the United Nations International Children's Emergency Fund (UNICEF), primarily to meet the distress of children caused by widespread disasters (Fig. 1-1). In 1948 the World Health Organization (WHO) was established as the major international health organization. Since then the work of these organizations has been greatly expanded and is described in Chapter 20.

In addition to international organizations, various nations and individuals within nations have initiated projects to assist other peoples of the world. The Peace Corps, now a division of ACTION, is such a project. Paid for by United States taxpayers, technical advisors, medical personnel, and educators are sent into underdeveloped countries to work with the peoples to improve their lives. Project Hope, initially carried out aboard a hospital ship, is another such program (Fig. 1-2). It is devoted to medical teaching and treatment and is staffed and outfitted entirely by volunteers.

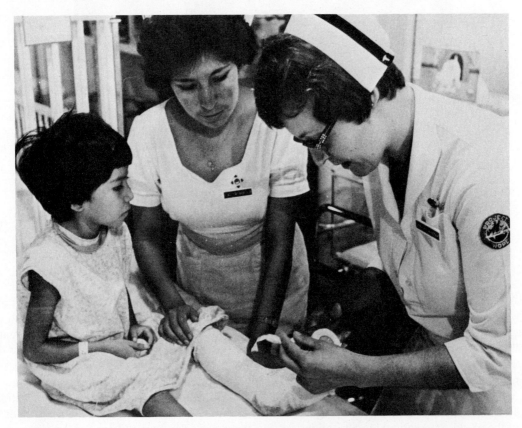

Fig. 1-2. An Ecuadorian nurse watches as her American counterpart bandages a young patient's leg aboard the S. S. HOPE at Guayaquil, Ecuador. (Courtesy Project Hope.)

DECLARATION OF THE RIGHTS OF THE CHILD
as approved unanimously by the Fourteenth General Assembly
of the United Nations, November 20, 1959

Preamble

Whereas the peoples of the United Nations have, in the Charter, reaffirmed their faith in fundamental human rights and in the dignity and worth of the human person, and have determined to promote social progress and better standards of life in larger freedom,

Whereas the United Nations has, in the Universal Declaration of Human Rights, proclaimed that everyone is entitled to all the rights and freedoms set forth therein, without distinction of any kind, such as race, colour, sex, language, religion, political or other opinion, national or social origin, property, birth or other status,

Whereas the child by reason of his physical and mental immaturity, needs special safeguards and care, including appropriate legal protection, before as well as after birth,

Whereas the need for such special safeguards has been stated in the Geneva Declaration of the Rights of the Child of 1924, and recognized in the Universal Declaration of Human Rights and in the statutes of specialized agencies and international organizations concerned with the welfare of children,

Whereas mankind owes to the child the best it has to give,

Now therefore,

The General Assembly

Proclaims this Declaration of the Rights of the Child to the end that he may have a happy childhood and enjoy for his own good and for the good of society the rights and freedoms herein set forth, and calls upon parents, upon men and women as individuals, and upon voluntary organizations, local authorities and national Governments to recognize these rights and strive for their observance by legislative and other measures progressively taken in accordance with the following principles:

I

The child shall enjoy all the rights set forth in this Declaration. Every child, without any exception whatsoever, shall be entitled to these rights, without distinction or discrimination on account of race, colour, sex, language, religion, political or other opinion, national or social origin, property, birth or other status, whether of himself or of his family.

II

The child shall enjoy special protection, and shall be given opportunities and facilities, by law and by other means, to enable him to develop physically, mentally, morally, spiritually and socially in a healthy and normal manner and in conditions of freedom and dignity. In the enactment of laws for this purpose, the best interests of the child shall be the paramount considerations.

III

This child shall be entitled from his birth to a name and a nationality.

IV

The child shall enjoy the benefits of social security. He shall be entitled to grow and develop in health; to this end, special care and protection shall be provided both to him and to his

Continued.

DECLARATION OF THE RIGHTS OF THE CHILD—cont'd

mother, including adequate prenatal and post-natal care. The child shall have the right to adequate nutrition, housing, recreation and medical services.

V

The child who is physically, mentally or socially handicapped shall be given the special treatment, education and care required by his particular condition.

VI

The child, for the full and harmonious development of his personality, needs love and understanding. He shall, wherever possible, grow up in the care and under the responsibility of his parents, and, in any case, in an atmosphere of affection and of moral and material security; a child of tender years shall not, save in exceptional circumstances, be separated from his mother. Society and the public authorities shall have the duty to extend particular care to children without a family and to those without adequate means of support. Payment of State and other assistance towards the maintenance of children of large families is desirable.

VII

The child is entitled to receive education, which shall be free and compulsory, at least in the elementary stages. He shall be given an education which will promote his general culture, and enable him, on a basis of equal opportunity, to develop his abilities, his individual judgment, and his sense of moral and social responsibility, and to become a useful member of society.

The best interests of the child shall be the guiding principle of those responsible for his education and guidance; that responsibility lies in the first place with his parents.

The child shall have full opportunity for play and recreation, which shall be directed to the same purpose as education; society and the public authorities shall endeavour to promote the enjoyment of this right.

VIII

The child shall in all circumstances be among the first to receive protection and relief.

IX

The child shall be protected against all forms of neglect, cruelty and exploitation. He shall not be the subject of traffic, in any form.

The child shall not be admitted to employment before an appropriate minimum age; he shall in no case be caused or permitted to engage in any occupation or employment which would prejudice his health or education, or interfere with his physical, mental or moral development.

X

The child shall be protected from practices which may foster racial, religious and any other form of discrimination. He shall be brought up in a spirit of understanding, tolerance, friendship among peoples, peace and universal brotherhood, and in full consciousness that his energy and talents should be devoted to the service of his fellow men.

The guiding principles behind all these efforts were set forth by the United Nations General Assembly in 1959 in the historic *Declaration of the Rights of the Child* (see pp. 13-14).

SUMMARY OUTLINE

I. The scope of pediatrics
II. Historical perspective
  A. Ancient world
    1. Prehistoric times (before 3000 BC)
    2. Ancient civilizations (3000 BC to 500 AD)
  B. Medieval world (450 to 1350 AD)
  C. Renaissance and early modern world (1350 to 1800 AD)
  D. Modern world (1800 AD to the present)
    1. Scientific and social advances
    2. Child care in the United States
      a. White House conferences
      b. Children's Bureau
    3. Child care throughout the world

STUDY QUESTIONS

1. Identify a medically significant event during each of the following time periods: ancient civilizations, medieval world, Renaissance, modern world.
2. What two facts of history, coming together, caused the remarkable advances in public health and welfare in modern times?
3. Compare *The Children's Charter* of 1930 and *The Declaration of the Rights of the Child* of 1959. What do they have in common? How do they differ? Why are they significant?

REFERENCES

Deloughery, G.L.: History and trends of professional nursing, ed. 8, St. Louis, 1977, The C.V. Mosby Co.

Johnston, D.F.: History and trends of practical nursing, St. Louis, 1966, The C.V. Mosby Co.

Shippen, K.B.: Pool of knowledge: how the United Nations share their skills, rev. ed., New York, 1965, Harper & Row, Publishers.

Sigerist, H.A.: A history of medicine, 2 vols., New York, 1951, 1961, Oxford University Press, Inc.

Growing, developing children and their health

2
Characteristics of growth and development

VOCABULARY

Maturation
Karyography
Pubertal spurt
Ossification
Dentition
Prehension
Mental age
Parallel play

The chief difference between children and adults is that the child is still growing. This fact influences every aspect of child care. For this reason a knowledge of human growth and development is basic to pediatric nursing, including the general principles that govern growth, the understanding of physical and psychological growth, and the role of play in the development of the child.

GENERAL PRINCIPLES OF GROWTH

Normal growth from birth to adulthood is characterized by certain general observations that have been found to be true for all healthy children. These principles may be stated as follows: Growth continues from the moment of conception in an orderly sequence, as a total process, involving the whole child; although growth is continuous, it occurs in spurts and rest periods, with each child following a unique timetable and with various body structures within each child growing at different rates. This general statement can be divided into four separate principles, as follows.

Continuous growth

Growth occurs continuously from conception onward, but it is not even or regular. There are spurts when growth is greatly accelerated, followed by rest periods when it is slowed. Growth is greatest during prenatal life and is still rapid during infancy and early childhood. It slows but continues during middle childhood; then there is a growth spurt during early puberty that tapers off in late adolescence. Growth never really stops until maximum size is reached.

Variable rates

Growth rates vary from child to child, from time to time, and from body structure to body structure. There are periods of rapid growth and periods of relatively little growth in each child, but all children have their own unique timetable and their own ultimate size. The tendency for children to be larger or smaller than other children their own age remains fairly constant. The body structures are likewise independent from one another in their growth patterns. The genitalia remain small and undeveloped until early puberty, whereas the brain attains its adult size when the child is about 7 years of age.

Orderly sequence

Normal growth follows an orderly sequence. The increase in size of children proceeds without interruption. Even if they may seem to grow rapidly, they never skip a stage. In like manner, children increasingly develop the capacity to use their bodies. They do simple things and then more complex ones. For example, they first learn to roll over, then to get up onto their hands, then to creep, then stand, and then walk. Even though they still know how to do the more simple things, they will go on to more and more complex activities.

Total process

Growth is a total process involving the whole child. All of the various parts of a child are growing at the same time. The mind and emotions do not grow one day and then the physical body the next. The child develops as a whole being, physically, mentally, emotionally, and socially. Physical growth affects interests and abilities, and the child passes from one stage of life to the next in a total progression of growth and development.

PHYSICAL GROWTH AND MOTOR DEVELOPMENT
Terminology

The word *growth* refers to the increasing size of the physical structure of the body. It is measured by inches and pounds or centimeters and kilograms. When growth stops, the ultimate size is called the *extent of growth* and depends on inherited traits, adequate nutrition, a balance of hormones, and a number of environmental factors.

The *rate of growth* is the amount of growth measured within a given time. Growth is a continuous process, but all normal children experience well-defined periods when the growth rate changes. These are called *periods of growth* and include the rapid growth of prenatal life, the still rapid growth of infancy and early childhood, the period of slow but uniform growth during middle childhood, the growth spurt of early puberty, and the period when growth tapers off in a late puberty. When a series of growth periods in a given child is considered at one time, the total picture is called a *growth pattern*.

All the body tissues and systems follow the general pattern described by these periods of growth, with three exceptions: (1) the nervous system grows most rapidly during infancy and reaches maximum size by puberty, (2) the reproductive system grows very slowly until the pubertal spurt that accompanies sexual maturity, and (3) lymphoid tissue grows at a greatly accelerated pace until the child is 12 years of age when it gradually shrinks to adult proportions.

The word *development* refers to the increasing capacity of children to use their bodies. It is inseparable from growth because the two go together, growth having to do with the physical structure of the body, development with its function. The *extent of development*, or the ultimate degree of achievement, depends on genetic inheritance, adequate nutrition, normal hormone activity, and a favorable emotional environment where the child can have satisfying experiences.

The *stages of development* are general divisions of life that are based on a consideration of the physical, emotional, intellectual, and social maturity of the child. There are a variety of names and groupings for these stages. One of the more detailed classifications identifies six stages of development as follows: (1) prenatal, from conception to birth; (2) infancy, from birth to walking alone; (3) toddler, from walking alone through 3 years of age; (4) preschool, 4 and 5 years of age; (5) early school age, from 6 years of age to puberty; and (6) adolescence, from puberty to adulthood.

Maturation is the total process whereby a child grows and develops according to individual inherited patterns of physical, mental, and emotional potential. *Maturity* means full or complete growth. It may be used in a general way to mean that a person is fully grown or mature in every area of life or it may refer to a single area of growth such as sexual maturity. Physical maturity is normally complete by 20 to 25 years of age. Emotional maturity and intellectual maturity are not as easily measured as the physical body, so assigning an age when such maturity is reached is more difficult. In normal individuals, however, it is generally expected that a certain level of emotional and intellectual maturity will have been attained by about the age of 25 years.

Measurement

Because growth is a highly individual process, the comparison of a child with others and with the child's own past growth is a valuable means of evaluating progress. One common method is to measure the child in various ways and to plot the results on graph paper. The resulting picture is usually an upward curving line called a *growth curve*. *Growth norms* are standardized average measurements that have been determined as a result of measuring thousands of children. These figures allow for a normal range of variation from the strict mathematical average. When growth norms are plotted on graph paper, the picture that results is called a standardized growth curve, or a growth chart. (Figs. 2-1 to 2-4 are standardized growth charts for full-term infants and healthy girls and boys. Fig. 11-1 is standardized for low birth weight infants.) The pediatrician uses growth charts to compare the growth of an individual child with the normal range indicated on the chart.

Growth is measured in a number of ways, including weight, height, body proportion, bone development, tooth development, and motor development. See Tables 2-1 and 2-2 for conversion of weight and height measurement systems. The nurse is expected to make these measurements and to understand their significance and what is considered normal for children of various ages.

Weight

Weight is influenced by all the other increases in body size and so is probably the best overall indication of nutrition and growth.

At birth most infants weigh between 6 and 9 lb (2.72 and 4.09 kg). After an initial weight loss of ½ to 1 pound during the first week of life, there is a steady gain of about 1 ounce (28 gm) a day. By 6 months of age the birth weight has doubled, and by 1 year of age it has tripled. After the first year the rate of gain drops and remains a steady 4 to 6 lb (1.8 to 2.72 kg) per year until preadolescence. Diet and exercise have a pronounced effect on the relative weight to height.

Rapid weight gain occurs in both boys and girls during puberty, corresponding to the gain in height. Girls begin their preadolescent growth spurt at about 10 to 12 years of age, reaching adult proportions about 16 to 18 years of age. Boys follow girls by 2 years, growing to be heavier and taller than girls as adults.

Text continued on p. 26.

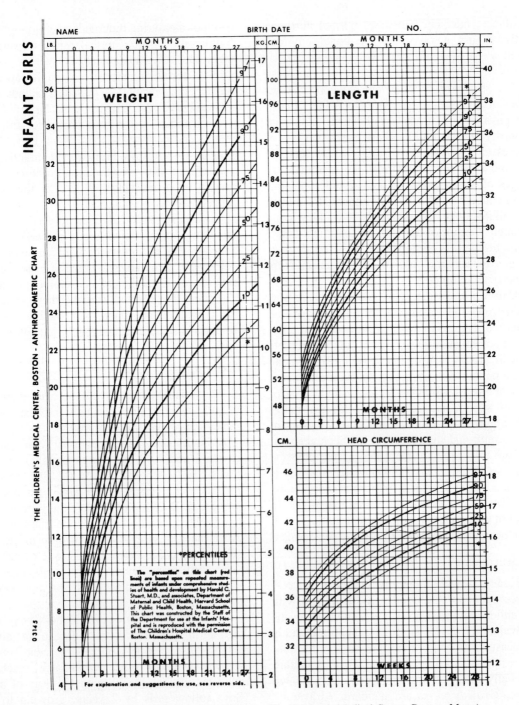

Fig. 2-1. Growth chart for infant girls. (Courtesy The Children's Medical Center, Boston, Mass.)

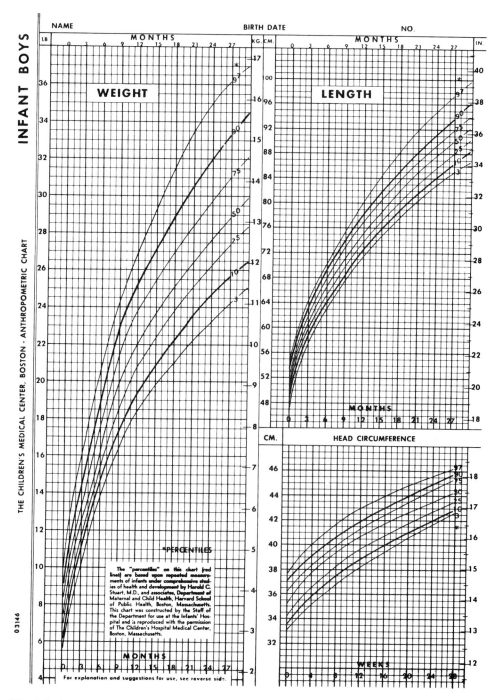

Fig. 2-2. Growth chart for infant boys. (Courtesy The Children's Hospital Medical Center, Boston, Mass.)

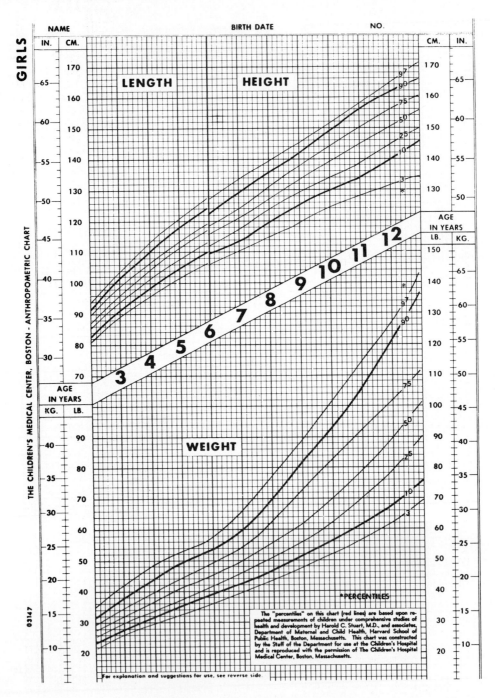

Fig. 2-3. Growth chart for girls. (Courtesy The Children's Hospital Medical Center, Boston, Mass.)

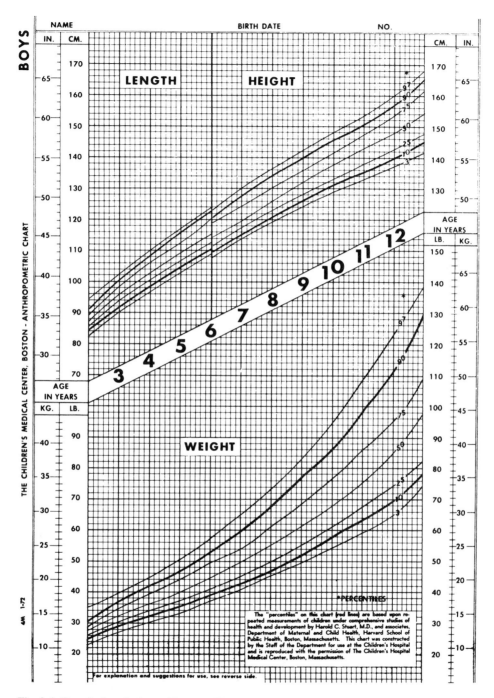

Fig. 2-4. Growth chart for boys. (Courtesy The Children's Hospital Medical Center, Boston, Mass.)

Table 2-1. Conversion of grams, kilograms, pounds, and ounces

| Grams | Kilograms | Avoirdupois | |
		Pounds	Ounces
1	0.001	22/10,000	35/1000
10	0.01	22/1000	35/100
28*	0.028	1/16	1
280	0.28	625/1000	10
454	0.454	1	16†
1000	1	2²/₁₀	35
4540	4.54	10	160
10,000	10	22	352

*28 grams = 1 ounce in the avoirdupois system. 30 grams = 1 ounce in the imperial system. 32 grams = 1 ounce in the household system.
†16 ounces = 1 pound in the avoirdupois system. 12 ounces = 1 pound in the imperial system.

Table 2-2. Conversion of centimeters, meters, inches, and feet (imperial system)

Centimeters	Meters	Inches	Feet
1	0.01	39/100	325/10,000
2.54	0.0254	1	12
30.48	0.304	12	1
100	1	39	3¼

Table 2-3. Typical growth pattern of height in children

Age (years)	Height increases
Birth to 1	10 in (25.4 cm)
1 to 2	5 in (12.7 cm)
2 to 6	3 in (7.6 cm) per year
6 to 10	3 in (7.6 cm) per year
10 to 20	A total of 5 to 16 in (12.7 to 40.6 cm) added during the pubertal spurt

Height

The average length of a newborn infant is about 20 inches (50.8 cm). The periods of most rapid growth are during infancy and puberty. Although there is a great variation between children, Table 2-3 shows the typical growth pattern of height in average children.

Birth height is usually doubled by 4 years of age and tripled by 13 years of age. In general, the height of an adult is about twice what it was in the same individual at 2 years of age. Men tend to be somewhat taller than this and women somewhat shorter.

Body proportions

One of the most obvious ways in which "a child is not a miniature adult" is in body proportions (Fig. 2-5). At birth the head is one fourth the total body length, whereas in the adult it is about one eighth the total body length. The arms and legs are relatively short and the chest and abdomen more barrel shaped. As growth proceeds, the midpoint of the total height moves from the umbilicus to the pubic bone, the chest flattens, and extremities grow longer.

During puberty, adult proportions are attained and the characteristic male and female contours develop. In girls, the hips become rounded, the breasts develop, and the skinny legs become more curved. In boys, the hips remain small, while the chest and shoulders broaden, and the abdominal fat of childhood disappears.

Body build varies from person to person so that one may be stocky, another tall and lanky, another petite, and still another large. Regardless of the body build, changes in the proportions of the body follow the same general pattern in all children.

Bone development

Of all the tissues in the body, bone exhibits the most dramatic changes; beginning in early fetal development as simple connective tissue, it later becomes cartilage. By about the fifth month of gestation, calcium and other minerals begin to

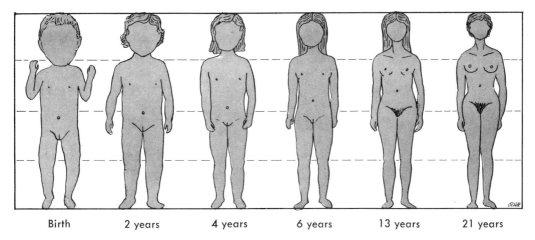

| Birth | 2 years | 4 years | 6 years | 13 years | 21 years |

Fig. 2-5. Changes in body proportions from birth to adulthood.

be deposited in certain areas of cartilage, called *ossification centers*, and the cartilage is gradually changed into bone. In the long bones, ossification begins in the shaft, or *diaphysis*, and moves out toward the end, *epiphysis*. Growth takes place at the ends by a continual thickening of the cartilage. Bone development is complete when the epiphysis and diaphysis fuse. See the discussion on bone formation on p. 446.

"Bone age" is the average osseous development for children of a given chronological age as determined by x-ray examination. By comparing an individual child's bone development with standardized bone-age studies, the child's skeletal growth can be evaluated.

The first ossification centers to appear after birth are those of the small bones of the wrist. These bones appear at about 6 months of age. Bone development is complete in girls at about 17 years of age and in boys at about 19 years of age.

Tooth development

Early in fetal life the foundations of the child's tooth structure are formed. At birth all the *deciduous*, or baby teeth, and the first *permanent* teeth, or 6-year molars, are developed in the child's jaw and covered by a fleshy gum. There

is great individual variation in the ages of *dentition*, or tooth eruption, but usually the lower center incisors erupt first at about 6 months of age. They are followed by the upper incisors, and by 2½ years of age all 20 deciduous teeth have usually appeared. A dormant period precedes the eruption of the first permanent teeth, the 6-year molars, during which all the permanent teeth are growing and maturing and the roots of the baby teeth are gradually absorbed and disappear. Only the crowns of the baby teeth are left when the permanent teeth fill the spaces. All 32 of the permanent teeth usually erupt by the age of 20 years.

It is important to maintain the health and retain the presence of each of the deciduous teeth because their condition directly affects the permanent teeth lying under them and their presence helps maintain spaces for the permanent teeth to fill.

Motor development

Motor development is the process whereby children learn to control and integrate their muscles in purposeful action. It is an indication of the degree of maturity of the nervous system.

When children are born they are uncoordinated and helpless. Soon they learn to roll over,

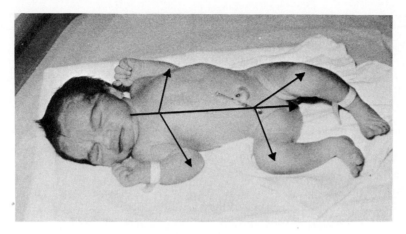

Fig. 2-6. Motor development is cephalocaudal and proximodistal.

sit up, stand alone, walk, reach out, and grasp objects. As with other aspects of growth, motor development proceeds in an orderly sequence, moving from the simple to the more complex. It characteristically begins in the head region and moves downward toward the feet in a *cephalocaudal* direction. Development also tends to proceed from the center of the body toward the extremities in a *proximodistal* direction (Fig. 2-6). Motor development is similar for all children, but each one progresses at an individual rate.

There are many motor skills that do not need to be taught; they just develop naturally as children gain increasing awareness of their surroundings and an increasing ability to control their muscles. Two of these skills are the ability to reach out and grasp an object and then do something with it called *prehension*, and the ability to move the body from place to place, called *locomotion*. Both of these skills proceed from the simple to complex, in an orderly sequence, and are usually accomplished by the time a child is 14 months of age. Mental retardation, nerve damage, or disease may delay the development of these motor skills.

The Denver Developmental Screening Test is a way of estimating the motor skills, language, and personal-social development of children up to 6 years of age. It is most useful with English-speaking children from the cultural mainstream of America (Figs. 2-7 and 2-8).

Influences on growth

As has already been indicated by the definitions of both physical growth and functional development, there are a number of factors affecting both the potential and the ultimate extent of a child's development. These include factors that are the result of inheritance, intrauterine life, birth environment, nutrition, and endocrine function. It should be remembered that the growth and development of a child from conception to adulthood is not simply the result of a single factor, but that it is the result of a combination of factors, including the child's reaction to and the result of interaction with these influences.

Inheritance

Inheritance plays an important part in the future growth and development of the child. It is responsible for many disorders. An understanding of its basic theory and practical application is of value to the nurse.

Transmission of traits. All the inherited characteristics and sex of a baby are fixed at the

DATE

NAME

DIRECTIONS   BIRTHDATE

HOSP. NO.

1. Try to get child to smile by smiling, talking or waving to him. Do not touch him.
2. When child is playing with toy, pull it away from him. Pass if he resists.
3. Child does not have to be able to tie shoes or button in the back.
4. Move yarn slowly in an arc from one side to the other, about 6" above child's face.
   Pass if eyes follow 90° to midline. (Past midline; 180°)
5. Pass if child grasps rattle when it is touched to the backs or tips of fingers.
6. Pass if child continues to look where yarn disappeared or tries to see where it went. Yarn
   should be dropped quickly from sight from tester's hand without arm movement.
7. Pass if child picks up raisin with any part of thumb and a finger.
8. Pass if child picks up raisin with the ends of thumb and index finger using an over hand
   approach.

9. Pass any enclosed form. Fail continuous round motions.
10. Which line is longer? (Not bigger.) Turn paper upside down and repeat. (3/3 or 5/6)
11. Pass any crossing lines.
12. Have child copy first. If failed, demonstrate

When giving items 9, 11 and 12, do not name the forms. Do not demonstrate 9 and 11.

13. When scoring, each pair (2 arms, 2 legs, etc.) counts as one part.
14. Point to picture and have child name it. (No credit is given for sounds only.)

        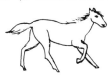

15. Tell child to: Give block to Mommie; put block on table; put block on floor. Pass 2 of 3.
    (Do not help child by pointing, moving head or eyes.)
16. Ask child: What do you do when you are cold? ..hungry? ..tired? Pass 2 of 3.
17. Tell child to: Put block on table; under table; in front of chair, behind chair.
    Pass 3 of 4. (Do not help child by pointing, moving head or eyes.)
18. Ask child: If fire is hot, ice is ?; Mother is a woman, Dad is a ?; a horse is big, a
    mouse is ?. Pass 2 of 3.
19. Ask child: What is a ball? ..lake? ..desk? ..house? ..banana? ..curtain? ..ceiling?
    ..hedge? ..pavement? Pass if defined in terms of use, shape, what it is made of or general
    category (such as banana is fruit, not just yellow). Pass 6 of 9.
20. Ask child: What is a spoon made of? ..a shoe made of? ..a door made of? (No other objects
    may be substituted.) Pass 3 of 3.
21. When placed on stomach, child lifts chest off table with support of forearms and/or hands.
22. When child is on back, grasp his hands and pull him to sitting. Pass if head does not hang back.
23. Child may use wall or rail only, not person. May not crawl.
24. Child must throw ball overhand 3 feet to within arm's reach of tester.
25. Child must perform standing broad jump over width of test sheet. (8-1/2 inches)
26. Tell child to walk forward, ⊂🔲⊃⊂🔲⊃➡ heel within 1 inch of toe.
    Tester may demonstrate. Child must walk 4 consecutive steps, 2 out of 3 trials.
27. Bounce ball to child who should stand 3 feet away from tester. Child must catch ball with
    hands, not arms, 2 out of 3 trials.
28. Tell child to walk backward, ⬅⊂🔲⊃⊂🔲⊃ toe within 1 inch of heel.
    Tester may demonstrate. Child must walk 4 consecutive steps, 2 out of 3 trials.

DATE AND BEHAVIORAL OBSERVATIONS (how child feels at time of test, relation to tester, attention
span, verbal behavior, self-confidence, etc,):

Fig. 2-7. Denver Developmental Screening Test items. The child's capacity to perform each of the 28 tasks is compared with standardized norms given on the scoring sheet. (Courtesy William K. Frankenburg, M.D., University of Colorado Medical Center, Colo.)

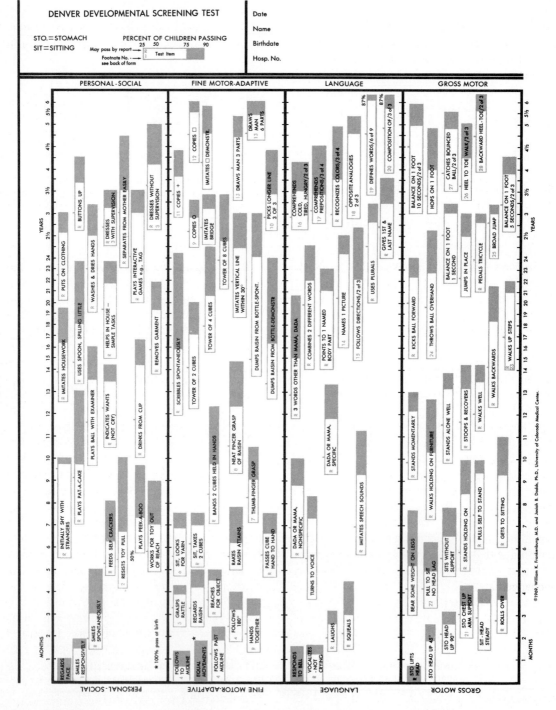

Fig. 2-8. Denver Developmental Screening Test scoring sheet. The child's capacity to perform each of the 28 tasks is compared with standardized norms given on the scoring sheet. (Courtesy William K. Frankenburg, M.D., University of Colorado Medical Center, Colo.)

moment of conception when the male sex cell, the sperm, enters the female sex cell, the ovum. At that time the two cells, with their 23 chromosomes each, fuse to form the first cell that will later divide into trillions of differentiated cells that will make a new individual. Each one of those trillions of cells, whatever its function, will contain a nucleus with 46 chromosomes that are exactly like the original 46. The chromosomes, or colored bodies, are the means whereby inherited traits are passed from generation to generation. The basic units of the chromosomes are the genes. The genes are arranged along the chromosomes like beads on a string, each occupying a definite and constant position called a *locus*. Every human characteristic is produced by a pair of genes, one from the mother and one from the father. At cell division the 23 chromosomes from the mother pair off with the corresponding 23 chromosomes from the father, causing the pairs of genes to lie opposite each other. If the two genes produce exactly the same characteristic, such as blue eyes, the genes are called *homozygous* and the child will have blue eyes. If the genes are contrasting, such as one for blue and one for brown, the genes are called *heterozygous* and the brown one will assert itself as being dominant over the recessive one, thus causing the child's eyes to be brown. The child, however, will be a carrier of the recessive blue eye gene and can pass that gene on. In this manner a defect may be passed from generation to generation, never appearing until, by chance, it is paired with a similar gene from the other parent. This phenomenon of the genes remaining unchanged and being passed on in a predictable pattern was first reported by Gregor Johannes Mendel (1822-1884), an abbot in a monastery in Moravia, and has since been called Mendel's law. By this law, when the father and mother carry a recessive gene, one fourth of their children will have a trait, two fourths will be carriers but not exhibit the trait, and one fourth will not carry the gene at all. A later geneticist, R. C. Punnett, developed a square to portray graphically Mendel's law (Fig. 2-9).

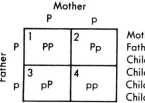

P = enzyme-producing gene, no disease (dominant)

p = no enzyme-producing gene, disease (recessive)

Mother: Pp (no disease)
Father: Pp (no disease)
Child 1: PP (no disease)
Child 2: Pp (no disease)
Child 3: pP (no disease)
Child 4: pp (PKU diseased)

Fig. 2-9. Punnett square demonstrating the application of Mendel's law of inheritance to the recessive trait that causes phenylketonuria (PKU) when both parents carry the trait but are not diseased. (PKU is discussed in Chapter 14.)

Genetics. In recent years geneticists have been able to photograph the nuclei of human cells and to enlarge them sufficiently to visualize the 46 chromosomes. This technique is called *karyography*, or "nucleus picturing." When the scrambled 46 chromosomes are clipped from the photograph and arranged into matching pairs from the largest to the smallest, the resulting picture is called a *karyogram*. An artist's drawing of this picture is called an *idiogram* (Fig. 2-10). A normal person has a karyogram that shows 22 pairs of chromosomes called *autosomes*, and one pair of *sex chromosomes*. In the female, pair 23 appears as XX. In the male, pair 23 consists of one X about the size of pair 12 and one Y, and the pair is designated XY.

Abnormalities. Karyogram studies have demonstrated that a number of serious birth defects are caused by abnormal forms or numbers of chromosomes (Fig. 2-10). One of the first autosome or nonsex chromosomes defects to be identified was a disorder called *trisomy 21*. This means that three chromosomes occur in the twenty-first place instead of two. Trisomy 21 causes a condition characterized by mental retardation and a typical oriental appearance, called Down's syndrome, or mongolism. Other autosomal defects have been identified, including trisomy 18, trisomy D_1, and mosaicism, a mixture of abnormal forms. All of these cause severe developmental defects.

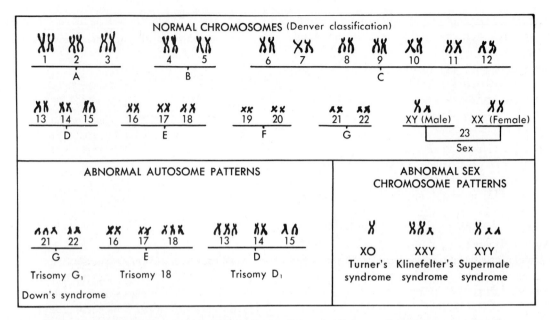

Fig. 2-10. Idiogram of normal chromosomes and some abnormal autosome and sex chromosome patterns.

Defects of the sex chromosomes are numerous. Among them is Turner's syndrome, a condition in which the second sex chromosome is missing and the person has a total of 45 instead of the normal number of 46 chromosomes. In these persons is neither XX as in girls, nor XY as in boys, but just one X. As a result the person has the body of a prepuberty girl throughout life, never maturing sexually.

Another well-known sex chromosome defect is called Klinefelter's syndrome. In this condition there may be a variety of abnormal sex chromosomes including XYY, XXY, XXYY, XXXYY, and so forth. The individual seems to have a male physique but does not develop normally. There are a great many other defects of the reproductive system that are the result of abnormal sex chromosome forms.

Another type of inherited characteristic is *sex linked*. This term means that the genes that cause these conditions are carried on the sex chromosomes. It has been found that the X sex chromosome carries a large number of genes whereas the Y of the male carries almost none. As a result recessive traits carried by the mother could appear in a son, because he does not have a matching X chromosome to carry a dominant gene. Hemophilia and color blindness are examples of sex-linked defects.

Genetic counseling. Scientific information about genetics and the causes of specific birth defects is increasing rapidly. Soon it will be possible for geneticists to study the genes and chromosomes of individuals and to diagnose those who are the carriers of defects and disease. Someday it may become standard practice for each person to have a genetic typing or chromosome study made. When these persons consider parenthood, they and their prospective mates would have a counseling session with a geneticist to discuss the potential offspring that might result in their union. The couple then would have the responsibility to decide whether they should bring children into the world. Such counseling is now available to a limited extent in large research centers (Fig. 2-11).

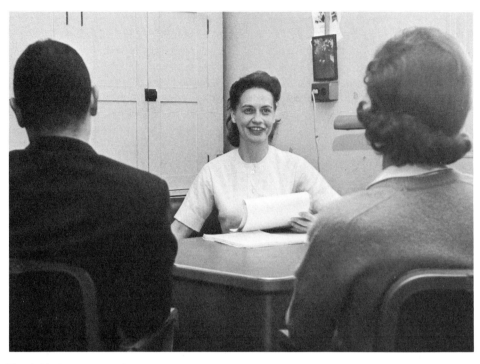

Fig. 2-11. A young married couple, who have had an infant with a major birth defect, confer with a genetic counselor physician over the advisability of having another child. (Courtesy The National Foundation–March of Dimes.)

Grouping of people. All humans are composed of the same biological stuff, all normally possess the same number of chromosomes, and all are classified by biologists as of the genus *Homo* and the species *sapiens*. The fact of human oneness is not universally understood. People are classified by their superficial physical differences into three major groupings called races—Negroid, Mongolian, and Caucasian. Further subdivisions are made according to nations, classes, and families. The similarities of those persons within their groups and their differences from people in other groups, however, are the result of inbreeding caused by geographic and social isolation rather than by any basic genetic difference between them. At the present time there are still large groups of people with very different physical characteristics from one another, but as people become more mobile and

mate freely, an infinite variety of human characteristics will result and the superficial differences between humans will be lessened.

Influence of sex. The influence of sex on the normal child is profound, not only regarding physical growth but also psychological and social development.

Boys are generally physically larger than girls from birth until about 10 to 12 years of age. At that time girls experience accelerated growth and approach their maximum height at about 16 years of age. Boys mature approximately 2 years later than girls but catch up with the girls by 16 years of age, and, passing them, continue to grow until about 21 years of age.

The social and psychological development of boys and girls is greatly affected by the culture in which they grow to maturity, because the roles of men and women may be defined in different terms. For example, the amount of physical exercise, outdoor activity, physical risk, and even the type of diet may be different for boys than for girls. Educational opportunity and social development, especially in the non-Western world, are frequently quite different for boys and girls.

Intrauterine life

A number of factors can affect the embryo after conception while it is still growing and developing within the mother. Such factors are placental defect, drugs taken, or diseases afflicting the mother.

Placental defects. During intrauterine life the developing fetus depends on the placenta for its supply of oxygen and nutrients and as a means to excrete wastes. Any defect or problem associated with the placenta directly threatens the life of the growing embryo. A number of such conditions may occur, including the inadequate or abnormal development of the placenta, its premature aging before the pregnancy has reached full term, and premature separation of the placenta before delivery.

Maternal effects. The "marking" of an unborn infant by the mother's thoughts or actions is an ancient belief. In recent years specific deformity-causing biological and chemical agents have been identified. These teratogenic agents are transported by way of the mother's bloodstream to the placenta and then to the embryo. They include many otherwise harmless drugs and some relatively minor pathogens. The embryo is most vulnerable during the first few weeks of development, when even a single dose of some drugs or a mild maternal infection may cause severe deformities. The virus of rubella was one of the first biological teratogenic agents to be recognized, but there is increasing evidence that implicates the pathogens of mumps, influenza, hepatitis, syphilis, and many others. The potential danger of drugs to a developing embryo has been widely recognized since 1961, when hundreds of babies were deformed as a result of their mothers' taking the tranquillizer thalidomide (Fig. 2-12). Dozens of other drugs have since been found to be teratogens. Endocrine disturbances in the mother (especially diabetes mellitus), blood type or Rh factor differences between the fetus and the mother, malnutrition, and cigarette smoking all affect the growth and development of the unborn child.

Birth

Although the birth process is an arduous experience for the infant, the effects are normally only temporary and future growth and development are not affected. Those few exceptions are related to oxygen deprivation and nerve injuries. If brain cells are without enough oxygen for even a few minutes, they die and permanent brain damage results. If the birth is difficult, there may be permanent injury to nerves causing muscle paralysis and a variety of serious developmental problems (see Fig. 18-6).

Environment and nutrition

When infants are born, they bring with them an inherited potential, a physical body, and an undeveloped personality. The environment into which they arrive and the diet they receive profoundly affect growth and development.

Environment is that which surrounds a child: the air, home, family, the presence of disease or danger, the emotional climate, and religious and social customs. All these influence a child's growth and development.

Adequate nutrition is essential to normal physical growth. This means enough of all the necessary dietary nutrients, the quality of the diet, not just enough food to fill an empty stomach. The essential nutrients and the result of an inadequacy are discussed in detail in Chapter 3.

Endocrine function

The endocrine glands play an important role in growth and development. These small ductless glands secrete their powerful hormones

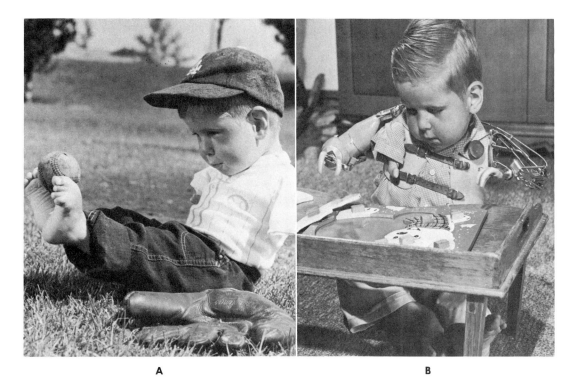

A   B

Fig. 2-12. Four-year-old congenital amputee. Birth defect was caused by drugs taken by the mother in early pregnancy. **A,** Note the abnormal formation of the toes and small vestige of a right arm. **B,** Using his prosthetic devices (arms), the child is putting a puzzle together. (Courtesy The National Foundation–March of Dimes.)

directly into the bloodstream. The hormones are carried to every part of the body where they control and integrate cell metabolism and the growth process. Any imbalance of too much or too little seriously disrupts normal development.

PSYCHOLOGICAL DEVELOPMENT

The physical development of the child, from conception to adulthood, is a miracle of chemical and biological interaction. Because it is physical, it can be seen and felt, measured and studied. Psychological development is equally complex and is interrelated to physical development, but it is far more difficult to measure, nourish, protect, and treat when ill. It is constantly influenced by forces over which there is little control.

For the sake of understanding and study, the psychological development of the child is divided into at least three areas—mental, emotional, and social. In life these are not separate entities but are parts of the whole person, each one revealing a different facet of the personality; each part interacting with all others.

Mental development

Mental development is demonstrated by the ability of the child to solve problems and to react to a situation in a way that shows general understanding. It is continuous, may be more rapid at one age period than another, and may deteriorate with disuse. It is dependent on inherited mental potential (intelligence) and environmental factors that foster its growth.

Measurement of intelligence

Potential mental ability, called *intelligence*, is inherited and fixed at birth. Intelligence can be defined as the ability to adjust to new situations, to think abstractly, and to profit from experience.

Tests. A number of tests have been devised to measure intelligence, including the Wechsler Intelligence Scale for Children, the Stanford-Binet, and the Bayley Mental and Motor Scales. During infancy and early childhood such tests are of the performance type in which the child is asked to manipulate objects or to demonstrate motor development by picking up blocks, and so forth. When the child is able to understand speech, verbal tests may be given; when the child is able to write, individual or group written tests may be used. From 5 years of age and onward, intelligence tests begin to be more reliable. All tests that use language as a basic tool are limited to the cultural group for whom the test was devised, because words may have different meanings to different groups of people.

When a child takes an intelligence test, the score is compared with the scores of thousands of other children to determine *mental age*. For example, if the score of a 10-year-old child was in the range of the scores of average 12-year-old children, his mental age would be designated as that of a 12-year-old child. The intelligence quotient (IQ) is the ratio between the mental age and the chronological age times 100 as expressed in the following formula:

$$\frac{\text{Mental age} \times 100}{\text{Chronological age}} = IQ$$

$$\text{EXAMPLE:} \quad \frac{12 \times 100}{10} = 120 \text{ IQ}$$

When the IQ was first devised it was believed that mental maturity was reached between 16 and 21 years of age, so the mental age of the adult was arbitrarily set at 16 years. We now know that a person's IQ can increase or decrease during life depending on mental use or disuse. An IQ between 90 and 109 is considered to be average-normal. Children with an IQ of over 140 are called gifted; those with an IQ below 90 are retarded in various degrees.

Piaget's theory of intelligence

According to Jean Piaget's theory, intelligence is the regulating force that provides balance between a person and the environment. As children interact with the world, they organize sensory input, assimilate it into themselves, and adapt to it in sequenced structures or thinking-processes called *schemes* and *operations*. Intelligence develops in stages characterized by *sensorimotor reactions, concrete operations*, and *formal operations*. Each stage issues out of the preceding one reconstructing it on a new level and later surpassing it. At first the child reacts to the environment with sensorimotor reflexes and innate reactions. Then the child moves into the first stage of "operational" intelligence where groupings, or processes of thinking about concrete, real objects are developed. These groupings are called concrete operations. Finally, the child develops processes to engage in abstract thought about real objects as well as forms and ideas. These processes are called formal operations. This final stage results in the accomplishment of equilibrium with the environment whereby the social world is thought of as a whole unit with laws, regulations, roles, and functions; self-centeredness is replaced by moral concern; a sense of equality supercedes submission to authority; and, throughout the remainder of life, exchange of ideas with other persons produces personal development. A greatly condensed description of Piaget's stages of intellectual development is given in Table 2-4.

Influences on mental development

Inherited intellectual potential is something like a bank account from which each person may

Table 2-4. Piaget's stages of intellectual activity*

Stages and phases	Approximate age	Knowledge activities
Sensorimotor stage		
Phase 1—sensorimotor	Birth to 1 month	Reflex and innate reactions
Phase 2—primary circular reaction	1 to 4 months	Only reality is that which affects the body; repetition by recognition; first habits
Phase 3—secondary circular reaction	4 to 8 months	Actions are object centered, intentional, and involve a means and a goal
Phase 4—coordination of secondary schemes	8 to 12 months	Perceives cause and effect relationships; problem solving develops
Phase 5—tertiary circular reaction	12 to 18 months	Instead of repeating the same action, child examines object to see what else it will do
Phase 6—invention of new means through mental combinations	18 to 24 months	Intentional invention of new means to an end; insight; make-believe emerges
Stage of preoperational concrete operations	2 to 7 years	Increasing ability to use symbols to represent the environment, but only in a set pattern as they relate to experience; "centering" of attention on a single factor in solutions to problems
Stage of concrete operations	7 to 11 years	Ability to order and relate experiences to an oragnized whole; egocentricism; ability to take into account another's point of view; conservation of weight and volume
Phase of preoperational formal operations	11 to 15 years	Ability to form ordering structures or groupings and to form connections between groups
Stage of formal operations	15 years and onward throughout life	Ability to operate solely through symbols; problem solving develops; ability to conceptualize, to center on "forms" of thoughts and experiences; equilibration between the world and the individual

*Modified from Piaget, J., and Inhelder, B.: The Psychology of the Child, New York, 1979, Basic Books, Inc.

draw. Some have limited resources and are able to make full use of all they were given by inheritance; others have large intellectual endowment but are able to use only a fraction of their wealth. What happens to a child's intellectual potential depends in large measure on the environment in which maturation takes place. Such an environment is more likely to be found in homes where the basic physical and emotional needs of the child are met and where the child is allowed to recognize and solve problems appropriate to the given age.

The various causes, classifications, and management of mental retardation are discussed in Chapter 18.

Nutrition. Recent studies show that when a child does not receive adequate nutrition, especially protein, during infancy and the toddler years mental capacity is permanently damaged. This may account in part for the cycle of poverty that grips large numbers of people from generation to generation.

Environment. Mental development is fostered in homes where learning is respected, where there are cultural advantages such as music and books, where language is used to express ideas, and where the child is allowed "room" to think. Within the limits of safety, the child needs to be allowed to experiment, make mistakes, recognize problems, and attempt to solve them. In fact, problem solving helps develop creativity, a unique ability not necessarily related to IQ scores. If every need of the child is instantly met by an overprotective parent, the child is deprived of the motivation to find answers and mental development is stunted.

Emotional development

Emotional development is closely related to physical, motor, and mental development. It involves the child's feelings in relating to other persons and to stressful situations in an expanding world.

Measurement

Emotional development is not easily measured objectively, although a number of evaluative tests have been devised. Many of these depend on language and are not useful for young children. Most depend on a subjective comparison between the child's responses to the test situation and those described in established norms. Perhaps the most common means of evaluating emotional development is to compare the child's progressive development in the family setting to that of other children.

For the first few weeks of life an infant's chief drives are to satisfy basic needs for survival and security. The child rapidly gains an increasing degree of neuromotor control, and learns to follow a moving object with the eyes and to hold an object placed in the hand. The child smiles. During the many repetitions of feeding, bathing, and diaper changing the child comes to know the mother. By about 3 months of age the child stops crying when she approaches because the child has learned that the needs of the moment will be supplied. This is believed to be the earliest evidence that an infant is now aware of self and of the difference between self and others and the surrounding world.

The infant's mother becomes the central person in life. She represents security, gratification of needs, and relief of discomfort. Her rejection and hostility or acceptance and affection is felt by the child, who responds in kind. These attitudes are called *life positions* by Eric Berne and are identified as: "I'm OK, you're OK," "I'm OK, you're not OK," "I'm not OK, you're OK," "I'm not OK, you're not OK." The basic foundations of emotional security are laid down in the first year or so of life. So too are the basic patterns for interpersonal relationships.

Prolonged hospitalization of the child during these early months may cause apathy, listlessness, and underdevelopment. The child may have permanent emotional scars that become evident years later when there arises an inability to establish warm relationships with others.

In early childhood, as the child explores and learns about the world outside, horizons widen and relationships with people become more complex. By the end of infancy and the beginning of childhood the child is walking well and improving language skills and conception of self. Then the child feels clearly distinct and begins to socialize to a much greater degree. During these early years the child develops a unique mind. The child learns to say "yes" and "no," although the meaning may be confused at first. The child is more independent and is ceaselessly curious and exploring.

By 3 or 4 years of age, children begin to understand that they are either girls and boys. It is important to children's future self-concept that they become identified with their own sex. This identification helps avoid confusion and possibly serious psychiatric difficulties in the future.

By the age of 5 or 6 years the patterns of inner life are well established. Children enter the outside world by way of the school, reacting and interacting with the many forces of life they find there. Their ability to adjust successfully is largely affected by the basic emotional foundations laid during infancy and early childhood.

Influences on emotional development

Some of the important factors that influence the development of the personality of a child are (1) whether the basic emotional needs of the child are gratified, (2) the attitudes of the parents and other adults toward the child, (3) the psychological environment of the home, (4) the relationship of the child to others inside and outside the home, and (5) the effects of illness on the child's personality.

Basic emotional needs. Eight basic emotional needs of the child have been identified as love and affection, security, acceptance as an individual, self-respect, achievement, recognition, independence, and order and control.

Love and affection. The most important emotional need of the child is to be loved unconditionally and to experience physical tenderness. Without love the child may become isolated, apathetic, aggressive, or sullen; or the child may take refuge in physical complaints. The child may even be so emotionally damaged that warm human attachments will never be formed, and the child may become cold and distant.

Security. During growth the child experiences many threats to a sense of security. Perhaps the first of these is the threat of bodily discomfort, such as hunger or cold. Later on, the threats are to emotional comfort. The child constantly runs headlong into all of the restrictions of the family and society because of restraints and the demands of conforming to authority. This places the child in conflict with those from whom love and approval are desired and arouses concern about whether the child is liked or disliked. As a result the child experiences insecurity. If basically sure of family love, the child will learn to cope with both physical and emotional discomfort.

Sometimes illness or death of a parent may cause insecurity, especially in the young child. Other causes include physical handicaps, sibling rivalry, social ineptitude that prevents warm friendships, obesity or skinniness, moving from place to place, lack of skill in sports, and chronic illness. Whatever the causes for insecurity, the effects on the emotional and mental development of the child are far reaching. Every effort should be made to identify them, remove them, or help the child cope with them.

Acceptance as an individual. Every child is unique and different from any other, physically, mentally, and emotionally. For this reason it is important to help the child develop into the best person possible within individual potential. Some parents do not understand this and try to force children into preconceived ideals. They reject what the child is in favor of what they want the child to become. Although no child is perfect and all children need correction and direction in the general areas of self-control, personal habits, and social niceties, children cannot develop talents that are not latent, nor can they change their appearance or sex. When children feel acceptance, they are free to benefit from parental guidance.

Self-respect. Children need to feel valuable. If they are compared unfavorably with other children by parents, or are made fun of, they begin to feel inferior. Children may respond by becoming aggressive, retreating into seclusion, or simply giving up an effort to succeed. Children are more sensitive to criticism than adults realize. Harsh criticism and ridicule crush the spirit and destroy self-esteem.

Achievement. Achievement of one skill after another is the normal way children develop. They learn to sit, to walk, to run, to ride a tricycle then a bicycle, and, later on, to drive a car. They are challenged by the many attainments of others and are active, adventurous, and curious. Children are not satisfied to remain babies but want to go on to greater and greater accomplishments. This drive to achieve is thwarted by overprotective or critical parents. Happy are the children whose parents encourage independent accomplishments and place only necessary protective boundaries about them, while allowing maximum freedom to push on toward maturity.

Recognition. Praise for work well done is encouraging at any age, but for children it is a necessity. They need to be recognized by parents and playmates. Recognition is a food (for the soul) that stimulates the child to future effort. Parents, or nurses, for that matter, may not realize how important this need is. They may provide children with the best physical care but never give a word of approval. If children only receive correction and reproof and never praise or commendation, they will become discouraged and may even give up trying. On the other hand, if effort is rewarded by recognition, children will not spare themselves to accomplish goals. This kind of positive motivation is practiced with great success by the Boy Scouts, Girl Scouts, and other such organizations.

Independence. The ultimate goal for each child is to experience self-realization and to become a self-reliant, mature adult. Such independent responsibility is not a gift that arrives on the twenty-first birthday. It is the result of a gradual process whereby the child assumes increasing self-responsibility. This normal desire for independence can be frustrated by overprotection and needless supervision. It can be crushed by an arbitrary domineering parent or by older sisters or brothers. Some children give in, but harbor deep resentment to all authority; some rebel in angry outbursts until the first opportunity to leave home. Realizing this, wise parents foster the gradual development of independence, at the same time maintaining the steady discipline and kind authority that is necessary for the child's well-being. They realize that the job of parents is to work themselves out of their job.

Order and control. Children, like all living things, need the stabilizing effect of order. Order in human relations is maintained by rules and by a system of authority. Children's first introduc-

tion to authority comes in the home from parents. Attitudes children form there will affect their responses to the rules of school and the community. The purpose for discipline and authority in the home is to prepare children for accepting restrictions on behavior that they will encounter the rest of their lives.

A wise exercise of authority is perhaps the most difficult task faced by modern parents. They may be weak and vacillating or severe, unfair, cruel, and unforgiving. Those who seem to be the most successful set sensible rules, expect reasonable compliance, keep their word, remember that punishment is a means to an end, not an end in itself, fit the punishment to the crime, and reward good behavior with praise. They do not resort to unimaginative beatings that build resentment and fear. Instead, they use appropriate means of correction such as sending the young child from the room to return when behavior has improved or depriving the older child of the television or family auto. Time spent motivating children to want to behave, and approving of them when they do, is well invested.

Home environment

Parental attitudes. Some surveys of families in America reveal that over 50% of all pregnancies were unwanted. Fortunately, most parents love the new baby after it arrives, but some do not. These parents may openly demonstrate their rejection by cruel abuse or may secretly reject such children but pamper or overprotect them to ease their guilt feelings. In either instance, rejected children are tragic victims of circumstances. They might well envy the child of an unwed mother who with sacrificial love gives her baby up to adoptive parents.

Influence of brothers and sisters. Although parents are the central figures in the young child's life, other children in the family play an important part. Each child occupies a certain place in the family in relation to the other children. Oldest children may be expected to assume parental responsibility and so may become leaders; youngest children may be kept in the "baby" role because they were the last; middle children may feel that they "also ran" and that they are of little value. These early roles which children experience within the family group have a significant effect on their later social development in school and in the community.

Illness. All children experience acute illnesses, but usually they recover rapidly and their emotional development is not affected. During these illnesses they may regress to infantile behavior such as thumb-sucking or bed-wetting, but when the illness has passed, they return to their former level of emotional development with no apparent ill effects. If, however, children are ill for prolonged periods of time, seriously neglected, or told that their illness is a punishment for some misdeed, they may suffer severe psychological damage.

Social development

Social development begins at birth and is an integral part of the total growth of the child. It can only be measured as it compares with that of other children of similar age.

During the first few weeks of life the infant sleeps most of the time, only awakening when feeling physical discomfort. Awareness of self is at an instinctive level. Gradually, by 3 months of age, the child begins to recognize the mother. At this time it is believed that the child also becomes aware of a separate identity.

In time, the child notices others who come and go and "talk." By 9 months of age the child recognizes familiar persons and shows fear of strangers.

During the second and third years of life the child feels a kinship of size to other toddlers, likes to play near them, but does not play with other children as yet. Vocabulary grows from 300 to 900 words, and the child is able to communicate simple ideas to others, but is still mother-centered.

During the fourth and fifth years the child becomes a truly "social creature." Vocabulary grows at a rate of about 600 words per year, and

the child uses it to ask questions about everything. The child learns to play with others, enjoys group activities, and now father shares a place with mother. The child notices the relationships of others and may display rivalry with brothers or sisters. The imagination is so real that the child can combine truth and fancy without questioning, often enjoying the friendship of an imaginary playmate.

When a child enters school, the center of social life is transferred from home to school. Children of the same age, called peers, become increasingly important. By 8 years of age the child prefers to be with others of the same sex. The ages of 9 to 11 years might be called the "gang" years, for this is the period of clubs and hero worship, when boys hate girls and girls hate boys, and blood-brother friendships are formed between buddies.

About 12 to 14 years of age, girls begin to titter about boys. An increasing awareness of the opposite sex develops. The boys "show off," the girls flirt, but both are more at home with their own sex. About this time adolescents may have mixed feelings toward parents and insecure questions about self. They may confide all these to an adult outside the family whom they feel they can trust.

By late adolescence individuals begin to feel secure about themselves and as a result are comfortable with members of both sexes. They no longer need to cling to the family, a buddy, or a gang for support. They are independent of others, yet are sure enough to move freely in any social situation. When they have reached this level of social development, they are adults.

In review, personality development proceeds in a natural sequence from infancy to adulthood (Fig. 2-13). These steps to maturity have been described by Erik Erikson as:

1. Trust in others; developed during the first year of life.
2. Autonomy, a mind and will of one's own; developed during the toddler period.
3. Initiative, inner controls, and a con-

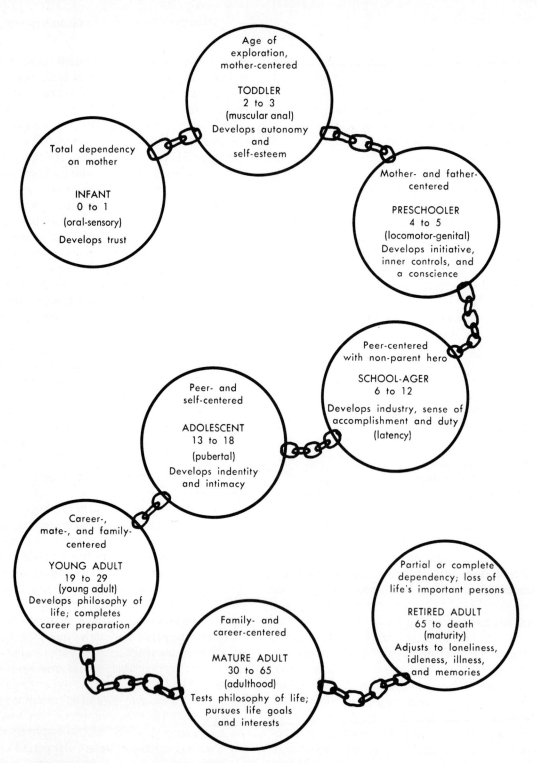

Fig. 2-13. The chain of life from infancy to old age. (Adapted from the developmental theories of Freud and Erikson.)

science, a desire to learn to do what they see others doing; developed during the preschool years.

4. Industry, duty, and accomplishment of tasks; developed during school age.
5. Identity, answers questions "who am I?" and "what do I believe?"; developed during the adolescent years.
6. Intimacy, the ability to form a relationship of deep and lasting concern for another person; developed during late adolescence.

PLAY IN THE DEVELOPMENT OF THE CHILD

Play is serious business to children. It is their vehicle for development. Through play children learn about themselves and the world in which they live. Play serves several specific functions, and as children grow and mature, play changes in form or type, fitting appropriately into the increasingly complex needs of each child.

Functions of play

Physical and motor development. Physical and motor development is the immediate and continuing result of play. The activities of play serve to exercise the muscles and teach motor coordination. The whole body is involved in play as the child bends and twists, jumps and runs, lifts and handles objects, pushes and pulls. Surplus energy can be worked off and general good health enhanced by active play.

Social development. Social development occurs as a result of play with other children. At first the child is satisfied to be near others, and then begins to play with them. The child learns to share, to take turns, to communicate, to enjoy the friendship of others, to compete, to be a "good sport," and to relate to individuals and groups. In play the child has an opportunity to practice the art of interacting successfully with others, thus preparing for adult relationships.

Emotional expression. Emotional expression is a valuable function of play. The toddler can relieve anger by hammering pegs through a peg board. The preschooler can supply the need to act out deep feelings by imaginative play. The school-aged child and adolescent may use competitive sports to vent hostility. Play can be as flexible as the child's need. It is, therefore, a valuable part of the maintenance of mental health in children.

Intellectual education. Intellectual education could be called "play" if it were not made "work" by schoolmasters and zealots. All the bodily senses are involved in the process of learning, which to the young child is play. As the child feels, sees, tastes, hears, and smells, the information gained, is put together to form concepts. This process of gathering information, putting it together, and coming to conclusions is called "education." When it is enjoyed, it is called "play."

Development of moral values. The development of moral values takes place as children interact with other children at play. They begin to learn that good actions help others and that bad actions hurt others. At first their sense of right and wrong is limited to simple situations, such as taking a toy from another child or playing roughly. As children grow they learn about telling the truth and lying. Later on they learn about gossiping and hurting the feelings of classmates. Adolescents learn about paying debts, honesty, loyalty to friends, and sexual responsibility; thus moral values evolve as a result of interaction with others and with the code of ethics taught by meaningful persons in the society.

Types of play

As children grow and develop, the types of play characteristic for their age change (Table 2-5). Babies play by themselves with objects that they move about. Toddlers still play by themselves but enjoy playing near other children. This is called *parallel play.* By 3 years of age they begin to play together in simple direct ways. By the preschool years children begin to play together in a more complicated way, such as one child being "doctor" and the other being "pa-

Table 2-5. Interests and activities of children according to age

Age	Interest	Activities (toys, crafts, games)	Music and books
Infant, 0 to 1 year	Objects that attract eye and ear but go into mouth	Bright mobiles, bells, rattles, rings, rubber squeaking toys	No books Enjoys being sung songs
Toddler, 1 to 3 years	Play things that allow parallel play and muscle coordination and give attention and security	Sand, pail and shovel, peg board and mallet, kiddie car, jumping horse, pull toys, cuddly animals, large dolls	Likes large print cloth books, to hear the same story over and over, to hear stories about animals Sings to self
Preschool child, 3 to 5 years	Toys; equipment that stimulates imaginative, creative, and active play	Play houses, tinker toys, trains, trucks, magnets, building parts, dolls, finger paint, tricycle	Enjoys familiar stories about fire engines, trains, action; likes to "read" books with pictures Enjoys singing action songs in group
Early school-aged child, 5 to 9 years	Activities that use mental and physical skills; plays with others of same sex; enjoys surprises	Crafts: metal, beads, leather, spool knitting Games: board games, old maid, rook, puzzles Play: hide and seek, swimming, riding tricycle and bike, imaginative play with mother's clothes, trains, slot cars	Still enjoys hearing stories; reads for self; enjoys fairy tales, adventures, and think-do books Enjoys group sings; may begin solo instrument
Middle school-aged child, 9 to 12 years	Activities that use mental and physical skills; does things with the gang; enjoys team play, has "buddy"; works for awards, prizes	Active team sports: baseball, soccer, basketball Swimming, bicycling Boy Scouts, Girl Scouts Crafts: metal, leather, modeling, carving Games: checkers, chess, board, cards	Enjoys adventure stories, biographies, comic books Group singing Solo instrument
Early adolescence, 12 to 15 years	Budding interest in opposite sex; activities that require skill in body and mind; wants to earn spending money	Active sports—every kind More advanced hobbies: photography, radio, telescope, microscope, complicated models Cosmetics for girls Games: monopoly, chess, checkers, cards	Adventure and love stories, technical or specialized books in interest area Popular music, some group singing, solo instrument
Adolescence, 15 to 21 years	Recreational activities much like adults; opposite sex; vocational	Active sports, autos, boats, motor bikes, swimming, team sports Games: adult kinds Dances, dating, relaxing	Reads or writes any type of book Perform or audit popular, classical, or folk music

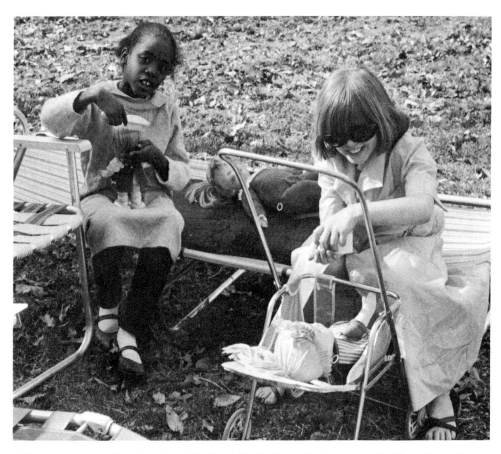

Fig. 2-14. Make-believe play of neighborhood friends. Lawn furniture makes the "house"; sunglasses, high-heeled shoes, lady's dresses, and dolls turn these girls into "mothers."

tient." During the school years play usually involves a group of children in such activities as hide and seek, baseball, board games, and clubs. "Make-believe" play serves a special need for 8- to 10-year-old children (Fig. 2-14). Solitary play has a place at every age, including fishing, making models, painting, and just walking alone. Adolescents usually do not consider these activities "play" anymore, even though they serve the same purposes as before. Adolescents tend to think of work and school as separate from recreation, the adult word for "play." When adolescents play baseball, go skin diving, or attend a dance, they think of these activities as recrea-tion, and so they are. They also serve to provide physical, motor, social, and moral development, emotional expression, and education.

SUMMARY OUTLINE

  I. General principles of growth
    A. Continuous growth
    B. Variable rates
    C. Orderly sequence
    D. Total process
 II. Physical growth and motor development
    A. Terminology
    B. Measurement
      1. Weight
      2. Height
      3. Body proportions

4. Bone development
5. Tooth development
6. Motor development
C. Influences on growth
    1. Inheritance
        a. Transmission of traits
        b. Genetics
        c. Abnormalities
        d. Genetic counseling
        e. Grouping of people
        f. Influence of sex
    2. Intrauterine life
        a. Placental defects
        b. Maternal effects
    3. Birth
    4. Environment and nutrition
    5. Endocrine function
III. **Psychological development**
    A. Mental development
        1. Measurement of intelligence
        2. Piaget's theory of intelligence
        3. Influences on mental development
            a. Nutrition
            b. Environment
    B. Emotional development
        1. Measurement
        2. Influences on emotional development
            a. Basic emotional needs
                (1) Love and affection
                (2) Security
                (3) Acceptance as an individual
                (4) Self-respect
                (5) Achievement
                (6) Recognition

(7) Independence
(8) Order and control
    b. Home environment
        (1) Parental attitudes
        (2) Influence of brothers and sisters
        (3) Illness
C. Social development
IV. **Play in the development of the child**
    A. Functions of play
        1. Physical and motor development
        2. Social development
        3. Emotional expression
        4. Intellectual education
        5. Development of moral values
    B. Types of play

STUDY QUESTIONS

1. List the four general principles that characterize growth.
2. Define the following terms as they relate to growth: extent, rate, periods, patterns, curves, and norms.
3. Define the following terms as they relate to development: extent, states, maturation.
4. Compare the weight, height, body proportion, bone, tooth, and motor development of a boy or girl at 1 month, 1 year, and 6 years of age.
5. Using the information given about inherited traits, show how the trait of diabetes might appear in a family of four children where both mother and father carry the recessive gene.
6. Give two examples of teratogenic agents.
7. Discuss eight basic emotional needs of children.
8. List the five functions of play for a child.

3
Ensuring healthy growth and development

VOCABULARY

Metabolic rate
Calorie
Antibody
Passive immunity
Vaccination
Booster dose
Antidote
Pedodontist

The practice of pediatric medicine has two sides—prevention and treatment. If there is truth in the old adage "an ounce of prevention is worth a pound of cure," then the practice of preventive pediatrics is of greater importance, for its purpose is to ensure the healthy growth and development of children. Nurses play an important part in making this goal a reality. They act as health teachers to parents and children; they assist physicians in immunization programs and regular physical examinations; and they support safety programs. Thus, their role in advancing preventive pediatrics is significant.

PREVENTIVE PEDIATRICS

Prevention of disease and defects starts before conception, continues through intrauterine life and delivery, and proceeds throughout the childhood years.

Before conception. Recent genetic studies have revealed that many defects and diseases are caused by inherited traits passed from generation to generation in a predictable pattern. As the ability to identify persons who are the carriers of defective traits increases, so responsible decisions by prospective parents should increase and the number of children born with serious defects decrease. The genetic counseling involved in these decisions thus provides an important form of preventive pediatrics.

Prenatal period. During intrauterine life the fetus depends on its mother for its supply of life-giving nutrients and on the placenta as the means whereby it receives these essentials. If the mother cannot supply it with adequate nutrients or if her blood carries harmful substances, the fetus can be seriously damaged. If the placenta is defective, the fetus cannot receive necessary nutrients. In either case the growth and development of the growing baby are affected. To prevent such damage to the baby, it is important that the mother have an adequate diet and that she avoid harmful drugs which might deform the developing infant. Although defects of the placenta are not as easily overcome, prenatal medical supervision of the mother provides the baby with a maximum chance for health.

Parturition. The most serious and permanent birth injuries are those that affect the central and peripheral nervous systems of the infant. The practice of modern obstetrics is geared to the prevention of these injuries. Early prenatal care and careful and continuous medical supervision during labor and delivery all help to assure the infant a safe arrival.

Immediate newborn infant care. The paramount needs of the newborn infant are for adequate respiration and for a warm environment. Modern hospital delivery rooms and nurseries are equipped with suction devices, oxygen equipment, and controlled environmental units for infants. In addition, they are staffed with highly skilled professionals to provide specialized care. If an infant is born in a modern hospital facility, the chances for survival are greatest because of the advantage of all these resources to assure an opportunity to live.

Infancy, childhood, and adolescence. Ensuring the health of the child through the growing years is accomplished in the following six general ways: (1) by providing adequate nutrition for physical needs, (2) by providing for dental health, (3) by meeting basic emotional needs, (4) by immunizing against infectious diseases, (5) by protecting from harmful accidents, and

(6) by giving continuous medical supervision. These six areas have been classified as preventive pediatrics. They are of vital concern to all who work with children and are of equal importance to the child born with defects as to the apparently normal child.

ADEQUATE NUTRITION

Good health depends on good eating habits. Good nutrition promotes a healthier body and mind. It provides greater personal vitality and resistance to disease. A well-nourished body repairs itself faster than it would otherwise and grows at its optimum rate and capacity. The child who eats well feels better, has a good appetite, digestion and elimination, has good posture, and sleeps more soundly. It is important that pediatric nurses understand the basis for judging just what a "good diet" really is so that they will be able to advise parents and to encourage children in their eating habits.

Foods in the diet

There are three major functions of foods in the body: to build and repair tissue, to regulate the body processes, and to provide heat and energy. For the body to perform these important functions it must be supplied with the components that make them possible. These components are oxygen, water, protein, minerals, vitamins, carbohydrates, and fats. The first one, oxygen, comes from the air; the others are found in the fluids and foods that are ingested. A balanced intake of these nutrients that meets the current needs of the body is considered a "good diet" (Fig. 3-1).

Components

Oxygen. Oxygen is essential to all of the complex chemical processes that enable the body to make use of food. It is freely available to the body by means of the respiratory system from the fresh air of the atmosphere. Inspired air consists of 20% oxygen, 0.04% carbon dioxide, and 79% nitrogen. Expired air consists of 16% oxy-

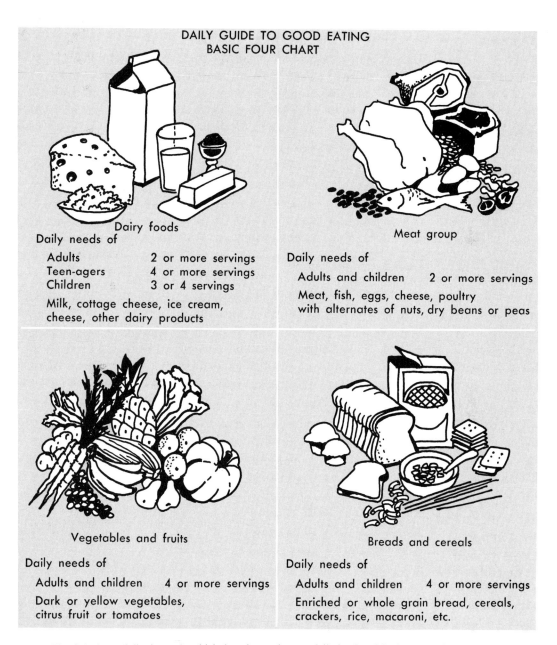

DAILY GUIDE TO GOOD EATING
BASIC FOUR CHART

Dairy foods

Daily needs of

Adults	2 or more servings
Teen-agers	4 or more servings
Children	3 or 4 servings

Milk, cottage cheese, ice cream, cheese, other dairy products

Meat group

Daily needs of

Adults and children   2 or more servings

Meat, fish, eggs, cheese, poultry with alternates of nuts, dry beans or peas

Vegetables and fruits

Daily needs of

Adults and children   4 or more servings

Dark or yellow vegetables, citrus fruit or tomatoes

Breads and cereals

Daily needs of

Adults and children   4 or more servings

Enriched or whole grain bread, cereals, crackers, rice, macaroni, etc.

Fig. 3-1. A good diet is one in which there is an adequate daily intake of the four basic food groups.

gen, 4% carbon dioxide, and 79% nitrogen. This continuous supply of fresh oxygen is used by the body to oxidize, or burn, the fuel of the other components of food. Through the respiratory system, oxygen enters the bloodstream and is carried to every living cell, in which it enters into the life-sustaining processes that utilize all of the other nutrients taken into the body. Without oxygen the cells die in a few minutes.

Water. Water is the second most necessary substance for life. Without it, death occurs in a few days. The adult body is 60% water; the newborn infant body is 77% water. Water is the major constituent of all cells, blood, lymph, spinal fluid, and the various body secretions of urine, mucus, and sweat. *Dehydration*, or too little water in the body, occurs when there is inadequate fluid intake or when there is unusual loss of body fluids from vomiting, diarrhea, or high fever. The chemistry of the body is normally held in a state of balance, with water playing an important part. In small children the balance of body chemistry is especially delicate; dehydration can seriously disrupt it, causing grave consequences. The body normally eliminates excess water. If, however, the normal means of eliminating fluid from the body is disrupted, such as occurs in serious heart or kidney disease, water is retained in the tissue and a condition called *edema* results.

Protein. Every living cell and most body fluids contain protein. Protein builds and repairs body tissue and is an important part of enzymes, hormones, and immune bodies that help the body resist infection.

Before protein can be used by the body, it must be broken down in the digestive process into smaller units called amino acids. The body needs about 30 gm of new protein each day. If more is taken in than is needed, the excess is stored in the liver and tissue cells as body protein. If less is taken in than is needed, then the body protein splits into amino acids again and is released into the blood for use. Of the 23 amino acids, 10 are known as essential, because the body cannot manufacture them from its stored body protein but must take in these acids from a continuous supply in the diet.

Proteins that contain all of the essential amino acids in sufficient amounts are called *complete*. Examples of complete proteins are meat, fish, eggs, and milk products. *Incomplete proteins* are those that do not contain all of the essential amino acids or are lacking in sufficient amounts for growth and repair purposes. Cereals, beans, peas, and nuts are examples of incomplete proteins. Even though some products may be 100% protein, such as gelatin, they may not contain all the essential amino acids and so are not complete proteins. Soybeans contain all the essential proteins but in insufficient amounts and so are considered only partially complete. Stunted growth, poor resistance to infection, and emaciation (marasmus) result from a chronic deficiency of complete proteins.

It should be remembered that proteins also furnish energy to the diet, supplying 10% to 15% of the daily calorie requirements. When heavy demands for body protein occur, as during growth spurts, burns, and fever, additional protein should be added to the diet.

Minerals. Mineral salts form the essential framework of the body and make up 4% of the total body weight. They form the greater portion of bones, teeth, and nails and are essential constituents of all the cells, especially of the blood, lymph, and glands. They influence or promote muscle and nervous activity, digestion, and oxidation, and they regulate the acid-base and water balance of the body. More than 20 elements are found in the body, some only in minute quantities, but all are necessary for growth and health. Included are calcium, phosphorus, chlorine, sodium, iodine, iron, potassium, sulfur, copper, fluorine, manganese, arsenic, cobalt, and silicon.

Most of these mineral salts are readily available in a well-balanced diet. Sodium, potassium, and chlorine are found in all natural foods. Calcium, phosphorus, iodine, and iron may need to be added because the usual diet does not always meet body requirements. Minerals are normally excreted in the urine, sweat, and feces. Excessive mineral loss may occur through diarrhea or vomiting. Harmful chemicals in pesticides may contaminate food crops and water supplies, so must be strictly monitored.

Calcium and phosphorus. Calcium and phosphorus function together in many chemical processes in the body and are naturally present in many of the same foods. Together with vitamin D, they are needed to build strong bones and teeth. In addition, they are essential for normal heart action and muscle contractions, for nerve function, and for the clotting mechanism of blood. Insufficient amounts of these minerals cause deformed bones and muscle spasms. Insufficient blood calcium, called *hypocalcemia*, may cause muscle twitching and convulsions. The best source of calcium and phosphorus is found in milk products.

Iron. One of the most important elements in the body is iron. The great majority of the body iron resides in the hemoglobin, the oxygen-bearing part of the blood. Most of the remainder is stored in the liver as *ferritin* and in muscle as *myoglobulin*. A lack of dietary iron leads to a lack of hemoglobin and thus to nutritional anemia, called iron deficiency or second anemia. It is most common in infants and young children, because by 3 weeks of age the iron stored before birth is depleted and both cow and human milk contain insufficient iron to meet the infant's needs. If iron is not added to the baby's diet, and the infant receives only milk, iron deficiency anemia results. These infants are sometimes called "milk babies." Baby cereals with supplementary iron or vitamin-mineral medications may be used to supply this need.

Iron is needed throughout childhood for growth; the amount varies according to the growth pattern. During growth spurts the diet should include iron-rich natural foods such as meats, liver, egg yolks, and dark green leafy vegetables.

Iodine. In some regions of the world iodine is lacking in the soil; vegetables grown there are iodine poor. Although the thyroid gland needs only a tiny daily amount of iodine to manufacture sufficient thyroxin for normal metabolism, persons living in those regions may develop goiters, or enlarged thyroid glands, from iodine deficiency. Through the widespread use of iodized salt, table salt with iodine added, this condition is now rarely seen. Natural sources of iodine include drinking water, vegetables, and seafoods.

Vitamins. Vitamins are organic compounds found in tiny amounts in foods. By regulating the many chemical reactions within the cell, they promote growth, sustain life, and maintain health. A lack of any of the vitamins causes a disturbance in the metabolism. As a result, the growth pattern and development of the child are affected. Vitamins A and D are the only two vitamins stored in the body. Excessive intake of them will cause skin lesions, liver enlargement, and bone abnormalities. For this reason, taking vitamins indiscriminately can actually be harmful.

Although the precise mechanism by which most vitamins work in the cells is still not fully understood, all the known vitamins have been isolated and synthesized in the laboratory. They are usually categorized according to their solubility in water or fat. The fat-soluble vitamins are A, D, E, and K. The water-soluble vitamins are the eight members of the B-complex group and vitamin C. The best sources of vitamins are natural foods, although doctors sometimes prescribe vitamins to supplement the diet of infants and young children. A well-balanced diet normally provides an adequate supply of vitamins without any additional supplement (Table 3-1).

Carbohydrates. Carbohydrates provide the body with heat and energy. They are the sugars and starches of the diet and include such foods

Table 3-1. Some essential vitamins

Vitamin	Function	Deficiency effects	Sources
Fat soluble			
A (retinol)	Promotes good eyesight, helps maintain skin and mucous membrane, helps form bone and teeth	Night blindness, dry mucous membrane allows microbe invasion, poor tooth formation	Yellow and dark green vegetables, dried fruit, liver
D (calciferol)	Regulates calcium and phosphorus metabolism, vital to tooth and bone growth and maintenance	Rickets, retarded growth, abnormal bone formation, decay of teeth	Fish oil, egg yolk, irradiated foods, milk, liver, sunshine
E (tocopherol)	Promotes normal growth, normal reproduction	Sterility	Green vegetables, seed germ, oils
K (menadione)	Essential to blood clotting mechanism, promotes normal liver function	Hemorrhages, impaired liver function	Green vegetables, oils, tomatoes
Water soluble			
B_1 (thiamine)	Vital to nervous system health, essential to carbohydrate metabolism, aids muscle tone	Beriberi, fatigue, anorexia, impairment of neuromuscular, digestive, and cardiovascular systems	Lean pork, meats, milk, whole grain and enriched cereals
B_2 (riboflavin)	Essential to protein and carbohydrate metabolism, aids normal growth, aids eye adaptation	Skin and mouth lesions, impaired blood cell formation	Meats of all kinds, milk, eggs, green leafy vegetables
Niacin (nicotinic acid)	Essential to protein and carbohydrate metabolism and normal growth, aids function of digestive and nervous system	Digestive disturbances, general poor health, mucous membrane of mouth ulcerates, anorexia, mental disorders	Meats of all kinds, whole grain cereals, peanuts, eggs
Pantothenic acid	Related to fat, protein, and carbohydrate metabolism, synthesis of cholesterol and steroid hormones	Lowered resistance to disease, gray hair	Meat, fish, egg yolk, cauliflower, peanuts, peas
Biotin	Participates in metabolism of fatty acids, amino acids, and carbohydrates	Dermatitis, anorexia, and nervousness	Synthesized in intestine of humans, all foods
B_6 (pyridoxine)	Essential to protein, fat, and carbohydrate metabolism	Consulsive seizures, nausea, dizziness, kidney stones	Whole grain cereals, organ meats, peanuts, tomatoes
Folacin (folic acid)	Essential to maturation of megaloblasts into mature red blood cells	Megaloblastic anemia, diarrhea, glossitis	Liver, green leafy vegetables, asparagus

Table 3-1. Some essential vitamins—cont'd

Vitamin	Function	Deficiency effects	Sources
Water soluble—cont'd			
B_{12} (cyano-cobalamin)	Essential to iron use and hemoglobin formation	Pernicious anemia, iron deficiency anemia	Liver, kidney, milk, cheese, lean meat, eggs, fish
C (ascorbic acid)	Works together with vitamin B_{12} and folic acid in iron use; essential to growth, wound healing, bone and tooth and collagen tissue formation	Skin hemorrhages, weakness, fatigue, delayed wound healing, faulty bone and tooth development, scurvy	Citrus fruit, tomatoes, raw cabbage, dark green vegetables (cannot be stored by body, must be taken fresh daily)

as bread, rice, honey, candy, corn, potatoes, and milk products. More than half of the body's energy requirements are met with carbohydrates. Chemical digestion changes them into glucose, the sugar of the body. As the glucose circulates in the blood, it may be used by cells to produce heat and energy, stored in the liver and muscles as glycogen, changed into body fat, or retained in the body fluids. The normal level of sugar in the blood is 70 to 100 mg per 100 ml. Insulin plays an important role in the transport of glucose into the cells where it is converted into useful energy. When the blood level of glucose drops below normal, epinephrine, which is secreted by the adrenal gland, causes the stored glycogen to be split back into glucose. A lack in either insulin or epinephrine disrupts the normal balance of glucose in the body. The waste products of carbohydrate metabolism are carbon dioxide and water.

Fats. Fats are concentrated sources of heat and energy. They constitute an important part of the diet, providing flavor to foods and a vehicle for the fat-soluble vitamins A, D, E, and K. They assist in protein metabolism, normal growth, and the maintenance of healthy skin. Stored fats act as padding around vital organs and glands and aid in keeping body temperature static. Fatty foods digest more slowly and delay hunger pangs.

Fats can be found in both vegetables and animal foods. Butter, egg yolks, meat, soybean oil, olive oil, and corn oil are good sources of the essential fatty acids. At least one of these fat sources should be included in the daily diet because one of the essential fatty acids, linoleic acid, cannot be synthesized from other fats. The waste products of fat metabolism are carbon dioxide and water.

Fatty tissue in the body is synthesized from excess protein, glucose, and fat that are eaten as food but that are not needed at that time. If the intake of food is not sufficient for body needs, the body converts its stored fat back into usable energy. This is why overeating causes one to become fat and eating too little makes one thin. Some children develop layers of excess fat during the preadolescent years but burn it up in the growth spurt and the increased activity of adolescence.

Functions

Building and repairing body tissue. Although all of the nutrients taken into the body are used by the body in a complex interdependence, the chief building materials of the body tissues are proteins and minerals. Proteins are changed by the digestive process into amino acids. These small units form the building blocks for the cells. Minerals are used throughout the body in its structural and cellular growth. Calcium forms the main part of bone. So, then, the

Table 3-2. Recommended daily dietary allowances for children*

Age (years)	Boys Height in	cm	Weight lb	kg	Protein (gm)	Calcium (gm)	Daily calorie needs	Girls Height in	cm	Weight lb	kg	Protein (gm)	Calcium (gm)	Daily calorie needs
0 to 1	19-34	48-86	7-29	3.2-13.2	10-32	0.7	700-1,300							
1 to 3	34	86	29	13.2	32	0.8	1,300	Same as for boys						
3 to 6	42	107	40	18.2	40	0.8	1,600							
6 to 9	49	124	53	24	52	0.8	2,100							
9 to 12	55	140	72	32.7	60	1.1	2,400	55	140	72	32.7	55	1.1	2,200
12 to 15	61	155	98	44.5	75	1.4	3,000	62	157	103	46.8	62	1.3	2,500
15 to 18	68	173	134	60.8	85	1.4	3,400	64	163	117	53.1	58	1.3	2,300

*Modified from the Food and Nutrition Board–National Research Council: Recommended daily dietary allowances, Washington, D.C., 1963, National Academy of Sciences, U.S. Government Printing Office.

prime function of protein and minerals is the building and repairing of body tissue.

Regulating body processes. The regulators of the body processes are vitamins and minerals, in addition to water and oxygen. Vitamins are involved in the chemical reactions within the cells in a still-mysterious way to influence growth and to maintain normal cell activity. Minerals are also important in maintaining the delicate balance of the body's chemistry.

Providing heat and energy. The body is a living organism and as such must have fuel to maintain itself and to perform work. Food is the body's fuel, and carbohydrates and fats are the first components of food that are converted into heat and energy to do work.

Because the energy released in the body ultimately appears as heat, the rate at which that heat is produced provides the most accurate measure of metabolism and is called the *metabolic rate*. The unit of heat in metabolism is called the *calorie*. A calorie is defined as the amount of heat needed to raise the temperature of 1 liter of water 1° C. The *basal metabolic rate* (BMR) is the minimum amount of heat produced by body cells when the body is at rest. The *total metabolic rate* is the total amount of heat produced by the body during a given period of time, usually 24 hours, under normal conditions. It represents the total amount of food that the child needs to replace what was used up in the process of living during that period of time. Some typical recommended daily dietary allowances are shown in Table 3-2.

To determine what the total fuel, or food, needs of the child are, the following individual fuel values of energy-producing foods must be known:

Carbohydrates	4 calories per gram
Proteins	4 calories per gram
Fats	9 calories per gram

If the number of grams of carbohydrate, protein, and fat in foods is known, the caloric value can be determined by multiplying each by the appropriate fuel value. For example, the calories of a 5-gram soda cracker, a carbohydrate, are calculated by multiplying 4 calories times the 5 grams of the cracker, for the total value of 20 calories. Dietitians have calculated the carbohydrate, protein, and fat contents of many different natural foods, have determined the caloric value of each, and have published these findings in calorie charts. These charts are of great help to parents and others who care for children with nutritional disorders, such as obesity and diabetes.

A number of factors increases the metabolic rate and causes the body to burn its fuel more rapidly. Exercise can double the rest metabolic rate. Fever, or an elevation of the body temperature above normal, causes an increase in metabolism and in the need for fuel and water. Thus a feverish child resting in bed may burn up many more calories than a healthy one at play.

Three potent hormones, thyroxin, insulin, and epinephrine, have a profound effect on body temperature. Thyroxin, produced by the thyroid gland, increases the metabolism in all of the tissues. A lack of thyroxin can lower the rate by 50% and an increase can cause a 300% rise. Insulin plays an important part in glucose and fat metabolism. Any disturbance in the normal secretion of this hormone seriously disrupts metabolism. Epinephrine, a hormone produced by the adrenal gland, stimulates metabolism in crisis situations.

The balanced diet

Children are not given minerals, proteins, and fats. They are served foods. These foods must be chosen to include all the necessary components so that children will grow properly and have energy and body heat. When these daily needs are translated into foods, children's diets are said to be *balanced*. This means that total dietary needs are met by the foods they eat.

A number of charts have been devised to help parents select the foods for their families that will provide a balanced diet. One of these is the "Basic Four Chart," recommended by the U.S.

Department of Agriculture. This chart recommends both food items and numbers of servings that should be included in the diet each day (Fig. 3-1).

Planning a balanced diet of foods within a fixed income that will be attractive to a family of various ages is something of an art. It requires knowledge and considerable skill. Parents may need help in this important, but difficult, task, If pediatric nurses find that they cannot provide the needed help, they should seek the assistance of dietitians whose training especially prepares them to give meal-planning advice.

Principles of pediatric nutrition

The feeding of infants and children has been the focal point of much debate. Just about every aspect of the subject has been argued, from breast versus bottle, to force feeding 4-year-old children, to teenage diets. Everyone seems to have an opinion, including grandmothers, preachers, doctors, and scientists. Out of all this controversy, what general truths can be found that will apply in all cultures to all children? What guidelines can the pediatric nurse follow that will be universal and nutritionally sound?

At least three principles apply to the feeding of infants and children: (1) the diet should meet the current nutritional and caloric needs of the child, (2) the foods eaten should be of an appropriate consistency and form to suit the age of the child, and (3) eating should be separated from emotional stress, pressure, and pain, thus making it a pleasant experience.

Nutritional and caloric needs

As the child grows physically, so do nutritional needs. The child needs more of all the essential nutrients and a greater amount of fuel (calories) to meet increased activities and size. These nutrients and fuel are especially important during growth spurts. The daily allowance shown in Table 3-2 demonstrates the rather dramatic increase in both nutrient and calories needed by the child during the growing years.

Appropriate foods

The consistency and form of the foods offered to infants and children must be appropriate to their physical development. At first when babies have no teeth and have a strong sucking reflex, they need liquid foods fed through a nipple. Later when they learn to place food in their mouths but have no teeth, they need soft foods. When the molars come in so they can chew, children can manage solid foods.

Pleasant experience

From the beginning of life the process of taking food into the body is closely associated with emotions. The baby who is held and cuddled while nursing is more contented than the one left in the crib with a propped bottle. The young child who sees and hears pleasant conversation during meals comes to look forward to mealtime as a happy occasion. Attitudes toward food are developed during childhood and continue to influence individuals throughout their entire lives. If a child is punished for not eating or forced to eat some particular food when nauseated, negative attitudes may be formed that persist for years. Studies have shown that a child, given a variety of foods from which to choose for a period of several consecutive days, may overindulge on one favored dish for a while, but after a few meals will begin to select a well-balanced diet. No adult direction, bribes, or threats are needed. In general, one can say that the best environment for the child to develop eating habits is one that is free of tension, where foods are served on a take-it-or-leave-it basis, and where the prevailing attitudes are positive.

DENTAL HEALTH

Health of the mouth and teeth is of utmost importance to the growing child. It affects emotional, social, and physical well-being. Like all other areas of health, prevention is of greater value than cure. Four ways by which dental health can be promoted are (1) good nutrition and eating habits, (2) oral hygiene, (3) fluorida-tion of the drinking water or topical application of fluoride to the teeth, and (4) regular dental examinations and care.

Good nutrition that includes adequate protein, fresh fruits, and vegetables is particularly important to dental health. Equally important is the restriction in the diet of concentrated sugars and starches. If these foods remain around the teeth they create an excellent medium for the growth of cavity-producing bacteria. For this reason, candy and sugar-gum should be avoided. The child should be taught to rinse the mouth with water after drinking milk or eating concentrated foods.

Oral hygiene is closely associated with eating habits. It includes all measures that will promote health in the mouth and teeth. Keeping the teeth clean and free from bacteria that would eat away the enamel is an important part of oral hygiene. Regular brushing of the teeth and flossing between them should begin early in the child's experience (Fig. 3-2). Many dentists recommend the use of the electric toothbrush and the water-jet cleaner, which not only encourage use because of their novelty but also clean the teeth more thoroughly. Successful hand brushing can be accomplished by using a circular, vigorous stroke. If the child is not able to do this, parents should see that the teeth are brushed properly.

Thumb-sucking in a small infant does not disrupt the normal alignment of the teeth. Prolonged thumb-sucking during the toddler, preschool, and school years can seriously affect normal development of the oral structure. The tongue may grow very large from overuse and the teeth may be pushed out of line affecting both speech and appearance. Some dentists find that special exercises that encourage the child to draw the tongue back into the mouth and to align the jaws and teeth are of value in overcoming such deformities. Because thumb-sucking is a strong habit, born of oral satisfaction needs, the child may need special help to overcome the habit after emotional and physical needs are satisfied.

Fluoridation is an added aid to dental health.

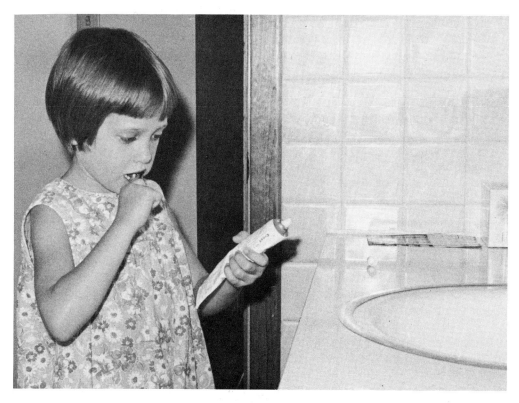

Fig. 3-2. Regular brushing of the teeth should begin early in the child's experience.

Recent studies indicate that the amount of tooth decay in children is less if fluoride-bearing water is consumed from birth through 8 years of age. This is the period when tooth enamel is being formed. The benefits continue throughout life. These children have two thirds less tooth decay than children who have drunk water deficient in fluoride. Because of this finding, many communities add what is considered to be the optimum amount of fluoride to the public water supply. This is 1 part fluoride to 1 million parts water. It has also been found that topical or painted-on applications of fluoride further protect teeth from decay. For this reason current practice recommended by pedodontists (children's dentists) is to clean and then paint the teeth with either stannous fluoride or sodium fluoride every 4 to 6 months throughout childhood. Some dentists recommend that this practice continue throughout life.

Regular dental examinations should be as much a part of the child's medical supervision as general physical examinations. Dental examinations should begin at about 2½ to 3 years of age. A friendly relationship between the dentist and the child should be established in these early visits to eliminate the fear that so often leads to postponement and dental neglect. During each examination the dentist inspects the gums, tongue, and teeth. Over 150 symptoms of various systemic diseases can be observed in the oral cavity. The dentist cleans the teeth, treats any decay, paints them with fluoride, and discusses home care with the child and the parents. Positive information and attitudes established during childhood continue throughout life.

PROVISION FOR EMOTIONAL NEEDS

To ensure the emotional and mental health of children, their basic emotional needs must be met. This area of preventive pediatrics has been ignored or considered to be outside the province of medicine for too long. Recent public concern for mental health gives hope that this most vital area will soon receive rightful attention. Although great strides have been made in the treatment of mental illness, the best solution is prevention, and such prevention must take place during childhood. The basis of mental illness begins early in life. If children live with hate, insecurity, and neglect, they will be permanently damaged by the time they reach adolescence. Doctors and nurses who work with children and their parents should be especially alert to symptoms that suggest that the child's basic emotional needs are not being met.

The eight basic emotional needs of children have been identified as love, security, achievement, acceptance, self-respect, recognition, independence, and order and control. Their importance in influencing the growth and development of the child is discussed in greater detail in Chapter 2.

Because every child and family unit is different from every other one, the manner and degree by which the basic emotional needs are met may be quite different. The important thing is not *how* they are met, but that they *are* met. This difference is difficult to judge. If there is a question about the adequacy of a child's daily protein intake, the answer can be calculated rather easily. But how does one decide if a child is receiving "enough" acceptance, especially when no one knows what the daily recommended allowance is or even how it is measured? It cannot be measured. What *can* be seen and evaluated are the reactions a child has to others and to frustrations. Emotional responses may reveal how well the needs of the child are being met. The child may react with temper tantrums, aggressive behavior, cruelty, lying, tattling, showing off, with-drawal, or sugary-sweet compliance. All such behavior is manifested by most children at some time. If any one of these behaviors becomes habitual, however, something is wrong and needs attention. Pediatric nurses are frequently the ones who hear parents describe such adverse behavior or who see children under stress when they manifest these symptoms. Nurses should be alert to the importance of these responses and report them to the physician, who may then seek to counsel the parents or refer them for more extensive psychological counseling.

IMMUNIZATION AGAINST DISEASE

Only two or three generations ago contagious diseases threatened the life of every child. Almost every family lost children to diphtheria, whooping cough, and other infections, sometimes suffering the loss of many children in a single epidemic. In those days quarantine, or isolation, was the only means available to control the spread of such diseases. In recent years such measures have been changed as a result of widespread immunization of the population, particularly children. Immunization has proved to be the safest, most effective, and most inexpensive method of preventing illness. It has become a routine procedure in preventive pediatrics.

Mechanism of immunity

Immunization is the process whereby a person becomes immune, or is able to resist disease. Immunity to specific diseases is possible because within the body substances called *antibodies* destroy or injure the disease-producing agent or neutralize its toxins. When antigens are injected into the body, the body produces specific antibodies against the antigens and is then able to resist future attacks by those same antigens. This resistance is called *active* immunity because the person's own body produced the antibodies. Sometimes ready-made antibodies are injected into an individual to provide immediate immunity to some disease. This resistance is called *passive immunity*, and since the person's own body did not make the antibodies, it is only temporary.

Antigens may be pathogenic organisms and their poisons, or they may be ready-made vaccines and toxoids. Antibodies may be formed in the human body or may be formed in animals and given to humans to provide a passive immunity (Fig. 3-3).

Types of immunity

Fig. 3-4 provides a graphic picture of the kinds of immunity present in humans. *General immunity* refers to the many built-in defense mechanisms in the body. The skin, the secretions of the digestive tract, the circulatory system with its lymph and white blood cells all serve to protect the body against general infections. Good nutrition and positive mental attitudes contribute

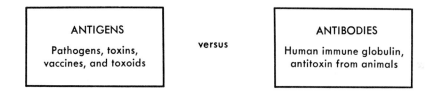

Fig. 3-3. Antigens and antibodies.

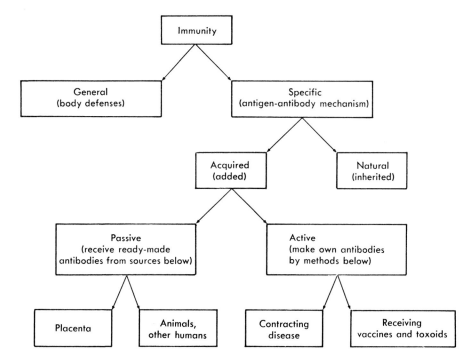

Fig. 3-4. Types of immunity.

Table 3-3. Immunization and tuberculin testing schedule for normal infants*

2 months	Diphtheria, tetanus, pertussis (DTP)
	Trivalent oral polio vaccine (TOPV)
4 months	DTP, TOPV
6 months	DTP, TOPV optional in areas of high poliomyelitis endemicity
12 months	Tuberculin test optional, depending on exposure risk
15 months	Measles-mumps-rubella
18 months	DTP, TOPV
4 to 6 years	DTP, TOPV
14 to 16 years and thereafter every 10 years	Tetanus and diphtheria toxoids, adult type (Td)
At time of contaminated injury if more than 5 years since last dose	Tetanus toxoids (T)

*Recommended by the American Academy of Pediatrics in Report of the Committee on Infectious Diseases, Evanston, Ill., 1977, American Academy of Pediatrics.

Table 3-4. Immunization and tuberculin testing schedule for children not immunized in early infancy*

Under 6 years of age	
First visit	Diphtheria, tetanus, pertussis (DTP)
	Trivalent oral polio vaccine (TOPV)
Interval after first visit	
1 month	Measles, if child over 15 months; mumps, rubella
2 months	DTP, TOPV
4 months	DTP; TOPV optional unless in area of high poliomyelitis endemicity
10 to 16 months or preschool	DTP, TOPV
Age 14 to 16 years and thereafter every 10 years	Tetanus and diptheria toxoid, adult type (Td)
6 years of age and over	
First visit	Td, TOPV, tuberculin test
Interval after first visit	
1 month	Measles, mumps, rubella
2 months	Td, TOPV
8 to 14 months	Td, TOPV
Age 14 to 16 years and thereafter every 10 years	Td

*Recommended by the American Academy of Pediatrics in Report of Committee on Infectious Diseases, Evanston, Ill., 1977, American Academy of Pediatrics.

to this reinforcement of all defense systems. *Specific immunity* involves the complex antigen-antibody mechanisms described previously. Some persons seem to inherit an inborn resistance to certain diseases that is called *natural immunity*. All normal persons are able to become immune to certain conditions in a process called *acquired immunity*. One can acquire immunity passively or actively. Passive immunity is always temporary because it results from the "gift" of someone else's antibodies, either by injection or through the placenta during intrauterine life. Antibodies manufactured by the mother against specific diseases pass into the fetus and provide immunity for about 4 to 6 months after birth. Because there is no passive immunity to pertussis (whooping cough) and because the mother may not have all types of antibodies, immunization of infants is begun as early as possible, sometimes by 2 or 3 months of age.

Active immunity can be acquired by contracting the disease in a mild or severe form or by receiving the attenuated or inactivated pathogen or toxin by means of injection. The controlled solutions of these pathogens or toxins are called *vaccines*, and the injection of them into an individual is called *inoculation* or *vaccination*. Vaccines have been produced for a number of contagious diseases, including smallpox, diphtheria, pertussis, tetanus, typhoid, poliomyelitis, cholera, and most recently mumps, rubella, and rubeola. Research continues, with the goal that one day all the major infectious diseases can be conquered.

Current practice

Currently the immunization of infants is started at 2 to 3 months of age when the combined vaccines of diphtheria, pertussis, and tetanus are given in a single injection (Tables 3-3 and 3-4). At the same time an oral feeding of polio vaccine is given to the infant. This feeding is repeated at 1-month intervals for a total of two or three times. During the interval the baby is

manufacturing antibodies against all four diseases. After the initial series of three doses, booster or recall doses are given to stimulate added antibody production and produce maximum immunity. Booster doses of individual vaccines may be given at any age after the initial series if there is an epidemic. Tetanus toxoid boosters are given if there has been a skin wound. An injured person who has not had the tetanus toxoid series is given an injection of tetanus antitoxin (in horse serum) or human globulin containing tetanus antitoxin. Because of possible reaction to horse serum, a skin test using a minute amount of the vaccine may be done before administering the full dose. A skin test for tuberculosis may also be done at 2-year intervals throughout childhood and adolescence. This is not a vaccination but is a sensitivity test to see if the body has developed antibodies against the tubercle bacillus. Other vaccines such as cholera, smallpox, and typhoid may be given if the child is living in or traveling through an area where these diseases are common.

Contraindications

Immunization procedures must be deferred or altered in the following special circumstances:

1. When the child has an acute respiratory infection or other infection, the body's defense mechanisms are under maximum stress and the addition of a potent antigen could be overwhelming. The interval between injections does not interfere with final immunity, and so deferring one of a series of injections up to 6 months is acceptable.

2. A child with eczema, impetigo, or any other form of dermatitis should not be vaccinated against smallpox because of the danger of *eczema vaccinatum*, a widespread skin infection caused by the vaccine. The child should be isolated from other children who have been vaccinated to prevent cross contamination.

3. The brain-damaged child or one with convulsive disorders should not receive immuniza-

tions until age 1 year, and then the immunizations should be begun cautiously in fractional doses.

4. Children who are receiving any of the steroid drugs have a diminished antibody-manufacturing response. For this reason routine immunization procedures should be deferred until the steroid therapy is completed, or the routine should be altered so that the child will be able to cope with those vaccines given.

Clinic procedure and precautions

Immunization procedures are done regularly in doctors' offices and in the outpatient clinics of hospitals. In mass immunization programs they may be carried out in schools, churches, and other public places. The nurse is responsible to see that the equipment and supplies are set up and that proper records are kept for each individual immunized. Although a doctor may administer the vaccine, the nurse is frequently authorized to do so. Ideally, the waiting room should be separated from the room where the injections are administered. The equipment should

be arranged in a convenient manner on a table with a chair for the parent and one for the doctor. The child stands or is held by the parent (Fig. 3-5).

The following precautions should be carefully observed:

1. Needles and syringes must be sterile. The practice of using one syringe with a change of needles between injections is not considered safe.

2. The injection site and rubber stopper of the antigen container should be cleansed with an antiseptic solution.

3. Toxoids and vaccines that contain alum should be given intramuscularly, preferably in the midlateral thigh or deltoid muscle.

4. Vaccines should be stored according to the directions printed on the containers. Outdated, discolored, or abnormal appearing vaccines should not be used.

5. An emergency stimulant such as epinephrine should be available in the event of an untoward reaction to the vaccine or antitoxin.

6. Systemic or severe local reactions follow-

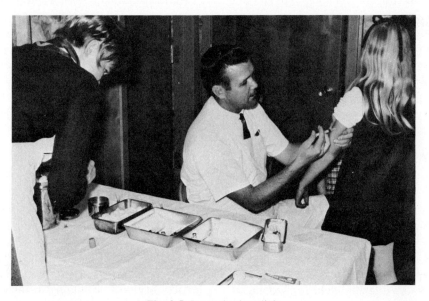

Fig. 3-5. Immunization clinic.

ing an injection should be brought to the attention of the doctor, who may order a delay or decrease in the next dose. The nurse should ask the parent about reactions to the former injection.

Attitudes of the child and the public

Many children begin to cry when there is even mention of a doctor visit. They remember the painful injection they received at the last visit and want no more. Although it is impossible to remove all the physical discomfort of a potent vaccine, much of the psychological pain can be relieved if the parent and nurse work together. A doctor visit or an injection should never be used as a threat or a punishment. The trauma of the experience can be lessened if it is not preceded by worry and if the injection is done quickly and skillfully. It is best not to tell the child in advance when the next immunization will be given but to simply go for a ride and end up at the doctor's office. When the moment of truth does come, if the needle is sharp and the injection done without hesitation, pain is lessened.

Although medical records are kept by the doctor or clinic, parents should be encouraged to maintain one at home for each child. This record should include all immunizations with the dates given and all contagious diseases with the dates symptoms appeared. This information is needed for future applications for school, camp, international travel, and other activities.

Once there was a great deal of public resistance to immunization programs. The dramatic success of the Salk and Sabin vaccines against paralytic poliomyelitis softened public attitudes. Now resistance has changed to apathy. Immunization is now largely ignored and left to public health departments and private physicians. For this reason nurses should seize every opportunity to educate the public about the need for continuing programs of immunization to the end that every child and every adult will be protected. Parents of newborn infants should be encouraged to take the child to a physician or to a well-child conference for follow-up care and immunization. Some school districts require immunization for every pupil. Adults should also be encouraged to maintain their immunity.

PROTECTION AGAINST ACCIDENTS

The tremendous progress made in the prevention and treatment of infectious diseases and nutritional disorders has resulted in a distinct decline in child mortality. Today, the greatest threat to the health and well-being of the child is accidents. Approximately 47,000 children under 25 years of age die annually in the United States from accidents. Another 5 million, or one third of all children in the country, suffer nonfatal accidents, some of which are disabling for life. According to U.S. National Center for Health Statistics, accidents kill more children than the next five leading causes of childhood deaths, which include: homicide, cancer, congenital anomalies, pneumonia, and heart disease.

These tragic accidents can be explained, if not excused, by the fact that infants and children are both physically and mentally immature, that they have a natural curiosity that is not tempered with experience or fear, that the modern world is filled with powerful, rapid machines, and that every home contains literally thousands of potentially lethal chemicals and physical forces. All these factors contribute to the increasing dangers to children in this modern, hurried world.

Some of the measures that can be taken to reduce the numbers and severity of accidents are (1) education of parents to potential home hazards, (2) promotion of safer manufacturing standards for children's toys, clothes, and furniture, (3) encouragement for early and universal swimming instructions, (4) promotion of fire prevention programs, (5) use of poison control centers, (6) support for driver education and safety programs, and (7) support for legislative action of accident prevention. The public must become aware of the magnitude of the accident problem before they will be willing to take the needed steps to curb it.

Accidents

An accident, by definition, is "an unexpected event of an injurious nature." By far the most accidents involve violent trauma, with motor vehicles leading the group that also includes falls, piercing wounds, and animal bites. Burns, drowning, and poisoning complete the sorry picture. The tragedy is greater when one realizes that the numbers of self-inflicted "accidents" leading to suicide and to child abuse are high.

Influencing factors

Certain factors seem to influence the incidence and occurrence of accidents. Some of these are age, sex, race, season, place, and proneness. They are of great importance because 90% of all accidents and 98% of all poisonings are considered preventable.

Age. Most home accidents occur when children are 1 to 1½ years of age. They have just learned to walk but have not become aware of the dangers of the world around them, so fearlessly and trustingly they stumble into all manner of harm. Adequate supervision in a safe environment could prevent most of these injuries. The adolescent years are also accident filled. Unresolved conflicts and unstable hormonal levels of youth cause depression and aggression that lead to suicide, drug abuse, and vehicle accidents. Counseling and crisis intervention services could help prevent much of this waste.

Sex. Boys have a much higher accident rate than do girls in the years beyond babyhood. This increase is probably caused by cultural factors that encourage more active and daring play.

Race. The nonwhite population has a higher incidence of accidents than the white population caused by factors that stem from poverty: poor housing, dangerous unsupervised play areas, and inadequate medical care.

Season. There are far more accidents in the spring and summer months than in the other seasons. This fact reflects the dangers found in the outdoors—heights, water, animals, insects, and vehicles. Children must be allowed to play outdoors and thus to risk some kind of injury, but they should not be exposed needlessly to danger. This risk of injury is why all children should learn to swim at an early age and should be taught safety precautions when handling matches, firearms, vehicles, and other potentially dangerous devices.

Place. A high percentage of accidents occurs in or near the home, especially with preschool children. As children increase their sphere of activity, the range of accident sites also increases.

Proneness. It has been found that more than half of all accidents occur to one tenth of the population and that this accident proneness begins to appear in the preschool years. It is associated with certain personality traits, including anxiety, insecurity, and the need for attention. Adults need to be alert to children who have repeated accidents, and should provide special help for them.

Traumatic accidents

Traumatic accidents include the many cuts from knives, broken glass, and other sharp objects (Fig. 3-6), piercing wounds from sticks and metal objects, broken bones from falls or blows, and tears from jagged metal or animal teeth.

Motor vehicle accidents produce the great majority of traumatic accidents. Automobile accidents are caused by driver error, mechanical failure, weather conditions, or a combination of these. The enormous loss of life and property that results from auto accidents has caused nationwide concern. As a result, large-scale efforts have been made in three areas: (1) Driver education classes have been started in high schools across the nation where the principles of "defensive driving" are taught. (2) Better roads and highways are being built with particular emphasis on safety features. (3) Legislative acts have been passed to reduce allowable speeds and to force automobile manufacturers to meet certain minimum safety standards in all makes of cars and to recall any auto proved to have a manufac-

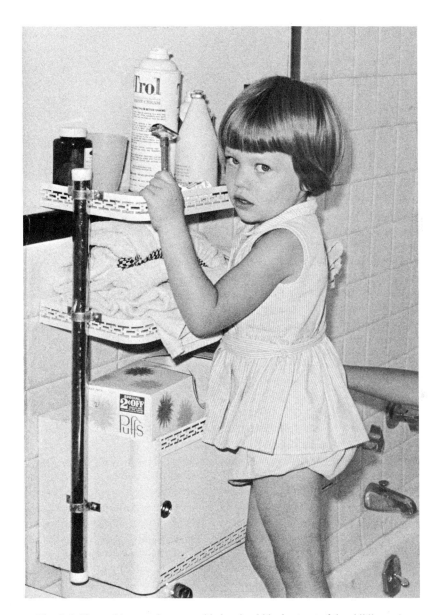

Fig. 3-6. Sharp objects such as razor blades should be kept out of the child's reach.

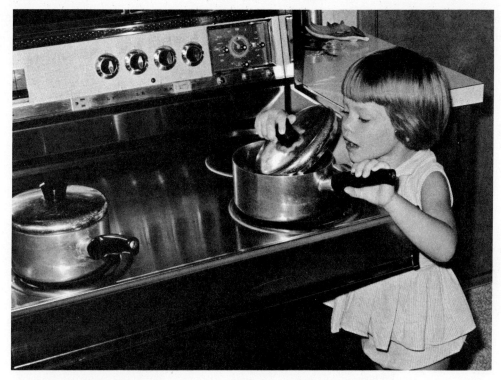

Fig. 3-7. Hot liquids can cause serious burns. If the handles of pots are turned in, there is less danger that little hands will reach them.

turing defect. (4) Public education to promote the use of safety belts and childseats for children. It is hoped that these combined efforts will reduce motor vehicle accidents.

Adequate supervision of the young child, teaching the older child reasonable judgment and safety, and leash laws to control dogs could prevent most traumatic accidents.

Burns and explosions

Burns from fires and explosions are almost all preventable. Open flames are always hazardous, whether they be from a fireplace, cooking stove, campfire, lit matches, or gas heaters. Combustible materials such as gasoline, kerosene, natural gas, and trash are potentially dangerous in all circumstances and should be treated with the ut-

most caution. Hot liquids, such as water from the tap or from pots overturned from the stove, can cause serious burns (Fig. 3-7). Because we live with potential fire hazards daily, fire safety should be observed at all times and taught at an early age to every child. Small children should never be left alone in a home. Babysitters should be given specific instructions about what to do in case of a fire. Some cities have annual voluntary fire inspection of homes, and school programs stress the need for constant vigilance.

Drowning

Swimming is an excellent activity for adults and children alike, but it is never entirely safe, even for the experienced swimmer. For this reason children should learn water safety as soon as they can learn to swim. All children should learn to swim; they can in fact, learn to swim before they learn to walk. Children are not "naturally" afraid of water, but learn this fear from adults and other children. Recent work with toddlers shows that children 6 to 24 months of age can learn to swim with daily lessons over a 6-week period.

Although children *can* learn to swim at an early age, not all do. Thousands are exposed to possible drowning every year. Some are saved because someone knew how to administer cardiopulmonary resuscitation (CPR). Many more would be saved if everyone learned CPR. See Chapter 12 for a discussion of this life-saving technique.

First aid priorities

If the nurse comes on an accident victim with unknown injuries, action should be taken according to the following list of priorities:

1. Evaluate the safety of the immediate environment and take steps to prevent greater injury or numbers of injured. (For example, turn off electricity in an electrocution; get someone to slow or stop traffic at the scene of an auto accident.)
2. Evaluate the nature and extent of injuries and treat in the following order:
   a. Stoppage of breathing—establish an airway; restore and maintain respirations.
   b. Hemorrhage—control by direct pressure, or in extreme cases, tourniquet.
   c. Poisoning—establish respirations, rush child and poison container to emergency room of hospital.
   d. Wounds—control bleeding; cover with clean cloth; do not attempt to clean.
   e. Burns—do not attempt to remove clothing if stuck to burn; cover loosely with clean cloth and take child to emergency room of hospital.
   f. Fractures and dislocations—immobilize the affected part; improper movement

can cause serious additional injury, particularly if the spinal cord has been fractured; move these patients with help; avoid twisting.
3. Keep the patient warm and quiet and treat for shock; avoid letting patient see the injury; avoid nervous chatter.
4. Send someone for help; keep the curious away and stay with the injured person.
5. Never give liquids to an unconscious person or alcohol to an accident victim.

Poisoning

Children will swallow almost anything, no matter how it tastes. The variety of poisonous substances children have been known to swallow is amazing. Many poisons are found at home in the medicine cabinet or under the kitchen sink (Fig. 3-8). The majority of accidental poisonings are preventable and only occur because of ignorance or negligence.

Each year more than 2,000 children die from accidental poisoning in the United States. The majority are in their second year of life. For each death, there are an additional 100 to 150 nonfatal cases, many of whom suffer permanent disabilities such as esophageal stricture or kidney or liver damage. This tragic waste could be largely prevented if reasonable precautions were taken.

Precautions

1. Never leave toddlers unattended. Expect them to explore. Anticipate their curiosity.

2. Keep all drugs, poisonous substances, and household chemicals out of the reach of little hands. Get rid of all animal poisons.

3. Never give a child a bottle of medicine or poisonous substance to play with, no matter how tightly stoppered it may seem to be.

4. Do not use food containers for medicine or poisonous substances.

5. Label all medicines in bold print and read the label carefully before administering.

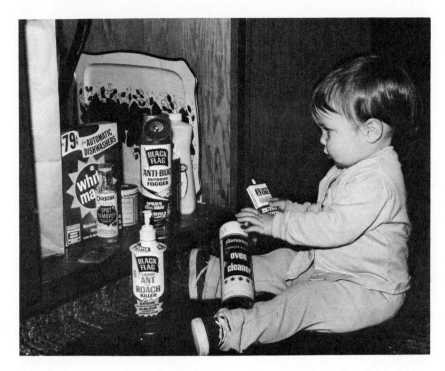

Fig. 3-8. Poisons lurk under the kitchen sink in the form of common household chemicals.

6. Never tell children that flavored medicine is candy.

7. Used bottles and cans which have contained poisons should be removed from the home and discarded.

8. Keep a bottle of ipecac with emergency supplies to induce vomiting when it is safe to do so. (See later discussion for safe conditions.)

Immediate care

Any accidental poisoning should be treated as an emergency. Read the label of the substance. Unless contraindicated, induce vomiting, then call the physician and take the child and poisonous substance to the nearest emergency room. If the child is unconscious, the airway should be kept open. If breathing has stopped, resuscitation should be commenced at once. The child should be kept quiet, warm, and dry.

Emergency management

When the child arrives in the emergency room, the following action should be taken at once: (1) remove the poison, (2) identify the poison, (3) administer the antidote, and (4) administer other supportive treatment.

Remove the poison. The stomach should be emptied as soon as possible, except in the case of corrosive agents such as lye, where further damage could be done to the mucous membrane, or in the case of petroleum distillates such as gasoline, which might be aspirated into the lungs. Vomiting can be induced by mechanically stimulating the gag reflex (sticking a finger down the throat) or by the use of an emetic drug such as ipecac. Gastric lavage (washing out the stomach) is perhaps the most effective method. A gastric tube is inserted and about 200 ml of tap water is injected and aspirated as many times as

Table 3-5. Universal antidote

Ingredients	Chemicals provided	Action of chemicals
Two parts burned toast	Activated charcoal	Absorbs or inactivates substances
One part milk of magnesia	Magnesium hydroxide	Neutralizes acids
One part strong tea	Tannic acid	Precipitates metals, alkaloids, and glucosides

necessary to remove any trace of the poison. Lavage should not be attempted when a corrosive agent has been swallowed; instead, a neutralizing chemical should be used to nullify the corrosive.

Identify the poison. Specific antidotes can be given as soon as a poison is identified. The poison container should be brought with the child to the emergency room. Many products have the ingredients listed on the label. If there is a question about the poison or antidote, a telephone call to a Poison Control Center may be necessary. At these centers information about the chemical composition, toxicity, and recommended treatment is readily available.

Administer the antidote. Immediately after the stomach has been emptied, antidotes are given to neutralize any remaining poison and to prevent its absorption. Specific antidotes for the particular poison are of course preferred. If they are not available certain general antidotes can be used, such as BAL (British anti-lewisite), which is effective against heavy metals such as lead, mercury, and antimony. The so-called "universal antidote" may be given when the poison is unknown or when a specific antidote is unavailable (Table 3-5).

Supportive treatment. Vomiting or gastric lavage is a physically and emotionally exhausting experience. After the initial treatment the child needs to rest and to be kept warm and dry. The vital signs are checked at regular intervals, signs of shock observed, pain relieved, airway kept open, and fluids and nutrition maintained.

Poison control centers

Because time is of such great importance to the successful treatment of poison victims, the need for immediate information about poisons and their treatment is urgent. To meet this need, a network of Poison Control Centers has been established across the United States with 24-hour answering service. Information about over 250,000 toxic and potentially toxic trade name products is as near as the telephone. These centers are usually associated with medical schools or large hospitals. Besides offering emergency information, the centers serve as treatment centers and are engaged in public information and education programs to prevent accidental poisoning.

Principles of accident prevention

Three general principles that emerge from any study of accidents among children are (1) protection from danger must be provided for helpless infants and inexperienced children, (2) dangerous environmental conditions should be changed to promote safety, and (3) safety education needs to be provided for all children so they will know how to assume self-responsibility.

Protection from danger. The naïve trustfulness of children is one of their most delightful traits. It is also one of their greatest hazards. During the years while infants develop awareness, toddlers learn a healthy respect for danger, and adolescents learn restraint, adults must assume responsibility for their safety. Although it is true that advancing age of children usually reduces the need for close adult supervision, adults should not take too much for granted but must continue watchful protectiveness.

Environmental safety. A large percentage of accidents are caused by unsafe conditions such as burns from unprotected flames, drownings from open wells, automobile accidents from dangerous roads, poisonings from accessible chemicals, and gunshot wounds from loaded firearms. All adults must become safety minded, that is, they must seek constantly to prevent accidents by removing environmental causes.

Safety education. One of the aims of child rearing is that children should become responsible for themselves, particularly in the area of safety. As children grow and develop, they should be taught safety in every area of life.

MEDICAL SUPERVISION

Medical supervision means that professionally trained members of the medical team work together to supervise the physical and emotional health needs of the child. The team includes the physician, dentist, nurses, and all other related health personnel. This team does not replace the parents, but it does provide specialized services in prevention, diagnosis, and treatment of abnormal conditions that may affect the health of children. It is important for parents to understand that consultation with members of the medical team should not wait until the child is obviously ill. It should go on continuously, beginning at birth. Medical supervision is provided through a variety of means, including visits by the public health nurse to the home, well-child conferences, immunization clinics, school health programs, telephone consultation with informed medical sources, and examinations by the physician, pediatric nurse practitioner, and dentist.

Every child needs regular physical examinations to safeguard health. A recommended schedule of examinations is as follows:

Birth to 12 months	Every month
12 to 18 months	Every 2 to 3 months
18 months to 5 years	Every 6 months
5 or more years	Every year

Every child needs regular dental examinations, beginning at about 2½ to 3 years of age and continuing throughout life. Abnormal conditions of the mouth or teeth need special attention promptly. A recommended schedule of examinations and care by the dentist is:

Birth to 2½ years	No visits unless a problem
2½ to 18 years	Every 4 to 6 months
18 or more years	Every year

SUMMARY OUTLINE

I. Preventive pediatrics
  A. Before conception
  B. Prenatal period
  C. Parturition
  D. Immediate newborn infant care
  E. Infancy, childhood, and adolescence

II. Adequate nutrition
  A. Foods in the diet
    1. Components
      a. Oxygen
      b. Water
      c. Protein
      d. Minerals
        (1) Calcium and phosporus
        (2) Iron
        (3) Iodine
      e. Vitamins
      f. Carbohydrates
      g. Fats
    2. Functions
      a. Building and repairing body tissue
      b. Regulating body processes
      c. Providing heat and energy
    3. The balanced diet
  B. Principles of pediatric nutrition
    1. Nutritional and caloric needs
    2. Appropriate foods
    3. Pleasant experience

III. Dental health

IV. Provision for emotional needs

V. Immunization against disease
  A. Mechanism of immunity
  B. Types of immunity
  C. Current practice
  D. Contraindications
  E. Clinic procedure and precautions
  F. Attitudes of the child and the public

VI. Protection against accidents
  A. Accidents

1. Influencing factors
   a. Age
   b. Sex
   c. Race
   d. Season
   e. Place
   f. Proneness
2. Traumatic accidents
3. Burns and explosions
4. Drowning
5. First aid priorities

B. Poisonings
1. Precautions
2. Immediate care
3. Emergency management
   a. Remove the poison
   b. Identify the poison
   c. Administer the antidote
   d. Supportive treatment
4. Poison control centers

C. Principles of accident prevention
1. Protection from danger
2. Environmental safety
3. Safety education

VII. **Medical supervision**

STUDY QUESTIONS

1. What are six general ways a child's health can be ensured?
2. List the three major functions of food in the body.
3. List the seven components of food. Why is each necessary for life?
4. Discuss the pros and cons of thumb-sucking and fluoridation as they relate to dental health.
5. Define immunization, antibodies, antigens, active immunity, passive immunity, vaccines.
6. List the first aid priorities at an accident scene.
7. When a child has been poisoned, what should be done by the parent at the scene? What should be done in the emergency room?

4
Infancy

VOCABULARY

Physiological resilience
Atelectasis
Protective reflexes
Icterus neonatorum
Supplementary feedings
Pacifier
Cradle cap
Hand-mouth coordination

The newborn infant is a miracle of nature, the result of 40 weeks of never-to-be-equaled growth and development. At birth the process of moving from total dependence to independence begins, though for some time the child will continue to rely on the immediate environment for physical care, mental stimuli, and emotional support.

All newborn infants are unique. Their genetic inheritance makes them different in size, shape, and appearance; their 9 months of intrauterine life were unique in nutrition, oxygen supply, and other factors; the delivery and immediate care after birth were unlike that of any other infant. In spite of this uniqueness, all babies share common needs and follow similar developmental patterns. It is important for the nurse to know what the average, or representative, infant is like so that each baby may receive special attention if there should be too much deviation from the normal.

The period of infancy extends from birth until the child learns to walk at about 12 to 18 months of age. It is characterized by a 1-month period of initial adjustment and growth called the newborn period, followed by the dramatic emotional, physical, and motor development that culminates in the independence of walking alone. Because the process of growth is gradual, each stage of development merges into the next stage.

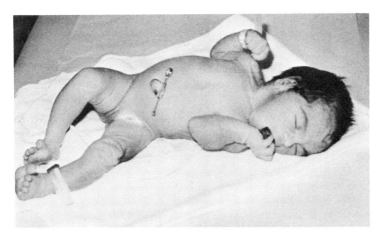

Fig. 4-1. The newborn infant.

THE NEWBORN INFANT
(birth to 1 month)
Characteristics

Proportion of boys to girls. Statistically, there are 106 male infants born to every 100 female infants. The genetic reasons for this difference in proportion of boys to girls are still unproved, but male infants are more fragile and have a higher mortality rate.

Physiological resilience. All normal newborn infants of both sexes possess a certain physiological resilience, which is a kind of passiveness to both internal and external stress. This resilience protects the infant during the first hours and days after birth from reacting too greatly to the new and hostile world outside and to the physiological revolution taking place inside the body. Because of this resilience, the newborn infant can survive extremes of cold and heat, abnormal levels of substances in the blood, and a lack of food and water. There are, however, limits to the normal infant's reserve that should not be risked. The premature infant does not have this resilience and so must be protected from as many stresses as possible.

A week or so after birth, when the regulating mechanism and the body systems of the infant begin to function in their intended way, this special physiological resilience is no longer needed and disappears. Then the baby reacts more acutely to cold and heat and to an imbalance of the body chemistry.

Immunity. If the mother has antibodies for certain infectious diseases, they pass through the placenta from the mother to the infant. Among these antibodies are those for smallpox, mumps, diptheria, and measles. This passive immunity lasts from a few weeks to several months. Few, if any, antibodies are passed on for chickenpox or pertussis, and so young infants are easy prey to these diseases. Because all contagious diseases are more severe in newborn infants than in older children, particularly pertussis, immunization measures should be commenced as early as 2 to 3 months of age.

Body shape and size. Newborn infants seem to be all head and abdomen, with small, bowed legs and little hips; their necks are short and creased, the nose is flat, and they appear to be chinless. Their tiny feet look impossibly inept and flat because of the pad of fat on the sole. The genitalia, though small, seem swollen and out of proportion. Their little arms are dwarfed by the large protruding abdomen (Fig. 4-1).

As a general rule, boys tend to be longer and weigh more than girls. White infants are larger than nonwhite ones. The first-born child is likely to be smaller than siblings and small parents tend to produce small children. The normal ranges of body measurements at birth are as follows:

Head circumference	12 to 14 inches
	(30 to 35 cm)
Chest circumference	11 to 13 inches
	(27.5 to 30.5 cm)
Length	18 to 22 inches
	(45 to 55 cm)
Weight	6½ to 9 pounds
	(2,900 to 4,000 gm)

Vital signs. Temperature, pulse, and respirations of newborn infants vary in response to the environment. Because of physiological resilience, they can withstand a rather wide range of body stresses, but when the limits of tolerance are exceeded, infants may suddenly become ill. For this reason nurses must constantly observe their small charges and seek to provide them with as optimum an environment as possible.

Temperature. At birth the temperature of infants is about the same as their mothers', but because they have little fat insulation, a large body surface, relatively poor circulation, and do not sweat or shiver yet, their ability to regulate body temperature is poor. Because excessive cold may overload the heart and excessive heat causes "prickly heat," a pinpoint rash called *miliaria*, the nurse must regulate the environment to provide constant body temperature near 98.6° F. (37° C).

Pulse. The pulse rate of newborn babies is 90 to 180 per minute, depending on activity. It may become irregular from any one of a number of physical and emotional stimuli such as being startled, crying, or undergoing a sudden temperature change. The temporal artery is the most convenient place to count the pulse with the fingers, and the apical cardiac pulse the most convenient to count with the stethoscope.

Respiration. Respirations of newborn infants are irregular in depth, rate, and rhythm and vary from 32 to 48 per minute. Like the pulse rate, respirations are affected by such things as crying. Normally, respirations are gentle, quiet, rapid, and shallow. They are most easily observed by watching abdominal movements, because newborn respiration is carried on mainly by the diaphragm and abdominal muscles.

Retraction, or pronounced sucking in of the chest with each inspiration, is not normal and indicates respiratory distress. Dyspnea and cyanosis may occur suddenly in an infant who has been breathing normally. These signs may be the first indication of a congenital anomaly or some other serious condition. The nurse should notify the physician if respirations drop below 32 or exceed 48 per minute when the infant is at rest.

Blood pressure. The blood pressure of the newborn infant is characteristically low and difficult to measure accurately with the conventional sphygmomanometer. When a cuff 2.5 cm wide is used, pressure ranges from 55 to 80 mm Hg systolic to 40 to 45 mm Hg diastolic. As the child grows older blood pressure gradually rises and pulse and respiration rates drop.

Skin. At birth the delicate skin of the newborn infant appears dark red because it is thin and the layers of subcutaneous fat have not yet covered over the capillary beds. This redness shows through even heavily pigmented skin. It becomes even more flushed when the infant cries. Some common characteristics of the skin of newborn infants follow.

Vernix caseosa. During the months of intrauterine life the fetus floats in amniotic fluid. Its tender skin is protected by a cheeselike, cream-colored paste, called *vernix caseosa*, that is secreted by the sebaceous glands and the epithelial cells (Fig. 4-2). At birth some infants are covered thickly while others may have deposits only in the body creases. Many physicians prefer that a minimum of the vernix be removed so that it may continue a protective function. Others pre-

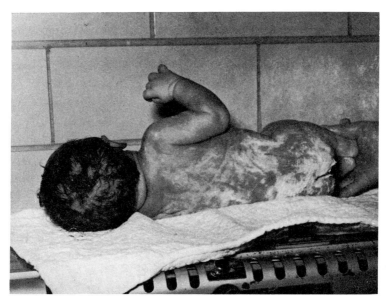

Fig. 4-2. Vernix caseosa protects the tender skin of the fetus as it floats in amniotic fluid during intrauterine life. (From Hamilton, P.M.: Basic maternity nursing, ed. 4, St. Louis, 1979, The C.V. Mosby Co.)

fer that it be thoroughly removed to prevent the possibility of its harboring bacteria. In any case, the vernix usually disappears in 2 or 3 days.

Lanugo. Lanugo is a soft, downy hair that covers the skin of the fetus beginning about the sixteenth week of gestation and continuing until the thirty-second week, when it begins to disappear. Thus the more premature an infant is, the more lanugo is present at birth. It is distributed over the entire body but is more dense on the shoulders, back, extremities, and temple. Lanugo tends to disappear during the first week of life.

Desquamation. Desquamation is the peeling of the skin that occurs normally during the first 2 to 4 weeks of life. It may be pronounced or quite minimal and is most common in low birth weight infants.

Erythema allergicum. Erythema allergicum is a kind of "allergic redness" that appears as red blotches on the skin of otherwise normal infants.

It may appear on the day of birth and may persist for many weeks. The red blotches may become raised and even develop blisters before they gradually disappear. There is no known cause or cure; it is not contagious and most often affects healthy, vigorous babies.

Mongolian spots. Occasionally, bluish black pigmented areas occur on the buttock or lower portion of the back of infants with yellow, brown, or black skin. They are of no permanent significance because they usually disappear during the first 5 years of life.

Petechiae. Petechiae are tiny "blood bursts" or miniature spiderlike dots that are the result of capillary breakage. They may appear on the face after a traumatic delivery or they may be associated with a more serious blood disease. In either case they should be brought to the attention of the physician.

Milia. The tiny whitish dots commonly seen on the nose, forehead, and cheeks of the newborn infant are called milia. They are clogged sweat and sebaceous glands that have not yet begun to function. After about 2 weeks, when the sweat begins to be secreted, the milia gradually wash away and disappear.

Birthmarks (nevi). There are a number of types of birthmarks—some temporary, some permanent, some from birth trauma, and some from structural abnormalities, such as pigment, blood vessels, hair, or other kinds of tissue. They may be elevated or flat and of any size or shape, may occur any place on the body, and may even develop days or weeks after birth, as does the "strawberry mark." Cosmetic surgery, if attempted, is usually delayed for a number of years to allow for possible fading. In Chapter 19 a more detailed discussion is provided.

Jaundice. Jaundice is a yellow discoloration that may be seen in the skin or in the sclera of the eye. It is caused by excessive amounts of free bilirubin in the blood and tissue. Complex enzyme processes within the liver are responsible for the maintenance of bilirubin levels in the body. Because of the immaturity of the newborn infant's liver, there is an excessive amount of bilirubin in the blood at birth. During the first week there is a further breakdown of hemoglobin from the reduction of red blood cells. As a result, about the second or third day approximately 60% of all infants begin to show some jaundice. By about the seventh day it usually disappears. This is called physiological jaundice, or *icterus neonatorum.*

If jaundice occurs before the third day, it indicates abnormal blood cell destruction. This condition is called pathological jaundice and may be caused by Rh factor or blood group A, B, or O incompatibility. It is discussed in greater detail in Chapter 13. Any jaundice should be reported promptly, but particularly that which appears soon after birth.

Hair and nails. The infant may be born with long, thick hair or may be bald. It may be quite different in color, coarseness, and curliness from what it will be in later life. The eyelashes and eyebrows are normally present at birth. The fingernails may be long and sharp enough to make deep scratches. To prevent scratches, some nurseries use shirts with closed long sleeves. The nurse should not attempt to cut the fingernails; the danger of cutting the fingertips is too great.

Head. The newborn infant's head is proportionately much larger than it will be in adulthood. It represents one fourth the infant's total body length, whereas an adult's head is only one eighth the total height. The circumference of the baby's head ranges from 12 to 14 inches (30 to 35 cm) and equals or exceeds that of the chest. During delivery, for the large head to pass through the small birth canal, the skull bones may actually overlap, reducing the diameter temporarily. This strange-looking elongation usually disappears a few hours after birth as the bones assume their normal relationships. Caput succedaneum and cephalohematoma are relatively common injuries that result from birth trauma and are discussed in Chapter 18.

The bones of the infant's skull are separated from one another along the suture lines. Where more than two bones come together, the space is called a *fontanel*, or "little fountain," because the pulse is sometimes visible there. The anterior fontanel is the largest and is called the *bregma*, or soft spot. It normally is closed in with bone by the eighteenth month. The posterior fontanel closes in about 2 months. If closure occurs too soon, there is inadequate space for brain growth. During infancy the anterior fontanel provides valuable information about the baby's condition. A sunken fontanel indicates dehydration; a bulging fontanel indicates increased intracranial pressure.

Breasts. The breasts of both boys and girls may be enlarged at birth because of high levels of female hormone in the mother's blood. They may even secrete a substance similar to colostrum, but the response disappears soon after birth in the absence of continued hormone stimulation.

Genitalia. The genitalia of the newborn infant should be examined carefully for defects. In boys, the testes normally descend during intrauterine life and are present in the scrotal sac at birth. Failure to do so is called *cryptorchidism*. Surgery may be required in later years, before puberty, if descent does not occur spontaneously. *Hydrocele*, an accumulation of fluid around one or both of the testes, is fairly common and in most cases is absorbed in a few months. A condition called *phimosis*, where the foreskin or prepuce cannot be retracted to expose the glans penis, is also common and usually is self-corrected by growth by the first year. Tiny glands located under the prepuce secrete a cheeselike matter called *smegma*. To promote cleanliness, prevent continued phimosis, or fulfill a religious rite, the foreskin may be cut or removed in whole or in part. This operation, called *circumcision*, is most frequently performed during the first week of life and sometimes immediately after birth.

In girls the labia minora and the clitoris may be swollen at birth as a result of the high female hormone levels in the mother's blood. A white mucoid discharge may fill the vagina. Occasionally this discharge is tinged with blood as a result of the sudden withdrawal of female hormones from the mother, and so is called *withdrawal bleeding*.

Genitourinary system. At birth the kidneys function at 30% to 50% of adult capacity and are not yet mature enough to concentrate urine. The dilute urine, however, is collected in the bladder. The infant usually voids within 24 hours. It is important to record the time of the first voiding. Complete anuria should be reported. It may indicate a congenital anomaly of the urinary system.

Respiratory system. During intrauterine life the fetus does not need the lungs to obtain oxygen because it is supplied from the mother's blood by means of placental circulation. Long before birth, however, the mechanism of respiration is established. As early as the fourth

month of gestation, prerespiratory movements begin. The lungs develop but their air sacs are in an almost total state of collapse, or *atelectasis*. At birth placental oxygen is cut off, carbon dioxide builds up in the infant's blood, and the infant is suddenly exposed to a shocking new environment. In response the baby draws a first breath, fills the lungs with air, and utters a robust cry with the first expiration.

It is important that mucus and amniotic fluid be removed from the air passages so that the infant will not aspirate them and breathing will not be blocked. During the first weeks of life the respiratory rate may be irregular because of the immaturity of the respiratory center in the brain. The rate should not drop below 32 or rise above 48. Abdominal breathing is normal; sternal retraction, or chest breathing, and cyanosis are abnormal and indicate dyspnea. They should be reported promptly.

Circulatory system. During intrauterine life the fetus receives its oxygen and nutrients from the mother by way of the placenta. At birth the umbilical cord is severed, the infant takes a first breath, and momentous changes occur that reroute the flow of blood from fetal circulation to independent circulation. A detailed description of these changes is given in Chapter 13 in connection with the disorders that result if they fail to occur.

Blood. During intrauterine life and for the first few postnatal days before the lungs expand fully, a relatively high number of red blood cells and level of hemoglobin are needed to provide the fetus with adequate oxygen. During the first 2 weeks after birth, oxygenation improves and large numbers of red cells are no longer needed; so hemolysis occurs. Fetal hemoglobin differs chemically from adult hemoglobin. The red cell count and fetal hemoglobin continue to fall for the first 3 months of life, resulting in a physiological anemia (Table 4-1). Gradually new red blood cells with adult-type hemoglobin replace the hemolyzed cells.

As was mentioned earlier in connection with

Table 4-1. Hemoglobin content in blood according to age

Age of child	Grams of hemoglobin per 100 ml of whole blood
At birth	17 to 20
3 months	10.5 to 12 (physiological anemia)
1 year	11 to 12.5
5 years	12 to 13
10 years	13 to 14
Adult	14 to 16

jaundice of the skin, the bilirubin levels in the newborn infant's blood are high at birth and rise still higher to 18 to 20 mg per 100 ml of serum. When the liver matures sufficiently, this level drops to the normal level of 1 mg per 100 ml. Continuing high levels of bilirubin beyond the first 2 weeks indicates a pathological condition such as obstruction, abnormal blood destruction, or serious infection.

During the first few days of life the prothrombin level decreases and the clotting time in all infants is prolonged. This process is most acute between the second and fifth postnatal days. It can be prevented to a large extent by giving vitamin K to the mother during labor or to the infant after birth. If this condition is untreated, clotting time returns to normal within a week to 10 days.

Digestive system. The newborn infant's lips should be pink and the tongue smooth and symmetrical. It should not extend or protrude between the lips. The connective tissue attached to the underside of the tongue (frenulum of the tongue) should not restrict the mobility of the tip of the tongue. If this restriction interferes with feeding, it is called "tongue-tie" and the doctor may cut it. The gums may have tooth ridges along them, and rarely a tooth or two may have already erupted. The roof of the mouth (hard palate) should be closed, and the uvula, or soft palate, should be present. Sometimes there are white glistening spots along the hard palate, called Epstein's pearls, where the two halves of the hard palate fused. They will disappear in time.

At birth the capacity of the infant's stomach is about 1 to 2 oz (30 to 60 ml), and increases rapidly. The infant is fed formula from a bottle or milk at the mother's breast. As the infant sucks the nipple, air, as well as milk, may be swallowed. This creates a false feeling of satisfaction from a full stomach. If the baby is not lifted to a head-up position so that the air can escape by rising (burping), it will remain in the stomach for some time. When it does escape, it may force the milk out with it (regurgitation). After being burped, the baby can then take more milk. As the feeding continues, the milk leaves the stomach almost immediately, passing through the pyloric sphincter into the small intestine. Occasionally this valve is stenosed, or too tight, and instead of the milk passing through, it is vomited with great force immediately after the feeding. Such projectile vomiting should be reported promptly since it may indicate a pathological condition, called *pyloric stenosis* that may require surgical intervention.

The baby's first stool is a blackish green, odorless, sticky substance called *meconium*. It consists of amniotic fluid, vernix, digestive tract secretions, bile, lanugo, and waste products from the body tissues. As soon as the baby begins to take milk, the stool begins to change to what is known as *transitional stool*, then typical milk curd stools follow. The stool of the breast-fed infant is greenish yellow, watery, and acid in reaction. As a result, the baby's buttocks may become excoriated. The stool of a cow's milk–fed infant is usually bright yellow, formed, less frequent, and neutral to slightly alkaline.

Normally there is some type of defecation within the first 24 hours after birth. The absence of any stools during this period may indicate a congenital defect and should be reported.

Skeletal system. The bones of the newborn infant are soft because they are composed chiefly of cartilage in which there is only a small amount

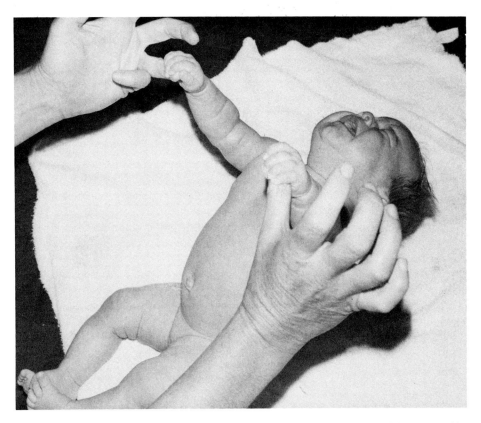

Fig. 4-3. The grasp reflex, one of the protective reflexes, causes the infant to hold so tightly to any object placed in the hands that the whole body weight can be lifted up.

of calcium. The skeleton is flexible and the joints are elastic to ensure a safe passage through the birth canal.

The infant's back is normally flat and straight. The spinal curves develop later when the infant sits up and begins to stand. The legs are small, short, and bowed. The hands are plump and fingers relatively short.

A number of common defects affecting the extremities of newborn infants are clubfeet, dislocation of the hip, and webbed fingers and toes (see Chapter 17).

Neuromuscular system. At birth, the infant's muscles are firm and resilient. They have tonus, the ability to contract when stimulated, but the infant lacks the ability to control them. The in-

fant wriggles and stretches. Movements are uncoordinated. When the nurse picks a newborn up, she must support the heavy head because as yet the newborn lacks the strength to hold it up. Normally, the infant is not limp in the nurse's hands, nor do the muscles twitch or jerk. There is, instead, a certain normal resistance to gravity that makes the child "hold together." Any lack of this may indicate brain damage or narcosis from drugs given to the mother during labor. The muscular development of the infant awaits the further development of nervous control.

The nervous system of the newborn infant is characteristically immature. Bodily functions and responses are mainly carried on by the lower centers of the brain and reflexes in the spinal

Table 4-2. Reflexes and special senses

	Description	Presence and duration
Protective reflexes		
Startle (Moro)	Sudden stimulus causes arms to fly out and up, tremble, and slowly relax	At birth; fades at about 2 months of age
Tonic neck	Postural "fencing" response; head, arm, and leg turn to one side, slowly relax	At birth; fades at about 2 to 3 months of age
Grasp	Infant grasps any object put in his hands firmly enough to hold his body weight, relaxes	At birth; fades at about 2 months of age
Eye blinking	Eyelids close and open when stimulated by touch or light	At birth; lifelong
Crying	Sudden pain, cold, hunger cause air to pass through vocal cords	At birth; lifelong
Feeding reflexes		
Sucking	Lips pucker, tongue rolls, inward pull or sucking caused by hunger, lip stimulation	At birth; 6 to 8 months of age (as a reflex movement)
Rooting	Touch of cheek or lips causes head to turn toward touch	At birth; 6 months
Swallowing	Throat muscles close trachea, open esophagus when food is in mouth	At birth; lifelong
Gag	At stimulation of uvula, esophagus opens; reverse peristalsis occurs	At birth; lifelong
Breathing reflexes		
Respiratory motion	Chest and abdominal muscles cause inspiratory and expiratory muscle movement	At birth; lifelong
Sneeze	Violent reverse flow of air from nose and throat	At birth; lifelong
Cough	Violent reverse flow of air from throat and lungs	1 year; lifelong
Conditioned reflexes	Learned responses to various stimuli such as to stop crying when mother comes	2 months; may begin and end throughout life
Special senses		
Touch, pain, pressure	Infant's lips most sensitive	At birth; lifelong
Smell	Odor perception	At birth; lifelong
Taste	Sweet and sour; flavors learned later	At birth; lifelong
Hearing	Loud noise perception	2 to 3 days when eustachian tubes clear
	Voice recognition	6 months
Sight	Light sensitive	At birth; lifelong
	Perceives light, follows it	At birth; lifelong
	Focus and tear formation	At birth; lifelong

cord. Gradually, nervous control from the higher centers develops, making possible more complex and purposeful behavior.

Reflexes and special senses. Reflexes are responses to stimuli that do not have to be consciously directed by the brain. The infant is born with a number of life-preserving reflexes. Some of these reflexes will disappear during development and will no longer be needed; others will remain throughout adult life (Fig. 4-3).

The special senses have not had an opportunity to mature in the newborn infant nor the capability of interpreting the meaning of all of these senses. The infant does feel pain, temperature change, and pressure and responds in appropriate ways (Table 4-2).

Psyche. The emotional and intellectual aspects of the newborn infant are as immature as the body. The mechanisms are all potentially present but are as yet undeveloped. The most basic emotional need of all humans, to feel secure, is present at birth, as evidenced by the infant's positive response to fondling. The infant derives obvious satisfaction from sucking, and communicates feelings of discomfort by crying. Psychologists believe that these early associations of the infant to the surrounding world have a profound influence on future adjustment to life.

Sleep. The newborn infant sleeps, or rests tranquilly, for 18 to 20 hours each day. The infant is awakened by internal stimuli such as hunger or pain and remains awake for short periods, usually until these wants are met, then returns to sleep. Even if these needs are not met, the infant becomes fatigued from crying and falls asleep.

The periods of wakefulness gradually lengthen and the periods of sleep become shorter so that by 1 month of age the infant is sleeping 15 to 18 hours each day, often with a longer period during the night when external stimuli are reduced.

Care

The dramatic transition of the infant from a dependent parasite to an independent individual begins at birth. Up to that time the fetus has been floating comfortably within the mother's womb, warm, protected, largely unrestricted, and free of pain and want. Then labor begins and it is pushed and pounded, squeezed, and twisted through the narrow birth canal until free. But this freedom is full of pain and shock. The baby is anoxic, cold, wet, and restrained. With the first gasp of air the baby protests with a robust cry. The umbilical cord is cut, fetal circulation ceases, and the infant is at the mercy of those nearby. The moment of birth is recorded as the time when the entire baby is separated from the mother regardless of the position of the cord or placenta.

The internal changes that begin within the infant at birth have been described in the preceding portion of this chapter. The effect of the environment on the newborn infant and immediate and continuing care have a profound influence on infant well-being, for the neonate is totally dependent on others for fulfilling needs.

Environment

When the baby is born, little subcutaneous fat is present to insulate from the cold and the body tends to become the temperature of the surrounding air. The hospital delivery room is usually about 70° F, whereas the intrauterine temperature was about 100° F. This sudden cold first shocks then chills the baby, and causes the blood pressure to fall. At first, this chilling acts to help close the ductus arteriosus in the heart but continued cold becomes harmful. Unlike the young of other species, the human child has no natural covering and is dependent on others for clothes and warmth. Providing a warm, safe environment becomes one of the life-preserving factors in the care of the newborn infant.

Alternate delivery sites

In recent years, an increasing number of mothers have chosen to deliver their babies at home or in an out-patient delivery suite located in a hospital. In these situations the family is more involved in the event, but principles of safe care are the same as in the hospital.

Immediate care

In the delivery room

Airway. The first and most important care given to the newborn after birth is to clear the nose and mouth of mucus and amniotic fluid so that the airway is open. This step is usually done by the physician or midwife moments after the baby is born. A rubber bulb syringe or soft rubber catheter with electric suction may be used. The baby's head should be placed below its body and turned to one side so that any regurgitated amniotic fluid will not enter the lungs. If breathing is not satisfactory, more extensive resuscitation measures are begun at once.

Umbilical cord. The baby remains attached to the umbilical cord until it is severed. Under certain circumstances clamping the cord may be delayed and the infant lowered to permit additional placental blood to flow into the baby. Such placental transfusion can increase the baby's blood volume by one half. The baby may then be placed on the mother's abdomen, in a pan of warm water, or on the back table while a cord clamp or tie is fastened securely around the cord near the baby's abdomen. A variety of cord-clamping devices are in current use; regardless of the type, all must be fastened securely to prevent fatal blood loss. If the second clamp attached to the section of cord leading to the placenta becomes loose, no serious blood loss will occur because the mother's blood vessels are not connected through the placenta. Occasionally it is desirable to obtain a blood specimen from the newly delivered baby to test for such conditions as syphilis or erythroblastosis fetalis. In these cases the cord blood is allowed to flow from the placenta into a waiting test tube before it begins to clot.

Evaluation

General condition. A standardized means of evaluating the condition of a newborn infant is of great value. Although a number of systems have been devised, the one Dr. Virginia Apgar first proposed in 1953 has been widely accepted. It consists of five observations made when the infant is 60 seconds old and again when 5 minutes old. A value of 0 to 2 is given for each observation and the five values are then added, giving a total Apgar score (Table 4-3). A baby in excellent condition would score 9 to 10; a dead baby would score 0. Most babies score 7 or better. Generally, premature babies, those born after long labors, and those born in breech or abnormal positions have lower scores than those full-term babies born in the occiput anterior position after normal labors.

Parent-baby interaction. Recent concern with the roots of child abuse has led to studies of the interaction between parents and infants, called *bonding.* This early claiming process is affected by the expressed attitudes of staff members, the physical environment of the delivery suite, and the parents' feelings about their new baby. Observations of how the mother looks, what she says, and what she does in the perinatal period have proved to be accurate predictors of child abuse or nurturance. A standardized means of evaluating parent-child bonding was devised by Jane Gray and associates in 1975. It consists of three observations made in the delivery suite during and immediately after the infant's birth and again during the first 2 or 3 days of the postpartum period. A value of 1 to 4 points is given for each observation, and the values are scored for each period. A highly positive interaction would score 10 to 12 for each period. A strongly negative interaction would score 3 to 6. Follow-up counseling for low-scoring parents is indicated to prevent child abuse and teach nurturant parenting (Table 4-4).

The physician or any other person in the delivery room may make the observations. The score should be recorded on the delivery room record and the baby's chart.

Resuscitation measures. Once the umbilical cord is cut, the baby's only source of oxygen is from the air. If, for some reason, the baby does not attempt to breathe or if the airway is blocked, oxygen cannot reach the bloodstream by way of the lungs and the baby will soon die. Even if the

Table 4-3. Apgar scoring chart for newborn babies

Sign	Score		
	0	1	2
Color	Blue, pale	Body pink, extremities blue	Completely pink
Heart rate	Absent	Below 100	Over 100
Respiratory effort	Absent	Irregular	Good, crying
Muscle tone	Limp	Some flexion of extremities	Active motion
Reflex irritability (catheter in nostril)	None	Grimace	Cough, sneeze

Table 4-4. Scoring chart for parent-baby interaction*

Bonding score	How the mother acts regarding her baby		
	Looks	Says	Does
1 Strongly negative, inappropriate 2 Mildly negative, inappropriate 3 Mildly positive, appropriate 4 Strongly positive, appropriate	General appearance: depressed, fearful, angry, apathetic ↓ Joyful, exuberant, happy, enthusiastic, serene, beaming	Makes disparaging remarks about baby and husband, expresses hostility or disappointment in baby's sex or looks ↓ Talks directly to baby, using baby's name, expresses positive reactions	Focuses attention on self, turns away from baby, cries ↓ Reaches out for, cuddles, examines, establishes eye contact with baby

*From Gray, J., Cutler, C., Dean, J., and Kempe, C.H.: Perinatal assessment of mother-baby interaction. In Helfer, R.E., and Kempe, C.H.: Child abuse and neglect: the family and community, Philadelphia, 1976, Ballinger Publishing Co.

baby survives, sensitive brain cells may be permanently damaged if deprived of oxygen for more than 5 minutes.

Resuscitation efforts are aimed at overcoming the three following problems of newborn asphyxia: (1) clearing the blocked airway of mucus and fluid, (2) forcing oxygen or air into the collapsed lungs, and (3) stimulating the baby to breathe. These efforts are continued for every baby until breathing is established or the heart stops beating and the baby is pronounced dead. Usually the anesthetist, attending physician, or specially trained nurse institutes these measures at once if the baby does not breathe spontaneously.

Clearing the airway. The baby's head should be lowered, but the body does not necessarily have to be held upside down. Mucus, amniotic fluid, vernix caseosa, and meconium should be removed from the mouth and trachea. This is done by putting a finger in the infant's mouth or by gently milking the trachea; a rubber bulb syringe or electric suction with a soft rubber catheter may also be used. To prevent the baby from aspirating (breathing in) vomitus, the stomach may be emptied with suction. Great caution should be taken to prevent injury to delicate tissues. Occasionally, it is necessary for the anesthetist to insert a tube into the larynx to provide an airway. This procedure is called *intubation*.

Forcing oxygen into the lungs. If the baby still does not breathe spontaneously after all obstructing mucus and fluid has been removed, it may be necessary to force air or oxygen down into the collapsed lungs. Forcing can be done by mouth-to-mouth positive pressure or by specially designed intermittent positive-pressure equipment. In either case, the lungs are filled by a positive force.

Stimulating the baby to breathe. Artificially filling the lungs at intervals is only a temporary measure until the baby begins to breathe independently. If the baby is sleepy because of certain drugs that were given to the mother during labor, the doctor may order stimulants. These must be carefully chosen or an opposite effect may result. A variety of physical ways to stimulate respiration may also be used. They include rubbing or snapping the feet or spine, performing nasal suction, and stimulating the rectal sphincter. It should be remembered, however, that the baby should not be allowed to become chilled.

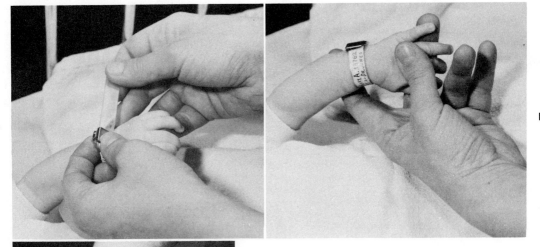

A B

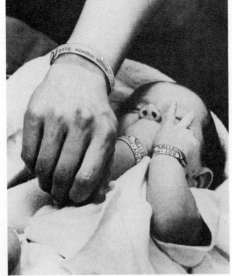

C

Fig. 4-4. Identification bands are attached in the delivery room. **A,** Ident-A-Band is locked in place with thumb pressure. **B,** Each band shows the mother's name and admission number, date, time of birth, and baby's sex. **C,** Bands are placed on the infant's wrists and that of the mother. (Courtesy Hollister, Inc., Chicago, Ill.)

If extensive resuscitation was required, the baby is usually placed in an incubator in the neonatal intensive care nursery where continuous observation is possible and where complete resuscitation equipment is available for emergency use.

Environment needs. It is important to conserve the baby's body heat. As soon as the normal baby is born it may be placed in a pan of warm water or directly against the skin of the mother. When the cord is cut, the baby is wrapped in a blanket and placed in the preheated crib in the delivery room or next to the mother's body. There the baby remains until the delivery room care is complete and it is time to be moved to the newborn nursery.

Identification. Proper identification of the newborn infant in a hospital setting is most important from a legal standpoint. The American Academy of Pediatrics recommends that "while still in the delivery room two identical identifi-

cation bands be placed on the infant's wrists or ankles showing the mother's full name, admission number, sex [of infant], date and time of [infant's] birth, and that the mother be fingerprinted and the infant's foot, palm, or fingers be printed." Many hospitals have adopted the Hollister Ident-A-Band, which provides three identically numbered soft plastic bands for each infant delivered, one for the mother and two for the infant (Fig. 4-4). Responsibility for preparing and attaching these bands rests with the nurse in charge of the delivery room.

Prophylaxis. Ophthalmia neonatorum is a serious gonorrheal infection of the conjunctiva of the newborn baby and may be acquired as the baby passes through an infected birth canal. Because this disease may cause blindness, all states have laws that require the prophylactic (preventive) instillation of a bactericidal agent in the eyes of all newborns (Fig. 4-5). Silver nitrate 1% drops (Credé prophylaxis) are effective

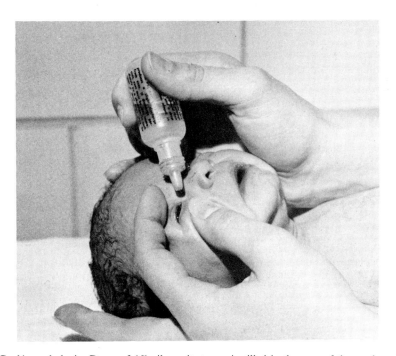

Fig. 4-5. Credé prophylaxis. Drops of 1% silver nitrate are instilled in the eyes of the newborn baby followed immediately with a saline solution irrigation. (From Hamilton, P.M.: Basic maternity nursing, ed. 4, St. Louis, 1979, The C.V. Mosby Co.)

against *gonococcus*; however, silver nitrate may cause severe irritation and even damage. For this reason, some hospitals require an immediate wash of saline solution after use. Great care must be taken to check the strength and freshness of the silver nitrate before instilling it into a baby's eyes.

In some hospitals it is the practice to give every newborn an injection of vitamin K to assist the clotting mechanism. Because there is some risk involved in giving so small an infant an intramuscular injection into the buttocks, the preferred site is the outer thigh. A physician's order and specific instruction as to injection technique are absolutely necessary before a nurse administers this or any other drug.

Recording. The newborn's chart usually originates in the delivery room and may include a copy of the mother's delivery record. Although each hospital uses its own forms, the record should include accurate and significant information about the infant, including time and type of birth, sex, Apgar and bonding evaluation scores, color, cry, general condition, obvious abnormalities or birth injuries, medications and treatments such as silver nitrate 1% in the eyes, Ident-A-Band number if used, oxygen, resuscitation measures, and weight if done, how the baby is to be fed (breast or bottle), and when, how, and in what condition the infant leaves the delivery room. The chart usually goes with the newborn to the nursery. The newborn, as any other patient in the hospital, must be under medical supervision. It is important, therefore, that the responsible physician be indicated on the newborn's record.

In the newborn nursery. The immediate care of the newborn on arrival at the nursery from the delivery room includes initial cleansing and observation, measurement, clothing, cord care, environmental control, and rest. In addition, the infant must be protected from harm and observed carefully and continuously.

Initial cleansing and observation. The newborn's hair frequently is matted with dried blood from passing through the birth canal, and the body may have areas where vernix caseosa is deposited heavily. It is not considered necessary to remove all of this sebaceous gland secretion, just the excess. Some nurseries dispense with water bathing as such and simply wipe off the excess vernix and sponge away the dried blood. Others use oil. Regardless of the procedure, this initial cleansing is an excellent time to observe the baby closely. The first temperature usually is taken rectally to ensure that the anus is open. Great care must be taken, however, to avoid perforation if the anus is not patent. Pulse and respiration may also be measured at this time. The nurse should work quickly to avoid unnecessarily chilling the baby's body.

Weighing and measuring. Although some delivery rooms are equipped with scales, a great many are not, and the newborn is first weighed on arrival at the nursery. The scales should be balanced with a protective cloth or paper on

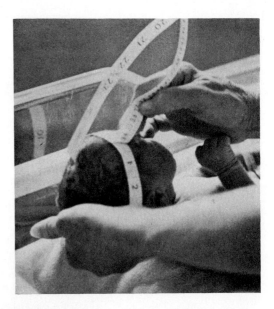

Fig. 4-6. Measurement of the circumference of the baby's head provides a basis for future comparison. Too rapid enlargement may indicate hydrocephalus. (From Hamilton, P.M.: Basic maternity nursing, ed. 4, St. Louis, 1979, The C.V. Mosby Co.)

which the naked infant is carefully placed. Great care should be taken to protect the infant from falling from the scales. The birth weight is important to the family and as baseline data for those who will care for the infant. Accuracy is vital. Most babies lose several ounces during the first week of life and then begin to gain it back. Weight gain or loss gives a general indication of the infant's condition and progress. The initial weight is therefore especially important.

Measurement of the circumference of the head and chest and of the length (heel to crown of the head) of the newborn baby are also made at this time (Fig. 4-6). These measurements are not done for idle curiosity but as a standard from which to make future comparisons. For instance, a rapidly enlarging head might indicate hydrocephalus. Unusual growth in length or size might indicate excessive anterior pituitary secretion.

Cord care. When the newborn first arrives in the nursery, there will be approximately 2 inches of umbilical cord extending from the abdomen with some type of clamp, pin, or tie fastener. In a few days this cord will shrink and darken, and in a week or so it will fall off, leaving a small granulation area that will eventually heal and be covered by skin cells, with only a small, contracted scar called the umbilicus or naval remaining throughout life.

Immediately after birth the umbilical vessels are still capable of allowing fatal hemorrhage if the clamp or tie should become loose. For this reason, the cord should be checked initially and at frequent intervals for the first 24 hours after birth. If bleeding occurs, a second tie or clamp should be applied at once and the baby watched closely.

Occasionally bacteria invade the area before healing has occurred. As a precaution against such an infection, the American Academy of Pediatrics recommends that some measure to reduce bacterial growth be taken, such as application of triple dye or 70% alcohol daily until it is completely healed (Fig. 4-7). These drugs both disinfect and dry the tissue. A small, dry sterile gauze strip may be placed around the cord ini-

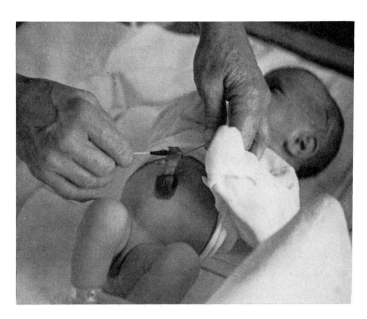

Fig. 4-7. Umbilical cord is painted with triple dye during initial care as a precaution against infection. (From Hamilton, P.M.: Basic maternity nursing, ed. 4, St. Louis, 1979, The C.V. Mosby Co.)

tially to protect the abdominal skin from the wet cord. However, the elaborate belly bands and dressings of yesteryear are no longer used because it was found that they harbored bacteria and kept the stump moist, thus hindering healing. The metal clamp or pin may be removed on the second or third day because the umbilical vessels are sealed off by then and there is no danger of hemorrhage.

Clothing and cover. Although the newborn must be kept warm, it is not desirable to constrict movement with heavy clothes or blankets. For this reason normal infants are dressed in a diaper and a single shirt or gown and bundled in lightweight cotton wrapping blankets. Every piece of clothing and linen must be washable and is often sterilized before being used in the newborn nursery.

Positioning and environment. When all the initial care has been given and the newborn is clothed, the baby is placed in a preheated crib or incubator, usually on the side with the head slightly lower than the rest of the body. This helps drain out any remaining amniotic fluid or mucus from the stomach and nasopharynx. Extra oxygen is not administered routinely unless there is definite anoxia as indicated by cyanosis and respiratory difficulty, and even then it is rarely given in concentrations of over 40%. *Retrolental fibroplasia*, a condition producing blindness, may result from excessively high oxygen concentrations.

After a few hours the baby of normal size and development does not need extra heat and is warm enough in a regular bassinet in the warm air of the newborn nursery.

Feeding and rest. The newborn does not need food or fluids immediately after birth. The chief need is for rest. For this reason nothing is given by mouth for 12 to 16 hours after birth. Infant feeding is discussed in a later section in this chapter.

Recording and identifying. All of the observations, measurements, and care given to the newborn after first arriving in the nursery should be carefully recorded on the chart. Because each baby's crib is kept separate from all the others, it is important to label it with a clearly marked card. The crib card should have the mother's name and her room number, the baby's sex, birth time and date, and the doctor's name. The crib card is usually made at the time the initial care is given. It is customary to give the card to the mother when she takes her baby home.

Continuing hospital nursing care

Nursery. One of the most carefully regulated areas of the hospital is the newborn nursery. The staff is specially qualified and trained, and the facilities are uniquely equipped and inspected frequently. The American Academy of Pediatrics published recommended standards that are reflected in the regulatory laws of each state. These laws govern the personnel and the physical facilities of all licensed hospitals.

Staff. Nurses who staff newborn nurseries must have specific training, and a definite aptitude for their work. They must be able to work in a team in which everyone shares the responsibility for every infant in the nursery. They must fully understand the principles of aseptic technique and maintain personal cleanliness and orderliness. Nursery nurses must enjoy working with tiny, helpless infants and their sometimes helpless mothers. Not all nurses are suited for this kind of nursing, but for those who are, the newborn nursery is a special world.

Physical facilities. Nursery facilities vary according to the size of the hospital. Ideally, the physical facilities should include the following: (1) regular nursery, equipped with as many bassinets as there are postpartum beds, hand-scrubbing sinks, covered waste cans, scales and work table, charting area, examing area, soiled-linen hampers, clean linen and supply closets, and chairs; (2) observation unit where babies who have been exposed to or suspected of infection may be observed; (3) isolation unit in which infants with a definite diagnosis of infection can receive care (they are never returned to the observation or regular nursery); (4) ritual circumcision unit in which the Jewish rite of ritual circumcision is performed; (5) demonstration room where mothers may observe demonstrations in feeding, bathing, and dressing an infant; and (6) formula room in which infant feedings are prepared (may be in a different area of the building or even in another community as long as strict aseptic technique is maintained).

Principles and practice. Procedures are ways of putting principles into action. Each newborn nursery develops its own procedures, but the principles of newborn care are quite universal because they are based on scientific facts. For example, it is known that infection occurs because pathogenic organisms invade the body. If the body could be separated from such organisms, infection would be prevented. A principle of newborn care that comes from this fact is that newborns should be isolated from as many pathogenic organisms as possible.

To implement this principle, the following practices have become almost standard in hospitals across the nation:

1. Any person with an infectious disease is barred from the obstetric-nursery area, including visitors, nurses, doctors, and auxiliary persons.

2. All supplies, especially linens, that are to be used in the newborn nursery are handled separately and sometimes sterilized before use.

3. Any infant suspected of infection, including those infants born out of asepsis, is removed from the regular nursery. No infant is returned to the regular nursery after having had a diagnosed infection.

4. Every newborn is kept separate from every other one by the practice of barrier technique. The nurses wash their hands between handling of babies and mothers.

5. Personal cleanliness is required of all personnel. Hair is covered; clean clothing is worn; gowns are placed over nursery dresses when the nurse leaves the nursery; and scrupulous handwashing technique is observed before touching each baby.

6. The air, all cribs, the walls, and all equipment are made as free of bacteria as possible by every means available, including disinfectant lamps and chemicals.

Another principle of newborn care grows out of the knowledge that the infant is weak and helpless, needs extra body heat, and is in a dangerous period of life. The principle that follows these facts is that the newborn should have a protected, regulated environment under constant observation. To implement this principle, the following practices are followed:

1. The newborn nursery is never left unattended.

2. All newborns are kept in unobstructed sight of the nurse.

3. Humidity and heat are carefully controlled (humidity of 50% and a temperature of 74° to 76° F).

4. A baby is never left unattended on a table or on the scales.

5. Babies are held for every feeding, never left with propped bottles.

Daily care. Every day each newborn is examined, cleansed, and weighed and the temperature is taken. All of the information thus obtained is then recorded. This provides the doctor with valuable facts about the infant's progress.

The nurse must handle the infant gently, avoiding unnecessary exposure, and check general appearance, nose, eyes, mouth, ears, skin, cord, genitalia, and the character of stools. This is all done before morning feeding so that the handling will not cause newly ingested milk to be regurgitated.

Nurses should care for only one infant at a time and wash their hands after each baby is handled. Each baby is kept completely separate from the others. An individual thermometer, hair brush or comb, and linen pack is needed for each baby. A typical procedure is as follows:

1. Cleanse the eyelids with water, wiping from the inner canthus outward.

2. Inspect the nostrils; if there is mucus or milk curd in them, remove it with a small, moist piece of twisted cotton.

3. Wipe the face.
4. A mild soap may be used to wash the hair.
5. Remove the shirt; inspect and wash the hands, arms, and axillae.
6. Inspect the cord and cleanse the base with 70% alcohol.
7. Remove the diaper; cleanse and inspect the feet, legs, groin, genitalia, and buttocks.
8. Turn the infant, and cleanse and inspect the back.
9. Take the rectal or axillary temperature, depending on hospital policy. Taking it rectally may stimulate the infant to defecate. Cleanse as needed.
10. Place a clean paper or cloth on the scales, balance them, and weigh the infant.
11. Dress the infant in a shirt and diaper, being sure that the pin is inserted at right angle to the baby's body; then, if the pin should open by accident, the baby would not be injured.
12. Place the infant on the bassinet tray and change the linen.
13. Replace the infant in the bassinet, and cover with a top cover.
14. Wash hands and record nursing observations in the baby's record.

Infant feeding. At delivery the mother indicates whether she wishes to breast- or bottle-feed her infant. Because this is a highly personal decision and because neither breast nor bottle can truly be called better in all cases, the nurse should support the mother's choice without undue involvement.

Usually newborn babies are given nothing by mouth (NPO) for the first 12 hours of life. This allows time for the mucus and amniotic fluid to leave the oral passages and for the baby to rest. Practice varies, but in some hospitals all babies are given glucose water after they are 12 hours old and milk formula or breast feedings after 24 hours. Full-term babies are fed every 4 hours for the remainder of their hospital stay.

Breast feeding. The mother who indicates her intention to breast-feed should be given special instructions on the care of her nipples and breasts. The first time the baby goes to breast an experienced nurse should bring the baby to the mother to provide her with assistance and encouragement. The following steps should be followed to ensure the mother and infant of safety and success in the nursing experience:

1. The mother should have a daily shower or bath to provide general cleanliness.
2. Before touching her breasts or the baby, the mother should wash her hands thoroughly with soap.
3. The mother needs to find a comfortable position, either sitting or lying down, using pillows for support.
4. The baby should be held in a natural position with the nipple extending well into the mouth. Breast tissue should be pressed in near the infant's nose so that breathing will not be obstructed (Fig. 4-8).
5. At first both breasts should be nursed for brief periods of time. After the nipples have toughened and the milk flow has become established, nursing time at each breast can be lengthened and alternate breasts may be nursed.
6. Breast feeding requires patience, skill, and a certain degree of discomfort. It is easy for a young mother to become discouraged. If the mother shows signs of fatigue or frustration at a feeding, the nurse should return the infant to its crib and allow the mother to rest.

At first the infant receives very little nourishment from the mother. The infant may cry a great deal in the nursery but fall asleep in the mother's arms. Opinion varies regarding extra feedings for a breast-fed infant. Some physicians order "p.c. feedings" of formula (p.c. = after feeding), called complementary feedings. Others order only water between feedings. The theory behind giving only water is that the baby will eventually become hungry enough to take the breast. The theory behind the complementary feeding is that the infant needs the nourishment and that in 4 hours will again be hungry enough to nurse.

By the third day the milk usually "comes into the breast," meaning that the glands begin to produce milk. Often there is much more than the

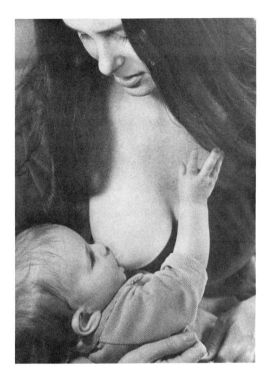

Fig. 4-8. Baby at breast. Mother is a Member of La Leche League, an organization devoted to helping mothers breast-feed their children.

infant can use. This situation can be relieved by partial or complete expression of milk. Sometimes the engorgement is so great that the infant cannot grasp the nipple. A nipple shield may be necessary for a few days until the vascular congestion recedes. In about 4 to 6 weeks the milk supply is adjusted to the infant's needs and the mother experiences less "leaking" between feedings. Most mothers learn the art of breast feeding by that time and experience no further difficulty.

Supplementary feedings are formula feedings given to babies who normally nurse but whose mothers must be away from them for one or more feedings. They allow the mother more freedom without neglecting her infant.

Bottle feeding. Babies who are not breast fed are given formula in a nursing bottle. A great variety of nursing devices have been invented, each seeking to duplicate the human breast as closely as possible and still be safe, economical, and easy to use. Generally speaking, the breast-fed infant must suck harder and longer to obtain the same amount of milk as the bottle-fed infant. To provide bottle-fed infants with more sucking time, some persons recommend that they be given a pacifier between feedings.

A formula is an infinitely variable recipe that can be made to precise specifications as to caloric, carbohydrate, protein, fat, mineral, vitamin, and water content. The amount may also be adjusted and the temperature varied.

Most hospitals have a "house" or standard formula that they either order from a commercial formula company that makes regular deliveries or make in their own formula kitchen. There are a large number of companies that prepare and sell their own standard formula. Special formulas are also made on the specific order of the doctor.

All formulas, regardless of their content must be sterile, fresh, and clearly labeled. Formula prepared for the newborn nursery is usually put in 4-ounce bottles because few newborns can tolerate more than that amount at one time. The formula may be given chilled, at room temperature, or warmed, depending on hospital practice. Outdated formula is discarded, as is any unused portion in an opened bottle.

Bottle-fed babies are usually started on a dilute house formula by the time they are 24 hours old. Four ounces of this formula is offered every 4 hours until the baby is 3 days old. The formula is usually increased in concentration at that time. Many newborns are discharged from the hospital about the third day, and the mother is given a formula that provides 6 ounces at each feeding. As the infant grows and nutritional needs increase, the formula will be altered and solid foods added to the diet.

The mother of the bottle-fed infant is encouraged to hold her baby for every feeding, just as a breast-fed infant is held. Before feeding her infant, the mother should wash her hands and find a comfortable position. The baby should be held in the crook of one arm, and the bottle held in the other hand. The nipple should be placed in the infant's mouth at the angle of the tongue. When an ounce has been taken, the newborn should be burped to allow swallowed air to escape from the stomach. Then a second ounce may be given, followed by burping. Two ounces is usually enough at the beginning. Overfeeding may cause hiccoughs or regurgitation and should be avoided. Most babies stop sucking and go to sleep when they have had enough.

Feeding routines. In some hospitals, it is the practice for all mothers, using breast or bottle, to feed their babies for all feedings except at 2 AM, when the nursery nurse feeds them water or formula. In other hospitals, breast-fed babies go to their mothers every 4 hours around the clock. Regardless of this policy, most nurseries follow a rather typical pattern of nursing care at each feeding time.

The formula is made ready for use. Each newborn is then prepared for feeding. The infant is diapered and cleansed according to individual need and is then wrapped in a blanket. In some hospitals, each wrapped infant is carried to the mother in a nurse's arms. In others, several infants are placed on a cart specially made for the purpose, and in still others, each individual infant unit is wheeled right to the mother's bedside. If the infant is to be bottle fed, the formula is taken along. If the infant is to be breast-fed, nipple-cleansing sponges are taken.

After 20 to 30 minutes the infants are returned to the nursery. The amount of formula taken by bottle babies is recorded. In some nurseries all breast-fed babies are weighed just before and just after feeding. Any increase in weight is caused by ingested milk. This increase is then recorded as the amount of milk received. All warmed and open bottles of formula are discarded, because only fresh ones will be used at the next feeding. The infants are all checked to see that they are dry and clean and are turned on a side to sleep until their next feeding.

Medical supervision. Every infant born in a hospital must have a doctor who is responsible for individual medical supervision. If the mother is under the care of an obstetrician, she usually indicates the name of the pediatrician who will be responsible for her baby. If the mother is delivered by a general practitioner, responsibility for the infant may be assumed by that physician or by a pediatrician.

Within a few hours after the baby's birth the doctor comes to the nursery and examines the baby carefully. The doctor checks the baby for any abnormalities, including the head and scalp, nose, mouth, eyes, ears, heart, lungs, umbilicus, groin, genitalia, hip joints, and extremities. The doctor also checks for normal reflexes as well as general condition and color. The attending nurse should remain nearby in case the doctor needs assistance.

After examining the infant, the doctor writes specific orders for the infant's care, including the feeding, any medications or treatments to be given, and special orders for laboratory tests. The doctor will check daily thereafter to find out how the newborn is feeding, if there is weight loss or gain, and general condition. The baby's doctor orders dismissal from the hospital. Unless there is some contradiction, babies are dismissed at the same time as their mothers.

Blood testing. On the second day of life infants are screened for three congenital disorders of metabolism: phenylketonuria, hypothyroidism, and galactosemia. These tests are important because early diagnosis is critical for successful treatment (see Chapter 14). It is the responsibility of the nursing staff to see that these tests are performed before the infant is dismissed.

Birth registration. Each of the 50 states has a department or division of vital statistics, with which all births, deaths, marriages, divorces, and so forth, are registered. It is the legal responsibility of the one who attends a birth to see that it is properly registered. Often the registration is channeled through a local county seat or township and then to the state office. When a baby is born in a hospital, the form is usually made out by the medical record department and then signed by the mother and her physician.

Information included on a typical birth certificate includes the mother's name, her address, a description of her pregnancy and delivery, the newborn baby's name, information about the birth, the father's name and address, and the attendant at the birth.

A clerk from the medical records department of the hospital usually comes to the obstetrical ward to obtain information for the birth certificate. When the certificate has been typed the clerk returns for the mother's signature. The physician or whoever attended the birth must also sign the certificate; it is then sent to the county and state where it is officially registered. A photostatic copy may be obtained thereafter from the state department of vital statistics. This certificate is not to be confused with the "hospital birth certificate" sometimes given as a memento to the mother.

Discharge. A normal, healthy newborn is usually discharged from the hospital at the same time as the mother. The baby's doctor examines the infant and writes dismissal instructions, including the formula for the feedings and when the mother should bring the baby for the first office visit. This visit is normally scheduled in about 1 month. Frequently the doctor will spend some time in consultation with the mother to answer her questions and establish rapport. If the mother is especially fearful of her new responsibility, the doctor may suggest that a public health nurse call on the mother to instruct and assist her with infant care.

When the mother is ready to go home, the nursery is notified and the infant is prepared for dismissal. The discharging nurse checks the identity of the infant with the supervising nurse and then takes the baby to the mother's bedside.

The mother checks the baby's Ident-A-Band number with her own, and if it is identical, she knows that this is indeed the baby she delivered. She signs the infant's record to that effect. One of the two Ident-A-Bands from the infant is removed and fastened to the chart. The other is left on the infant.

The baby is then dressed in the clothes that the mother provides for dismissal. The nurse should take advantage of this opportunity to instruct the mother regarding dressing and diapering the infant, as well as about cord and genital care. Usually the cord has not dropped off, and the mother may be concerned about its care. She should be instructed to paint the base with 70% alcohol until it is fully healed and warned not to use belly bands and pressure dressings.

The crib card is usually given to her, as well as photographs, certificates, and other mementos provided by the hospital. If the baby is receiving formula, some hospitals provide one or more courtesy feedings.

When all is in readiness, the mother is seated in a wheelchair, the baby is placed in her arms, and she is wheeled to the exit. The mother should not walk from the maternity ward with the baby in arms; a fall would be disastrous. At the exit, the discharging nurse lifts the baby out of the mother's arms while she gets into the auto and then places the baby in her arms.

Home care

It may seem to the other children in the family that all the new baby does is eat and sleep, and, indeed, this is just about true. The primary needs of the new baby are for sleep and food and to be bathed, held, and protected from sickness.

Sleep. At first the infant sleeps about 18 to 20 hours a day. The bed at home may look quite different from the one in the hospital, but the basic requirements are the same. It should have a firm mattress, be easy to clean, have sides high enough so the baby will not roll out, and if the sides are made of slats, they should be close together so that the baby's small head will not become wedged between them. The first crib need not be elaborate; even a dresser drawer will do. After being fed most babies sleep best on their abdomen. This position helps prevent aspiration of regurgitated milk, and if they always lie on their back the bones of the skull become flat.

Feeding. If the baby has been breast-fed in the hospital, the mother will probably continue to do so at home. The mother should have been properly instructed in breast feeding before she left the hospital. At home the baby can be fed on demand, which means whenever hungry. This may be from every 2 to 5 hours. After a few weeks the baby will usually take more at each feeding and will go longer between feedings. In about 4 weeks most babies begin to sleep through the night. The mother is given guidance by her pediatrician as to when and what foods to introduce into the baby's diet.

If the baby is being fed formula, the mother must have certain supplies and equipment, depending on how much preparation is needed. Usually the formula is made of milk, water, and some form of sugar. The recipe, or formula, is given to the mother by the doctor before she goes home. Some formula is premixed and packaged in disposable bottles. Other formula is premixed but must be poured into sterilized bottles. Still others are measured, mixed, bottled, and sterilized in the home. For this most involved process, besides the ingredients, the following items are needed for formula preparation: eight nursing bottles and nipples (two for water and six for formula), a large pan or sterilizer, and a mixing pitcher.

Formula must be sterilized to protect the newborn from unnecessary infection. There are two methods of sterilizing formula—concurrent and terminal. In the concurrent method the bottles and ingredients are all presterilized and then carefully combined to prevent contamination. In the terminal method the ingredients are mixed together and poured into clean bottles and then sterilized in a water bath or a sterilizer. Terminal sterilization ensures that the formula is indeed safe; it is, therefore, the recommended method.

Bacteria multiply rapidly in warm, sweet milk. For this reason formula should be made fresh daily and partially used bottles of formula discarded.

Bathing. Most mothers bathe their babies before the midmorning feeding each day, although there is no "correct" time. It is not necessary to have an expensive bathing unit. A plastic tub on the kitchen table is perfectly acceptable. The room should be free of drafts and the infant protected from falling.

The baby's bath should begin with the face and head, then upper torso, arms, abdomen, back, legs, and finally buttocks. When the navel is healed, the baby can be soaped and carefully placed down into the warm water. The baby should be supported on the mother's arm until able to sit up unaided. The bath should not be prolonged, nor should the baby be chilled. The baby should be dressed promptly and wrapped in a warm blanket for feeding.

A daily routine many mothers find satisfactory is to make the daily batch of formula, bathe the baby, and then sit or lie down to feed the baby; this gives the mother a chance to rest and ensures that the baby is held during feeding. After the feeding, the baby should be placed in bed for a long sleep while the mother cleans up.

Handling and holding. The new baby needs to be held but not handled; that is, excessive wrestling about could cause fretfulness, tiredness, and even regurgitation of food. On the other hand, the baby should not be left in the crib with a propped bottle. To develop emotionally, the baby needs the comforting security that comes from being held while eating.

Medical supervision. The infant was under continuous medical supervision by various members of the hospital staff until leaving the hospital. Unless ill, the baby usually does not see the doctor again until about 1 month of age. In the interim, a visiting public health nurse may be available to provide continuing medical supervision for both the mother and the infant.

Ideally, the visiting nurse first visits the home of the new baby the morning after discharge from the hospital. Follow-up visits are made according to need. Two aspects of the medical supervision are provided by the nurse—teaching and observation. The nurse teaches by demonstration and discussion with the mother, sometimes giving a demonstration bath or formula preparation. The nurse must also be an astute observer, alert to signs or symptoms that may indicate a potential medical problem. If problems are found, the nurse may make arrangements for the mother and baby to be seen immediately by a physician.

There is a wealth of literature available to new mothers on the subject of infant care. Many commercial baby product companies provide free materials. The U.S. Government Printing Office in Washington, D.C., publishes a number of excellent, inexpensive pamphlets about infant care. There are both paperback and hardcover editions of baby care books. Private doctors and many clinics publish their own information and instruction leaflets. All these are available to mothers who wish to increase their knowledge about baby and child care.

Disorders of the newborn infant

The possibility of death is greater during the first month of life than in any later period. The reason for this possibility is the frailty of the infant and the relative magnitude of afflicting conditions. The disorders that appear during the newborn period are caused by prematurity, congenital defects, birth injuries, infection, and respiratory disorders. Prematurity is the only one of this group unique to the newborn period and that affects all the body systems and their functions. It is discussed in Chapter 11. The other disorders affect specific body systems and may continue into later periods of the child's life. For this reason they are discussed in the ensuing chapters devoted to the various body systems.

Some newborn infant disorders are more common than others. These common conditions are listed below according to the five general causes of newborn disorders:

Prematurity
Retrolental fibroplasia
Hyaline membrane disease
Vomiting
Diarrhea
Dehydration
Jaundice
Convulsions

Congenital defects
Respiratory system
    Laryngeal stridor
    Choanal atresia
    Tracheoesophageal fistula
Circulatory system
    Heart and vessels
    Hemolytic disease
Musculoskeletal system
    Anomalies of the extremities
    Clubfoot
    Dislocated hip
    Osteogenesis imperfecta
Gastrointestinal system
    Cleft palate and harelip
    Esophageal atresia
    Pyloric stenosis
    Intestinal obstruction
    Diaphragmatic hernia
    Omphalocele
    Imperforate anus
Neurosensory system
    Spina bifida
    Encephalocele
    Meningomyelocele
    Down's syndrome
Genitourinary system
    Obstructions of the urinary tract
    Wilm's tumor
    Hypospadias
    Epispadias
    Polycystic kidney
    Exstrophy of the bladder
    Hermaphroditism
Integumentary system
    Nevi

Birth injuries

Caput succedaneum
Cephalohematoma
Intracranial hemorrhage
Brachial plexus palsy
Facial nerve paralysis

Infections

Gonorrheal neonatorum
Thrush
Congenital syphilis
Umbilical infection
Epidemic diarrhea
Impetigo

Respiratory effort

Anorexia of the newborn
Atelectasis
Pneumonia

THE INFANT (1 month to advent of walking alone)
Characteristics and care
One to 3 months

Physical and motor development. At 1 month of age the infant's weight is about 8 pounds. The infant gains 5 to 7 ounces per week for the first 6 months of life. Height at 1 month of age is about 20 to 22 inches. The infant grows about 1 inch per month for the first 6 months of life. The infant can raise the head unsteadily at 1 month of age, hold it high at 2 months of age, and raise the head and chest off the bed by 3 months of age. By then the infant can also sit up with support (Fig. 4-9). The infant pushes with the toes, makes a crawling movement at 1 month of age, and can turn from side to side by 3 months of age. At birth infants perceive light and follow it. By 2 months of age they actually follow and interact with the world around them (Fig. 4-10).

Emotional and social development. The 1 month old smiles and cries when hungry or uncomfortable, usually without tears. Tears are formed by the second month. By 3 months of age the infant smiles, laughs, and coos, cries less, and sleeps about 16 to 18 hours a day.

The infant's need to suck is greatest during the first 3 months of life. It is believed that if the need to suck is met during the first 3 months of life the infant will grow out of the oral, sucking stage without becoming a thumb-sucker. To satisfy these needs, nursing mothers may be able to allow the infant to suck longer at the breast and mothers of bottle-fed infants can see that old soft nipples are replaced with new ones. Some find that the pacifier, a blind nipple on a large disk, is useful in supplying this need. If pacifiers are used, they should be washed and inspected frequently for wear.

Care. During these early months the infant's day is divided between long periods of sleep and brief feeding times that come every 3 to 4 hours. Most infants begin sleeping through the night feeding in their second month of life. Although there is no "right" schedule, many mothers follow the one established in the hospital that began the day with a milk feeding about 6 AM, followed by a midmorning bath and feeding, an early afternoon feeding, an evening feeding, and a late feeding just before the parents retire. As the child matures, periods of wakefulness grow longer and periods of sleep shorter.

In handling the infant, the mother or nurse must support the head until the infant is strong enough to do so unaided. The infant should be allowed freedom to exercise the legs and arms and should not be bound tightly in blankets. Too many blankets may overheat the infant and produce a heat rash called "prickly heat." A personal bed, equipped with a firm mattress and no pillow, is recommended by most pediatricians.

The tender skin of the baby may become excoriated from strong soaps left in the diapers or from ammonia formed in urine and fecal matter. Diapers should never be left unwashed for long periods of time but should be rinsed immediately and washed daily. The baby's buttocks should always be washed between diaper changes. Antiammonia ointments are available without prescription and are recommended to prevent diaper rash.

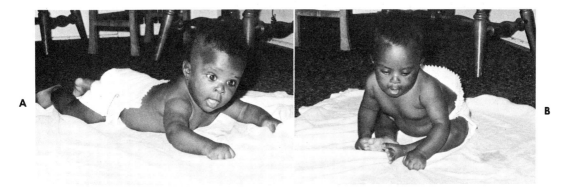

Fig. 4-9. A, By 2 months of age the infant can hold the head high, and by 3 months can lift the head and chest off the floor. **B,** This 2½-month-old child is not yet strong enough to sit up without support.

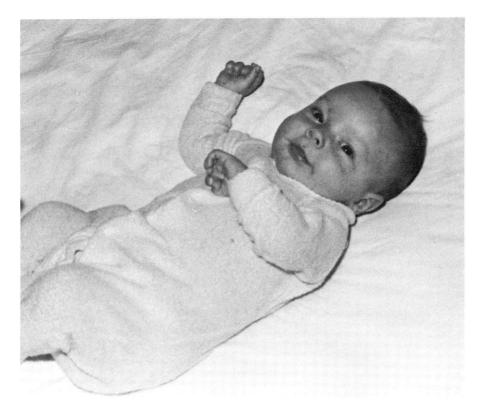

Fig. 4-10. This 2-month-old baby actively follows the movement of people around him.

Some infants are troubled by painful episodes of acute abdominal pain, called colic, during which they draw up their legs and scream in anguish. No particular cause can be identified, and treatment is symptomatic. The episodes usually follow a feeding. Sucking a pacifier, lying on the abdomen, and warm applications seem to help. Colic usually stops by about 3 months of age.

Sometimes mothers are afraid to shampoo the infant's head because of the soft spot. As a result, an accumulation of sebaceous oil, old skin, and blanket fuzz builds up on the baby's scalp. This condition alone is not a disease but can harbor bacteria and may aggravate seborrhea, a common condition found in newborn infants. The "cradle cap" should not be scraped or peeled but should be softened with baby oil and washed away with a gentle detergent shampoo. Daily shampoos help prevent it from returning.

Hiccoughs are a common problem in small babies. They may be triggered by overfeeding or failure to burp the infant. Although they are distressing, they are not a serious condition.

Nutrition. During the first month the infant's nourishment is usually supplied by breast milk or formula with supplementary vitamins and iron. Thereafter, recommended feeding patterns vary greatly. Some pediatricians recommend a diet of mother's milk only until the child is 6 months of age. Others recommend that solid foods, such as cereals and pureed fruits, be added the second month and pureed vegetables and meats by the third month. If the first solid foods are given at the late evening feeding, they remain in the stomach longer and help prolong that period of sleep. During these early months the sucking reflex is strong and infants try to suck the food from the spoon rather than close their lips around the food and swallow. As a result, nearly as much food "toothpastes" out of the mouth with each spoonful as is swallowed. With time and much patience, both mother and infant learn how to make more go in than out.

Medical supervision. During the first year of life the infant should be seen by the doctor every month because development and needs are changing so dramatically. At these visits the baby is examined, weighed, and measured. Diet is adjusted according to needs and the immunization procedures are carried out. Usually the first DPT injection and first oral polio feeding are given at the end of the infant's second month. The second DPT injection and oral polio feeding come at the end of the fourth month. A more extensive discussion of current immunization practices is given in Chapter 3.

One of the important functions of these monthly doctor visits is to provide the mother with an opportunity to ask questions and to discuss infant care. It may be helpful for the mother to make a written list of questions when they occur to her between office visits.

Four to 6 months

Physical and motor development. By the fifth month the infant has doubled the birth weight.

During the fourth month the infant begins to drool because saliva has begun to appear, but the infant does not know how to swallow it. The first of the 20 baby teeth erupt during this period. Usually the lower incisors appear first, followed by the upper incisors. By the fourth month the infant can hold the head steady when held in a sitting position. By the sixth month the infant can roll over and pull unaided to a sitting position and sit without support momentarily. By the sixth month many of the neonatal reflexes, such as grasp, Moro, and tonic neck have faded (see Table 4-2).

By the fifth month the infant can grasp handed objects and by the sixth month reaches for the objects, grasps them with the whole hand, and may bang them against the table or floor.

Emotional and social development. Between the fourth and sixth months the infant initiates social play by smiling. The infant coos and babbles in "angel talk" and enjoys being near other members of the family. By the fifth or sixth month the infant notices strangers and cries if frustrated or deprived of a personal desire.

Between the third and fourth month the infant sleeps through the night and takes a long morning and afternoon nap. By the sixth month the nap times may become shorter.

Care. During the weeks when the infant is constantly drooling and teething it may be helpful to tie on an easily laundered bib to absorb the saliva. The infant may be irritable and cross just before the new teeth erupt and may derive some comfort from chewing on a hard rubber or plastic teething ring. High fevers and convulsions are *not* caused by teething but are symptoms of more serious conditions for which a physician should be consulted.

Babies enjoy being propped in a sitting position even before they are able to sit alone, but they should not be left until they are tired. Early displeasure at being wet and exposed during the bath changes to pleasure during the fourth to sixth month when infants can sit and splash in the water. They should not be left alone even for a moment because of general instability.

The newborn infant usually has three to four stools a day. As solid foods are added to the diet the number of stools per day gradually decreases and the quantity, consistency, and odor change so that by the age of 6 months most infants defecate once or twice a day. Frequently these come with considerable regularity at about the same time of day. The infant audibly strains and pushes so that an alert mother can usually change the diaper soon afterward with a minimum of bother for both herself and the infant. Toilet training at this early age is of no lasting value and may create future problems.

Nutrition. By 6 months of age the infant usually is offered a variety of nonspicy pureed fruits, vegetables, meat, cereals, and milk products. New foods should be introduced individually and at a time when the child is hungry, not when teething or irritable. The doctor may recommend that certain foods such as egg white and orange juice be withheld from the diet of allergy-prone children until they are older. Force and punishment only do harm if associated with the introduction of new foods; so if the baby refuses a certain food, it should be omitted temporarily and tried again later. Mealtime should be pleasant. Fresh milk is often substituted for formula by this time. Normally diet additions and changes are made by the doctor at the monthly visit.

Medical supervision. During the sixth month the series of three DPT injections and polio feedings is usually completed. The mother should be encouraged to continue the monthly visits for consultation and supervision of the infant. She may have questions about the infant's diet, teething, and developmental progress.

Seven to 9 months

Physical and motor development. During the second 6 months of life the infant gains 3 to 5 ounces a week and grows about ½ inch per month in height.

By the seventh month the infant sits alone with more steadiness and by the ninth month shows good coordination and control. The backward crawling, called hitching, of the latter part of the sixth month is replaced by a forward movement accomplished by raising the chest and head and moving the arms while the legs drag. This is called crawling. Creeping, which occurs when the legs support the trunk and move along with the arms, is a more advanced type of locomotion than crawling. Not all infants follow this pattern of hitching, crawling, and then creeping. Some skip a stage (Fig. 4-11). By the age of 9 months infants can pull themselves up to their feet, if assisted.

By 7 months of age the infant can grasp a toy with one hand and transfer it to the other. By 8 months the infant uses the thumb to grasp things, and by 9 months prefers the use of one hand over the other. At 7 months the infant plays with the

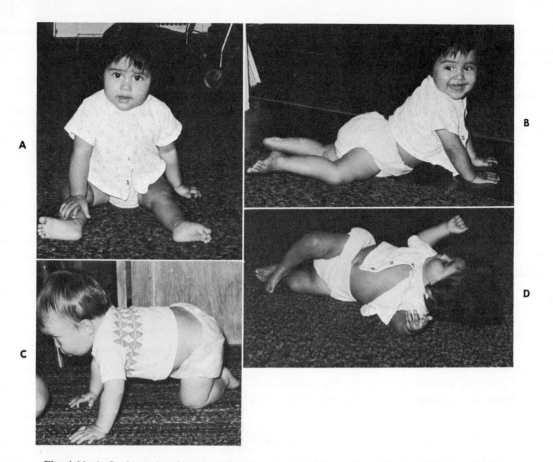

Fig. 4-11. A, By 9 months of age the infant can sit up and has good coordination. **B,** In crawling, the infant raises the chest and head and pulls the body along with the arms while the legs drag. **C,** In creeping, the infant uses both arms and legs. This is a more advanced type of locomotion than crawling. **D,** Rolling over requires considerable coordination. Note the crossed right leg.

toes and puts them in the mouth; by 9 months hand-mouth coordination is perfected and the infant can put a nipple in and take it out of the mouth at will.

Emotional and social development. By 7 months of age the infant shows fear of strangers and recognizes and enjoys the affection of the family group. The infant changes quickly from tears to laughter. By the ninth month the infant begins to show imitative expressions by saying "Da-da" and other such sounds, cries when scolded, and responds to approval.

Some infants begin the practice of head-banging or rocking rhythmically to and fro while they are in the process of going to sleep. Although it is frightening to the parents, it does not seem to harm the child, who normally outgrows the practice by 2 or 3 years of age.

Care. After learning how to crawl, the infant is not satisfied to remain in the crib. At the same time the infant is becoming more social and wants to be where the action is. The wise parent provides a safe, relatively clean area where the baby can see and hear the family and where there is enough room to move about. This is the ideal playpen age. After learning to walk, the infant will not be satisfied with so small a space (Fig. 4-13). Small toys that are just right for the hands to grasp but not small enough to swallow, such as blocks and animals with protruding legs, are ideal for this age.

By 9 months of age the infant's sleeping pattern is more like that of the other family members. The infant still needs long naps, but sleeps about 10 hours through the night.

Occasionally infants have a "different" day, when they do not follow their usual pattern of sleep and wakefulness. This is perfectly normal and should not cause alarm.

Nutrition. The infant with teeth enjoys chewing on finger foods. By 9 months of age the infant has learned to handle semisolid food and can swallow liquids from a cup. The strong sucking reflex has faded. These physical changes affect the diet. The infant can be fed soft nonpureed foods such as chopped meats and vegetables, may be ready to give up the bottle and drink from a cup, and is usually satisfied with three meals a day of solid foods.

Medical supervision. The baby should continue to be examined by the doctor at monthly intervals during the first year of life even though the initial immunization series has usually been completed by this age.

Ten to 12 months

Physical and motor development. By 10 months of age the infant can pull up to a standing position and makes stepping movements with the feet and legs. By 11 months the infant can stand erect when holding onto some support, and by 12 months can stand for a moment alone without support. The infant can walk with help and moves about by holding onto chairs and stepping sideways (Fig. 4-12), and can sit down from a standing position without help. Until this time the back was relatively straight, but when walking begins the spinal curves appear.

The 10 month old can bring the hands together in a "pat-a-cake" motion and can grasp and release objects. By the twelfth month the infant can pick up food and place it into the mouth and can eat from a spoon and drink from a cup. If given a crayon, the infant can hold it and make a mark on a paper.

By the twelfth month the infant has tripled the birth weight, is about 29 inches tall, and has six teeth.

Emotional and social development. The 10 month old has learned its name, plays games, says "bye-bye," and can repeat one or two words and imitate an adult's vocal inflection. By 12 months of age the infant can say two words besides "Ma-ma" and "Da-da." The infant uses jargon to communicate with others, recognizes the meaning of "no," loves rhythm, and shows jealousy, affection, anger and other emotions. The infant loves an audience and cries more often with frustrations than before.

Care. The tenth through the twelfth months are especially exciting for parents because the child is beginning to communicate with jargon and some language. The child is active and aware and is developing a unique personality. The child no longer needs the morning nap and follows the family's pattern of eating and sleeping.

The increasing mobility of the 10 to 12 month old creates more susceptibility to danger. The child is less satisfied with the confinement of the playpen and wants more freedom to roam.

If the child's sucking needs have not been met during the early months of life, thumb-sucking may have become a well-established habit, especially when the child is tired, bored, or feels rejected. It is usually too late to substitute a pacifier. Parental threats, punishment, and application of bitter flavors or restraints seldom stop it. Fortunately, damage to the mouth structures is not serious for most children because thumb-sucking usually stops before the permanent teeth come into the mouth.

Closely associated with thumb-sucking is weaning the child from the bottle. Some time

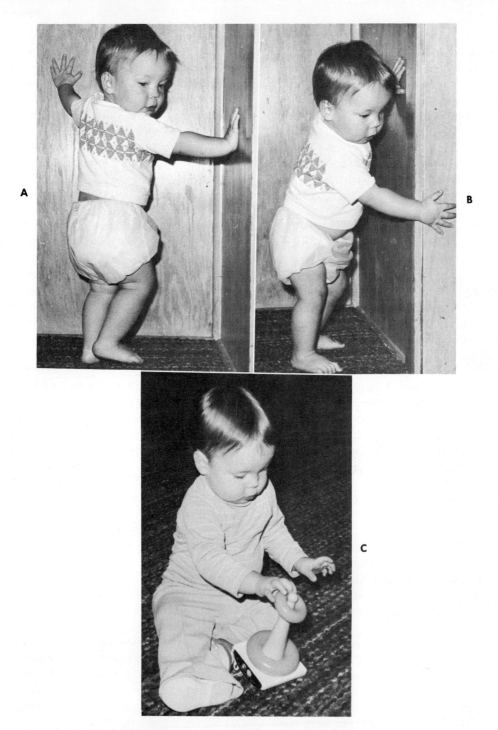

Fig. 4-12. A and **B,** Before walking alone, the infant cruises sideways, cautiously holding onto walls and furniture for support. **C,** By the age of 12 months the child can grasp and release objects with considerable accuracy. (Note the intense concentration.)

between 10 and 12 months, most children learn to drink fluids from a cup. At that time they could give up the bottle as a means of taking fluids. If, however, they use the bottle much as the thumb-sucker uses the thumb, they will not be weaned easily. If the mother tries to remove the bottle and it causes extreme anxiety for the child, it may be better to give it back for a few months than to have the child begin thumb-sucking. Here again, it is more often the parents' pride than the child's development that is at stake. Weaning should never be attempted when the child is ill or hospitalized. The newly weaned child may regress to thumb-sucking during illness.

Nutrition. By the twelfth month the child can be given a full range of foods, including fish and some of the food withheld previously because of possible allergy. These foods should be introduced with caution, one at a time.

Many mothers become concerned because about the time they are weaning the child to the cup and fluid intake decreases, so does an appetite for solid foods. This decreased interest in food is normal and not a cause for alarm.

Medical supervision. Some time between 10 and 12 months of age the infant may be given a tuberculin test. This skin test is usually negative unless the child has been exposed to tuberculosis. If positive, a chest x-ray examination and careful medical history are necessary for the child and all members of the family.

Thirteen to 15 months

Physical and motor development. The anterior fontanel, or soft spot, closes by the fifteenth month.

By the thirteenth to fifteenth months most infants learn to walk alone. Their balance and pacing may cause them to fall frequently, but this does not seem to hurt or hamper them (Fig. 4-13).

The child can take part in dressing and uses a spoon ineptly and drinks from a cup with increasing skill (Fig. 4-14).

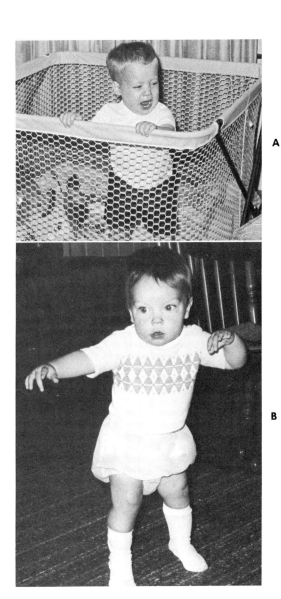

Fig. 4-13. A, The playpen is too confining. **B,** The first fearful steps.

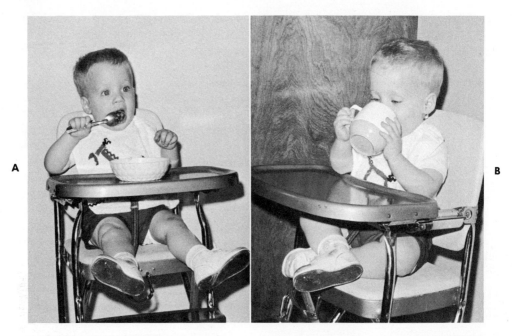

Fig. 4-14. A, Thirteen-month-old children want to hold the spoon, but they may not get it to the mouth bowl-side up. **B,** The 13-month-old child drinks from the cup with increasing skill.

By this time the child can place objects into a container and build a tower with two blocks.

The child usually has the front eight incisors at 15 months of age.

Emotional and social development. By the fifteenth month the child's vocabulary has increased to six words. The child is curious and searching and understands commands but has such a short attention span that the child may forget the command before it can be carried out.

Care. The 15-month-old child who can walk, has left infancy, become a toddler, and entered the period of life when there is a higher incidence of accidents than at any other time. Parents should go through the house and discard all insect and animal poisons; they should place all medicines and chemicals in inaccessible places. Sharp instruments such as knives and ice picks should also be put in inaccessible places. The handles of cooking pots on the stove should be turned inward, and electrical outlets should be covered or concealed. Even with all these pre-

cautions, the child should not be left unattended even for a brief time.

Nutrition. Small, attractive servings of foods should be offered—finger-foods, such as crackers and fresh fruits and vegetables, are especially suitable. No fuss or punishment should be made if the child does not want to eat.

Medical supervision. During these months if the child has received all the scheduled immunizations and has no acute infections, the primary role of medical supervision may be that of an information source. The mother may have questions about weaning, thumb-sucking, toilet training, and eating habits at this time. She should be reminded about the dangers of accidents.

Disorders common to the infant

Disorders that commonly affect the child from 1 to 15 months of age can be best described as short-term care conditions and long-term care conditions.

Short-term care conditions

Respiratory conditions
    Acute nasopharyngitis (common cold)
    Otitis media
    Acute bronchiolitis
    Interstitial pneumonitis
    Lipoid pneumonia
    Aspiration of foreign bodies
    Sudden infant death syndrome
Gastrointestinal conditions
    Foreign bodies
    Diarrhea
    Vomiting
    Pyloric stenosis
    Intussusception
    Inguinal and umbilical hernia
Genitourinary conditions
    Hydrocele
    Pyelonephritis
Generalized infections
    Roseola infantum

Long-term care conditions

Nutritional conditions
    Malnutrition
    Rickets
    Scurvy
Gastrointestinal conditions
    Celiac syndrome
    Cystic fibrosis
    Prolapsed rectum and sigmoid
    Biliary atresia
    Megacolon
Blood conditions
    Blood formation disorders
    Iron-deficiency anemia
    Sickle cell disease
Endocrine conditions
    Cretinism
Inborn errors of metabolism
    Phenylketonuria
    Galactosemia
    Tay-Sachs disease
Skin conditions
    Infantile eczema
Central nervous system conditions
    Tetany and convulsions
    Subdural hematoma

Skeletal defects
    Craniosynostosis
Emotional disturbances
Battered-child syndrome

SUMMARY OUTLINE

I. **The newborn infant (birth to 1 month)**
    A. Characteristics
        1. Proportion of boys to girls
        2. Physiological resilience
        3. Immunity
        4. Body shape and size
        5. Vital signs
            a. Temperature
            b. Pulse
            c. Respiration
            d. Blood pressure
        6. Skin
            a. Vernix caseosa
            b. Lanugo
            c. Desquamation
            d. Erythema allergicum
            e. Mongolian spots
            f. Petechiae
            g. Milia
            h. Birthmarks (nevi)
            i. Jaundice
        7. Hair and nails
        8. Head
        9. Breasts
        10. Genitalia
        11. Genitourinary system
        12. Respiratory system
        13. Circulatory system
        14. Blood
        15. Digestive system
        16. Skeletal system
        17. Neuromuscular system
            a. Reflexes and special senses
            b. Psyche
            c. Sleep
    B. Care
        1. Environment
        2. Alternate delivery sites
        3. Immediate care
            a. In the delivery room
                (1) Airway
                (2) Umbilical cord
                (3) Evaluation
                (4) Resuscitation measures
                    (a) Clearing the airway
                    (b) Forcing oxygen into the lungs
                    (c) Stimulating the baby to breathe

      (5) Environmental needs
      (6) Identification
      (7) Prophylaxis
      (8) Recording
   b. In the newborn nursery
      (1) Initial cleansing and observation
      (2) Weighing and measuring
      (3) Cord care
      (4) Clothing and cover
      (5) Positioning and environment
      (6) Feeding and rest
      (7) Recording and identifying
  4. Continuing hospital nursing care
   a. Nursery
      (1) Staff
      (2) Physical facilities
      (3) Principles and practice
   b. Daily care
   c. Infant feeding
      (1) Breast feeding
      (2) Bottle feeding
      (3) Feeding routines
   d. Medical supervision
   e. Blood testing
   f. Birth registration
   g. Discharge
  5. Home care
   a. Sleep
   b. Feeding
   c. Bathing
   d. Handling and holding
   e. Medical supervision
 C. Disorders of the newborn infant
II. The infant (1 month to advent of walking alone)
 A. Characteristics and care
  1. One to 3 months
   a. Physical and motor development
   b. Emotional and social development
   c. Care
   d. Nutrition
   e. Medical supervision
  2. Four to 6 months
   a. Physical and motor development
   b. Emotional and social development
   c. Care
   d. Nutrition
   e. Medical supervision

  3. Seven to 9 months
   a. Physical and motor development
   b. Emotional and social development
   c. Care
   d. Nutrition
   e. Medical supervision
  4. Ten to 12 months
   a. Physical and motor development
   b. Emotional and social development
   c. Care
   d. Nutrition
   e. Medical supervision
  5. Thirteen to 15 months
   a. Physical and motor development
   b. Emotional and social development
   c. Care
   d. Nutrition
   e. Medical supervision
 B. Disorders common to the infant

STUDY QUESTIONS

1. Describe a normal infant giving the following information: proportion of girls to boys; measurement ranges of head, chest, length, weight, temperature, pulse, respirations, blood pressure, and hemoglobin; condition of skin, breasts, genitalia, digestive system, skeleton, and reflexes.
2. What immediate care should be given an infant after birth? Give priorities.
3. What care should be given the newborn infant in the nursery during the first 24 hours of life?
4. Discuss the advantages and disadvantages of breast and bottle feeding. What nursing measures can be taken to help the mother with cracked nipples, engorgement, and inverted nipples?
5. Describe the physical and emotional development and care needed by the child during infancy.

REFERENCE

Gray, J., Cutler, C., Dean, J., and Kempe, C.H.: Perinatal assessment of mother-baby interaction. In Helfer, R.E., and Kempe, C.H.: Child abuse and neglect: the family and community, Philadelphia, 1976, Ballinger Co.

5
The young child

VOCABULARY

Ritualistic behavior
Ambidextrous
Enuresis
Masturbation
Negativism
Fantasies

The child's life is divided by certain major developmental and social milestones. The break between infancy and the toddler stage is marked by the advent of walking and talking. These skills produce an independence that separates the infant from the young child. During the next 4 or 5 years the child develops increasing motor and verbal skills, expanding, elaborating, and refining them. The next major break comes when the child enters school and enlarges the social world beyond the family. The training and education received by the child during the toddler and preschool years are extremely important in preparing for future periods of development.

TODDLER (advent of walking to 3 years)
Characteristics

Physical and motor development. Birth weight triples during the first year of life, and then the rate of gain slows to 4 or 5 pounds (1.8 or 2.3 kg) per year until 5 years of age. For example, the child weighing 7 pounds (3.17 kg) at birth would weigh about 21 pounds (9.5 kg) by 1 year of age, 26 pounds (11.8 kg) by 2 years of age, and 31 pounds (14 kg) by 3 years of age.

The height increases about 5 inches (12.7 cm) between 1 and 2 years of age, and then the rate slows to a yearly gain of 3 inches (7.6 cm) until 6 years of age. The 2-year-old child is about 35 inches (89 cm) tall; the 3-year-old child is about 38 inches (96.5 cm) tall. At 2 years of age 16 teeth have erupted, and by 3 years of age all 20 of the baby teeth have appeared.

Most children walk alone by 14 or 15 months of age. By the time they are 18 months old they can run and seldom fall, and by the time they are 2 years of age they can climb stairs one at a time. The 3 year old can pedal a tricycle, walk backwards, jump from a low step, and walk upstairs with alternating steps (Fig. 5-1).

The 2 year old can build a tower of five or more blocks, open doors by turning the doorknob, scribble, and imitate a vertical stroke. The 3 year old can build a tower of nine blocks, string large beads, begin to use scissors, copy a cross or a circle, dress and undress unaided, and unbutton buttons on the front or side of clothing.

The 2 year old can drink well from a small glass with one hand and put a spoon into the mouth without turning it. Three year olds can feed themselves without difficulty.

Toilet training requires both a physical and a psychological readiness that most authorities agree does not occur until the second year of life. Bowel and bladder control is possible when the nerve tracts of the spinal cord are insulated with myelin down to the level of the anus. Although this neurological readiness is essential, the child must also want to exercise control, and so the will and the emotions become a part of the process. By 3 years of age most children can take themselves to the toilet both during the day and at night.

Emotional and social development. During the first year of life children learn to trust familiar adults. Moving through the toddler period, they begin to develop a sense of being individuals. This self-concept is greatly influenced by the way they feel significant persons think of them:

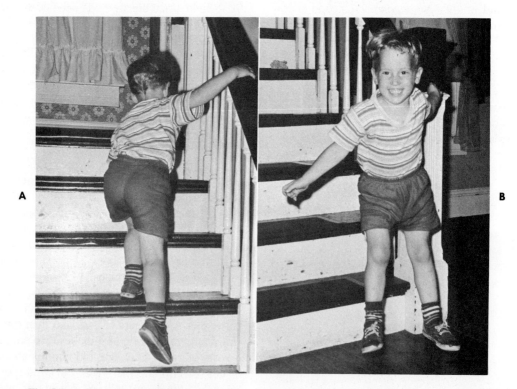

A

B

Fig. 5-1. A, Three-year-old children can walk up stairs alternately. (Although they may be too busy to remember to go to the toilet in time. Note wet clothing.) **B,** The 3-year-old child can jump from a low step.

as a thing of value and worth or as a burden to be tolerated or an object to be despised. The child also begins to be aware of being a separate person who is related to other individuals. When that individualism is challenged, the toddler reacts by becoming negative and opposite. If the toddler finds that there is no other course than to comply to the will of the stronger one, the reaction may be frustration and violent physical action called a temper tantrum.

Temper tantrums begin to appear about 18 months of age. They continue in varying degrees until the child's motor coordination, verbal skills, reasoning ability, and emotional control mature sufficiently to allow coping with frustrations brought about by conflict of wills. In time the child is better able to understand restrictions as a result of more experience. For example, the 2 year old might have a temper tantrum if removed from a jumping horse. By 3 years of age, the child might accept the idea that giving up the jumping horse allows going outside to play, a pleasure recognized as sometimes more desirable.

During the toddler period there is an enormous increase in the child's vocabulary from 10 words at 18 months of age to 900 words at 3 years of age. The ability to use language also develops, so that by 3 years of age children understand the plural form, make complete sentences, and speak fluently. They are able to verbalize displeasure by saying "I don't like you," rather than acting out dislike by striking as was done at an earlier age. Toddlers do not yet understand concepts such as truth and love or past and future. They live in the present, in a world of things.

By 3 years of age the children realize they are called a boy or a girl, but the fact does not take on special significance.

Ritualistic behavior is characteristic of the toddler, who makes a ritual of simple tasks such as putting away toys or hanging up a coat. Such behavior provides a means for self-mastery. Leaving the toddler period, the child has less and less need for a strict routine because of increased self-assurance, and the ability to adapt to changes better than when younger.

The 18 month old is happy to play alone. About the age of 2 years the child prefers to play near other children but does not play with them, an activity aptly called *parallel play* (Fig. 5-2). The child treats other children as if they were physical objects, hugging them or pushing them out of the way. By the age of 3 years the child recognizes them as playmates and learns to play simple games and to take turns (Fig. 5-3).

The young toddler is very tender and innocent, in many ways still a "baby." If a new baby comes into the home, the toddler needs special assurance of continued love (Fig. 5-4).

Thumb-sucking normally reaches its peak about 18 months of age. At about the same time the child may choose a favorite toy or blanket that is held when sleepy or in need of comfort. By the age of 3 years the thumb-sucking has usually decreased markedly and the original favorite object has worn out.

Recent studies indicate that left- or right-handedness is inherited and that 7% to 10% of the normal population are left-handed. Most children are ambidextrous; that is, they use both hands equally well until about 3 years of age. At that time maturing nerves of the brain become insulated with myelin and handedness develops. If myelination is disrupted by brain damage, function may shift to the opposite side of the brain and the 90% to 93% of children who would normally become right-handed become left-handed. This accounts for the higher percentage of left-handed epileptic and retarded persons and confirms the theory that hand-preference is an inherited trait. If handedness is indeed an inborn trait, punishment to force change is of questionable value.

The young toddler likes to manipulate play materials such as sand and clay. If left with a bowel movement in the diapers, the child may discover that it, too, is soft and pliable and may smear it about until discovered. The idea that fecal matter is considered "dirty" and not a play-

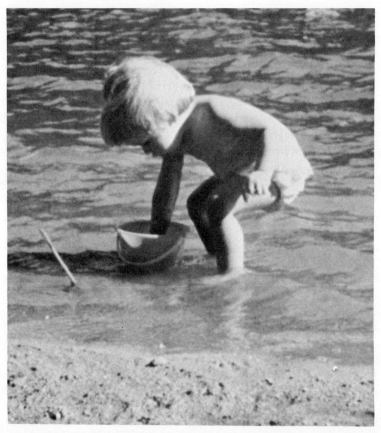

Fig. 5-2. This 2-year-old child is happy playing by herself, near others, but not with them, a typical example of parallel play.

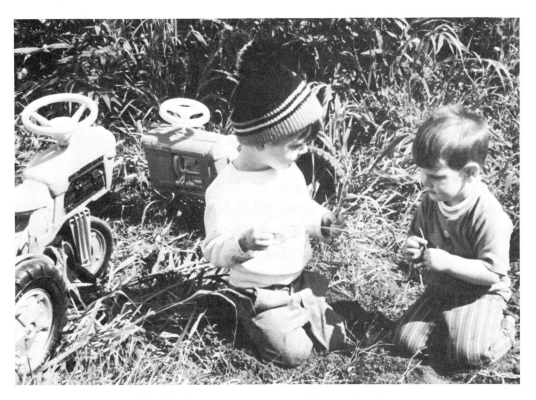

Fig. 5-3. Brothers sharing some special moment together.

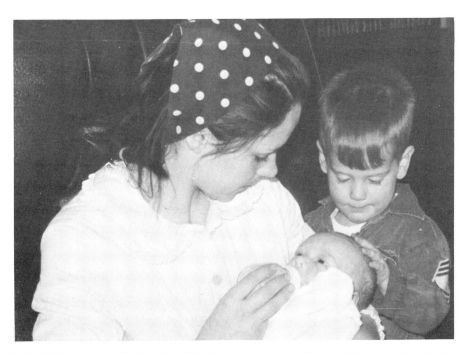

Fig. 5-4. The young toddler is still a "baby" in many respects. If a new baby comes into the home, toddlers need special help to understand that they are still loved.

thing is learned. As toilet training progresses, the child sees that it is a waste and not a part of the body and that it is flushed away.

Nutrition

Most children of 18 months have been weaned from the bottle as a means of gaining nourishment and are drinking fluids from a cup and eating foods from a spoon on a three-meal-a-day schedule with the family. By 2½ years of age all 20 baby teeth have erupted, so that the child can chew bites of reasonably soft foods.

Beginning with the second year of life, the child needs less food than during infancy because the growth rate has slowed considerably. The child's reduced appetite may worry the parents, who may resort to force and thus create needless future feeding problems. The following suggestions can help improve enjoyment of mealtime for both children and parents: (1) serve simple, unspiced foods that are easy to handle, (2) serve small portions that will not overwhelm a poor appetite, (3) eat meals as a group, observing courtesy and avoiding mention of dislikes, and (4) prepare for mealtime by avoiding appetite-dulling snacks, by alerting the child in advance that mealtime is near so that play is not spoiled, by toileting and hand washing, and by having a cheerful, everyone-is-doing-it attitude.

Attitudes toward foods formed during these early years tend to persist throughout life. Although it is important that children receive all the essential nutrients during these years, it is even more important that they learn to associate eating with pleasant rather than with painful emotional experiences. The nutritional needs of children are discussed in greater detail in Chapter 3.

Care

As attested to by the high incidence of child abuse, perhaps there is no period of a child's life that places such physical and psychological demands on parents as that of the toddler years. Parents must keep a constant watch on their actively curious child who still does not understand the meaning of danger and who is endlessly investigating the world. Parents must guide the child through this time of negativism and temper tantrums. They must see that the child receives proper nourishment even when appetite has decreased and must let the child know by word and deed of their love and respect. Their objective is to help the child establish self-controls and to find socially acceptable outlets for behavior. Difficult? Yes, but well worth the effort, because the ideas and attitudes the child gains about self and the world during these early years serve as a basis for all of the child's life.

During the later part of infancy the child takes the first step toward maturity by becoming weaned. The next major step comes during the toddler period, when the child learns bowel and bladder control. The child has yet to gain emotional control and is characteristically negative and reacts to frustrations by having temper tantrums, hence the term "terrible twos" used to describe the 2 year old.

The greatest single hazard to the toddler is innocent curiosity. The toddler climbs, explores, pokes, tastes, turns knobs, reaches for handles, and tries to imitate what others are doing. This is the period of life when most accidents occur. No amount of scolding, punishment, or "no, no"-ing will substitute for a home in which dangers have been anticipated and preventive measures taken. Someone must provide constant, visual supervision of the toddler. At the age of 18 months a child does not always understand the meaning of "no." It is usually better to remove the child physically from a dangerous situation than to expect obedience or to precipitate a temper tantrum.

There is considerable debate about the practice of spanking. Most parents believe that an occasional spanking, administered at the scene and time of the offense for violations of safety rules, may be the most effective means of education ("negative conditioning"). Everyone agrees that cruel beating is damaging. It may make the child docile and obedient for a time, but the long-term effect will be to create fear and hate, which distort and cripple the child's emotional development. The purpose of all punishment should be to teach self-control, not to produce guilt and fear; the child must know of parents' love and respect.

It should be noted here that discipline, or child training, is the legal and moral responsibility of the parent, not the medical personnel of the clinic or hospital. Although certain rules and restrictions must be made on the child's activities in the interest of safety, spankings by the medical staff are not permitted.

Temper tantrums are an expression of frustration. Most authorities agree that the best way to treat them is to isolate the child from an audience and to give the needed support to gain self-control. Many frustrations can be avoided by reducing conflicts. If a tantrum develops and parents give in to keep peace, the child soon recognizes this power and begins to rule the family by whim. Such a situation deprives the child of the opportunity to learn self-control and to accept the authority of others.

Negativism can be kept within reasonable limits in the same way as tantrums. The parents can simply reduce the number of situations that require a "yes" or "no" response. For example, instead of asking, "Do you want to come to dinner?" the parent can simply say, "It is time to eat. Let's go wash our hands."

The awake toddler appears to be in constant motion (Fig. 5-5). The child gets cross and fret-

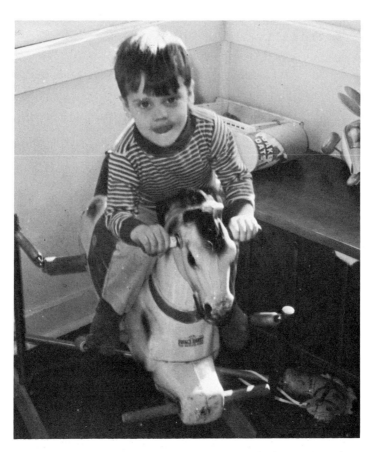

Fig. 5-5. When the toddler is awake, he appears to be in constant motion.

ful when tired, and needs 12 to 14 hours sleep a day. Although most toddlers still take an afternoon nap, some sleep only at night. The process of going to sleep in the evening can become a prolonged series of toileting, bathing, story reading, drinking of water, and on and on with the toddler in command. By establishing reasonable limits and by using the child's love for ritual, parents can make bedtime pleasant for everyone.

Brushing the teeth should begin as soon as the deciduous teeth have erupted. By about 2 years of age a child should be taught to use a toothbrush, and be encouraged to brush the teeth regularly after meals and at bedtime.

Toilet training should not be attempted until there is evidence that the child is ready. Bowel control usually comes first because the child has some warning, and it usually occurs only one or two times a day at about the same time. The child should be placed on the potty chair or training seat without a distracting toy. When successful, the child should be praised and rewarded by being allowed to flush the toilet. Punishment for failures and accidents serves no purpose. Bladder control comes later. When the weather is cold or the child is excited or too involved in play, urinary accidents may occur. Boys are slower to train than girls and may continue to have enuresis, or incontinence, longer than girls. The correct names for bodily functions and parts of the anatomy should be taught to children. "Toilet," "go potty," "BM," and "urine" are unmistakable and easily pronounced. Secret code names make it difficult for the child to tell nonfamily members of needs. When a child is admitted to the hospital, however, the nurse should ask the parents what names the child uses for these functions.

The toddler likes to do things independently, dressing, feeding, and placing toys in certain places, all unassisted. Although it tries parents' patience because they could do these things faster and more skillfully, they should allow these acceptable ways for children to develop independence.

Medical supervision

During the toddler and preschool years regular doctor visits should be made every 6 months. The child's growth and development can be evaluated and early diagnosis made if any abnormal conditions appear. A booster dose of DPT and oral polio vaccine are given at 18 months of age and again at 4 to 6 years of age. A skin test for tuberculosis may be made at 12 months of age and at 14 to 16 years of age and thereafter every 10 years when exposure is suspected (see recommended immunization schedule, Chapter 3).

Dental examinations should begin at about 2½ to 3 years of age or sooner if any unusual conditions appear. The dentist examines the oral cavity, cleans the teeth, paints them with fluoride, and discusses nutrition and home dental care with the parents. The establishment of a good relationship between the dentist and the child is of utmost importance in the initial dental examination, so that fear will be reduced for future dental care.

Disorders common to the toddler

The disorders that commonly affect the toddler can be classified as short-term care conditions and long-term care conditions.

Short-term care conditions

Accidents
 Poisoning
 Burns
 Fracture of the femur
 Foreign bodies in the nose and ear
Respiratory system
 Retropharyngeal abscess
 Croup
 Laryngotracheobronchitis
 Pneumococcal pneumonia
 Staphylococcal pneumonia
Intestinal parasites

Long-term care conditions

Cleft palate
Nephrotic syndrome (nephrosis)
Acrodynia (erythredema)

Lead poisoning
Cerebral palsy
Deafness
Blindness
Emotional disturbances

PRESCHOOLER (3 to 6 years)
Characteristics

Physical and motor development. The preschool years are characterized by a slowed rate of physical growth and an increased rate of motor coordination. The preschooler enjoys active, energetic play but may also settle down to tasks that require finer motor skills. During this period the child gains less than 5 pounds in weight and 3 inches in height per year. Baby chubbiness

seems to disappear as the child becomes more sturdy and muscular.

The 5 year old begins to lose baby teeth in the same order as they first appeared—the lower incisors first, followed by the upper incisors (Fig. 5-6).

The 4 year old can jump, go up and down stairs without holding onto the railing, throw a ball overhand, use scissors to cut out pictures, copy a square, button buttons on the front of clothing, lace shoes, and brush teeth. The 5 year old can jump rope, play games well, skip on alternating feet, roller skate, use a hammer to hit a nail on the head, copy a triangle, draw a recognizable picture of a person, and dress without help, and may be able to tie shoelaces. The child

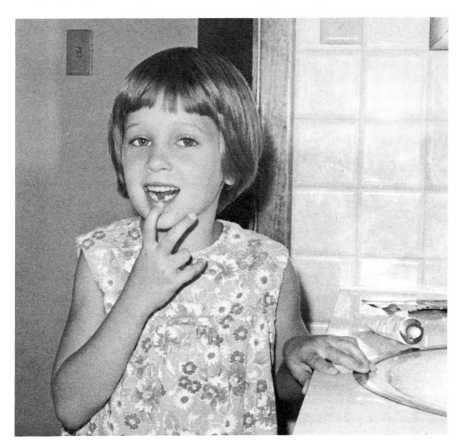

Fig. 5-6. The lower incisors usually come out first.

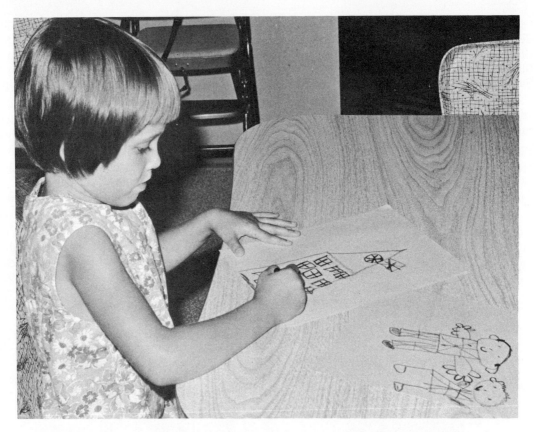

Fig. 5-7. The 5-year-old child draws recognizable pictures of people and houses. Note the five fingers on the man.

has good posture and excellent motor control (Fig. 5-7).

Emotional and social development. During infancy the child learned to trust others; during toddler days the child recognized individuality; the preschooler is ready to find out about individual abilities. The child wants to learn about the world and the other people in it, and watches adults and imitates what they do. When not able to participate in the adult world, the child pretends, sometimes by making up elaborate, make-believe stories and other times by means of imaginative play. The child may use simple equipment to represent articles used in real life, so that a series of blocks may become a train

and a few cardboard boxes a playhouse.

The vocabulary of the preschooler increases at the rate of about 600 words per year as a result of endless questioning and searching for explanations for a curious environment. The 4 year old can count to 4, know his or her age, and can name one or two colors. The 5 year old can name four colors and is interested in the relationship of relatives such as aunts, uncles, and cousins. The 5 year old enjoys storybooks, both to look at personally and to hear read (Fig. 5-8). During the preschool years the child begins to develop a conscience, and accepts those values learned from the family, a process called *internalizing*, and at the same time becomes aware of the in-

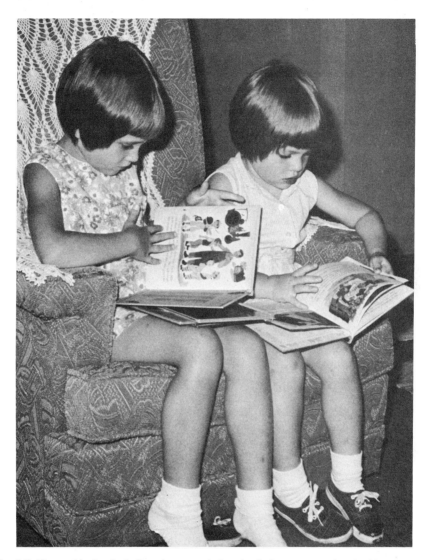

Fig. 5-8. The world of make-believe is very real. Storybooks become more loved with repeated use.

ability to always live up to those ideals. This development of conscience is demonstrated by the fact that the child sometimes feels deeply guilty for improper actions or fantasies.

If given the opportunity, the 4 year old notices the differences between boys and girls and accepts this difference without difficulty. A child is quick to notice adult attitudes of shame or disgust and gets the idea that there is something immoral or bad about sex. In the absence of correct information the child may create bizarre explanations for the absence or presence of a penis. Healthy attitudes result when adults give direct, simple, matter-of-fact answers to preschoolers' questions.

During infancy and toddlerhood children of

both sexes love and are dependent on their mothers. According to Freud, a change occurs between the ages of 3 and 6 years. The little girl becomes more interested in her father; the little boy remains in love with his mother. This change in the love-object influences behavior. Girls tend to be jealous of their mothers and boys of the father, yet at the same time try to imitate their mothers, and boys try to be like their fathers. At the end of the preschool period the boy no longer wants to replace his father, he wants to be like him. The girl wants to grow up to be like her mother. The family unit then becomes the love-object and the conflict is resolved. This stage of development when boys love their mothers and girls love their fathers is called *oedipal* from the Greek play entitled *Oedipus Rex*.

If the father is absent from the home during this period, a boy will not have a male model with whom he can identify nor will he find it necessary to give up his love for his mother. This unfortunate effect may also occur when the girl is without a mother or mother substitute. These children may find it more difficult to take the next steps in emotional development beyond this preschool level and may need guidance in later years to change their immature relations with their parents.

Nutrition

The preschooler does not have a large appetite, preferring plain foods served attractively in separate dishes. The child prefers finger-foods such as bread sticks, sandwiches, and celery sticks to creamed or highly flavored dishes. Simple but imaginative touches by creative parents can make mealtime more pleasant. Bite-sized food such as cheese squares are more fun to eat with a colored toothpick. A well of gravy in the mashed potatoes makes a lake in a tiny mountain, the pancake batter pours into all manner of animal shapes, and a drop of pink food coloring in the milk makes it special. The preschool child should eat regular meals of small

portions in the family group. When appetite gradually increases with increased growth, food intake will be adjusted upward to meet needs. Although parents may complain that their preschooler "eats like a bird," most children manage to take in all the needed nutrients and to show a modest weight gain (see the discussion on nutrition in Chapter 3).

Occasionally a preschool child is diagnosed as having a "feeding problem." If no organic reason can be found, the child may be placed in a nursery school setting where meals are eaten with other children the same age. Many dramatic changes in attitude and habits have been observed in these children as they learn to eat in a tension-free atmosphere, in which meals are a normal, social part of everyday life (Fig. 5-9).

Care

The preschool child requires less continuous supervision. The child is usually toilet-trained, can feed and dress alone, and prefers independence and outdoor active play. But in spite of this increased independent ability, the preschooler has certain special needs. These needs are to be loved, to feel secure, to accept limits to activities without feelings of guilt, to develop language skills, to gain information about the surrounding world, and to learn moral values. All these areas require considerable devotion, wisdom, and skill on the part of the parents.

Some of the special problems of the preschool child include anxiety, thumb-sucking, bad language, destructiveness, hurting others, and masturbation.

Anxiety in the preschool child may be caused by separation from the parents and by fear of pain. To the child, separation from the parents means loss of love. Most hospitalizations are only temporary, but long-term hospitalization, or being orphaned, or losing a parent by divorce or death may deeply hurt the child, who may go through a period of mourning for the parents. Being less verbal than the adult, the child may

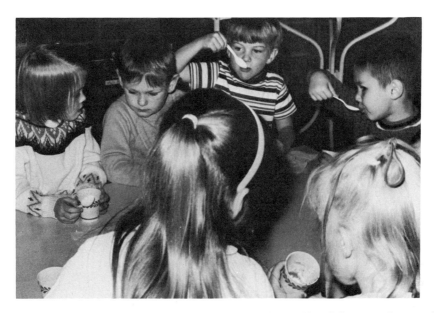

Fig. 5-9. Nursery school children eating together. Many "feeding problems" disappear when everybody is eating and no one is nagging.

respond in nonverbal ways such as regressing to infantile behavior or being uncooperative and naughty. The child may vomit or have diarrhea. The nurse should treat the child with kindness and encourage talking about the parent who has gone away. The child may feel guilty because of angry feelings toward the parents before and may feel responsible for the death or departure of the parent. The child should be helped to understand that a mere wish was not the cause of the parent's leaving.

Fear is a common experience of preschoolers. It may be fear of the dark, of thunder, or of real pain. The adult can help the child overcome these fears with reasonable explanation and reassuring presence, for the child is more fearful when alone.

Thumb-sucking in the preschooler is more of a problem for the parents than the child. To help the child, the parents should note the occasions of thumb-sucking and provide a demonstration of love and security for the child at those times.

Bad language and *naughty words* usually have more meaning to the shocked adult than to the preschool child who uses them. If this use of language gains attention and generates an emotional response, the child is more likely to repeat the offense than if the response is a bored, matter of fact reply such as "I'm tired of hearing that."

Destructiveness is seldom intentional in the energetic, curious preschool child. Parents should remove valuable objects that might be broken or damaged and should provide space for the active child to play where harm will not be done to the household furnishings. Adults should set up certain restrictions so that the child will learn to value personal possessions and the possessions of others. The loving child is often deeply sorry if something of value gets broken, even if the child knows that punishment will not be forthcoming.

The intentionally destructive child is an unhappy child unable to control feelings of anger, jealousy, or helplessness. The child may feel unloved, disliked, or bored and may even seem to want to be punished. The cause of such destructiveness must be recognized and remedied. The child should be helped to direct energy into appropriate activities.

Sometimes children get hurt in the normal rough and tumble of their play. A child who repeatedly *hurts others* by pulling hair, biting, scratching, or hitting, however, is a troubled child and needs help to learn self-control and needs to be prevented from injuring others. The child may be jealous or frustrated, and violent behavior may result from this mental state. The child needs to know that such behavior cannot be tolerated and that a loving person will take control. The child should not be punished with the same injury, or scolded as bad. Instead the child should be helped to feel a part of the group, praised for acceptable behavior, and isolated for antisocial acts.

Masturbation is an almost universal experience in children. The infant first discovers that a pleasant sensation occurs when the genitals are handled. In the preschool child masturbation may increase and be accompanied by fantasies. In the adolescent years it serves to fulfill sexual urges that the youth cannot otherwise release. Masturbation is not in itself bad or abnormal. It does not cause mental illness or physical disorders, as was once believed. Excessive masturbation, however, may mean that the child is failing socially and so turns to the self for pleasure. Shaming or punishing the child for normal genital pleasure sensations may cause lifelong psychological harm. Helping the child to relate satisfactorily with other children will meet the greater need and reduce this practice to normal limits.

Medical supervision

Except for a possible tuberculin skin test if exposed, or booster doses of tetanus following an injury, most healthy preschool children do not require any additional immunizations or medical tests. They should be examined regularly by a physician every 6 months during this period, however, so that early diagnosis and treatment of abnormal conditions can be made. Dental examinations and care should be given regularly every 4 to 6 months.

Parents of preschool children may need special consultation and help in meeting the particular needs of their children. They may need help in solving such problems as thumb-sucking, hurting others, destructiveness, masturbation, feeding problems, anxiety, toilet training, and bad language. Personal consultation and appropriate literature should be offered to the parents by the medical personnel.

Disorders common to the preschool-aged child

The disorders that commonly affect the preschool child can be classified as short-term care conditions and long-term care conditions. Listed are some common disorders that affect preschoolers.

Short-term care conditions

Communicable diseases
Acute glomerulonephritis
Vulvovaginitis
Gonorrheal vaginitis
Strabismus (cross-eye)
Tonsillectomy and adenoidectomy

Long-term care conditions

Leukemia
Hemophilia
Purpura
Allergy
Asthma
Allergic rhinitis
Serum sickness
Anaphylactic reactions
Epilepsy
Mental retardation
Phobias
Temper tantrums
Child schizophrenia
Autism

SUMMARY OUTLINE

I. **Toddler (advent of walking to 3 years)**
   A. Characteristics
      1. Physical and motor development
      2. Emotional and social development
   B. Nutrition
   C. Care
   D. Medical supervision
   E. Disorders common to the toddler
II. **Preschooler (3 to 6 years)**
   A. Characteristics
      1. Physical and motor development
      2. Emotional and social development
   B. Nutrition
   C. Care
   D. Medical supervision
   E. Disorders common to the toddler

STUDY QUESTIONS

1. Describe the physical and emotional development of the preschool child.
2. Discuss thumb-sucking, toilet training, temper tantrums, accident proneness, and masturbation. What attitudes, approaches, and techniques would you use to help the child mature? Would your expectations about the chronically ill child be modified? If so, how?

6
The school years

THE YOUNG SCHOOL CHILD
(6 to 12 years)
Characteristics

Physical and motor development. During the school years the rate of growth in height is decreased and the rate of gain in weight is increased. Children tend to lose the thin, wiry appearance and their frames become solid and sturdy. Their posture changes, with the disappearance of the typical lordosis (swayback) of preschool years, and motor coordination improves steadily. Movements become more graceful as they engage in active, large-muscle play, and their manual dexterity becomes more complex. These are the years when boys and girls excel in body movement activities.

The typical toothless smile of the 6 and 7 year old signifies the beginning of the gradual loss of the baby teeth and their replacement by the permanent ones. The 6-year molar also appears about this time.

During the early school years the lymphatic tissue of the body reaches the height of its development and then it slowly diminishes.

Between the ages of 10 and 12 years girls begin to develop sexually. This period, called prepubescence, or the period just before sexual maturity, is characterized in girls by a growth spurt, widening of the hips, budding of the breasts, pubic hair growth, and occasionally the beginning of menses. Boys are 2 or more years slower than girls in sexual maturity.

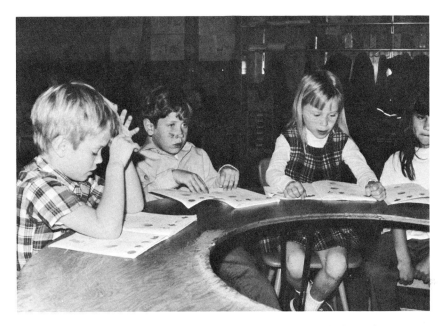

Fig. 6-1. A reading circle in which each child receives individual attention.

Emotional, intellectual, and social development. By the time children begin school at about 6 years of age, they should have developed a sense of trust, a sense of individuality, an ability to get along with others, a degree of personal initiative, and a conscience that provides inner control. They should have passed through the girl-loves-father and boy-loves-mother stage to the stage in which they identify with parents of the same sex and and want to be like some hero of the same sex. During the school years loyalties shift from the family to members of the same age group. They may become very sensitive to the conduct of family before friends and shun public displays of affection. They may be highly critical of their parents and seek out the confidence of some other adult whom they feel they can trust. In spite of criticism of the family, children internalize, or accept as their own, the attitudes and ideas that the family expresses. If the parents hold respect for formal education, civil authorities, and individual differences in race, religion, and politics, children are more likely to make these positive attitudes their own.

If the parents hold prejudices against various institutions and persons, children are more likely to make these negative ideas their own.

During the early school years children may become interested in religion and the idea of God. As they move on through the childhood years, their concern for these matters seems to wane but is renewed in early adolescence when moral questions about human relationships become important.

Children 6 years of age recognize that the wonderful world of make-believe they enjoyed as preschoolers is gone, but its memory is sweet, and so they join in the fun of maintaining such myths as Santa Claus for younger brothers and sisters.

School-aged children are increasingly able to manage their own personal care, although their standards may not be as high as their parents'.

Children of 6 to 12 years are naturally curious and eager to learn. As they move through their formal education, they become more and more skillful with oral language (Fig. 6-1). Their writing skill also increases, from the block printing

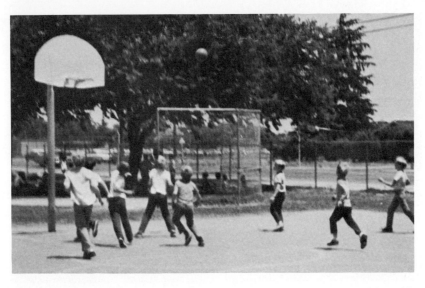

Fig. 6-2. Active sports provide a healthy outlet for pent-up energy and a competitive spirit.

of the 6 year old to the scrawled handscript of the 9 year old to the neat, smaller writing of the 12 year old. Children 6 and 7 years of age can perform simple addition and subtraction. As they progress, they learn to tell time, multiply, divide, and work with mathematical concepts. Creativity and special musical and artistic talents emerge during these years. Inherited intellectual potential, emotional stability, and cultural and educational opportunities all influence children's ability to learn.

School-aged children are highly competitive in sports, academic achievements, and within the family group. They thrive on pitting themselves against some opponent or goal (Fig. 6-2). Rewards and recognition for achievement serve to motivate them to accomplish difficult feats and to complete tasks that have lost their novelty. In the home this competitive spirit shows itself in strong sibling rivalries wherein brothers and sisters compete for leadership and parental attention. Excessive competition creates unhealthy tensions but reasonable amounts challenge and motivate children toward greater accomplishment.

The later school years are the years of the gang, the secret club, and close friendships between children of the same sex. Boys "hate" girls and tease them, girls have no use for boys and shun them. Children who are exceptions to this behavior are called "sissies" and "tomboys." These are the years when children are most cruel to one another. They sometimes choose a child who is slightly different and focus their collective hostility on that one. Because victims are thus ostracized, their life becomes miserable because acceptance and approval of their age group are of utmost importance.

Nutrition

During the first 6 years of school, caloric requirements of children continue to decrease and their need for adequate protein, fresh fruits, and vegetables increases. School children usually have better appetites and fewer food fads than preschool children, but because they are away at school all day, their noon meal may not be balanced or adequate. Breakfast and evening meals should be planned to make up for these inadequacies. Ideal between-meal snacks are celery and carrot sticks, fresh fruits, hot bouillon, dill pickles, and cold meat, served in small portions and not too close to mealtime.

Six year olds have good appetites, are talkative, stuff their mouths, and grab for their food. Seven year olds talk less during meals, may still bolt their food, but are quieting down. Eight and 9 year olds eat more neatly, mimic their elders, and are likely to use better table manners in public than at home. Ten to 12 year olds have table manners more like their parents, both at home and in public.

Care

The aim of child care during the school-age period is threefold: (1) to help children develop qualities of industry, self-motivation, and creativity so they will be able to make full use of educational and cultural opportunities offered them, (2) to instill attitudes of respect for self and other individuals and groups, and (3) to provide stable, loving homes to which they can come and go as they broaden social relationships outside the family.

Before the days of automatic heat, dishwashers, clothes driers, and garbage disposers there were many tasks about the home that children could do to develop industry, self-motivation, and creativity. Now these tasks are performed by machines, and the time they save has been filled with television viewing. Concerned parents must consciously counteract the effect of this modernization by providing work experiences and responsibilities for children and by limiting the number of television hours.

Parental attitudes, spoken or unspoken, profoundly affect growing children, who do not need to be told that their parents are proud of them and their achievements or that they value education. Children sense it from the interest parents take in school reports, their participation on school visiting day, and their positive cooperation with school authorities. In the same way children gain respect for other persons of various political and religious persuasions and national-ities by the obvious verbal and nonverbal actions of their parents.

Children need a stable home in which there is a loving relationship between the parents and the children. It becomes a secure haven from the new and threatening forces that children face each day. Although they usually make new friends and form new loyalties outside the home, children need the security and reassurance that the home provides. When the home is divided by divorce, sickness, or death, children are deprived of the security and strength it normally gives and need special guidance and help.

Medical supervision

Every child should have a preschool health examination including weight, height, posture, hearing, and vision. Defective hearing or vision can seriously affect a child's learning ability and should receive special attention at this time.

At 4 to 6 years of age children should receive a booster dose against diphtheria, tetanus, and pertussis and at 14 to 16 years and thereafter every 10 years a booster dose of tetanus-diphtheria toxoids, "adult type." After entering school, the child no longer needs immunization against pertussis because the disease is milder and vaccine reactions more frequent.

School-aged children should have an annual physical examination and a semiannual dental examination. Corrective orthodontic care for improperly aligned teeth may be recommended for both cosmetic and functional reasons. This commences soon after the badly aligned permanent teeth erupt.

School health programs are an important part of the national health program. Their purpose is to maintain, improve, and promote the health of every child. Services provided by the school health program include supervision of the physical, mental, emotional, and social aspects of school life, planning course content in health education and nutrition, and providing preventive services, health appraisals, and follow-up for individual children in the school.

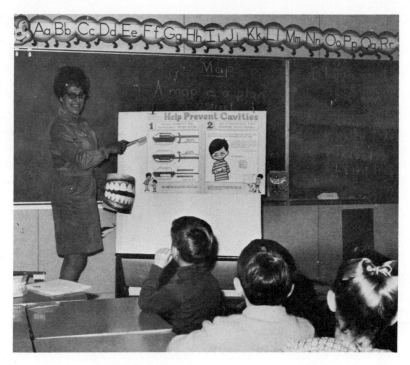

Fig. 6-3. The school nurse teaches dental hygiene.

The school nurse is usually the person who provides the leadership for the school health program (Fig. 6-3). The nurse works with the parents, teachers, administrators, school or private physicians, social workers, psychologists, and special education staff to carry out the broad health program of the school.

The three most common health problems that directly involve the school are communicable diseases, physical and mental handicaps, and problems related to sexual maturation.

Communicable disease information and education is provided to the parents so that needless exposure of other children will be prevented. Parents are instructed to keep children at home when they have a rash, fever, or cold symptoms.

Special education programs for handicapped children are being offered in communities across the nation. Information about these programs is available through local school districts.

Sex education, personal counseling, and medical examination, diagnosis, and treatment are necessary to meet the problems related to sexual maturity. Sex education in the schools is not uniform. Some school districts provide an integrated course of sex information that begins in the early school years and progresses through the high school years; others provide no formal sex education. The trend is toward providing this information as a normal part of health education.

Disorders common to school-aged children

Disorders that affect school-aged children can be classified as short-term care conditions and long-term care conditions.

Short-term care conditions
Epistaxis
Respiratory infections
Communicable diseases

Ringworm (tinea)
Pediculosis
Scabies
Osteomyelitis
Appendicitis
Meckel's diverticulum
Cryptorchidism

Long-term care conditions

Rheumatic fever
Rheumatoid arthritis
Diabetes mellitus
Abnormal sexual development
Head trauma and skull fracture
Cerebral concussion
Extradural hematoma
Brain tumor
Perthes' disease
Neurotic symptoms
Conduct disorders
Stuttering
Anorexia nervosa
Overeating
Chronic ulcerative colitis
Enuresis
Constipation

ADOLESCENCE (12 to 18 or more years)

Adolescence is a period of transition from childhood to adulthood. It is characterized by the dramatic physical changes of puberty and the complex emotional and social adjustments necessary to become an adult.

Characteristics

Physical and motor development. Puberty is that time of life when the reproductive system matures. It is marked by a preliminary period of a year or more called *prepubescence* during which the secondary sex characteristics appear. At this time the endocrine glands, particularly the pituitary and the gonads, begin to produce greater quantities of their hormones. These powerful chemicals are distributed to every part of the body by means of the bloodstream after which they effect changes in the functioning of the body systems, in the body contour, and in the rate of growth. These prepuberty changes usually begin to appear between the ages of 10 and 15 years. Girls have a tendency to develop before boys do, and those living in warm climates before those living in cold regions.

Typical changes in boys are (1) an increase in the size of the genitals, (2) swelling of the breasts, (3) beginning of rapid height and weight growth and a broadening of the chest, (4) growth of pubic, axillary, facial, and chest hair, (5) producing of spermatozoa, and (6) nocturnal emissions (wet dreams).

Typical changes in girls are (1) broadening of the hips and pelvis, (2) growth of the nipples and breasts, (3) growth of pubic and axillary hair, (4) menarche (onset of menstruation), and (5) ovulation (follows menarche by 6 to 12 months).

Other physical changes that occur in both boys and girls are skin changes, body contour changes, and variation of growth rates of the body organs.

Changes in the skin of adolescents causes them to blush easily, develop pimples and blackheads, and produce strong-smelling perspiration. Flushing of the skin is caused by a sudden dilation of surface blood vessels in response to nervous stimuli. As youths mature, the vasomotor mechanism stabilizes and the incidence of blushing decreases. During adolescence the sebaceous or oil glands of the face, back, and chest become more active. If the pores are small or clogged, infections may occur, causing blackheads, pimples, and, in severe cases, acne. The sweat glands begin to function as a part of the excretory system and temperature-controlling mechanism, producing perspiration and body odor.

During adolescence the body contour changes as a result of the redistribution of fat and growth of the bony frame of the body. Boys become broad chested, small hipped, muscular, and lean. Girls become rounded in contour, with broad hips and full breasts. These changes are effected because of the adrenal and sex hormones.

The physical growth of adolescents occurs in every part of their bodies. This growth may occur at different times. Their hands and feet may grow faster than their legs and arms, causing movements to be poorly coordinated. As a result this stage of development is often called the "awkward age." Posture may be poor because large muscles tend to grow faster than small ones. The heart and lungs grow more slowly than the rest of the body, causing youths constantly to feel tired. Pains in the joints, especially during periods of relaxation and rest, are not normal. They may indicate rheumatic fever and so should not be dismissed as simply "growing pains."

Between the ages of 18 and 23 years the last four molars erupt. These so-called "wisdom teeth" complete the full set of 32 permanent teeth.

By the end of adolescence the physical bodies of young people are those of adults, and they are normally in the prime of physical health and vigor.

Emotional, social, and intellectual development

Personality development. Adolescence is the period of life when individuals must work out their own value systems and solve certain major issues that will affect their entire lives. This transition takes time and is often stormy. There are conflicting forces that pull youths one way and then another—drives produced by developing physical body and sexual maturity, pressures of social conformity, demands of moral and ethical training, and emotional needs for love, security, achievement, recognition, and independence from parental authority. Working out these conflicts does not follow a timetable. Each youth must find solutions to the problems at hand. The youth does this in a highly individual manner, depending on family constitution, attitudes, health, educational and vocational opportunities, social and cultural environment, and intellectual potential. In working through and resolving these conflicts, the youth establishes what psychologists call *identity*, or an individual answer to the questions "Who am I?" and "What do I really believe?"

According to Erikson, when youths find their identity, they are ready to move on to the final step of maturity—the ability to form a deep, caring relationship with another person, called *intimacy*.

In the process of arriving at a full personality development adolescents must resolve the following four major issues:

1. Emotional independence from parents.
2. Acceptance of sexual gender.
3. Identification of the principles by which to live and relate to others.
4. Decisions about a vocation.

This process sounds very reasonable until one realizes how big and complex these issues really are. Adolescents are expected to resolve them in only 6 to 8 years while they are under tremendous pressures to achieve academically and athletically and while their bodies are growing and changing in new and perplexing ways. Parents often resist the efforts of adolescents to think and act independently. The adult world gives youths almost no help at all except in the area of vocational guidance. To find satisfactory solutions to the four major issues confronting adolescents, they must find out what the real world is like, establish contact with it, and become functioning parts of it. These demands on youths are enormous. It is no surprise that so many people go into later life, immature in one area or another, incompletely prepared to meet the demands of an adult world. Some become delinquents or criminals, using antisocial means to solve their conflicts.

Social development. Next to the obvious physical changes of puberty, the social development of adolescence is perhaps the most noticeable and perplexing to both youths and their parents. During these years they identify more with peers than parents. They conform to peer standards and seek peer approval more than that of their parents as seen by the fads that come and go. They also must learn to adjust their growing sexuality to the social world about them and find satisfactory and acceptable solutions to the problems these needs present.

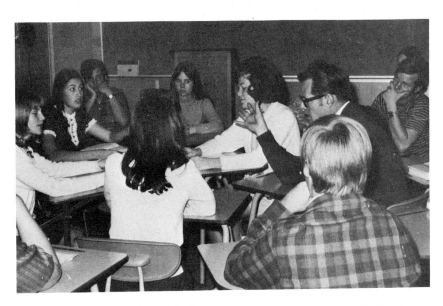

Fig. 6-4. Coeducational schools make social adjustments more natural because normal daily interchanges take place within the classroom.

In early adolescence youths still feel more comfortable with members of their own sex but enjoy group activities that include both girls and boys. At this time they usually have a special friend of their own sex with whom they share their innermost secrets and have a "crush" on someone of the opposite sex but be too bashful even to speak to that person. Gradually youths gain self-confidence, become comfortable in mixed groups, and no longer feel the need for so close a friend or to retreat from members of the opposite sex to the safety of a group of their own. Adolescents who attend coeducational schools are able to make these social adjustments more naturally because they have opportunities for normal daily interchanges between the sexes within the classroom (Fig. 6-4).

As adolescents mature, they become increasingly independent of any one person and have friends of both sexes, often developing "brother-sister" friendships with nonsiblings. They begin to date a number of different persons, eventually singling out one special person. This practice is of considerable value because it provides individuals with the opportunity to evaluate each other in terms of compatibility and to learn to share and care for another—a capacity called *intimacy.* Acquiring this capacity is the final step toward adulthood.

Intellectual development. Intelligence, or the ability to adjust to new situations and to think abstractly, increases at a relatively constant and rapid rate until about the age of 13 years, when it slows markedly. This leveling is of particular significance to the guidance counselor who, by measuring the intelligence of a youth in mid-adolescence, can provide realistic vocational guidance. Because of the many examples of "late bloomers," however, no one should be discouraged from higher goals than "tests indicate."

Care

The care of adolescents is on a different level from that needed by younger children. They no longer need direct physical care, because they are able to bathe, clothe, and feed themselves; they come and go to school on their own initiative; and they may earn their own spending money. Adolescents need to have their privacy respected. They also need maximum autonomy, a measure of their parent's trust. Adolescents should take care of their personal property and room and share with other family members in the maintenance of the home. In short, by adolescence youths should have assumed almost complete responsibility for their own activities of daily living and for their share of family living as well. So, then, the chief care that parents must give adolescents is not in the area of *doing for them* but rather in the area of setting the stage for the adolescents *to do for themselves*. It is true that parents must still provide food, shelter, clothes, educational opportunity, and medical supervision, but in recent years these things have become so expensive that the job of earning them has diverted the attention of the parents away from an even more important task—that of providing emotional support, information, and guidance for adolescents during the most critical period of their lives. This kind of healthy home environment provides youths with the psychological setting in which they can become responsible and independent.

Emotional support. Parents have a difficult task: they must work themselves out of a job. If the parents had an unhappy adolescence or grew up in a different culture or economic level, they may be baffled by their teenager and not sure of their own parental role. They may be too strict or too lenient. They may create needless conflicts by their ignorance of the long-term needs of the adolescent. Most parents sincerely want to be "good," but few have ever thought through what this means and even fewer have defined clear goals toward which they are working.

There are three general goals for child rearing: (1) children should enjoy maximum physical and emotional health, (2) they should become functioning, productive members of society, and (3) they should develop a system of values that is beneficial to themselves and others. These long-range aims seem especially important during adolescence when personality development becomes more fixed and the youths enter adulthood.

There are no pat answers for parents and oth-

ers to the question of how to rear an adolescent. The variables are legion. Every person, every home, every situation is different. Generally speaking, however, parents would find their job easier if they followed these recommendations:

1. Recognize the adolescent's need to resolve the major issues of life—separation from parents, determination of sexual role, development of a value system, and the choice of a vocation.
2. Set reasonable ground rules for the activities of daily living and family sharing. Expect occasional failures.
3. Make yourself available for communication. Listen, discuss, share ideas and activities. Solve problems jointly. Never preach or argue.
4. Trust and praise more; condemn and doubt less.
5. Respect the adolescent's need for privacy.
6. Permit maximum autonomy.
7. Relax and enjoy the freshness and vigor of adolescent youth.

Adolescents would find their lives more tranquil if they followed these recommendations:

1. Accept the authority of parents as a fact of life and make the most of it.
2. Recognize that parents and siblings are not perfect. Love and encourage them in spite of these defects. They are yours.
3. Communicate with your parents, discuss ideas, share plans, and ask questions. Parents are more likely to respect and trust a reasonable, thinking person than a secretive, silent bore.
4. Be helpful. Carry your share of the household load.
5. Control your temper and your tongue. Self-control is a sign of maturity.

Information and guidance. Adolescents need information about the physical changes going on within their bodies and guidance to adjust to these changes. They should understand that the rapid growth rate of early puberty makes them feel tired but that this fatigue is normal. The best solution for this weariness is rest.

Appearance is of special importance to teenagers. Both boys and girls want to dress like their friends regardless of the discomfort or oddity of the current fad. To them conformity is more important than comfort. If parents realized this desire, they might be more willing to go along with these fads knowing that the fads will pass soon and that in the long view these concessions to adolescents' need for group conformity are really minor. Their rapid growth may make difficult the task of keeping teenagers in well-fit clothing. Parents should be encouraged to buy fewer items more frequently throughout the year so that the teenager is not embarrassed by having to wear too-large sizes purchased "to grow into." Young adolescents may be self-conscious about their developing sexual organs. Girls should be provided with well-fitting brassieres and boys with athletic supports if they so desire.

Facial pimples and blackheads are the source of much concern, even though they are problems common to most adolescents. Because they are caused by oily skin and closed pores, the best treatment is regular cleansing and healthy, well-balanced diet. Pimples and blackheads should not be squeezed savagely, because doing so only damages the tissue and spreads infection. If healing does not occur promptly or if the general condition of the skin worsens, a physician should be consulted.

Bad breath and body odor are problems that adolescents may not recognize until someone tells them. They should be encouraged to brush and floss their teeth regularly, bathe frequently, and use an effective deodorant.

By providing adolescents with sympathetic, constructive guidance in these very practical areas of life, parents and others demonstrate their genuine concern and establish rapport with their teenagers.

Work, school, and recreation

Work, school, and recreational experiences are an important part of the learning process during adolescence. In most states, laws require school attendance for all children up to the age of 16 years. With few exceptions, national child labor laws prevent the employment of children under the age of 16 years for wages. The intent of both sets of laws is that children should receive a basic education in academic subjects before they go out into the working world. If work experiences do not detract from formal education, they can enrich it by providing valuable lessons in self-discipline, human relations, and the exploration of vocational interests. Some organizations such as Junior Achievement have been formed with the purpose of encouraging young persons to form and manage independent business ventures.

School has a central role in the life of adolescents, not only by providing information about a wide variety of academic subjects and a forum for the exchange of ethical, philosophical, and political ideas, but also by giving the opportunity for the development of athletic, artistic, and musical aptitudes (Fig. 6-5). The school also provides a kind of sheltered workshop in social and life adjustment. There adolescents learn to relate to the competitive group and other individuals, to members of their own and the opposite sex, to persons of different races, religions, economic status, and cultures. They develop loyalty to their class and school. They learn about the democratic process through elections and about organizational functions through committees and councils.

In recent years the services offered by the community high school have been increased greatly to include vocational and personal counseling, health services, psychological testing, family and health education, recreational, cultural, and social direction, and job and college placement. These services are all provided with the goal of assisting adolescents to make satisfactory emotional, intellectual, social, and physical adjustments to adult life.

Recreation plays an important part in adolescent development. Activities that use up energy and appeal to the adventuresome spirit of youths are especially healthful and desirable (Fig. 6-6).

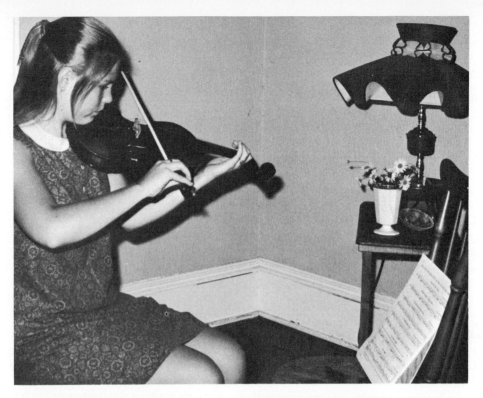

Fig. 6-5. Musical aptitudes and interests can be developed during the adolescent years.

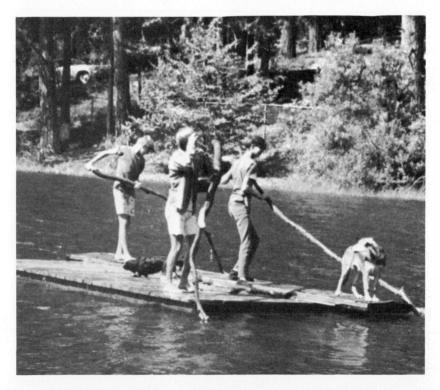

Fig. 6-6. Recreation plays an important part in the adolescent's development.

Nutrition

The need for energy-producing and body-building nutrients is at its highest level during adolescence. Caloric needs range from 2,300 to 3,400 calories per day. Protein intake should be about 15% of the total caloric intake. To maintain adequate nitrogen levels, an adolescent should receive up to 85 gm of protein per day. That boys have greater nutritional needs and enormous appetites to go with them is well known and accepted. Girls, too, need high protein and nutritious diets, but because they are weight conscious, they may go on unwise reducing diets and deny themselves the very nutrients they need most. If these crash diets are maintained for long periods, deficiencies can result. More often, however, girls tend to starve themselves for a few days, then overeat, and quickly regain the lost pounds. Repeated cycles of fasting and gorging only produce discouragement and prevent the individuals from attempting sound weight-control eating habits. Adolescents who believe they are overweight or underweight should be referred to a nutritionist for consultation rather than leaving them to experiment with crash diets.

Some adults disdain the favorite foods of American adolescents, such as hamburgers with fresh lettuce and tomatoes, french fried potatoes with catsup, pizzas made with cheese, meats, and tomato sauce, and milkshakes. Actually all of these foods are highly nutritious and if eaten regularly and in sufficient amounts would provide a balanced diet. It is true that sugary soda pop and chocolates may affect dental and skin health, but if the youth is also eating well-balanced meals, the extra calories added by the sweets may fill a special need for quick energy.

Both boys and girls need basic facts about good nutrition and foods in the diet. Recent studies indicate that men are particularly susceptible to cardiovascular diseases and that these conditions are affected by diet. Eating patterns established in youth could have a definite effect on the health in adult life.

Medical supervision

The medical needs of the teenager are different from those of either the adult or the child. They are unique, involving the interrelated psychosexual and physical changes of adolescence. A relatively new medical specialty has emerged in response to this need, named *ephebiatrics*, after the Greek word *ephébos*, "one arrived at youth." Ephebiatricians are concerned with the total adolescent, not just skin problems, or early or late growth, or a girl's menstrual irregularities. Another approach to the need for coordinated medical services for adolescents has been the formation of teen clinics in which a number of different specialists work together. In these clinics there may be a urologist, obstetrician-gynecologist, internist, dermatologist, endocrinologist, and psychiatrist. All these specialists are devoted to the total welfare of adolescents and are available to listen to their problems.

In addition to general medical supervision, adolescents need immunization against certain childhood diseases that may have worn off since the initial series were administered. Tuberculin skin tests should be made every other year or more often depending on the local incidence of tuberculosis. If the skin test turns positive, a year of prophylactic tuberculocidal drug is recommended, followed by annual medical checkups. A booster dose of diptheria and tetanus should be administered at 12 years of age and every years thereafter. If the person is wounded, an emergency booster of tetanus should be given according to the practice described in Chapter 3.

Dental care is of great importance during adolescence because the last of all the temporary teeth fall out and all of the permanent teeth appear. Because teenagers tend to practice irregular eating habits, dental hygiene may also be irregular and inadequate. Even if it is impossible to brush the teeth after taking food and drink, water should be swished around the teeth to help reduce the concentration of bacteria-encouraging nutrients. By late adolescence individuals should have well-established habits of dental hygiene and should assume responsibility for their own dental and medical care.

Beginning at menarche, many gynecologists recommend that girls have pelvic examinations and that a cervical scraping be taken to be examined for cancer. The test, called the Papanicolaou smear, should be repeated annually thereafter. Girls should be examined for cancer of the breast and taught to examine their own breasts monthly between menstrual periods for small lumps.

Both boys and girls need information about their reproductive systems, about venereal diseases, and about contraception. Such knowledge does not cause promiscuity; ignorance causes irresponsible sexual behavior. The epidemic of venereal disease and large numbers of teenaged mothers have underscored the need for such sex education. Public schools, parent groups, and church and civic groups are involved in meeting this need.

Accident prevention and safety education are especially important for the adolescent because a large proportion of automobile and water accidents occur during this age period.

Smoking, alcohol, and drugs have become serious threats to the health of adolescents. Laws have been passed to control their use, but these laws have not solved the problem. Group pressure for experimentation, the need to demonstrate independence, natural adolescent emotional conflicts, and ignorance have produced widespread misuse of these drugs. To combat the problem, many innovative programs have been instituted that include education, group and private counseling, and crisis intervention.

Disorders common to adolescents

The following disorders that affect adolescents fall into two general categories, those related to the process of growth and development and those that require long-term care.

Maturation disorders

Acne vulgaris
Postural defects
Fatigue
Anemia
Obesity
Menstrual irregularities
Hyperthyroidism
Neurotic symptoms

Short-term care conditions

Gonorrhea
Overdosages of drugs
Syphilis

Long-term care conditions

Tuberculosis
Scoliosis
Slipped femoral epiphysis
Malignant tumor of the bone
Osteosarcoma
Ewing's tumor
Abnormal sexual development
Juvenile delinquency
Psychoneuroses
Schizophrenic reactions
Substance abuse (drugs, alcohol, and others)

SUMMARY OUTLINE

I. **The young school child (6 to 12 years)**
   A. Characteristics
      1. Physical and motor development
      2. Emotional, intellectual, and social development
   B. Nutrition
   C. Care
   D. Medical supervision
   E. Disorders common to school-aged children
II. **Adolescence (12 to 18 or more years)**
   A. Characteristics
      1. Physical and motor development
      2. Emotional, social, and intellectual development
         a. Personality development
         b. Social development
         c. Intellectual development
   B. Care
      1. Emotional support
      2. Information and guidance
   C. Work, school, and recreation
   D. Nutrition
   E. Medical supervision
   F. Disorders common to adolescents

STUDY QUESTIONS

1. How would you characterize the physical development of the 6 to 12 year old?
2. What important steps in personality development take place during the 6- to 12-year period? The 13- to 18-year period?
3. Discuss the influence of peers, family, and teachers on the adolescent.
4. What can adults do to help adolescents cope with the stresses they experience during this period of life?

REFERENCES

Cronbach, L.J.: Essentials of psychological testing, ed. 3, New York, 1970, Harper & Row, Publishers.

Erikson, E.H.: Childhood and society, New York, 1963, W.W. Norton & Co.

Furth, H.G.: Piaget and knowledge, theoretical foundations, Englewood Cliffs, N.J., 1969, Prentice-Hall, Inc.

Gesell, A.L.: Studies in child development, Westport, Conn., 1972, Greenwood Press, Inc.

Gold, E.R., and Peacock, D.B.: Basic immunology, Baltimore, 1970, The Williams & Wilkins Co.

Goodenough, F.L.: The mental growth of children from two to fourteen years, Westport, Conn., 1970, Greenwood Press, Inc.

Hartlage, L.C., and Lucas, D.: Mental development evaluation of the pediatric patient, Springfield, Ill., 1972, Charles C Thomas, Publisher.

Piaget, J., and Inhelder, B.: The psychology of the child, New York, 1969, Basic Books, Inc., Publishers.

Schwartz, A.: Parent's guide to children's play and recreation, New York, 1965, The Macmillan Co.

Illness, children, and their hospital care

7
Pediatric illness and hospitalization

VOCABULARY

Debilitating
Febrile
Asymptomatic
Morbidity
Perinatal mortality
Separation anxiety
Compromise reaction

In spite of outstanding success in the field of preventive pediatrics, many defects, disorders, and diseases still afflict children. Pediatric nurses need a knowledge of the overall types, treatments, responses, and incidence of these conditions and an understanding of the effects of hospitalization, long-term illness, and impending death on the child and the parents.

PEDIATRIC DISORDERS
Types of disorders

Pediatric disorders are typified by terms that have special significance to those working with children. These terms may indicate the cause of a disorder, give a description, or indicate the course and outcome. Some of the most common types of disorders are described here.

Disorders by cause

Genetic, or inborn, disorders result from chromosomal defects. Some are inherited from the parents, such as cystic fibrosis; others seem to be accidents of cell division, such as Down's syndrome (mongolism).

Developmental disorders result from an interference with the normal process of growth and development both before and after birth. Cerebral palsy and dwarfism are developmental defects.

Infections account for a great many illnesses in children. They may be viral, bacterial, parasitic, amebic, or fungous in origin.

139

Nutritional disorders are those resulting from deficiencies of necessary nutrients or from an inability of the child to use the nutrients eaten. Rickets and scurvy are examples of these types of disorders.

Emotional disturbances result from factors that disrupt the normal psychological development of the child. Neurosis and antisocial behavior are examples of emotional disorders.

Malignancies such as leukemia and Wilms' tumor occur in children. Like malignant tumors in adults, they consume nourishment, interfere with normal organ function, destroy healthy tissue, and spread to other parts of the body.

Accidents such as burns, drowning, and poisoning cause many childhood and adolescent disorders. Because most of these conditions are preventable, they are particularly tragic.

Traumatic conditions are usually accidental, but sometimes they are the result of child abuse, of fighting between youths, or of suicidal self-abuse.

Disorders by description

Congenital anomalies are those abnormalities that are seen at birth, regardless of their cause. They include such conditions as cleft lip and club feet.

Disorders of the newborn are those that occur particularly during the first 4 weeks of life. Prematurity, erythroblastosis fetalis, and hyaline membrane disease are among these disorders.

Childhood diseases, in the broad sense, are all the conditions that affect children. Usually the term refers to the common communicable diseases such as chickenpox, measles, and mumps.

Adolescent disorders are those conditions associated with puberty, such as acne vulgaris, obesity, and menstrual irregularities in girls.

Mild or severe are terms used to describe the extent of symptoms; for example, cerebral palsy might be described in this manner.

Debilitating conditions are those that cause loss of strength. The muscular dystrophies cause progressive or increasing debility.

Febrile or *afebrile* are terms used to indicate the presence or absence of fever.

Asymptomatic stages of certain conditions are periods of time when there are no obvious symptoms, but the disorder is present. Syphilis and epilepsy have such stages.

Disorders by course and outcome

Acute conditions are those that have a rapid onset with severe symptoms but have a relatively short course. Bacterial infections of the nose and throat are typical of this kind of condition. Some long-term conditions such as rheumatic fever have acute stages.

Short-term care conditions are those that require only brief medical or surgical supervision. Acute infection, uncomplicated surgery, or minor emergencies are among this group.

Chronic or long-term care conditions are those that are drawn out over a prolonged period. Leukemia, cerebral palsy, and diabetes are examples of some childhood chronic conditions.

Terminal conditions are those that have so weakened or damaged the body that the child is near death. The final stages of such chronic conditions as leukemia and nephrotic syndrome are described as terminal.

Remissions and exacerbations are periods of time in the course of a disease when symptoms subside (remissions) and when they flare up again (exacerbations).

Treatment

The treatment of pediatric disorders begins by meeting the child's basic physical and psychological needs. Then the many specialized types of treatment are brought in to do battle with the particular disorder. These special therapies include surgical, medical, chemical, psychological, speech, and occupational therapy. They may be used to treat patients in the hospital, called inpatients, or those living at home but coming to the medical center for treatment, called outpatients. The place where treatment is given and the type of treatment used depend on the child's condition, age, and particular needs.

Surgical treatment involves operative procedures for the correction of deformities, repair of injuries, diagnosis and cure of diseases, relief of suffering, and prolongation of life.

Medical treatment involves the large area of nonsurgical treatment, such as treating pyloric stenosis with diet, infections with drugs, and hernias with supports. In some conditions both medical and surgical treatment is used.

Physical therapy involves the use of heat, cold, water, electricity, light, radiation, massage, and exercise to treat various conditions such as arthritis, cerebral palsy, and other types of nerve-damaging or muscle-weakening conditions.

Chemotherapy is the use of chemicals to treat diseases. Chemicals may be antibiotics, hormones, or any one of hundreds of drugs that have been developed to destroy invading organisms, correct deficiencies, or in some way protect the child from illness.

Psychotherapy is the treatment of emotional disturbances by such means as role playing, group therapy and individual counseling.

Occupational therapy is more than training for a vocation. In children it involves the application of physical and motor skills to specific problems of daily living, such as teaching children without arms to use their toes to hold a spoon and feed themselves.

Speech therapy is the process of helping a child overcome speech problems caused by brain damage or emotional or hearing disturbances.

Mortality and morbidity

Statistical information about sickness and death serves an important purpose. It provides a convenient tool for evaluating the health of a specific group of people during a definite period of time. The information can then be compared objectively to conditions during other years or to other groups. Progress, or the lack of it, can be noted and steps can be taken to make improvements.

Statistics are reported in two ways, by total numbers and by rates. For example, the total number of deaths for a population of 600,000 might be 6,000. The rate per 100,000 would be 1,000 deaths.

Morbidity is defined as the number of cases of a specific disease that occur during a given period of time among a definite number of persons of a particular group. For example, there were 393 cases of rheumatic fever reported to the Illinois Department of Public Health during 1966 among the population of 3.6 million persons in Chicago. Rheumatic fever morbidity was thus 10.8 cases per 100,000 population that year.

Mortality is defined as the number of deaths during a given period of time among a definite number of persons of a particular group. This rate is often given as deaths per population of 1,000, 10,000, or 100,000 and reported in the following age groupings: up to 4 years, 5 to 14 years, 15 to 24 years, 25 to 44 years, 45 to 64 years, 65 to 84 years, and 85 or more years.

Fetal mortality means the rate of deaths of fetuses after the twenty-eighth week of gestation and before birth.

Perinatal mortality refers to the rate of infants who die after the twenty-eighth week of gestation up until they are 1 month of age (fetal deaths plus neonatal deaths).

Neonatal mortality refers to the rate of deaths of infants at any time during the first month of life.

Infant mortality refers to the rate of deaths of infants at any time during the first year of life.

Maternal mortality refers to the rate of deaths of women as a direct result of pregnancy. Statistically, these deaths are often compared to live births. For example, in 1966 in Illinois the maternal deaths per live births were 2.8 per 10,000.

HOSPITALIZATION AND ITS EFFECTS

The hospitalized child feels alone, a stranger in an unfamiliar place, subject to painful and frightening experiences, and separated for the most part from mother and family. This aloneness and the apprehension it creates is called *separation anxiety*. It is experienced by all hospitalized persons at all ages to some degree, but is particularly common to children. It is the result of being deprived of certain basic emotional needs as a result of separation from the family unit. If this anxiety is unrelieved for long periods, the infant or child may fail to respond to medical treatment.

General measures to reduce anxiety

Members of the pediatric team have become increasingly aware of the adverse effects of separation on the hospitalized child. They have instituted a variety of measures of which the aim is to prevent or reduce anxiety. Some of these measures are as follows:

1. Programs of introduction to and preparation for hospitalization have been devised that include tours by young children of local pediatric units and illustrative booklets for parents and children in advance of hospitalization (Fig. 7-1).

2. A bed or large chair is provided so that a parent can remain near the child.

3. Playrooms have been established so that convalescent children can have a place to move about outside their bed in a more normal, non-sick environment.

4. Children are allowed their own familiar toy or blanket to give them the security and link with home it provides.

5. Visiting hours have been liberalized to reduce the number of hours that the child must be separated from the family.

6. Parents are encouraged to be present when their child awakens from anesthesia to eliminate the frightening experience of waking up alone in a strange world.

7. A supervised recreational program is becoming part of the regular care for every hospitalized child.

8. All of the family are encouraged to visit, including siblings, unless there are specific contraindications.

Individualized care

In addition to the measures just described to minimize the effects of separation, positive action can be taken to reduce the anxiety of children during their hospitalization. The pediatric nurse should seek to establish a relationship of trust with children and their parents.

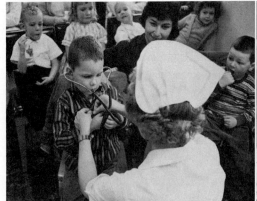 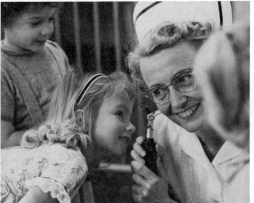

Fig. 7-1. A, A group of preschoolers are fascinated by a stethoscope during their prehospitalization tour. **B,** Instruments such as an ophthalmoscope will not be as frightening to this little girl if she is hospitalized in the future. (Courtesy Children's Hospital of the East Bay, Oakland, Calif.)

Meaning of separation

To the infant. Even though the hospitalized infant may have all physical needs fulfilled, the infant may be seriously deprived of emotional needs. Normally, the infant would be talked to, smiled at, held, and cuddled by family members. If these human contacts are lacking, the infant may develop a condition called "failure to thrive," characterized by listlessness and weight loss. To develop properly, the infant must feel loved and must interact with the loving ones.

To the 1- to 5-year-old child. The effects of separation on the child of this age are also serious. The child is restricted physically to a small crib, may be experiencing painful treatments, does not understand why hospitalization is necessary, and does not understand why the mother is not there. At first the child screams and cries, protesting violently. During this time the nurse only shows a lack of understanding by trying to stop the crying—the child's only way to protest such mistreatment. Gradually the child realizes that the mother is not responding to this crying and despairs of hope that she will return. The child becomes silent, depressed, and preoccupied with sorrow. If mother should return during this time, the child, who feels deeply hurt, might show this by denying that she has come back. Some mothers do not understand this behavior and spend the entire time trying to get the child's direct attention. Her very presence is what was needed most. Then, just when things begin to brighten, the mother leaves again and the cycle of protest, despair, and denial begins again. The mother may be quite distressed and think it would be better if she had never come. The nurse should help her understand that the initial protest of her going and denial of her when she returns are normal expressions of sorrow. The child may have waited all day for her visit, and her presence, especially her physical contact, has reassured the child she really does care.

To the 6- to 12-year-old child. The school-aged child is more accustomed to being away from mother and home than the preschooler. Ill-ness, pain, and weakness may, however, cause the child to regress to babylike ways, clinging to the mother like a 3 year old. Shaming or threatening the child serves no useful purpose; it merely demonstrates a lack of understanding. Sometimes school-aged children fear mutilation and pain but are too frightened to ask questions. The nurse should anticipate these fears and allay them by explaining procedures beforehand and by listening to remarks that might indicate a fear of nameless terrors.

To the adolescent. The adolescent may be more concerned about separation from friends, sports, and school activities than from the parents. The adolescent may worry about the expense of hospitalization, especially if it was caused by personal negligence, and may become depressed, lonely, and feel guilty and rejected. The nurse can encourage the adolescent to talk about interests and goals, can point out even small steps toward recovery, and can help find satisfactory means to cope with frustration.

Mechanisms for adjusting to anxiety

Although there are many undesirable and antisocial ways to react to frustration, there are a number of satisfactory mechanisms that can be used to handle the anxiety it causes. Because all these behavioral mechanisms are, as implied by the word, mechanisms, they should not be overused or misused to avoid all tension. Some tension serves a useful purpose because it motivates persons to become creative and productive.

The nurse can make use of at least three mechanisms to help the child cope with hospital separation. They are controlled aggression, withdrawal, and compromise.

Controlled aggression can be effectively used by the child to act out frustration and anger in such activities as pounding a peg board or playing with dolls. Older children can use the same mechanism by reading stories of wrongs made right.

Withdrawal from the real world of separation

and loneliness may be another means for the child to cope with anxiety. The child may act out happy fantasies in play and may settle into a small rocking chair and for a time enjoy the memory of being held and rocked in mother's arms. An older child may try to forget loneliness by reading or by active play.

There are a number of *compromise reactions* that the child can use to relieve anxiety, such as finding an alternative to the mother's presence in a nurse-substitute. An older child may compensate for feelings of defeat and rejection by seeking the approval of the hospital staff and may be especially brave or helpful. The school-aged child may project feelings of need for the mother onto some other lonely child and may become the "mother comforter." The child may relieve anxiety by identifying with the doctors and nurses and "join the team." The younger child can do this by being a "helper." The older child may do this by learning all about the disease; as a result, the advancing stages do not come as surprises and the child thus gains some control over it. Children (and adults) with serious long-term conditions frequently become almost authorities on their own disease as a result of this compromise reaction.

CHILDREN WITH LONG-TERM ILLNESSES

Happily, for most children, periods of illness are brief. Even if children must be hospitalized for a few days, their recovery is quick and neither they nor their family's lives are greatly disrupted. Unfortunately, some children have serious long-term conditions that require months and sometimes years of prolonged medical and, or surgical treatment. These children require special help if they are to develop physically, emotionally, socially, and intellectually. The pediatric nurse should understand the aim of care for these children, the principles that should guide that care, and the specific concerns related to implementing the aim and principles.

Aim of care

The aim toward which the care a child with a long-term condition is directed is twofold: to meet the special medical needs of the child, and to foster maximum growth and development of the child at as nearly a normal rate as possible.

Guiding principles

The guiding principles for care are as follows: (1) care should be individualized to meet the unique needs of the child because the medical problem, prognosis, age, sex, stage of development, and home environment are different for every child; (2) care should be family centered, with consideration of the total home environment, relationships with parents, other children or relatives, financial resources, and the actual house in which the family lives; and (3) care should involve maximum use of all the community resources available to meet the child's medical, educational, recreational, financial, and social needs.

Specific concerns

In caring for the child with a long-term illness the pediatric team is particularly concerned that the medical, physical, emotional, social, and intellectual needs of the child be met whether at home or in the hospital.

Medical care. The medical care of the long-term pediatric patient is of the utmost importance. Without it there is little hope for improvement, and the child's condition may deteriorate. For this reason medical orders for medications, treatments, exercises, or tests must be conscientiously carried out. In the hospital setting, with an experienced pediatric staff, medical procedures are performed with ease in an environment planned for medical care. In the home, however, the mother may be the only one to care for the sick child, and on a 24-hour basis. Space may be limited and facilities poor. In addition, other family members must share the space and mother's time. In such a situation the mother needs help in planning and in adapting procedures and treatments to the home. Public health nurses are especially trained to give just this help. They go to the home and work with the child, the family, and the medical team to ensure that the highest level of care is achieved.

Medical care, regardless of where it is given, should be adapted to the individual child with consideration for age, stage of development, personality, and need for safety precautions. For example, an injection of the same antibiotic drug might be ordered for two children, one 14 months old, the other 14 years old. Because of the age difference, preparation of the child, amount of restraint needed, dosage of the drug, and even site of injection may be different. Every area of medical care for children must be similarly adjusted to the individual needs of the child.

Medical treatment and hospitalization are extremely expensive. Many families have been impoverished as a result of the prolonged illness of one of their children. To help meet this need, a variety of local, state, and national funds have been established and are available, but families may not be aware of these resources. The nurse may be the one to whom the parents voice their concern. They should be referred to the supervisor, who will send them to the appropriate person in the hospital. Some institutions employ medical social workers who are prepared to assist families with financial arrangements.

Physical care. Meeting the physical needs of the child is closely related to meeting the medical needs. Pediatric nurses are concerned with nourishment, elimination, body cleanliness, dental hygiene, exercise, rest, and safety of the hospitalized child—particularly the one who is hospitalized for long periods of time. Their care is directed toward promoting good health habits and toward encouraging the child to assume maximum responsibility for personal needs. Chapter 8 is devoted to a discussion of this important aspect of hospital care.

Emotional and social development. The normal, healthy child has many problems associated with social and emotional development. These problems are multiplied for the child with prolonged illness. This becomes obvious when one considers the progressive steps toward maturity the child usually takes. The child learns to trust, to use an independent will, to develop initiative, industriously to accomplish goals, to discover individual identity, and finally, to love another person. For the weak child or the one isolated in a hospital bed or confined at home, these steps are extremely difficult to take, for they require the simultaneous development of the mind, body and emotions. It is not surprising, then, to find that children with long-term illnesses are frequently retarded in their emotional and social development. In some cases they actually regress, or go backward, during acute stages in their disorders. For children to progress toward maturity they must have their basic emotional needs fulfilled and have an opportunity to develop socially with others the same age.

Emotional needs during prolonged illness. The basic emotional needs of the child are for love, security, acceptance as an individual, independence, and order and control. These needs are discussed in greater detail in Chapter 2. Their application to children with prolonged illness is of special concern to the pediatric nurse.

An extra portion of love and security is needed by children with long-term illnesses and should be supplied at every opportunity. It is essential to the development of a sense of trust. Whenever it is possible, younger children should be held and cuddled. Older children may want to hold the nurse's hand, especially during painful or frightening treatments. A sense of security and continuity can be supplied if the same nurse is assigned to care for a child on several successive days. Something of the importance of this can be understood when the child says, "I won't cry if *my* nurse is with me." Nurses, however, must guard against becoming possessive of the child and using the relationship to meet their own emotional needs instead of those of the child. They must also guard against allowing their familiarity with the child to dull their capacity to make keen observations about the child's changing condition.

Acceptance as an individual can be demonstrated when nurses show that they really understand the child's problem and accept and respect the child as an individual. Ill children may not have much self-respect. They are weak, sometimes deformed or disfigured, and may feel they are a burden to the family. The nurse must find ways to build up the child's self-confidence by not scolding for crying or appearing shocked by angry outbursts. Embarrassing situations must be avoided. Adolescents are particularly self-conscious about being exposed, either physically or emotionally. For this reason care should be taken to respect their privacy. If a painful treatment must be done, the youth should be allowed the courtesy of a private room where peers cannot hear any cries. The nurse should look for ways to build the child's self-esteem and give recognition for real achievement. The child is not fooled by false praise, only mocked. Little accomplishments for effort or unselfishness can be noted and recognized. In all these ways the nurse lets the child feel valuable and worthy of attention and respect, and not like just another bed number.

For the nurse, finding ways to help the sick child develop independence is difficult. There are some means, however, that can provide the child with independence. The choice of toys, clothes, reading matter, arrangement of items on a side-table, and other small but significant matters can be the child's alone. Whenever possible, activities of daily living such as personal hygiene, eating, and elimination should be given to the child as a personal responsibility. In some cases, even treatment of a disorder can be assumed, in part, by the child: for example, the diabetic child who learns to administer insulin unassisted. Responsible independence builds

self-respect, good emotional health, and a sense of autonomy, initiative, and industry.

The child's basic need to learn respect for authority is greatly complicated by prolonged illness. Often these children become domineering, rude, selfish, frustrated by their restricted life, and hostile to everyone about them. A behavior modification treatment plan may be instituted to reward acceptable and curb unacceptable behavior. Whether they are sick or well, the purpose of all discipline is to teach children self-control and respect for the rights of others.

Social needs during prolonged illness. In recent years there has been an increasing awareness of the social needs of the long-term hospitalized child. A number of creative means have been devised to meet this need.

In some hospitals the pediatric ward is divided into units according to childrens' ages. Adolescents have their own "teen wing," younger children have their areas, and infants theirs. This division according to age allows children to develop socially with one another even though they may be confined to the hospital for long periods. It prevents some of the isolation and loneliness that might otherwise occur. In these age-grouped units, common playrooms and recreation areas are provided where the children can move about freely and play with each other. Play materials and equipment in each unit are appropriate to the age of the children who use the unit. (See Table 2-3 for play interest and materials.) There might be a television, record player, game table, and conversation-grouped furniture in the teen unit; crafts, juvenile books, and games might be in the unit for school-aged children; dolls, cars, picture books, and a playhouse may be in the toddler and preschool unit; and adult-sized rocking chairs and playpens may be in the infant unit.

In some hospitals a professional staff of recreation and occupational therapists work out a play and recreation program for every child. This is done in accordance with the child's medical, physical, emotional, and mental capabilities (Fig. 7-2).

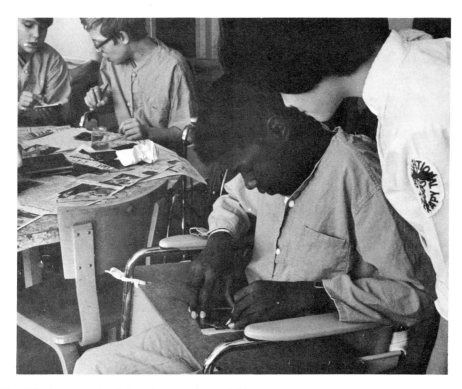

Fig. 7-2. An occupational therapist supervises activities appropriate to the age, interests, and needs of these school-aged boys. (Courtesy Children's Hospital of the East Bay, Oakland, Calif.)

In some regions there are convalescent hospitals devoted exclusively to the care of children with long-term conditions. In these facilities the children do not feel different from others or hopelessly odd; the atmosphere is more relaxed and homelike; and the whole orientation of the staff is toward rehabilitation. Some facilities are really special schools for children with physical handicaps rather than being special hospitals. Such facilities are the schools for deaf, sightless, or otherwise handicapped children. In other areas these physically impaired but healthy children are integrated into the regular public school programs where nonhandicapped children learn to accept their disabilities and include them in the social group.

Intellectual development. The people of the United States have endorsed the objective that all children should be given the opportunity to develop their intellectual capacity to the fullest extent. To this end taxpayers have assumed the responsibility of providing free public education for every child, regardless of race, religion, economic status, or handicap. To achieve this high goal, a variety of educational approaches are being used, including tutoring of hospitalized and home-bound children and using special schools and specialized programs within regular day schools. No child need be deprived of an education regardless of the problem, yet many are deprived because of lack of information or concern on the part of those who care for them.

Nurses are in a unique position to see that the intellectual development of hospitalized children is not neglected. They may be the first to note that the child has become bored or worried about loss of time in school. Parents, too, may voice their concern. As soon as the doctor indicates that the child is physically strong enough to undertake studies, necessary applications should be made so that an educational program may be tailored to the needs of the child.

Even after educational arrangements have been made, the child needs the same continued support and encouragement as at home. The nurse can provide much of this in daily contact by helping the child fix and keep a study time, discussing subjects the child is studying, and showing interest and offering congratulations for successes. In this way nurses reinforce their own efforts toward helping the child mature in every aspect of life.

CHILDREN WITH TERMINAL ILLNESSES

Death is filled with deep meaning and emotion. Few nursing assignments are more challenging than caring for a dying child and grieving parents. If nurses are to meet this challenge effectively, they must examine their own feelings about death and seek to understand its meaning. With this information the nurse will be better equipped to handle their own emotions and to give children and their parents the reassurance and support they need during the ordeal of a terminal illness.

Meaning of death

Death, by definition, is the cessation of life, but its meaning varies greatly from person to person. Those with spiritual faith believe that the nonphysical part (psyche or soul) of humans does not cease to exist when the physical body dies. Other persons believe that the physical and nonphysical parts are inseparable and that when one part dies, so also does the whole. Children grasp the significance of death with varying degrees of comprehension.

Meaning of death for the child. The meaning of death for a child is affected by age, intellectual development, and the concepts of death gathered from reading and the family's teaching.

The infant. The infant's world is small and self-centered. Because the infant has no understanding of time or of relationships between people and very little understanding of what separation means, death has no meaning at all to the infant.

The preschool child. The preschool child lives primarily in the "now." The attention span is brief, and the concept of time is limited. Each separation from the parents is a deprivation of love-support and so is like a death. One sees symptoms not unlike those of a grieving adult in a child experiencing separation anxiety. To the young preschool child there is no difference between separations, temporary or permanent; they are all painful. The concept of death as a permanent separation is not understood. As the child gets older and gains experience, the child finds that parents leave but they always return. Then the child learns that they return after a short time or a long time. When the concept of time has developed sufficiently, the child can understand the idea that some things come to an end whereas others do not. Then the child can understand that death is a permanent separation.

Because of a limited understanding of the consequences of death, the preschool child may take quite literally explanations of death regarding familiar persons who have died. When told that grandmother went to heaven the child may express a desire to go there, too. Death is thought of as a trip and heaven as a vacation place. Parents should not become alarmed but should realize that this is the child's interpretation of their words. It is not a suicide wish.

The young school child. By the age of 6 to 9 years, children are able to understand death as a permanent separation, but they do not think of it as an inevitable result of impersonal causes such as diseases or accidents. They think of death as the result of some personal act such as occurs when they play games like cops and robbers.

And, like that of the game, their feeling is that when it is over everyone should be able to get up and go home. If a loved one such as the mother should die, the child of this age feels that some person is responsible and that person could reverse the death. The child may even wonder if mother has not willfully left because she refuses to return.

Because a child of this age thinks of death as a kind of play acting, the child cannot conceive of being permanently dead. Even if the child talks of death, it is a temporary state from which one could recover at will.

Death, then, to the younger child with a fatal illness is not a frightening reality. It is an idea with only hazy outlines. For this reason the younger child does not need a formal pronouncement regarding life expectancy. The sick child accepts increasing restrictions and attention given as the disease progresses. The child is more troubled by the painful treatments, tests, and examinations, by separation from the mother, and by isolation from other children than by impending death. The nurses should do whatever they can to relieve the real problems that make the child's last days so difficult.

The older school child. After the age of 9 years the child is able to understand the idea of not being. The child is able to understand that death is a permanent separation, but is usually comforted by the belief that it is far off. Children between the ages of 9 and 12 years may be terrified if their mother becomes ill because they realize the permanence of death. Sometimes children of this age actually fantasize what it would be like to be orphaned, reveling in the thought of a heroic Peter Pan existence. If they think of themselves as dying, this, too, is idealized into some kind of comforting idea about returning to their families in a spiritual form.

The adolescent. The adolescent understands that death is a permanent separation from this familiar life, and also understands that it is caused by impersonal things such as auto acci-dents and cancer. The adolescent may take very literally religious teaching concerning an all-powerful God who plans and directs life and death. When unable gladly to accept such a ver-dict, the adolescent feels guilty for questioning God's wisdom. Although nurses should not im-pose their personal religious beliefs on the youth, neither should they ignore the need to find satisfactory answers to these philosophical questions.

Meaning of death for the parents. One of the most important parts nurses play in the care of a child with a terminal illness is in offering support to the grieving parents. By their words and deeds as they daily interact with parents, the nurses convey their understanding of the parents' grief and do what they can to help them cope with it.

The death of a child is a tearing, bitter experi-ence. For parents it is the opposite of their nor-mal expectation for a healthy growing child. Yet they are forced by circumstances to face this most painful reality. The gradual resignation of the parents to the death of a child is called the *process of mourning.* It follows a predictable pattern, much like the separation anxiety experi-enced by a child who is deprived of a parent, but it is more profound. When a child is killed ac-cidentally or dies from sudden illness, the period of mourning for the parents begins with the child's death. If, however, the child has a pro-longed fatal illness, the process of mourning may begin before death, during the terminal stages of the disease.

Mourning is divided by some observers into three phases—a time of protest, a time of despair and disorganization, and a time of rebuilding of hope.

Protest. The protest phase of mourning begins when the parents first take seriously the possi-bility that the child's condition is fatal. Parents may respond to this threat by denying it exists, by consulting another doctor, having more tests, or traveling to a different climate. They may become hostile, anxious, and critical of medical personnel and institutions. They may blame themselves and experience loss of appetite, feelings of emptiness, and sorrow. All these responses are natural ways to express grief and a normal part of the protest stage of mourning.

Parents should be allowed to express fears, to wonder whether they are guilty, to weep, and to seek all possible help. Nurses can provide support by listening to expressions of grief and dismay and by assuring the parents that they understand and share their concern.

The parents are greatly helped at this stage if they can become involved in the physical care of the child. They can bathe, feed, entertain, and go with the child to the x-ray department or to the laboratory. This effort helps them feel that they have done all they can for their child. They should be encouraged not to neglect their other children at home but to divide their time between them. The parents should take turns in this sharing.

As the parents participate in the child's care, they become integrated into the life of the ward and begin to trust the personnel and to communicate their feelings. This communication provides a means for the parents to share their heavy burden of sorrow. At first they only demonstrate concern for their own child but gradually begin to show interest in other children in the ward. When the parents do so, they demonstrate an increasing acceptance of the child's illness and ultimate death.

Despair and disorganization. During the phase of despair and disorganization the parents are floundering about emotionally. They may have periods of great discouragement and hostility. They may lash out at the nursing staff or the doctors and later give them exaggerated praise and sentimental appreciation. During this period their hope is less general and more specifically directed toward some scientific breakthrough by which their child will be cured. They recognize that only a miracle could save their child now,

whose general resistance is now failing.

In this stressful time the nursing staff must keep the behavior of parents in perspective. They should remain sympathetic and concerned, realizing the intensity of the parents' sorrow and the nature of their despair. The nurses can help the parents by encouraging them to talk about their child while they are away from the child's immediate presence. They can help the parents identify specific things they can still do for the child. During this period it is important that the parents see their continuing value to the child in spite of their feelings of helplessness.

As the child grows weaker, the parents' concern is diverted more toward relieving symptoms than toward overall cure. Thus, the parents are gradually accepting the inevitable course of the disease and are emotionally separating themselves from their child.

Hope and rebuilding. In the final stages, when the child is ravaged by the disease and its treatment, the parents' attitude gradually changes to one of calm resignation. They are able to place the needs of the ill child in perspective and consider the total needs of the family. For the first time they express the wish that the child would die to relieve the suffering. In effect, they give up the fight and recognize that the disease has won the battle for the child's life and that the child would be better off dead.

In long, debilitating conditions parents are more likely to reach the third phase of mourning during the child's illness, but many do not. There may be many days and weeks of numbness and loneliness after the child's death. During this time parents should be encouraged to talk about the lost child, to experience the loss, and finally, to let it go. This process of going back again and again and experiencing the loss is called "grief work." It seems to be a necessary step toward healing. When the loss is finally acknowledged and the depths of sorrow plumbed, the parents are able to reach out to others and to new interests and new activities.

The length of time involved in this third phase varies with the person and may take a year or more. When the parents are able objectively to look back on the lost relationship and realistically remember its joys and disappointments, the process of mourning is complete.

Meaning of death for the nurse. If nurses are to give the dying child and the parents the kind of sensitive, supportive care they need, they must arrive at a degree of understanding and control of their own feelings toward death. They can do this more objectively by considering death and its implications during a time when they are not faced with the crisis of a terminal patient.

Humans have made great strides toward extending life. They have developed vaccines and antibodies, invented surgical procedures, and transplanted major organs. They have devised safety programs and written peace treaties. Yet despite all these efforts, death is the ultimate conqueror, the one sure fate awaiting every living creature. Because humans find death (a state of not being alive) so difficult to comprehend they have used a variety of mechanisms for dealing with its mystery. Some invest death with importance by building great monuments to its victims. Some deny it, pushing all thoughts of death out of their consciousness and withdrawing from its presence. Others claim to have "conquered" it by explaining death as the portal to a superior spirit life. Some people react to death in a mass venting of emotions. Responses depend on personality, cultural, and religious training.

Nurses are not exempt from the fear and puzzlement of death. They are no less human because they are nurses. They fear and feel. Nurses need to recognize these strong emotions, gain some kind of control over them, and courageously go about their nursing duties with the welfare of the child and the parents foremost in their minds. Such courage is not a denial of feelings; it is the purposeful application of the will to act in spite of feelings. Nurses may feel strongly, but they must also function effectively.

Nursing the dying child

The goal of nursing the dying child is to make the last days more comfortable, both physically and psychologically, by relieving as much pain and anxiety as possible. Sometimes the child is greatly helped by the transference of attention away from the incurable disease to some specific curable problem, such as an upper respiratory infection. By directing attention toward treating the infection, the child is somehow distracted from the hopeless struggle against a major disease and is encouraged and reassured when able to "get well" from a minor one.

There are many painful treatments and tests that the dying child may undergo in the desperate effort to retard the advancing disease. The presence of a well-known nurse or the parents, may make these experiences more bearable for the weary child.

In addition to physical care and medical treatments, nurses must do all they can to provide the dying child with the psychological support needed. Such support includes, of course, supplying love and security and as many other basic emotional needs as possible. To this end parents should be allowed unlimited visiting privileges.

The dying child wishing to talk of sickness and death, should be allowed to do so. If the child wishes to pretend, to bargain, or to avoid, that should also be allowed. It does not help the child to answer despair with your own false hopes. But you should keep the child talking, maybe asking questions in response to questions, showing your genuine concern.

Religious faith is a source of comfort and strength to those who possess it, to the nurse, and to the dying child, and to the child's family. It is the responsibility of the nursing staff to consider the spiritual needs of families. Roman Catholics and most Protestants believe in a life after death and expect to see their loved ones again at a future time and throughout eternity. Prayers, readings, and administration of the Sacrament of the Sick by a priest for the dying person are comforting and important to the Catholic. Protestants appreciate the ministry of their own pastor with prayers and scripture readings. Those of the Jewish faith usually have a strong and comforting sense of family, especially in a time of crisis. The rabbi of their own congregation can bring a unique blessing at such a time.

When a child is in the terminal stages of an illness, it is difficult to provide privacy in a ward with many beds. Some hospitals move patients with terminal illnesses into a private room near the nurses' station. It is not long before the older children realize that anyone who goes into that room never returns. To avoid this problem, some of the newer pediatric facilities are arranged so that sufficient privacy and quiet are provided for each nursing unit so that when a child becomes critically ill there is no need to be moved to another place. If the child dies, the body can be removed at nap time or during the night.

There is growing recognition of the comfort dying persons obtain from being in their own home, surrounded by their own family. As a result, many physicians encourage families to take their terminally ill children to spend their last days in the security and love of their home.

SUMMARY OUTLINE

I. **Pediatric disorders**
  A. Types of disorders
    1. Disorders by cause
    2. Disorders by description
    3. Disorders by course and outcome
  B. Treatment
  C. Mortality and morbidity
II. **Hospitalization and its effects**
  A. General measures to reduce anxiety
  B. Individualized care
    1. Meaning of separation
      a. To the infant
      b. To the 1- to 5-year-old child
      c. To the 6- to 12-year-old child
      d. To the adolescent
    2. Mechanisms for adusting to anxiety

III. **Children with long-term illnesses**
  A. Aim of care
  B. Guiding principles
  C. Specific concerns
    1. Medical care
    2. Physical care
    3. Emotional and social development
      a. Emotional needs during prolonged illness
      b. Social needs during prolonged illness
    4. Intellectual development
IV. **Children with terminal illnesses**
  A. Meaning of death
    1. Meaning of death for the child
      a. The infant
      b. The preschool child
      c. The young school
      d. The older school child
      e. The adolescent
    2. Meaning of death for the parents
      a. Protest
      b. Despair and disorganization
      c. Hope and rebuilding
    3. Meaning of death for the nurse
  B. Nursing the dying child

STUDY QUESTION

1. Define and give an example of each of the types of pediatric disorders. Describe the type of treatment for various pediatric disorders.
2. Define mortality and morbidity.
3. What is separation anxiety? What does separation mean to the infant, young child, older child, and adolescent? What three mechanisms can the nurse use to help the child cope with anxiety?
4. What are the aims and guiding principles of care of the child with long-term illnesses? How would you implement these for a child with muscular dystrophy? diabetes?
5. Discuss the meaning of death to children of various ages from infancy to adolescence to parents, and to the nurse.
6. Discuss the "process of mourning," giving the three stages stages described in this chapter.

REFERENCES

Kubler-Ross, E.: On death and dying, New York, 1969, Macmillan, Inc.

Sahler, O.J.Z., editor: The child and death, St. Louis, 1978, The C.V. Mosby Co.

8
Hospital care of the child

VOCABULARY

Nursing process
Pathogen
Strict isolation
Apical pulse
Full liquid diet
Range of motion
Symptomatic treatment

When children become ill or have some disorder too serious to be treated at home, they are taken to the hospital, where the chief concern is to provide them with the quality of care that will allow them to recover maximum health in minimum time and to return to their homes and families. To that end nurses apply their knowledge of normal growth and development and specific disease conditions, together with an understanding of the pediatric unit and the hospital policies and practices that make it function.

THE PEDIATRIC UNIT

The pediatric hospital or pediatric unit within a general hospital is designed to meet the needs of children and their parents. It is staffed by a team of dedicated pediatric specialists.

The physical plant

Although there are many architectural plans for pediatric units, each one seeks to meet the needs of the children and the parents whom it serves. These needs have been identified as the need for psychological support, physical comfort and safety, and medical treatment and care.

Psychological support. The child needs cheerful, homelike surroundings with an opportunity to be near others the same age. In Chapter 7 various means of supplying the emotional, social, and intellectual needs of children hospitalized for long periods of time are discussed more fully. One of the means suggested is the design of the pediatric unit into age-grouped divisions, each with its own recreational area. Some of the newer hospitals use this plan.

Parents also need a cheery setting. If they are rested and relaxed, their anxiety will be lessened. Easy chairs should be near the bed so that parents may hold their child while caressing or reading to the child. Some hospitals have private rooms equipped with a cot or a bed for the parents. These rooms are reserved for the parents of especially ill children who need continuous care. If there is a positive parent-nurse-child relation, parents can be a great help, for there are some forms of care that only parents can give.

Physical comfort and safety. Furnishings in a pediatric unit are in children's sizes. In the nursery area, except for the adult-sized rocking chairs, there are small bassinets, cribs, playpens, potty chairs, and high chairs. Older children have larger beds and equipment. In the recreation areas, toys and furniture are appropriate to the age of the children who will use them.

Safety is a constant concern. Every area of the pediatric unit should be visible from many vantage points. Floors should be easily cleaned and kept free of anything that would cause falls. Electrical outlets should be covered when not in use; windows should be screened or permanently closed, fireproof materials should be used in construction, and gates and doors safely locked from little hands and easily unlocked by adults. Any broken item should be repaired at once, including crib slats, toys, high chairs, and medical equipment. Medicine and cleaning-supply closets and treatment rooms should be locked. Communicable disease areas should be completely separate from the "clean" areas. Children should have a place to play away from the halls and busy treatment areas. Every adult in the pediatric unit should feel personally responsible to keep a vigil for potential dangers.

Medical treatment and care. The child is hospitalized because of a need for special medical care otherwise not available. Pediatric units are designed to allow for this care. Isolation areas are provided for children with communi-

cable disease; emergency equipment is kept in running order; laboratory and x-ray departments are nearby to provide special diagnostic services; surgery departments and physical and occupational therapy departments are at hand to give specialized care. A nursing staff of specially prepared persons is provided on a 24-hour basis.

The pediatric team

A team is a group of persons working together for a common goal. Pediatrics has been an area that has developed a number of special roles within its "team," including the pediatric doctor, pediatric nurse practitioner, registered and licensed nurses, and pediatric aides. Other professionals join the team when their expertise is needed.

Of all the team members, pediatric nurses and aides are the ones most continuously in the presence of the child. Nurses receive the child from the anxious parents, carry out medical prescriptions for treatment, feed, bathe, clothe, comfort, observe the child, and report on progress. Pediatric nurses are not mother substitutes but they are the providers of expert care both day and night until the child returns to home and family.

To carry out so many duties, pediatric nurses, whether registered, licensed, or aides, must have special aptitudes and talents. They must have acquired competence to perform a great variety of nursing procedures with skill and efficiency and to understand the theory behind them. They must be alert, keen observers of subtle changes in signs and symptoms and be aware of the relative significance of these changes to the welfare of the child. Their awareness, however, cannot be limited to a single child but must include the many children committed to the care of the entire staff. Finally, they must be warm, caring human beings who like moms and dads as well as children. This special combination of expertise, energy, and compassion is a pediatric nurse. Their level of education and the degree of responsibility they assume on the pediatric unit determine the role they play on the nursing team.

Nurse-child-parent relationship

The relationship between nurses and parents greatly affects the child who is the reason for the relationship. If there is hostility and suspicion, the child will be affected. If there is mutual respect and trust, the child will feel more secure and loved.

Because the parents are under great stress, the task of establishing a positive relationship with the parents rests with the nurses (Fig. 8-1). If they think of themselves as godlike dispensers of all wisdom about child care, they will not be successful. Such a concept (once believed, but never true) is no longer acceptable. The role of modern pediatric nurses is that of specialists in the care and cure of ill children. They are not parent substitutes; they are parent helpers. They realize that the parents are specialists in the care of their own particular child and that they can learn much from parents about the child's personality and individual needs. When the nurses show respect for the parents, parents will be able to respect the judgment of the nurses.

In practice, this means that the nurse will welcome the parents at the bedside, will ask about the child's customary patterns of living, and will allow the parents to take over some of the important mothering tasks such as cuddling and feeding. If the parents show signs of fatigue and strain, they should be encouraged to rest and be assured that their child will not be neglected.

Nursing care organization

In pediatric units nursing duties are divided among the available personnel in a variety of ways including the individual, primary, functional, and team plans, or a modification of all four. Student nurses must learn to function within all of these plans and so must work closely with their instructor in understanding their particular role in any given situation.

When the *individual plan* is used, nurses are responsible for the total care of one or more children under the direction of a head nurse. They make assessments and concern themselves with the individual child's safety, hygiene, medications, nutrition, treatments, and records. The practical-vocational nurse may be assigned the individual care of children with stable conditions or those requiring uncomplicated care. This plan is frequently used for students, so that they might gain an understanding of the child's total needs.

Primary nursing is an extension of the individual plan. Each child is assigned to an individual nurse from admission to discharge. That nurse assesses the child's needs and designs and keeps current the nursing care plan, coordinates its implementation, and evaluates its effectiveness. The nurse is responsible for the child's care 24 hours a day, but delegates it to associates when not on duty. The nurse serves as the patient's advocate and the central source of information about the child for the physician, parents, and staff. In this system, a specially-prepared nurse serves as the primary care person. Practical-vocational nurses usually serve as associate nurses working closely with the primary nurse.

In the *functional plan*, various areas of nursing care are divided among the staff members according to the task rather than the patient. In this plan one nurse might be assigned to give all the medication to all the children, another might do all the treatments, and others give the hygienic care. The most complex tasks are usually assigned to the registered nurses and the least complex to the nursing attendants. This method separates the act from the acted on in such a way that continuity of care and close observation often suffer. It places extraordinary burdens of responsibility on one or two nurses and may not make full use of the abilities and skills of others.

In *team nursing*, there is a supervising or head nurse who is responsible to the hospital and to the doctor for the nursing care of all the children. The head nurse delegates responsibility to the leaders of nursing teams. At the beginning of each shift the team leaders receive a report from the former team leaders and then meet with their team and delegate specific nursing responsibilities to each member. The special problems,

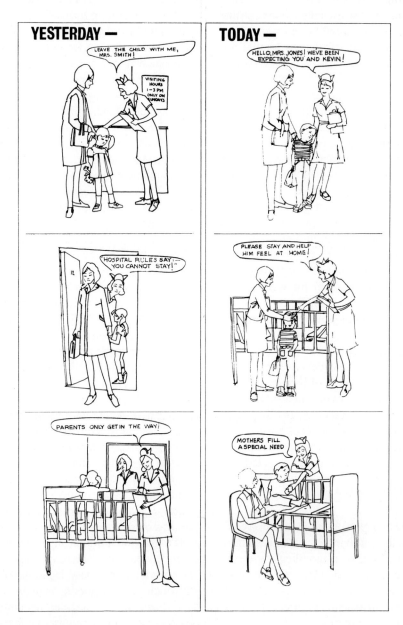

Fig. 8-1. The nurse-child-parent relationship has changed from one of suspicion and fear to mutual respect and trust.

needs, and concerns of each child are discussed and nursing goals are established. The team members then carry out their designated duties in continuous consultation with their team leader, reporting any changes that appear in each child's condition. The team leader is responsible for making written records and giving oral reports to the pediatric supervisor, who in turn reports to the hospital's director of nursing service, to the specific doctors of the patients, and to the nursing staff who follow on the next shift. This plan is a modification of the functional plan. It makes better use of personnel, but provides less continuity from shift to shift.

THE NURSING PROCESS

A *process* is a systematic series of actions directed to some end. The *nursing process* is the scientific method of problem solving applied to patient care. It consists of a series of actions used to deliver nursing care, including assessing the patient's status, planning appropriate nursing actions, implementing those actions, and evaluating their effects. The written document that describes the plan of care is called a *nursing care plan*. It must be changed continuously to reflect changes in the patient's needs.

Assessment

Assessment includes collecting data and making a nursing diagnosis. For example, a child is fretful, has pink, hot skin, a pulse of 118 beats per minute, a temperature of 103° F (39.4° C), an inflamed throat, and a medical diagnosis of streptococcal pharyngitis. The nursing diagnosis is "fever related to the medical diagnosis of streptococcal pharyngitis, as manifested by fretfulness, flushed skin, rapid pulse, elevated temperature, and streptococci cultured from a throat swab."

Planning

Planning nursing care is identifying a goal of care and developing a guide for actions to achieve that goal. For example, the goal of care

of the feverish child is to reduce the fever. Nursing actions, called interventions, are planned to accomplish that goal, such as giving the child a tepid sponge bath, increasing the fluid intake, and administering prescribed antibiotic medications.

Implementation

Implementation of the nursing care plan is carrying out planned nursing actions. In the case of the feverish child, implementation includes giving the sponge bath, offering juices or soda, and injecting the correct dose of antibiotic as prescribed.

Evaluation

Evaluation is judging how effective the nursing actions were in achieving the goal of care. For example, the temperature of the feverish child is measured after the sponge bath and it is 101° F (38.4° C). After 12 hours the temperature has gone down to 99° F (37.2° C). The evaluation is that the interventions were effective. If they were not effective, then the nursing care plan would need to be adjusted.

Responsibility for the nursing process

Responsibility for the total nursing process is that of the registered nurses. They must see that all steps of the nursing process are carried out for every patient entrusted to their care. They may, however, delegate elements of the nursing process to other members of the health team, such as ward clerks, nursing assistants, and practical-vocational nurses. For example, assessment data such as the temperature and pulse of the feverish child may be collected by a nursing assistant and recorded on the graph in the child's record by a ward clerk. Implementation of nursing actions such as giving a sponge bath or administering antibiotic medications may be carried out by licensed practical-vocational nurses acting within the legal boundaries of their license. This clear assignment of responsibility to registered nurses for the total nursing process has been made by the Joint Commission on Accreditation of Hospitals.*

ISOLATION TECHNIQUE

A high percentage of hospitalized children have infections or are especially susceptible to infection. The purpose of the isolation technique is to prevent the spread of infection from one person to another. To a large extent nurses are responsible for carrying out isolation technique. Therefore, they need to understand the terminology, concepts of the infection chain, categories of isolation, nursing roles in controlling infection, principles and practice of isolation technique, and its effect on parents and children.

Terminology

antiseptic a chemical substance used to retard or prevent the growth of microorganisms but not necessarily to destroy them

asepsis the absence of microorganisms; sterile

carriers persons who harbor disease-producing organisms but show no signs of the disease

clean a state of being free of gross contamination and filth, but not necessarily of all microorganisms

communicable or contagious diseases disorders caused by organisms or their toxins which can be passed directly from person to person, or animal to person

contaminated the soiling of an object, person, or air with disease-producing organisms or radiated particles

dirty a state of being contaminated with disease-producing organisms or radiated particles

disinfectant chemicals or physical forces, such as light rays, that destroy microorganisms and other living cells

medical asepsis, isolation, or barrier technique the procedure for maintaining separation between infectious and susceptible persons

nosocomial infections infections acquired in the hospital

pathogens disease-producing organisms

---

*Joint Commission on Accreditation of Hospitals: Accreditation Manual for Hospitals, Chicago, 1981, The Commission.

sepsis the presence of pathogens or their toxins

surgical asepsis strict sterile technique used when surgical procedures are performed

virulence the relative ability of a pathogen to cause infection

Infection chain

Infections are caused by living organisms that have life cycles of growth, reproduction, and spread. When a link in the chain is broken, the life cycle is interrupted and the infection is stopped. The links in the infection chain are the (1) infectious organism, (2) reservoir of infection, (3) portal of exit, (4) transmission means, (5) portal of entry, and (6) susceptible hosts. When a link in this chain is broken, the spread of infection stops. Nurses work to break the chain of infection and keep it from being rejoined.

Infectious organisms. Infectious organisms must be present to cause an infection. These pathogens may be bacteria, fungi, or viruses. Their virulence is measured by their ability to produce toxins and to invade tissue. They possess many characteristics to overcome the defenses of their hosts and protect themselves from destruction. Some organisms are encased in a protective covering. Some secrete damaging toxins (leukocidin), which destroys their host's white cells and produces pus. Each thrives when the host's resistance is lowered.

Reservoirs of infection. The places where pathogens multiply are called reservoirs. They may be human tissue, insect and animal intermediaries, or such inanimate things as food, water, and feces. These harbors of pathogens serve as sources for infection.

Portals of exit. The primary routes by which pathogens leave their reservoirs are called portals of exit. These include such things as the nose and mouth and open draining wounds.

Transmission means. The ways by which infections are spread are called the means of transmission. These may be direct means such as kissing and sexual intercourse, or indirect means such as by way of contaminated surgical instruments, food, and clothing and vectors such as mosquitoes and ticks.

Portals of entry. The route by which pathogens enter a new host often is the same as the portal of exit. Entry portals include such avenues as the mucous membrane of the mouth, urethra, or vagina and a break in the skin.

Susceptible hosts. Healthy people have a number of natural barriers to infection, including the unbroken skin and secretions of the mucous membranes. If pathogens gain entrance, there are phagocytes to consume them, antibodies to destroy them, and the general inflammatory response of the body to defend it. When persons are fatigued, malnourished, excessively stressed, or lacking specific antibodies they are more susceptible to invading pathogens.

Breaking the links of the infection chain

The chain of infection can be weakened or broken at each link, as follows:

Infectious organisms	Use antiseptics to inhibit growth, disinfectants to destroy, or antiinfectives to kill or weaken organisms.
Reservoirs	Use preventative measures, such as refrigeration of food, and active measures, such as disposal of contaminated wastes, to eliminate reservoirs.
Portals of entry	Cover nose and mouth, use flush toilets, and isolate infectious persons.
Transmission means	Avoid direct contact with infected sources, disinfect contaminated objects, wash hands, and filter air to prevent transmission of infectious organisms.
Susceptible hosts	Meet nutritional, emotional, and activity needs and obtain immunization against contagious disorders to bolster the defenses of potential hosts.

Categories of isolation

The categories of isolation have been standardized by the Center for Disease Control of the United States Department of Health and Human Services in their booklet, *Isolation Technique for Use in Hospitals, ed. 2* (1975). The categories are strict isolation, respiratory isolation, protective isolation, enteric precautions, wound and skin precautions, discharge precautions, and blood precautions. Degrees of isolation are indicated by the words *isolation* and *precautions.* Categories called "isolation" require more kinds of separation than those called "precautions." All categories require careful handwashing and limitation of visitors. To make a distinction between the various categories and to facilitate the practice of appropriate isolation measures, color-coded cards have been designed with the essential features of each category printed on them. These cards are attached to the door, bed, and record of the isolated person. Hospitals modify these cards to suit their needs. A summary of the precautions to be taken in each category follows.

Strict isolation (yellow card)

Private room—necessary; door must be kept closed.

Gowns—must be worn by all persons entering room.

Masks—must be worn by all persons entering room.

Hands—must be washed on entering and leaving room.

Gloves—must be worn by all persons entering room.

Articles—must be discarded, or wrapped before being sent to central supply for disinfection or sterilization.

Examples of diseases—anthrax, inhalation; *Staphylococcus aureus* or group A streptococcus infection of burns, wounds, skin, or pneumonia; congenital rubella syndrome; diphtheria (pharyngeal or cutaneous); disseminated neonatal herpes simplex; rabies.

Respiratory isolation (orange card)

Private room—necessary; door must be kept closed.

Gowns—not necessary.

Mask—must be worn by any person entering room unless that person is not susceptible to the disease.

Hands—must be washed on entering and leaving room.

Gloves—not necessary.

Articles—those contaminated with secretions must be disinfected.

Examples of diseases—rubeola, rubella, meningococcal meningitis, mumps, pertussis, tuberculosis.

Protective (reverse) isolation (blue card)

Private room—necessary; door must be kept closed.

Gowns—must be worn by all persons entering room.

Masks—must be worn by all persons entering room.

Hands—must be washed on entering and leaving room.

Gloves—must be worn by all persons having direct contact with patient. (Sometimes this is modified by substituting a 10-minute scrub, as for neonatal nurseries.)

Articles—sterilize all linen before use; keep such equipment as thermometers, sphygmomanometer, and stethoscope in room.

Examples of conditions—burns, noninfected but extensive; acute leukemia; lymphomas; agranulocytosis; dermatitis, noninfectious but severe.

Enteric precautions (brown card)

Private room—necessary; may place patients with same diagnosis in same room if each separated from one another.

Gowns—must be worn by all persons having direct contact with patient.

Masks—not necessary.

Hands—must be washed on entering and leaving room.

Gloves—must be worn by all persons having direct contact with patient or with articles contaminated with fecal matter.

Articles—special precautions necessary for articles contaminated with urine and feces. Articles must be disinfected or discarded after use.

Examples of diseases—cholera; gastroenteritis caused by *Salmonella*, *Escherichia. coli*, or *Shigella*; typhoid fever; hepatitis, viral, type A, B, or unspecified.

Wound and skin precautions (green card)

Private room—desirable.

Gowns—must be worn by all persons having direct contact with infected wound or skin areas.

Masks—not necessary except during dressing change.

Hands—must be washed on entering and leaving room.

Gloves—must be worn by all persons having direct contact with infected areas.

Articles—special precautions necessary for instruments, dressings, and linens.

Examples of diseases—skin infections other than *Staphylococcus aureus* and group A streptococcus that are not covered or contained by dressings; gas gangrene resulting from *Clostridium perfringens*; herpes zoster, localized; puerperal sepsis resulting from group A streptococcus; small, contained *S. aureus* or group A streptococcus infections of the skin.

Discharge precautions (oral and lesion secretions and urine and fecal secretions) (card color not designated by the Center for Disease Control; some hospitals use gray or lavender card)

Private room—not necessary.

Gowns—not necessary.

Masks—not necessary. Patients with oral secretions should cough or spit into tissues.

Hands—must be washed before and after caring for patient. Use "no-touch" dressing technique, that is, use instruments or gloved hands to touch contaminated dressings. When infection is in excrement, teach patient to use strict handwashing technique.

Gloves—use to change or touch dressings.

Articles—double-bag soiled dressings and equipment. Soiled tissues with oral discharge are placed in impervious bag for disposal. Excrement may be disposed of in standard sewage system.

Examples of diseases—oral secretions: *Streptococcus* pharyngitis; infectious mononucleosis; respiratory infection, acute. Lesion secretions: gonorrhea; syphilis, mucocutaneous; acute bacterial conjunctivitis. Excretions of urine and feces: amebiasis; poliomyelitis; tapeworm; food poisoning resulting from *Staphylococcus* or *Clostridium perfringens*.

Blood precautions (card color not designated by the Center for Disease Control; some hospitals use red card)

Private room—not necessary.

Gowns—not necessary.

Masks—not necessary.

Hands—wash before and after caring for patient. Take great care not to prick fingers with contaminated needles because disease is carried in patient's blood.

Gloves—not necessary unless nurses have break in skin and are handling needles or instruments contaminated by patient's blood.

Articles—label blood specimens and contaminated needles and syringes. Use disposable needles and syringes and place used ones in impervious puncture-resistant container for incineration or autoclaving.

Examples of diseases—serum hepatitis caused by hepatitis B virus, syphilis.

Nursing roles in controlling infections

Every hospital accredited by the Joint Commission on Accreditation of Hospitals must have an infection control committee to guide its program of infection control. Hospitals employ infection control nurses to assume leadership in implementing the policies of their committee. All nurses, however, are responsible for maintaining an environment that promotes health and healing. They do this by making accurate assessments of patients' signs and symptoms, by initiating and maintaining appropriate isolation technique, and by teaching patients and their families about infection control. No matter what their roles, nurses need to maintain high standards to prevent infections and their spread.

Principle of isolation technique

A principle is a general truth that serves as a guide for conduct. In the practice of isolation technique the guiding principle is *a clean, noninfectious item or area becomes contaminated if it comes in contact with anything infected.* A simple application of this truth is

Sterile to sterile, clean to clean, dirty to dirty;
But, dirty to any, dirties all.

Practice of isolation technique

When student nurses are first assigned to isolation areas they may be frightened, for they are faced with unseen foes—disease-producing organisms—and a whole array of gowns, masks, gloves, and other paraphernalia with which to implement an unfamiliar set of procedures called isolation technique. By remembering the general principle just stated, nurses can reduce some of their fear and practice effective technique.

General precautions. Infectious and highly susceptible patients can be placed in separate rooms and isolated from others, but nurses must travel between them. Even though they practice meticulous isolation technique, they may carry pathogens from room to room on their clothing, skin, and hair. To prevent such cross contamination, nurses are not assigned to care for both "clean" and "dirty" cases at the same time.

Infectious organisms also may be spread by so-called healthy carriers, persons who harbor the pathogen but show no symptoms. To identify such carriers, many hospitals require periodic throat and stool cultures of all personnel, particularly those caring for highly susceptible persons such as children with immune deficiencies.

Personal precautions. To guard their own health and that of their co-workers and patients, nurses should take the following specific personal precautions:

1. Maintain healthy living habits; get adequate rest, nourishment, and activity.
2. Do not care for sick and susceptible persons when ill.
3. Groom fingernails to prevent hangnails and wear gloves if the hands have open lesions or wounds.
4. Bathe and wash the hair frequently.
5. Do not touch the face with contaminated hands or objects.
6. Disinfect eyeglasses and hearing appliances periodically.
7. Avoid wearing jewelry of any kind. In strict isolation where no wall clock with a second hand is available, wrist watches can be brought into the unit in a plastic bag or placed on technique paper.
8. Wear only washable clothing in isolation units. Never wear sweaters!
9. Wash hands after touching the shoes. Shoes are the dirtiest of all clothing. Do not place them on sinks or table tops. It is best to leave them at the hospital to avoid bringing pathogens into the home.
10. Develop a sense of what is "clean" and what is "dirty."

Isolation unit. The isolation unit is the space and equipment set aside for an individual. It may be in a room with other children who need the same type of isolation, such as enteric or protective isolation. When an infection is especially virulent or the child is unusually susceptible, only one patient is assigned to a room at a time.

Isolation units are furnished sparingly with washable, disposable, or easily cleanable items. Water and sewage waste fixtures are available. Usually doors are kept closed but glass panels maintain visibility. Privacy is provided by screens if necessary. The isolated area should be cheerful, tastefully decorated, well-lit, and ventilated.

Isolation cart. The isolation cart is a four-wheeled metal chest of drawers that contains all of the special supplies needed to carry out isolation technique. Its surface provides a clean service table, and its side bins offer shelves for additional supplies. There is an isolation cart for each isolated child. It is parked just outside the isolation unit, maintained, stocked, and cleaned between use by the general supply service of the hospital.

Masks and gloves. Masks are used to intercept the passage of airborne organisms into or away from the nose and mouth of the nurse. They are used when the pathogen is transmitted by air-borne particles, in strict isolation of a highly infectious disease, or when protective isolation technique is employed to protect the child who is highly susceptible because of reduced resistance to disease.

Masks are made of disposable paper or many thicknesses of cloth. Those made of paper are used once and then discarded. Those made of cloth are placed in a special receptacle after use and then disinfected and laundered as is other contaminated linen.

If masks are not used correctly, they may become a source of infection rather than a protection against it. For this reason the nurse should observe the following precautions carefully:

1. Clean masks should be applied with clean hands before entering the isolated area. A clean supply is usually kept just outside the door if they are required. Strings remain clean unless they are contaminated.
2. To be of any value, the mask must cover both the mouth and nose.
3. The mask should never be touched after it is in place.
4. The mask should be changed at least every hour. A moist mask is worse than none.
5. To remove the mask, only the strings are touched with clean hands, untied, and the mask dropped into the waste can or, if the mask is to be laundered, into the soiled mask receptacle.

Gloves are not usually employed in the practice of routine barrier technique. Conscientious handwashing is effective in most cases. Occasionally gloves may be used to protect the nurse when there are infectious skin lesions or especially purulent dressings to be changed or when "strict isolation" has been ordered. In protective isolation, when the child is highly susceptible to infection, sterile gloves may be used for protection during such times as dressing changes for severe burns or skin grafts when surgical aseptic technique is employed.

Gowns. The isolation gown is a long-sleeved garment of paper or a closely woven, durable fabric. It has a tie at the back of the neck and one at the wrists. The knit cuffs on the sleeves give a snug fit around the wrists.

The isolation gown is worn whenever there is a possibility of contact with the ill child or any contaminated equipment. When strict or protective isolation is ordered, a gown must be worn by anyone entering the isolated area, whether they touch anything or not. The gown should not be worn outside the isolated area unless the nurse is transporting the child or contaminated furniture to or from the room.

When the isolated child must be taken to the x-ray department or some other area of the hospital, special precautions must be taken. The nurse should wear a fresh gown. The child is placed in a wheelchair, infant carrier, or on a gurney, and the whole is draped with a clean sheet. Clean tissues or towels should be brought along with which to touch doorknobs and elevator buttons, because the nurse's hands are contaminated. The nurse should bring a bag in which to discard these tissues. The child's chart should be handled only by clean hands. It should be placed in a clean bag for protection. When the child is returned to the room, the wheelchair, carrier, or gurney must be disinfected or kept in the isolated area. The linens and gown may be used in the isolation area unless they were soiled.

When the gown is used for the first time, it is clean inside and outside. If it is not soiled and care has been taken to keep the inside and neck and back edges clean, the gown can be reused.

Fresh gowns are taken at least every 24 hours to ensure safe technique.

Gowning and handwashing. Because gowning and handwashing techniques are so closely associated, they are described here together. But because handwashing is perhaps the most important measure in preventing the spread of infection, nurses will be washing their hands many more times than they will be putting on gowns. The handwashing procedure described here should be followed with or without a gown.

Before donning the gown the nurse's hands must be thoroughly cleansed. In the neonatal nursery a 10-minute scrub with antibacterial detergent is required. In other areas, a minimum of 2 minutes is recommended.

Donning the gown. (Remember the principle "clean to clean, dirty to dirty. . . .") The technique for donning the isolation gown (Fig. 8-2) is as follows:

1. With clean hands, grasp the neckband and open up the gown with the inside toward you.
2. Hold onto the inside of the top of the gown with one hand and slip the other arm into an empty sleeve and through the wristband.
3. With the first hand, reach up and grasp the neckband and put the other arm through the second sleeve.
4. When both hands are through the sleeves, reach up and tie the neckband.
5. Close the back according to the technique used in your pediatric unit. Two such techniques are as follows: (a) Pull the left-hand side of the back as far to the right as possible and lap the right-hand side over the left. Pull the belt around, cross it at the back; and tie it in the front. (b) Hold the left and right inner edges of the gown together and fold over the back part of the gown until it is snugly closed against the wearer's back. Pull the belt around, cross it at the back, and tie it in the front.
6. Push up the sleeves above the wrists; never roll them. This is done to avoid getting the sleeves wet during nursing care. A wet gown ceases to be an effective barrier.

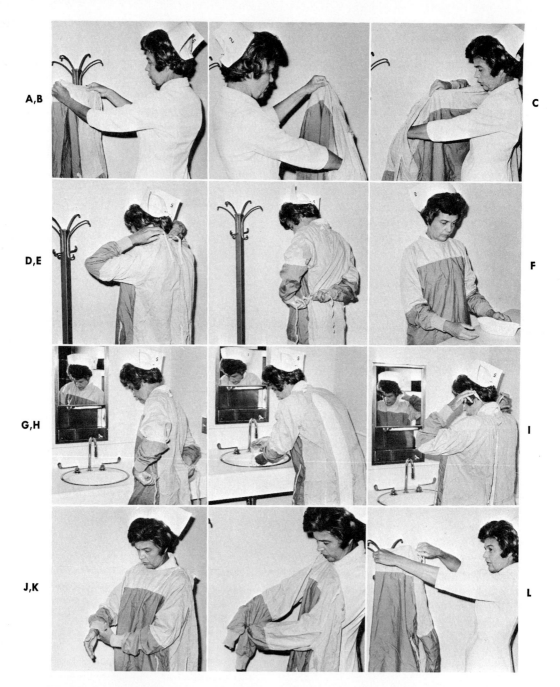

Fig. 8-2. Gowning technique. The inside and the neck and back edges should be kept clean. **A,** Grasp the neckband to remove gown from hook. **B,** Open gown with inside toward you and slip one arm into and through sleeve. **C,** Slip second arm into armhole and through sleeve. **D,** Tie clean ties at neck. **E,** Lap back edges and tie waistband (*Note:* In protective isolation, hands should cross in front rather than behind the body.) **F,** Proceed with care of infant. **G,** When ready to doff gown, untie waistband. **H,** Wash hands thoroughly. **I,** Untie neckband. **J,** Reach under cuff; pull it over hand. **K,** Using sleeve-covered hand, pull opposite sleeve down. **L,** Return gown to hook by holding clean neckband. (*Note:* In strict isolation technique, hair should be covered.)

Removing the gown and handwashing. When the isolation gown is to be removed, the nurse uses the following technique (hands are considered contaminated until properly washed):

1. Untie the contaminated belt; allow the ends to drop to the side.
2. Turn on the running water. Hand faucets, knee levers, and foot pedals are always considered contaminated. Foot pedals are operated with the always dirty shoes.
3. Carefully wash the hands and exposed portion of the arms for 1 minute with antibacterial detergent. Wash each finger and under each fingernail. Use considerable friction. A scrub brush may break or irritate the skin and so is not generally used. Rinse well with water. The hands should be kept below the elbows when washing to avoid wetting the sleeves of the gown. Pat the hands dry with a paper towel.
4. Turn off the hand faucet with a clean paper towel, or with the knee lever with the gown-covered knee or with a paper towel. The foot pedal requires no special concern because its operation does not involve the hands. For this reason it is preferred.
5. With newly clean hands, untie the neckband and drop the ties to the back.
6. Reach under the cuff of one sleeve with the clean fingers and pull it down completely past the other hand.
7. Reach over to the other sleeve with the covered hand and grasp it through the gown. Pull the second sleeve down over the hand, using special care to prevent contamination of the hand with the first sleeve. When both hands are clear of the sleeves, the clean neckband is grasped and the gown hung up for reuse or placed in the laundry hamper.
8. When a gown is to be reused, hang it on a hook. If the hook is inside the isolated (dirty) area, the gown is hung dirty side out.
9. Wash the hands again, using the same technique described above. If a hand faucet or knee lever is used, it is contaminated and must be turned off with a paper towel.

Leaving the isolation area. Before washing the hands and removing the gown, the nurse checks to see that all is in order in the room, that the child is safe and comfortable, and that in the case of an older child the calling device is nearby. The nurse makes one final visual check and is ready to leave the area, as follows:

1. Open the door with a clean paper towel used to turn off the hand- or knee-controlled water flow.
2. Walk through, brace the door open with the foot, and discard the paper towel in the wastebasket. If a mask was worn, remove it by the clean ties and discard.
3. Allow the door to close to maintain isolation of the contaminated area.

Technique papers and small plastic bags. The use of technique papers makes it possible for the nurse to carry out procedures with greater skill because they provide a temporary, flexible barrier that can be placed between clean and dirty items (Fig. 8-3). A clean paper towel folded double makes an excellent technique paper. When placed on a dry, contaminated area, it provides a safe, clean island on which clean items can be placed briefly while they are needed. If the paper becomes moist, organisms can pass through it and it is no longer a barrier.

Technique papers may also serve as temporary gloves with which to turn faucets or doorknobs.

A small, clear plastic bag is another useful, temporary, clean island in which a clean watch may be safely protected from contamination. When the watch is no longer needed in the isolation area, the nurse gently "pours" it onto clean technique paper, discards the plastic bag, washes the hands, reclaims the watch, grasps the paper by its clean side, and drops it into the wastebasket.

Meal service. Meal service for isolated patients in hospitals has been greatly improved by the introduction of attractive disposable dishes and utensils. The following procedure is commonly practiced:

1. The child is prepared for a meal by a gowned nurse; an overbed table or tray is put in place or a space cleared on the bedside table.

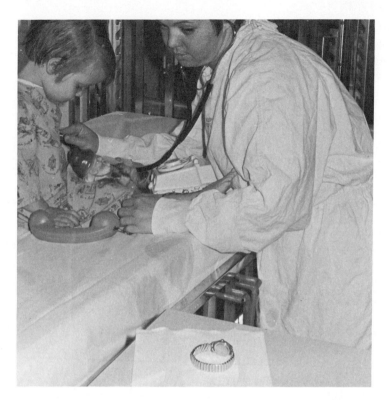

Fig. 8-3. A "technique paper" of a double-thickness paper towel keeps the wristwatch clean.

2. A clean worker brings the tray of food to the clean service table standing just outside the door of the isolated area. The food is served in disposable dishes. A new packet of disposable utensils may also be provided. If nondisposable utensils are used, they are washed after each use, stored in the isolated area, and placed on the child's meal tray as part of the preparations.

3. Food should be served immediately so that it will be appetizing. Hot things should be hot; cold things, cold. The gowned nurse goes to the door, opens it, lifts the individual dishes one by one from the clean tray without contaminating it, carries them to the child's tray, and then assists or feeds the child.

4. Uneaten food particles and liquids are disposed of in the same manner as bodily discharges, described later.

5. A record of intake and output is usually kept for all isolated children on a clean tally sheet kept just outside the door. When the nurse's hands are clean, these figures are recorded.

6. The clean, but now empty, tray is removed from the outside clean table by a clean worker and returned to the kitchen.

7. If china dishes and metal utensils must be used, they are transferred one by one to the child's tray from the clean tray. After use, wastes are discarded as described subsequently. The soiled dishes are then placed on a newspaper on the clean tray and carried to a large pan in which they must be boiled for at least 10 minutes, after which they are returned to the kitchen for normal washing. The contaminated newspaper is then folded in on itself and placed in the contaminated wastebasket.

Linen and diaper care. Laundry hampers or bags are provided in isolated areas to facilitate patient care. Linen is placed in the hamper as it becomes soiled. When the hamper is two thirds full, or at least every 8 hours, the top of the bag is closed and taken to the door of the isolated area by a gowned worker and placed upside down in a waiting, clean outer bag. A clean frame or a clean worker must hold the clean bag open. The top is then drawn closed; the bag is then plainly labeled "isolation" and sent to the laundry for special care. In some hospitals color-coded plastic bags are used for double-bagged linen, for example, red for inner, blue for outer. Each hospital modifies its procedure for linen care according to its own facilities.

The disposition of soiled diapers also depends on the hospital. In some, cloth diapers are placed in the general soiled-linen bag. In others, a diaper pail is provided. If paper diapers are used, soiled ones are placed in the waste basket. Regardless of practice, the principle of isolation technique is maintained.

Waste disposal. Wastes of urine, feces, emesis, and other bodily discharge can usually be placed directly into the sewage system. In some situations in which there is a case of typhoid fever or other such feces-borne disease, the excrement may be placed in a container with an equal amount of chlorinated lime for 1 hour before it is discarded into the public sewer.

Paper waste is collected in the liner bags of waste paper containers. These liner bags are placed in large, clean bags held open at the unit door and taken to an incinerator.

If there is no toilet inside the isolated area, bedpans and other liquid or semisolid wastes must be taken to a hopper outside the area. Some hospitals provide waste baskets in the room; others designate a "dirty utility room." If the latter is the case, the following procedure is followed:

1. The nurse completes the nursing care, washes hands, and removes the gown.
2. In one hand the nurse grasps the covered contaminated bucket handle and with the other a technique paper. The nurse moves down the hall cautiously, avoiding contact with any per-

son or thing. The technique paper gives the nurse a "clean hand."
3. In the dirty utility room the nurse empties the bucket or bedpan and returns to the isolation area immediately, replaces the bucket, and washes hands thoroughly.

Toys, books, and religious articles. The number of toys taken into an isolated area should be minimal. They should be of material that can be disinfected easily, such as plastic or wood, or else destroyed after use, such as paper dolls and coloring books. Valuable books should not be taken into an isolated area, but if they are, they should be sunned for several days before being returned to general use. Religious medals are easily disinfected, but they are so small that they are often lost. They can be taped onto the bedside stand or pinned to a curtain. Because there is a danger that small children might swallow them, it is best not to place them within reach of the child. The parents should realize that a medal may be lost if attached to a gown or bed linen.

Recording nursing observations. Medical records such as the child's chart should never be taken into an isolated area. When the nurse is caring for two or more children in the same isolated area, there may be difficulty in remembering the vital signs and other data until these are ready to be recorded in their charts. One solution is to make notes with clean hands on notepaper placed on technique paper. The notepaper can be taken out of the room if it has not been contaminated. Another solution is to make notes on contaminated paper, review them, and discard the paper just before leaving the area.

Disinfection. *Concurrent disinfection* is the term used for the killing of disease-producing organisms during the time when the child is still infectious. Contaminated articles are disinfected by either physical or chemical means. The most common types of physical disinfection are boiling and autoclaving (steam under pressure). Sunlight may also be used when autoclaving is not possible. When chemical disinfection is used, the item to be disinfected may be soaked in a chemical bath until pathogens are killed. Large articles may be wiped off with the disinfectant solution and then aired. Antibacterial detergents are used for handwashing.

When a child ceases to be infectious and is discharged, *terminal disinfection* of the unit is made. The unit is stripped of linen and all wastes are removed. The bed and other furnishings, walls, windows, and doors are cleansed with disinfectant solution, and the unit is left to air.

Organization of nursing care. Up to this point various aspects of isolation technique have been discussed. How do they all fit together? The following suggested organization of nursing care is given to help the nurse plan care:

1. All the known articles needed for nursing care should be assembled before gowning.
   a. Supplies from the linen closet—linens, clothes, diapers, and laundry bag
   b. Supplies from the kitchen—liquids or nursing bottles, as needed
   c. Supplies from the treatment room, as ordered
   d. Supplies from the utility room—fresh paper bags, towels, and personal hygiene items
   NOTE: Medicines are brought separately when it is time for them to be given.
2. If it is possible, two nurses should work together. This not only is more cheery, but it also makes for greater efficiency and sometimes better technique.
3. In some hospitals, the nurse is expected to do the housekeeping (wet mopping of floors, dusting, and emptying wastes) in isolated areas as well as nursing duties. If this is the case, the nurse must plan for this duty in the working schedule. Whether these duties are expected or not, the nurse should leave the unit tidy, with unnecessary articles disposed of or put away and the tabletop cleared.
4. Before removing the gown, the nurse should make sure that the child is comfortable and safe and that the room is in order.
5. Finally, the bedside nurse is expected to report to the team leader and usually to record important data on the child's chart.

Effects of isolation on children and their parents

Hospitalization is a stressful experience for both children and their parents. The anxiety is greatly increased when children must be placed in isolation, with its specter of masks and gowns and signs warning of contamination. Some of the fear can be relieved if nurses offer explanations and instructions in how to function safely within the restrictions of isolation, and if they are accessible and supportive.

ADMISSION
Preparation of the child and the family

General preparation. In the past, the feelings, needs, and individual differences between children were largely ignored. Children were to be seen and not heard. This social attitude was reflected in the treatment of children in hospitals as well as in other institutions. No thought was given to the need to prepare a child for the traumatic experience of hospitalization, much less the bewildered parents.

Of parents. In recent years the practice of no preparation has changed radically. Modern nurses recognize the child as an individual person and the family as an important part of the child's life. Nurses are not jealous of the parent's role; instead, they realize that when the parents are properly prepared and supported they can help the child adjust to hospitalization in ways that no one else can. To be prepared, the parents must be given sound information about their child's illness. They must have confidence in their doctor's judgment and have assurance of the intelligent care of devoted nurses. When parents are prepared in this way, they, in turn, will be better able to prepare their child for hospitalization.

Of children. The parents should tell their child *why* hospitalization is necessary. *What* might happen while in the hospital need not be described in frightening detail. The degree of explanation given depends on the child's level of understanding. A child given no explanation for the hospitalization may think it is a punishment. If told nothing of what will be done there, an active imagination may fancy a fate far worse than the truth. The parents will probably be the best judges of how much should be told, but whatever is told should be absolutely true. If the child has learned to trust the parents in the past, it will be easier to accept their judgment now. The parents' honesty in these matters can serve to further build the child's trust, thus making the hospitalization a potentially constructive experience in the child's development.

Methods. In response to widespread recognition of the need to prepare children and their parents for hospitalization, a variety of means have been developed by many groups and individuals. Pediatric units in hospitals across the country have prepared illustrative booklets for both parents and children. These booklets are distributed in doctor's offices, by schools, and in public agencies. Many pediatric hospital units offer tours and orientation parties for both individual families and groups of children (see Fig. 7-1). Hospital social workers, admission clerks, and others are ready to provide information and assistance to all who seek it. Doctors spend more time discussing hospitalization with the parents, often giving them printed instructions and pamphlets to ease their anxiety with information. Educational motion pictures, puppet shows, television programs, and children's library books are bringing information to large numbers of children and their parents about what happens when a child goes to the hospital. In all of these many ways children and their parents are being prepared for hospitalization.

Specific preparation. Unless a child's admission to the hospital is an emergency, the doctor usually makes arrangements for it in advance in consultation with the parents. A date is set and definite instructions are provided. If the pediatric unit has its own informational pamphlet for parents, it may be given to them at that time. The parents are able to ask questions, adjust themselves, make plans for the other members of the family, and prepare their child for hospitalization.

Preparation of the hospital

When a child's physician decides that the child must be hospitalized, the physician informs the appropriate person at the hospital either by telephone or in person. If the child is acutely ill, the physician may give verbal orders that should be written down by a licensed or registered nurse, read back for approval, and signed as soon as possible. If the child's admission is not an emergency, the child may be brought in for preadmission laboratory work. The physician may write admission orders and send or bring them to the hospital together with the child's medical history. When such information is sent to the hospital in advance, the staff has the maximum opportunity to be prepared to welcome the newcomer.

Procedure

No matter how well prepared the child and parents may be for hospitalization, the admission process is stressful. Admitting personnel should be warm, reassuring individuals who are able to establish rapport easily. By their calm control and sincere interest they are able to put the child and parents at ease. The actual admission process usually involves at least three steps. The first is an admission interview conducted by an admitting clerk in a private area near the hospital lobby for legal and financial purposes. The second step involves the admission of the child to the pediatric unit by an admitting nurse. The third step is a head-to-toe assessment made by a registered nurse and recorded. In emergencies, these steps are modified according to the situation.

Hospital admission and identification. If reservations have been made in advance by the physician, the admitting clerk will be expecting the child and the parents when they arrive in the hospital lobby and will invite them into an office.

There hospital records needed by the business office are filled out and permission for photographs, treatments, and operations are signed by the parents. An identification band is placed on the child's wrist. An information booklet about hospital policies and practices is given to the parents. The ward is then notified that the child and the parents have arrived and are ready to go to the pediatric unit. A volunteer hostess, nurse, or the admitting clerk then escorts them to the pediatric unit and introduces them to the admitting nurse.

Pediatric admission

Undressing and dressing. The child and the parents are taken to the nursing unit assigned to the child. The unit includes the bed, bedside stand, chair, and any other furnishings that may be provided. The child is undressed, weighed and measured, and dressed in hospital clothing. The parents should be allowed to assist in this if they wish. It is a good time for the nurse to learn more about the new patient by asking questions and making observations. Any abrasion, rash, or unusual condition should be noted. The child's clothing should be placed in a paper bag, sent home with the parents, and the fact noted on the record. If the clothing cannot be sent home at the time of admission, a clothing and valuables list should be filled out.

Establishing rapport. During this initial contact with the child and the parents, lasting impressions are being made. If the nurse is disorganized and confused, rough with the child, and cool toward their concern, the parents might well wonder about the care their child will receive. The nurse should seek to establish some rapport with the child and the parents but should not force the child. The nurse should address the child in a natural voice, by name. The parents should be encouraged to ask questions and to talk about their child. In some hospitals a personal record form is provided on which information about the child can be supplied by the parents, including such facts as the child's nickname, current habits of sleeping, eating, and toi-

leting, or special problems such as allergies to food and drugs. This information is invaluable to the nurse, and the fact that the nurse wanted it is comforting to the parents.

Weighing and measuring. All children, are weighed and measured during admission except those with severe injuries or fractures (Fig. 8-4).

Vital signs. The temperature, pulse, and respiration of all children should be taken. Blood pressure is taken when requested. (See discussion of vital signs later in this chapter.)

Restraints. Restraints should be applied if they are needed for safety. The nurse should explain the reasons for their use to both the child and the parents.

Urine specimen. A routine urine specimen should be obtained as soon as possible after admission. The nurse may enlist the parents' assistance in this if they seem eager to help. If they appear to be reluctant or excessively overwrought, the nurse should not urge their help.

Settling the child. When the child is safely settled in bed in hospital clothing, and the initial assessment is made, the nurse should introduce the child to other children in the ward. Depending on the child's age, the nurse should explain what to expect and how things work in the hospital, what to do when the child needs to use the bathroom or wants to call the nurse, how and when meals are served, and whether the child must stay in bed, or is allowed to be up in a chair or to play in the playroom. Older children may want to know how to operate the television set or use the telephone. Before leaving, the nurse should see that the child is provided with some diversional material such as a book or a toy.

Orienting the parents. The parents may wish to remain with the child. If they do, the nurse should see that they have a place to sit and are reasonably comfortable. In some hospitals parents are requested to remain in the hospital until the physician can interview them for recent information about their child. If this is the case, the nurse should see that they understand. The

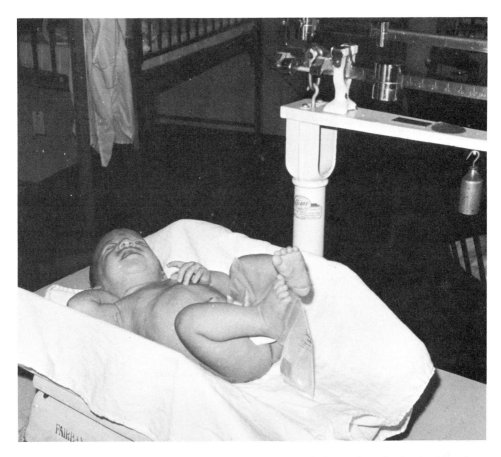

Fig. 8-4. All children, with few exceptions, are weighed on admission. Urine collection bag is in place. (The nurse is standing out of the picture, but an arm's reach away to ensure safety.)

parents may be given a brief orientation to the ward so that they will know where to meet the physician and where the bathrooms and cafeteria are located. If unlimited visiting hours are permitted, the nurse should explain about them and what general rules prevail. The nurse should answer as many questions as possible and introduce the parents to the head nurse or supervisor.

Hospital records. No admission procedure is complete until all the hospital record forms are assembled and filled out correctly. In some pediatric units the ward clerk assists in this task, but ultimately the nurse is responsible for seeing

that it is done correctly. Some of the most common forms are the following.

Bed card. The child's name and other identifying numbers should appear on the card. The nurse should add the child's nickname and attach it to the bed or unit.

Kardex cards. The headings of the Kardex card should be filled out. In some pediatric units a separate Kardex file is kept for diet, medications, and treatments. The supervising nurse usually notes physician's orders and sees that they are placed on the appropriate Kardex file.

Chart. The child's chart is the collected current record of hospital care. It includes a great variety of forms, permission slips, laboratory reports, graphic sheets, physician's and nurses' notes, and a nursing care plan. The chart contains specific information about the child's care and condition; it may be subpoenaed by a court order. For this reason it must be accurate in every detail. For the sake of uniformity, most hospital units keep all the forms included in the chart in a specified order.

On admission the nurses' notes and graphic sheet should include the following information:

1. When the child arrived
2. How the child came to the ward; for example, walking, wheelchair, carried by a parent
3. Accompanied by whom; for example, father, mother, guardian, Mrs. Lee
4. Room to which child was admitted
5. A head-to-toe assessment performed by a registered nurse describing physical and emotional findings
6. Restraints, if applied; for example, body restraint applied
7. Height and weight in space provided on chart
8. Vital signs: temperature, pulse, respiration, and blood pressure

Nursing care plan. A formal nursing care plan is required for all patients in hospitals accredited by the Joint Commission, except those who stay less than 48 hours, those cared for in long-term facilities, or patients in hospitals where problem-oriented records are used. The nursing care plan includes a data base, nursing diagnoses, interventions, goals, and evaluation (see discussion of the nursing process).

BASIC NEEDS AND DAILY CARE
Safety

In the first section of this chapter general safety measures were discussed as they relate to the physical plant of the pediatric unit, including such things as safe electrical outlets, nonslippery floors, and locking doors. In this section safe practices as they relate to the individual child are discussed. These include such measures as the use of restraints, cribs, side rails, and precau-

tionary signs; removal of dangerous toys and objects; and maintenance of continuous observation.

Restraints. Restraints are external means used for restricting movement so that the safety of the child will be ensured. They must never be used as a punishment or a substitute for careful observation. Improperly used restraints can cause physical and emotional damage. They should be applied in such a way that the child has maximum comfort and movement while still being restrained. When movement has to be restricted, the position of the child should be changed frequently and the restraint loosened whenever possible. The reason restraints must be applied should be explained to the parents and to children old enough to understand.

When restraints are applied, a notation should be made in the child's chart as to the time applied, the type of restraint used, the reason for application, and the child's reaction.

Some of the most common types of restraints, their special uses, and the techniques for applying them follow.

Waist restraints. Waist restraints are used to keep the child in bed. They may be applied in such a way that the child must lie flat in bed, or the ties may be left long so that the child may move about freely.

Sleeve restraints. Sleeve restraints are blind-ended sleeves with a tie at the closed end and other ties to attach the sleeve at the shoulder. They are used when it is necessary to control the child's hands or elbow movement.

Elbow restraints. The elbow restraint consists of a piece of material made with many long, narrow pockets into which tongue depressors can be inserted. It is fitted snugly around the elbow to keep the child from flexing it and then fastened securely to prevent slippage. Although it may still be possible for the child so restrained to rub the face with the upper arm, elbow restraints prevent the child from bending the elbow. It is often used in conjunction with a wrist restraint.

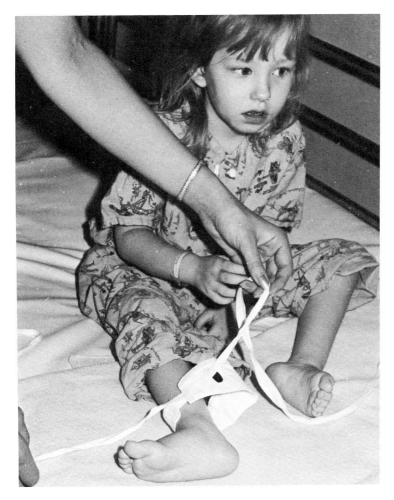

Fig. 8-5. An ankle or wrist restraint. The ties are pulled until the band fits securely; then a square knot is made and the long ends are fastened to the bed frame—never to the movable crib side.

Wrist and ankle restraints. Wrist and ankle restraints are made in various patterns and may be of disposable material (Fig. 8-5). Sometimes a padded clove-hitch rope tie is used for the same purpose. The restraint is fastened to the child's extremity, tightly enough so that it cannot be slipped over the hand or foot, but loosely enough so that circulation will not be impaired. The ends are fastened securely to the bed springs with bow knots. They should not be fastened to the movable side rails. These restraints are used for a variety of purposes and in conjunction with other types of restraints. For example, elbow and wrist restraints may be used after a child has had a cleft palate operation.

Mummy restraints. A sheet or blanket is wrapped around the child in such a way that the arms are immobilized temporarily. It is useful for examinations or procedures involving the head or neck (Fig. 9-3).

Jacket restraints. The jacket restraint is used to keep a child flat in bed or to allow a sitting position. It is applied instead of ankle restraints or crib-net restraints. It can also be used when the child is placed in a high chair or wheelchair.

Positioning-holds used as restraints. There are many occasions when the child must be held temporarily in a certain position for safety and the success of a treatment or examination. The "arm-leg hold" allows the thigh, groin, perineum, and abdomen to be examined. The nurse stands at the head of the table with the child on the back with legs spread apart in a froglike manner. The child's arms are held firmly against the nurse's body and the child's knee is held by the nurse's hand. This hold would be used for a venipuncture of the groin (Fig. 9-3).

The "head-leg hold" immobilizes the spine and is used for lumbar punctures. The nurse stands to the side of the examining table with the child lying on the side facing the nurse. The nurse places one arm over and around the child's neck and the other over and around the thigh. By drawing the arms firmly toward the body, the nurse can hold the child secure and produce the desired curve of the spine (Fig. 9-4).

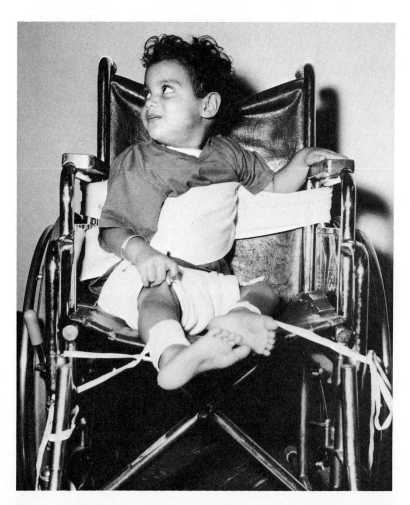

Fig. 8-6. Body restraint acts as a safety belt in wheelchairs. Ankle restraints may also be necessary.

Wheelchair and gurney restraints. When children are too large to be transported in infant carriers, they should be strapped safely into a wheelchair or onto a gurney, depending on their condition (Fig. 8-6). Infant carriers are like bassinets on wheels (Fig. 8-7). Because there is usually no way to strap a child into a carrier, any child large enough to crawl out should be attended constantly.

Bassinets, cribs, and side rails. It is customary to place children younger than 1 year of age in bassinets and children younger than 6 years of age in cribs. All cribs are made with side rails that can be moved out of the way while the child is receiving care. Never, under any circumstances, should the nurse leave a young child unattended with the side rails down—even for a moment.

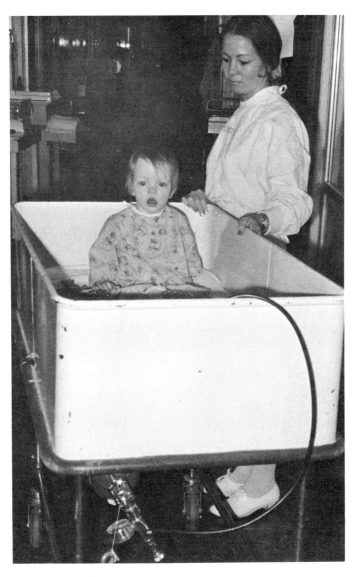

Fig. 8-7. Infant carrier. Emergency oxygen tank with opening wrench is available for immediate use.

When young children are agitated or potentially convulsive, bumpers may need to be positioned or the side rails padded to prevent injury. When infants are placed in full-size cribs, it may be necessary to place bumpers against the slats to keep baby's head from getting caught in the spaces between them.

In addition to side rails, children whose shoulders are above the crib side when standing should have safety belts, ankle restraints, crib nets, crib domes, or extended sides to protect them from climbing out over the crib's side rail.

Children over 6 years of age are usually assigned to youth or adult-sized beds. The side rails should be kept up if the child has had an anesthetic, is restless or irrational, has had sedation, or has a history of convulsions. Older children should be given an explanation for the need for side rails so that they will understand the reason for their use.

Precautionary signs. Precautionary signs such as "save all stool," "nothing by mouth," and "allergic to penicillin" are needed in any area of the hospital, but in the pediatric unit where many of the small patients cannot talk, such signs are of special importance. Pediatric nurses must be alert for and heed these signs at all times, especially when caring for children unfamiliar to them, such as at mealtime when they may be serving trays to less familiar children.

The responsibility to post the precautionary signs rests with the person noting the physician's order. If orders are to take effect at a certain time, such as "nothing by mouth after midnight," the person in charge of nursing care at midnight is responsible for seeing that the sign is posted. Such signs should be posted out of reach of the child.

It is important to remove signs as soon as they are no longer applicable. For example, as soon as the order to "keep bed flat" is changed, the sign should be removed or changed.

Toys and hazardous objects. The nurse must be constantly alert to the potential danger of toys and other objects within reach of the child. The nurse should see that the crib is at a safe distance from electrical outlets and other items that little hands might investigate. The nurse must also be alert for anything left with a young child by well-meaning visitors that might be hazardous. Some of these dangerous items are as follows.

Spark-producing toys. When oxygen is in use, spark-producing toys could start a fire.

Plastic bags. Plastic bags can asphyxiate a child in a few minutes. They should never be left in or near a child's crib.

Sharp objects or toys with sharp parts. Sharp objects can cause serious cuts or permanent eye injuries. Every toy should be checked for sharp edges or points.

Small objects. Small pieces that may come apart from larger toys, such as strings of beads that break and button eyes from stuffed animals, could be aspirated. Toys should be checked for loose parts.

Lead paint. Serious cases of lead poisoning have been caused by the ingestion of lead paint from toys and furniture over a period of time. If there is any question about a painted toy, it should be removed.

Toy stuffing. The material used to stuff toys may be contaminated with a variety of disease-producing organisms. Any toy that seems to be falling apart should be removed and given to the parent for repair.

Continuous observation. No matter how many safety rules, restraints, and plans are devised to promote safety in the pediatric unit, there is no substitute for continuous observation. Children are naturally curious, unpredictable, agile, and trusting. They pull wires, poke into holes, untie ties, turn switches, release levers, and reach the unreachable in an incredibly brief time. They do not do these things because they are naughty or bad but because they are inexperienced and inquisitive. Older children can understand more of the reasons for certain restrictions and rules and should be expected to cooperate. Younger children must be protected from harm because they cannot protect themselves. All the children on the pediatric unit, young and old, are the responsibility of all the persons who work there. Safety is everyone's business.

Personal hygiene and weight measurement

Although there may be some debate from a child's point of view as to the relative importance of cleanliness, there is no doubt that the comfort and effectiveness of medical treatment of the hospitalized child are greatly enhanced by the maintenance of personal hygiene. Oral hygiene, bathing, and shampoos are measures that provide this needed cleanliness. The frequency and method used depends on the age, medical condition, and needs of the child, as well as the facilities of the pediatric unit.

Oral hygiene. No matter how many teeth a child may or may not have, mouth care should not be ignored. Oral hygiene includes care of the teeth, gums, mucous cheek lining, tongue, and lips. It should always be appropriate to the needs of the child. A child who has had oral surgery should not be given a hard brush; if the child has only two teeth, swishing water in the mouth may be sufficient; if the tongue or gums are sore, special mouthwash may be ordered; if the lips are cracked, ointment or oil should be applied. If the child has no oral problem, the teeth should be brushed regularly, not only for current needs but also to teach good health habits. Symptoms in the mouth often provide valuable clues as the doctor assesses a child's medical condition. Any lesion, unusual appearance, or bleeding should be reported promptly.

Bathing. Regular cleansing of a child's skin prevents irritation, refreshes, and comforts. It also provides an excellent opportunity for observation and evaluation. The decision as to whether a tub or sponge bath should be given depends on the child's condition and the hospital facilities. Whenever it is possible, tub bathing is usually preferred over sponge bathing because it is more thorough and relaxing. If a daily weight check is ordered, the child is weighed just before the bath

on the same scales at the same time of day. (Fig. 8-8).

Tub bathing. Tub baths are given (1) when not otherwise contraindicated, (2) as a means for reducing elevated temperature, (3) as a means for treating certain skin conditions by prolonged soaking in water or with starch or drugs added to the water, and (4) as a means for softening skin crusts, casts, or dressings. The procedure for tub bathing is the same for children as for adults, and, as with adults, the degree of supervision depends on the bather. Small children should never be left alone. A small portable tub atop a worktable is convenient to wheel to the bedside (Fig. 8-9). Larger children can use a conventional bathtub. Teenagers require more direction but less supervision and appreciate privacy. Because some children fear tub bathing, feeling exposed and cold, the nurse should see that the room is warm and the bath pleasant and brief. To prevent scalding the child, turn off the hot water and move the spigot to the side. If a prolonged bath has been specifically ordered, the water temperature and child's reaction should be checked frequently to avoid harmful chilling.

Sponge or bed bathing. Sponge baths are given when the child (1) is quite ill or weak, (2) is in traction or using other special equipment continuously, (3) has casts or dressings that cannot be moistened, and (4) has skin lesions or incisions that must be protected from water. The procedure for giving a sponge bath is the same for a child as for an adult. A drape should be used to ensure privacy and prevent chilling. Infants are bathed similarly, from head to buttocks, with firm, rapid strokes.

Dressing. After the bath, the child should be dressed quickly. Most hospitals provide a variety of sizes of pajama sets and gowns. Whenever it is possible, the child should be given a choice about clothing, but the choice should be made before the bath when the bed linens are assembled. The nurse should try to avoid mismatched sets of pajamas and clashing colors. The sensitive child may be genuinely bothered

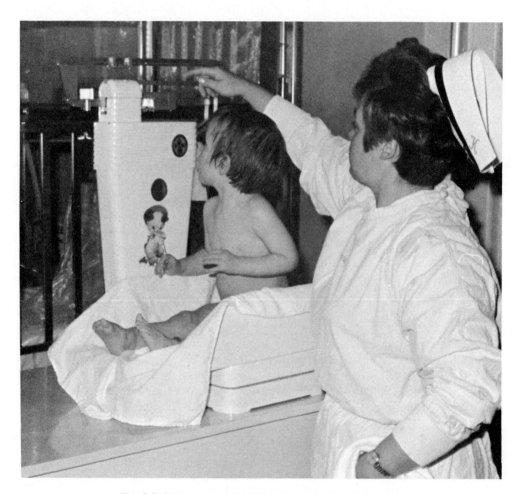

Fig. 8-8. Did you gain today? Child is weighed just before bath.

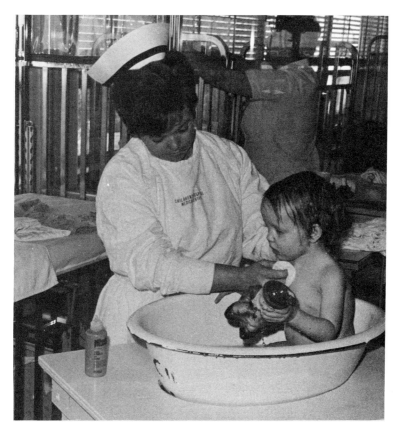

Fig. 8-9. The tub bath. The tub is secured to a movable table that is brought to the child's bedside. The nurse has laid out fresh clothing and a towel ready for use.

by such an insult to a personal esthetic sense. If the child has been toilet-trained before admission, diapers should not be used. A child dressed like a baby may act like one. Dressing, like everything else involving a child, can be turned into a fun game or a mean chore. It depends on how it is done.

Hair and scalp. Cleanliness of the hair and scalp is an important part of personal hygiene. It contributes to the health and feeling of well-being of children of all ages.

An infant's head should be shampooed daily as part of the bath. If the head is neglected, a white crusty layer of blanket fuzz, skin oil, and wastes may build up on the scalp. Such an ac-cumulation should not be scraped away but softened with oil and washed away with a cleansing agent.

Older children, too, need regular shampoos. Some hospitals require a special order from the doctor for this; others consider it a nursing judgment. The decision depends on the child's condition and the type of shampoo contemplated. If a soap-and-water shampoo cannot be used, one of the commercial, dry products may be substituted, although these are not as satisfactory.

There are a number of ways to give a hospitalized child a water shampoo. If a tub bath is given, the head can be washed at the same time. If the child can get onto a gurney, it can be rolled to a sink or tub and the head extended over the end while it is washed. If the child is bedfast, a trough can be formed from a rolled bed blanket formed into a curved U and draped with plastic to make it waterproof. This trough can lead off into a basin or tub beside the bed. Some hospitals use inflated Kelly pads and shampoo-only bedpans, whereas others have shampoo aprons similar to those found in beauty parlors.

Hair should be soaped at least twice and rinsed until it is squeaky clean. If it is tangled, a creme rinse may be helpful. After the shampoo the hair should be dried quickly between warm towels or with a hair drier and the child wrapped warmly to prevent chilling. When a child has an exotic hair style such as corn-rows the hair can be washed without undoing. Massage the scalp and pat to dry.

Daily brushing of the hair promotes circulation and gives a feeling of well-being. If this is neglected, the hair becomes tangled and matted with skin oils and wastes. Then it may be necessary to saturate it with vinegar or oil to untangle it. Long hair should be tied back and short hair brushed into its natural position. Daily hair care is a task ideally suited for the mother. It is a truly useful service she can do for her child more skillfully than anyone else. As the mother combs and brushes, the child feels her touch and experiences her care. If the mother cannot do the child's hair, the nurse must take time to do it.

The child's hair should never be cut without the parents' consent. But even with their permission, the hair that has been removed should be saved in a paper bag, clearly labeled, given to the parents, and the fact noted in the child's hospital record. All or most of the hair may be removed for surgical procedures or serious inflammation about the scalp. During the long growing-back period a boy may feel more comfortable with a cap and a girl with a wig.

Vital signs

The body temperature, pulse, respiration, and blood pressure are referred to as the "vital signs"
because of their importance as sensitive indicators of the child's condition. They are checked on admission and at frequent intervals throughout the child's hospital stay. If they are ever found to be abnormal or to have changed significantly, they should be checked again and reported to the nurse responsible for the child's care and recorded in the child's record.

Temperature. The body temperature is measured by means of a thermometer that is marked with either Fahrenheit (F) or centigrade (C) scales. There is no single "normal" temperature; instead, we speak of the "normal range" (Table 8-1). If a temperature falls below the normal range, it is called subnormal temperature; if it rises above the normal range, it is called a fever. A rise or fall of 1° from the previous reading should be checked with a second thermometer, and if the reading is confirmed, it should be reported at once.

The three most common methods of taking a temperature are by rectum, mouth, and axilla or groin. The most convenient place is the mouth or oral cavity. For this reason oral temperature readings have become standard. The most accurate readings are rectal; they are 1°F higher than oral readings (Fig. 8-10), but care must be taken to avoid damage to the rectal mucosa. The least accurate are axillary or groin readings; they are 1°F lower than oral readings. An indication of the method used should be made on the graphic sheet in the child's chart where temperatures are recorded.

A rectal temperature is usually routine for all children who cannot yet hold a thermometer in their mouths or for any others in whom, for the sake of safety or accuracy, the oral method cannot be used. These other cases include children who have seizures or poor muscular control and so might bite the thermometer, those who have difficulty keeping the mouth closed because of general weakness, oral surgery, or mouth breathing, and those receiving oxygen by any method. Rectal temperatures are contraindicated if the child has a rectal inflammation or has had rectal

Table 8-1. Body temperatures

	Rectal	Oral	Axillary or groin
Normal range	98.6° to 100° F (37° to 37.8° C)	97.6° to 99° F (36.4° to 37.2° C)	96.6° to 98° F (35.8° to 36.6° C)
Abnormal range			
Low-grade fever	100° to 101° F (37.8° to 38.4° C)	99° to 100° F (37.2° to 37.8° C)	98° to 99° F (36.6° to 37.2° C)
Moderate fever	101° to 104° F (38.4° to 40° C)	100° to 103° F (37.8° to 39.4° C)	99° to 102° F (37.2° to 38.8° C)
High fever	104° to 106° F (40° to 41° C)	103° to 105° F (39.4° to 40.6° C)	102° to 104° F (38.8° to 40° C)
Subnormal	Below 98° F (36.6° C)	Below 97° F (36.2° C)	Below 96° F (35.4° C)

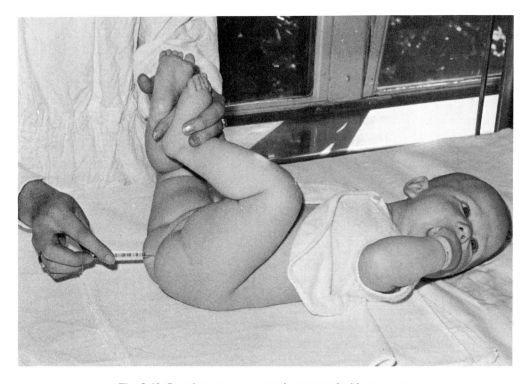

Fig. 8-10. Rectal temperatures must be measured with great care.

Table 8-2. Approximate heart rates, respiratory rates, and blood pressures of children at various ages

Age	Heart rate per minute	Respiratory rate per minute	Blood pressure (mm Hg) systolic/diastolic
Birth	140	40	70/50
6 months	110	30	90/60
1 year	100	28	90/60
3 to 4 years	95	25	100/70
5 to 10 years	90	24	105/70
11 to 15 years	85	20	110/70
Over 15 years	75 to 80	16 to 18	120/80

surgery. If neither oral nor rectal temperatures can be taken, an axillary or groin reading must be used, even though this method is the least reliable.

The specific technique for taking the temperature readings of infants and children varies with the hospital, but certain principles are true everywhere:

1. Never leave a small child while the thermometer is in place.
2. If there is any doubt about whether to take a rectal or oral temperature, take the rectal one. It is safer and more accurate. Broken thermometers are dangerous objects.
3. The oral temperature reading will be affected if cold or hot solutions have been in the cavity just before the insertion of the thermometer. Wait 10 minutes before taking the temperature.
4. Leave the thermometer in place until the reading remains constant, whether it is glass, electronic, or paper.
5. Cleanse soiled glass thermometers with firm friction in cool solution and shake down for reuse. In some hospitals soiled thermometers are cleansed in the supply room.

Pulse. Because the pulsations felt in the arteries radiate from the beating heart, they are an important indicator of the child's condition. The rhythm (pattern), rate, and force of the beat are affected by a number of factors, such as the following.

Age and size. Normally, the pulse rate slows as the child gets larger (Table 8-2).

Drugs. Certain drugs stimulate heart activity; others depress it.

Infections. When the body is invaded with infectious organisms, its usual reaction is to muster its resources to fight off the intruder. Often this reaction causes the heartbeat to increase.

Emotions. Strong emotion usually increases the heartbeat rate; depression slows it.

Activity. The pulse of the sleeping child is slower than that of the one who has just eaten or is playing.

Environment. Extremes of temperature cause the body to react in an attempt to normalize its temperature. This reaction makes the heart beat faster.

Because there are so many factors that influence the pulse rate, it should be counted under standardized conditions so that a representative count can be made. If the count must be made under other circumstances, the fact should be noted on the child's chart.

The procedure for taking the pulse is based on the knowledge that it can be best felt when the artery is pressed against a bone with even pressure. Commonly used pressure points are at the wrist (radial), on the temple, and at the ankle. The apical pulse is the heartbeat heard through a stethoscope directly over the apex of the heart

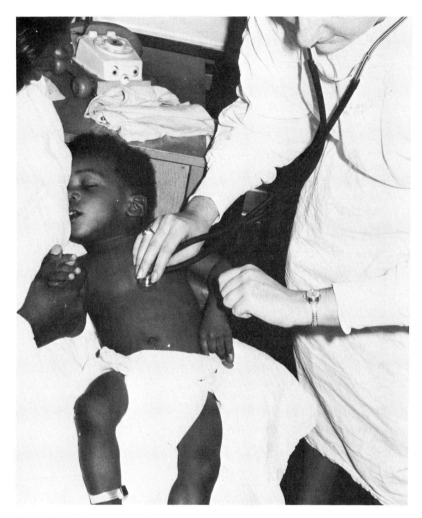

Fig. 8-11. Apical pulse. The comforting arms of his mother quiet this little boy and permit a more accurate count by the nurse.

(Fig. 8-11). The apical pulse is recommended for infants because their radial pulse is difficult to feel. The pulse is counted routinely for a full minute at the same time as the other vital signs on all children over 1 year of age. It is also counted for any infant receiving a drug or who has a disease affecting the circulatory system. The number of beats per minute, any irregularities, and the quality of the pulse should be recorded.

Respiration. The character and rate of the respiration give important information about the child's condition, because respiration is directly related to the body's need for oxygen. The factors that affect respiration are the same as those that affect the pulse, namely, age (Table 8-2), drugs, infections, emotions, activity, and environment. As with the pulse, the respirations should be evaluated under standardized conditions to give better information; that is, when the child is warm and relaxed.

The character of the respirations are particularly important. Some of the more important symptoms to note when observing respiratory effort are the following:

1. Noisy, crowing sounds as the expired air rushes over swollen obstructing tissue
2. Stertorous, snoring sounds made by air passing through secretions
3. Wheezing caused by narrowed passages that produce a whistle-like sound
4. Nasal flaring caused by inspiratory effort
5. Inspiratory stridor, or the restricted passage of air on inspiration
6. Labored, dyspneic breathing caused by oxygen hunger
7. Orthopneic breathing that requires a sitting posture
8. Cheyne-Stokes respiration, made when the critically ill child breathes rapidly and deeply for about 30 seconds, then stops breathing for about the same time, and then repeats the cycle.
9. Sternal retraction, causing a triangular indentation over the sternal area of the chest on inspiration; seen in infants with severe dyspnea
10. Shallowness or depth of the respiration
11. The amount of energy needed to breathe; the healthy child does not need to stop activity to breathe

The respirations are observed routinely at the same time as the other vital signs. The number per minute and unusual characteristics are recorded.

Blood pressure. Like the pulse and respiration, the blood pressure is affected by a variety of factors. For this reason the blood pressure should be taken when the child is warm and relaxed to give a representative reading. The child's blood pressure can be measured directly during such surgical procedures as heart catheterization or indirectly by means of the sphygmomanometer and stethoscope. Some facilities use electronic amplifiers to increase accuracy. (For children younger than 3 years of age and without an amplifer the indirect method is of little value.) The cuff size affects the accuracy of the reading. It should cover two thirds of the upper arm measured from the elbow to the shoulder. If the pulse sounds cannot be heard through the stethoscope, then the point at which the mercury column began to bounce or the needle began to twitch should be recorded and a notation made to that effect on the chart.

Food and fluids

The basic requirements for adequate nutrition are discussed in Chapter 3 and the feeding of newborn infants in Chapter 4. In this section we discuss the practical aspects of providing for the food and fluid needs of hospitalized children beyond infancy.

On admission of the child the physician leaves an order prescribing a diet. Common diets served in the pediatric area are clear liquid, full liquid, pureed, soft, high protein, high carbohydrate, low residue, diabetic with a stated number of grams of protein, carbohydrate, fat, and restricted salt with a stated amount or degree of sodium. Commercial preparations such as Justacal may be ordered to supplement the diet. The nursing leader sends the order to the dietitian with additional information about the child, including age, development, special handicaps, allergies, and any other facts supplied by the parents. The standard diets are then modified for each child. For example, a high-protein diet for a 1 year old who is allergic to milk would be quite different in texture, amount, and kind than would a high-protein diet planned for a 17-year-old football player.

The amount of food and fluids actually eaten by the child of that which is served makes up the *true* diet. Herein lies the important role of the nurse in carrying out the physician's orders and the dietitian's plan. In fulfilling this role the nurse must understand the vital part of hydration to the child's well-being and be skillful in mealtime management.

Hydration. Although the foods in a child's diet are important, the amount of fluids is even more so, especially for the young child or the one whose body loss of fluids is excessive. The amount of daily fluid intake depends on the size and condition of the child. An infant needs 70 ml of fluid per pound of body weight per day to maintain hydration, and needs more if suffering from excessive fluid loss or a preexisting dehydration. Older children need 1,500 to 2,000 ml per day, depending on their individual needs. Children who are immobilized in casts or traction apparatus and those with indwelling catheters need extra fluids because of their special elimination needs.

There are a number of ways to encourage a child to take fluids. The nurse should remember that small amounts taken frequently are retained better. Sometimes a special inducement such as a straw, a cup with a face at the bottom, or having a tea party will help a child increase intake. Older children respond to the challenge of drinking up to a certain goal, such as 2,000 ml during the day. In a negative way, the older child may respond to the fact that if not enough fluid is ingested, fluids must be given intravenously.

The kinds of fluids offered to a child depend on the diet order and any allergies the child may have. Clear fluids are any liquids that one can see clear through, such as water, strained fruit juice, soda, popsicles, gelatin, and bouillon. Full liquid diets include almost anything that can be swallowed without any chewing, such as creamed soups, milk shakes, milk products, sherbet, unstrained fruit juices, plus all of those listed for the clear liquid diet.

The child's fluid intake may be temporarily restricted for a variety of reasons. Infants with severe diarrhea and vomiting may be allowed nothing by mouth or only a limited amount to rest the gastrointestinal tract. Just before and just after surgery, fluids may be restricted to control the vomiting sometimes associated with an anesthetic. Fluids may be limited in connection with some heart and brain surgery to reduce total body fluids. When liquids cannot be given by mouth, they are usually administered parenter-

ally (see Chapter 10). The nurse can relieve some of the child's discomfort during these times by moistening or oiling the child's lips.

CAUTION: The child who is on restricted fluids may satisfy thirst by sneaking fluids. To prevent this occurrence, the child should be restricted to bed or watched very closely.

Because of the importance of fluids in the child's diet, *all* pediatric patients are routinely on measured fluid intake. This rule means that if a meal tray is removed, or any fluid is given to a child, including retention enemas, the nurse should be responsible for seeing that that amount is accounted for in the child's daily total. The administration of food and fluid by means other than by mouth is called parenteral therapy and is described in Chapter 10.

Mealtime management. Mealtime should be a happy time. Whenever possible, groups of children should be allowed to eat together, with adequate supervision, of course. If this is not possible, the nurse or parent should never just set a tray of food down in front of an ill child and walk away. The nurse or parent should stay nearby to encourage and, if weak or necessary, feed the child (Figs. 8-12 and 8-13).

When serving, the nurse should check each tray carefully to be sure it is the correct one for that child. Is there a salt shaker on a low-sodium diet, sugar on a diabetic diet, solid pieces of food for a toothless child, or cottage cheese on an allergic-milk diet? If so, the diet order should be checked and the offending item removed.

When the child has finished eating and wants no more, the tray should be removed promptly. Beets and carrots make bright-colored finger paints when they are no longer desired as food! The tray should be looked over to see how much was eaten. Fluid taken should be recorded on the child's daily total sheet. Diabetic trays are often returned to the kitchen for evaluation by the dietitian. The approximate amount eaten for that meal should be recorded as a percent. The food and fluid intake of the child is an important part of the treatment.

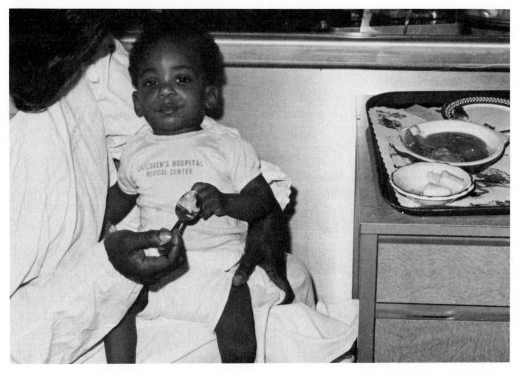

Fig. 8-12. Mealtime. Moms sometimes have the best success in patiently coaxing in one more bite of food.

Rest and positioning

The ill child needs rest. It is an important factor in the healing process. But rest is not necessarily assured just because the child is hospitalized. In fact, sometimes the pressured routines of the hospital actually prevent patients from getting adequate rest. They are bathed, fed, examined by the physician, and treated and medicated. By evening the ill child might well be exhausted if nurses are not conscientious about assuring that the child has adequate rest. The amount needed for each child depends on age and condition. To provide the proper amount, at least one nap time is set aside in the daily routine of all pediatric units; usually it is the hour following the noon meal. During this time ward activities stop, except for the most urgent ones. Shades are drawn, radios and televisions turned

off, playrooms vacated, and voices hushed, and every child, from the youngest to the oldest, is expected to rest quietly in bed. If parents are present during this time, they may be of help in cuddling and quieting their ill child.

Nap time is not the only time for resting. At home most children retire between 7 and 9 PM, and in the hospital a similar schedule is followed. Every effort is made to have the evening meal, tests, treatments, temperatures, and settling-down over early so that the children can get to sleep. An exception may be made for not-so-ill teenagers who normally keep later hours. One of the advantages of separating children in the pediatric unit according to age is that the older ones can have a different schedule from the younger ones. Even so, hospitalized teenagers should keep reasonable hours to ensure adequate rest.

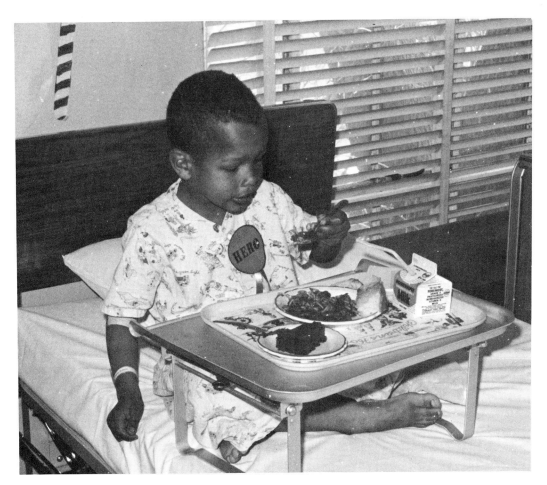

Fig. 8-13. This hungry boy just returned from the x-ray department where he won his "hero" badge for cooperation.

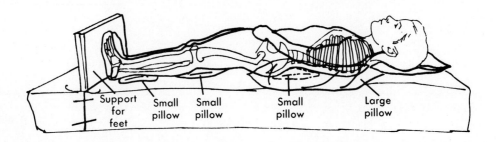

Support for feet — Small pillow — Small pillow — Small pillow — Large pillow

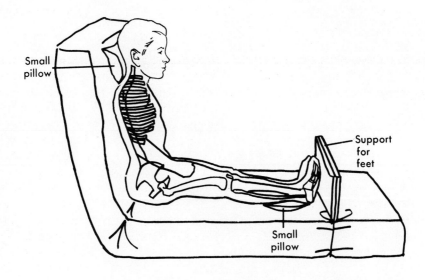

Small pillow

Support for feet

Small pillow

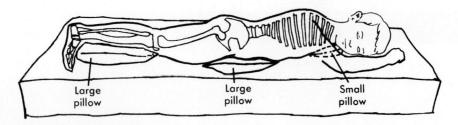

Large pillow — Large pillow — Small pillow

Fig. 8-14. Functional body positions showing how key body joints should be supported. Skin surfaces should be separated.

Rest and positioning are closely related. The comfortable child rests better because of good posture and can relax. Good posture means proper body alignment, whether the child is standing, sitting, or lying down. Both the ambulatory and the bedfast child should be encouraged (not nagged) to stand tall, sit up straight, and use all muscles to the maximum each day.

The bedfast child needs special help to maintain (1) proper body alignment, (2) range of motion of joints, (3) functional positions, and (4) healthy tissue for the whole body. Maintenance of all these measures takes conscious effort on the part of the nurse caring for children in every area of the pediatric unit, not just those caring for orthopedic patients.

Proper body alignment means that the bony frame of the body is holding the organ systems in their correct positions. In the "normal" posture the large muscles can relax, the lungs can expand fully, and the other organ systems can function properly.

The range of motion of each joint is that full, normal distance that it can move without stress. Because joints must be moved or they will become stiff, the major joints of the body should be put through their range of motion regularly. This can be done actively by the child moving the muscles and making the joints work, or it can be done passively by an outside effort that moves each joint through its range of motion. Unless there is a specific contraindication, range of motion exercise is a part of normal nursing care.

Functional positions are useful positions of the parts of the body in relation to other parts. These positions are of particular importance if a joint should become frozen (ankylosed). If the parts are immobilized in a useful relationship to one another, the condition is not as serious to the future life of the child as it would be if the joints ankylosed in a useless position. The key joints of the body where functional positions are of great importance are the neck, wrists, elbows, spinal column, hips, knees, and ankles. Fig. 8-

14 shows these areas, with notations for suggested ways to maintain them in functional positions.

Healthy tissue depends on general nutrition and adequate circulation of blood to the area. Weak, debilitated children are particularly susceptible, and pressure on a small area that prevents a constant blood supply may cause the cells to die, the tissue to slough away, and a decubitus ulcer, or pressure sore, to form. Improving the child's general nutrition, massaging the tissue to enhance blood circulation, and relieving pressure from bony prominences are important ways to prevent tissue breakdown.

Physical therapy

Physical therapy is the use of external physical means, such as electricity, water, radiation, light, diathermy, exercise, heat, and cold, to treat disease. Some of these forms of treatment have become so complex that they require special equipment and specially trained personnel, called physiotherapists, to administer them. When complex treatments are ordered, the child is transported to the physical therapy department or a therapist comes to the bedside. Some treatments are within the normal duties of the nurse, such as positioning and range of motion exercises discussed in the previous section and applications of hot and cold as they affect body temperature.

Body temperature alteration. Body heat is an evidence of life, a product of metabolism. In health the body temperature remains rather constant throughout life, rarely varying more than a degree or so. The mechanism responsible for this constant temperature is the body's thermostat, the *hypothalamus*. This remarkable nervous organ is situated in the brain and is constantly bathed in blood. It functions in the same way as any thermostat, "turning off" the heat when the blood around it gets too hot and "turning it on" when it gets too cold.

To turn on the heat, the sympathetic nerves of the hypothalamus stimulate metabolism and cause vasoconstriction, increased muscle tone, and piloerection (hairs standing on end). As a result body temperature rises until the preset level is reached and these activities are no longer stimulated.

Increased metabolism increases heat production.

Vasoconstriction conserves heat.

Increased muscle tone steps up the release of heat. The shivering so commonly associated with coldness is an evidence of this muscle activity.

Piloerection conserves heat by trapping large numbers of air molecules, thus giving the body insulation against the cold. (This is the same nervous response that makes the hairs stand on end in response to fright.)

To "turn off" body heat, the parasympathetic nerves in the hypothalamus are stimulated to do just the opposite of what the sympathetic ones did. They slow down metabolism, cause vasodilation, decrease muscle tone, and, in addition, cause the sweat glands to perspire, thus cooling the body surface by evaporation.

Fever indicates that all is not well within the body. It also acts to inhibit the growth of pathogens and to increase body repair by increased metabolism. It occurs when the body's thermostat has been reset in response to certain proteins released by pathogens or when body cells are damaged. The typical fever begins with chills and all of the other symptoms that occur when the body is too cold. When the fever "breaks," just the opposite occurs; the pores perspire profusely and vasodilation takes place. If the cause of the fever has been removed, the thermostat is reset to normal levels and the child again becomes afebrile, or without fever.

Brain tumors and other pressure sometimes disturb the normal functioning of the regulating mechanism, causing erratic temperature swings. All children tend to have more unstable temperatures than do adults and to respond more quickly and with higher fevers to infections, dehydration, and exposure to the sun or heat. A hard crying spell may even cause a temporary fever. One common response to fever in children is convulsion, called a "febrile convulsion" to denote its cause.

Because fever is so common among children, coldness may be ignored. There is a normal daily fluctuation in body temperature that is related to activity and metabolism. In the early morning after a night of sleep the body temperature is quite low. It increases slightly as the day progresses and then returns to its lowest point in the early hours of the morning. Afternoon fevers are typical of infections such as pulmonary tuberculosis. Abnormally low temperatures indicate circulatory collapse or a reduction of the basic body processes just before death.

The cold body has a lower metabolism and needs less oxygen. This principle is the basis for hypothermia, used with much success in recent years during and after heart surgery when the child's body temperature is lowered under controlled conditions to reduce his oxygen need. As the condition permits, the body temperature is increased to normal levels.

Body temperature is altered in a number of ways to produce certain therapeutic effects. Some of these methods include direct cooling of the blood as is done in open heart surgery, drug therapy, diathermy whereby deep penetrating high-frequency electrical current is applied, alteration of the total environmental temperature as in an incubator or chamber, and application of local heat or cold to the body.

Local application of heat. Heat is applied to the body to counteract cold, to relieve pain, and to localize abscess formation or hasten the drainage of an infected wound. The effects of the application of heat to the body are (1) a generalized body temperature rise, (2) increased metabolism, speeding up of bodily processes, (3) muscle relaxation, and (4) vasodilation, making the skin pink and warm.

Although these may be very desirable effects on some occasions, the application of heat is not without danger. The dangers are associated with the length of the application time, the patient's ability to react, the intensity, and the location of application. If the heat is applied for too long, the effects themselves may be reversed by a reflex nerve action that causes the blood vessels to constrict. In addition, the nerve endings may become less sensitive after a compress or lamp has been left in place for a while, and they may fail to relay pain stimuli until the skin has been badly burned. For these reasons the time of application should be limited to 1 hour and the interval between applications to at least 20 minutes. Paralyzed or young children are helpless to protect themselves from burning. Great caution and constant supervision are required if heat applications are ordered for these children.

The skin is damaged by temperatures over 110° F. Skin temperatures depend on the extent of exposure to the heat, the area exposed, the length of application time, the method used, and the temperature of the solution or the distance from the heat source. Fair-skinned persons and nontanned areas of the body are more sensitive to heat than those persons with more pigmentation. Because the goal of all heat treatment is to accomplish the desired effect without burning or damaging the child, the nurse should understand the purpose for the treatment and be constantly alert to any adverse symptoms.

CAUTION: When the child complains of a "tummyache," this might indicate inflamed appendix. If deep heat is applied, the inflammation could localize sufficiently to cause the appendix to rupture, with resultant peritonitis, a serious generalized infection. From this very real danger comes the rule: never apply heat to the abdomen for a "tummyache."

There are two general ways to apply heat locally—dry and moist. Dry heat provides continuous warmth without the problems associated with moisture on the skin or clothing, but moist heat is more penetrating and faster acting.

Dry heat. Dry heat may be administered by an electric heating pad, a pad through which warm water is circulated, or a blanket wrap to reduce

heat loss. Few hospitals allow electric heating pads because of the danger of electrical malfunction and the problems of disinfection. Hot-water bottles are not recommended either because of the instances of accidental burning that have resulted from their use. If hot-water bottles are used, the water temperature must be carefully measured, never being hotter than 115° F for infants or young children and 120° F for older children and adults. After being filled with water, the bottle should be emptied of excess air, its stopper tightened, tested for leaks, enclosed in a warm, dry cover, and then applied cautiously. Hot-water bottles should never be placed directly on the skin.

The most acceptable method for administering dry heat or for maintaining the temperature of moist heat has become the circulating water pad, known as the aqua pad. With this device, heat is applied to the patient by means of disposable pads of various sizes through which warm water is pumped at a preset temperature from a bedside heating unit. The apparatus uses distilled water that is periodically added to a reservoir at the top of the heating-pumping unit. The warm water flows through tubes embedded in the pad and returns to the heating unit. The pad is secured in place by means of ties, not bent so as to interfere with the circulation of the water, and *never* pinned. The disposable pads do not need to be covered to protect the child's skin. Manufacturer's instructions come with each unit.

Moist heat. Moist heat may be applied locally in the form of hot packs, soaks, or compresses. Hot packs involve the use of heavy, moist pieces of wool or flannel that have been spun or wrung very dry and applied to muscle groups to relieve spasm. When properly insulated, they hold the heat for long periods of time. Widely used during the days of the poliomyelitis epidemic, hot packs are seldom necessary today.

Hot soaks are the submerging of a part or the whole of the body in a solution for the purpose of providing local heat, cleansing, softening crusts or plaster casts, and facilitating drainage from a wound. The solution may be normal saline (0.9% salt), tap, sterile, or medicated water. Unless ordered otherwise, the temperature range should be between 95°F (35°C) and 105°F (40.5°C) and the duration of the soak 20 minutes. If a large area of the body is involved, the tub may be the most practical place; if a smaller area is involved, a basin or bowl may be used. The tub or basin should be cleansed well before and after use. To prevent infection of an open lesion, a sterile basin or a disinfected tub is recommended. If extensive hydrotherapy is ordered, the child is usually transported to the physiotherapy department where there are deep tubs, whirlpools, and other facilities.

Hot compresses are applied to specific areas of the body to speed abscess formation, promote wound drainage, and improve circulation. If the skin area to be compressed is broken, sterile gauze should be used. Because compress temperatures are 110° to 115° F, they must be wrung dry. Dripping solution of that heat might burn tender skin. Compresses should be changed when they cool, depending on the thickness and heat-holding capacity of the material used. Bedding should be protected from moisture. When continuous compresses are ordered, the involved part may be wrapped in an insulating towel and warmed by an overlying aqua pad or hot-water bottle. In some situations dry gauze is placed over the area to be compressed and warm solution is irrigated into the area with a sterile syringe, thus eliminating the need to wring out wet sponges in a bowl. When the skin is not broken, petroleum jelly may be ordered and applied to the skin to protect it from continuous moisture.

CAUTION: Small children should be protected from the hot solution used for compressing. Active young children must be supervised closely during any type of compress treatment to be sure the compress stays in the correct position.

Local application of cold. Cold is applied to the body to counteract fever, cool deeper tissue and muscle, give a temporary anesthesia to an area, reduce swelling, and slow down an inflammatory process. The effects of the local application of cold are (1) a generalized fall in body temperature, (2) a slowing of metabolism, thus slowing bodily processes, (3) vasoconstriction, reducing blood supply, and (4) numbing of the nerve endings. A lower than normal body temperature (hypothermia) can be just as dangerous to children as hyperthermia.

Like that of heat, the application of cold is not without danger. The dangers are associated with the length of application time, the degree of coldness, and the patient's ability to react. If cold is applied for too long, a reflex nerve action causes the vessels to dilate and the effects are reversed. For this reason cold should not be applied for more than 1 hour, with intervals that allow the skin's temperature and color to return to normal. Mottled skin signals danger. Cold applications to areas in which circulation is inadequate may produce frostbite, which may lead to gangrene. Because cold has a numbing or anesthetic effect on the nerves, a patient may be unaware of injury either from the cold itself or from other injurious factors. Regular inspection of the skin and supervision of the patient receiving cold therapy are essential to safety.

There are two general ways to apply cold locally—dry and moist. Moist cold is more penetrating than dry and its effects more rapid because it has the added cooling effect of evaporation. Dry cold can be used over a longer period of time. The two methods are often used together to enhance the total effect.

Dry cold. Dry cold may be administered by an ice bag, collar, or cap or by means of a hypothermia pad through which a coolant solution is circulated. Ice bags, collars, or caps may be of two types—those that must be filled with ice just before use and those that have a sealed-in coolant that are kept in the freezer ready for use. When filling the ice-chip variety, the nurse fills it only partway, adds some cold water, empties off excess air, stoppers it tightly, and tests for leaks. All ice containers should be enclosed in a cover to prevent condensation from wetting the bedding and to protect the child's skin. Every hour all cold should be removed for observation and the skin allowed to warm to its normal state, thus enabling the cold to continue its vasoconstricting action when reapplied.

A *hypothermia blanket* or pad is constructed like the aqua pad, with embedded tubes through which cold water or a mixture of alcohol and water circulates. Various sizes are available. Sometimes they are placed both over and under the child, depending on the degree of hypothermia desired. The temperature of the pad is adjusted to the temperature of the patient, either manually by the nurse or mechanically by a rectal probe that continually monitors the child's temperature and adjusts the pad temperature to a predetermined setting. A light blanket or sheet is placed between pad and patient. No pins should be used to secure the pad, nor should it be folded or bent. The child's general reaction and vital signs must be watched closely during hypothermia. If the child shivers violently, the effects of the cold are counteracted.

Moist cold. Moist cold may be applied locally in the form of compresses, soaks, ice packs, or sponge baths or internally by a cooling enema.

Cold compressing is ordered to relieve pain and reduce swelling. The materials used depend on the child's condition. If the child can tolerate the weight, a clean washcloth or towel is ideal; if not, light gauze squares may be used. After the bed is protected from moisture, a compress is saturated with ice cold water in a basin, wrung out well, and put in place. To take advantage of the cooling effect of evaporation and because the body heat soon neutralizes the cold, compresses are left exposed. They are changed when they become tepid. Soiled compresses should not be reused.

When the skin is broken in the area to be compressed, sterile technique is necessary. Sterile solution may be kept in a refrigerator or the container placed on ice at the bedside. For handling sterile compresses, sterile gloves are recommended over forceps because gloves are more

efficient and safer around the eyes and face of active children.

Cold soaks are the submerging of a part of the body, such as a sprained ankle, in cold water to reduce pain and swelling. Occasionally alternating cold and hot soaks are ordered to stimulate circulation. The cold-soaking period should not last longer than 20 minutes at a time.

Ice packs are the submerging of the entire body in ice and water to reduce body temperature. They are used when hypothermia blankets are not available and large amounts of ice are available. A tub is filled one fourth full of ice and covered with half the width of a bath blanket. The other half is rolled to the side to cover the child when placed in the tub. The child is wrapped in another bath blanket and lowered onto the blanket covering the ice. The upper half of the blanket is then folded over the child and covered with 2 inches of crushed ice. Water is then added to moisten the whole pack. Continuous nursing care is required, with checks for excessive shivering or irregularity of the pulse or respirations. The length of the procedure depends on the child's reaction. When the child's temperature is reduced sufficiently, the child is returned to bed.

Cooling sponge baths are given to increase evaporation and reduce body temperature. They are a frequent ally of the pediatric nurse in combating high fevers. Ice may be added to the water if desired. A waterproof sheet is placed under and a bath blanket over the child. Because convulsions are common with high fevers, an ice cap should be placed under the child's head to help reduce cerebral congestion and lessen the possibility of seizure. If excessive shivering occurs, the increased muscle activity may be enough to maintain the high temperature. To avoid this negative effect, the nurse should keep the half of the body not being sponged covered. In addition, some texts recommend a warm water bottle to the feet during the bath. Before beginning to sponge, the nurse should rub the skin of the child's extremities and torso with a dry washcloth to bring the blood to the surface. This decreases the shivering response and aids in heat reduction when the cool moisture is applied. The face and neck are washed. The side farthest from the nurse is then exposed. Two washcloths are wrung out so that they are not dripping and one placed in the groin and one in the axilla of the side being sponged. They help cool the blood as it passes near the surface of the skin in larger blood vessels. Using steady, long strokes, the nurse sponges the arm, chest, abdomen, and leg. The groin and axillary cloths are removed and that side covered, then the procedure is repeated on the near side of the child. The child is turned and the back sponged. Periodically during the sponge bath the child's condition is evaluated for color, irregularity of pulse and respiration, and excessive shivering. If these occur, the treatment is stopped, the child covered, and the symptoms reported to the supervising nurse. If no adverse reaction occurs, the skin is patted dry at the end of the sponge bath, the child dressed in a light gown, the waterproofing removed, and the child covered with a light sheet or blanket and allowed to rest. The child's temperature, pulse, and respiration should be taken 30 minutes after the sponge bath and reported to the supervising nurse or doctor.

Another method commonly used to reduce fever is the cooling enema, whereby cool tap water is administered intermittently into the rectum. It is effective in reducing fever and providing fluids to reduce dehydration by absorption through the rectal mucosa. Infants under 6 months of age usually do not tolerate more than 100 ml of fluid administered at one time. With increasing age, larger quantities can be used—up to 500 ml by adolescence. A small French catheter is less stimulating than a large rectal tube, and so is preferred. The child can be placed on the side or back and supported by a pillow so that the buttocks extend over a bedpan or curved basin. After expelling the air from the tubing, the nurse inserts the catheter into the rectum. The solution is introduced slowly with little force by either a gravity flow or a large syringe. Young children will expel the fluid immediately, whereas older ones may be able to retain it. The enema is repeated as ordered. Sometimes the fluid is drained off by means of a Y connection to a waste container and fresh cold solution introduced. The temperature should be checked after 30 minutes and any significant amount of fluid retained should be recorded as "intake."

Psychological therapy

All children undergo emotional stress as a result of hospitalization. The normal reaction to separation is discussed in Chapter 7. When a child is hospitalized for more severe emotional disturbances or if such disturbances should develop, the pediatric nursing staff needs the special guidance of the physician or a psychological consultant.

While being provided therapy, each child is cared for as an individual. Frequent conferences are held between the nurses and the doctor, during which the various manifestations of the child's disturbance, the reactions of the nurses to them, and the goals and plan for treatment are discussed.

Occupational therapy

Occupational therapy is a specialty that is primarily concerned with the stimulation and maintenance of manipulative skills in persons whose fine-muscle and joint coordination is hampered by injury or disease. Particular emphasis is placed on stimulating muscles that aid in carrying out the activities of daily living. The occupational therapist works closely with the doctor in setting goals for treatment, taking into consideration the child's age and disability. Special appliances are devised to help malfunctioning hands hold combs and eating utensils (Fig. 8-15). Many crafts and games are used to motivate and involve the child in such activities. The therapist must exercise great patience while working with these children toward more useful lives. The understanding and cooperation of the

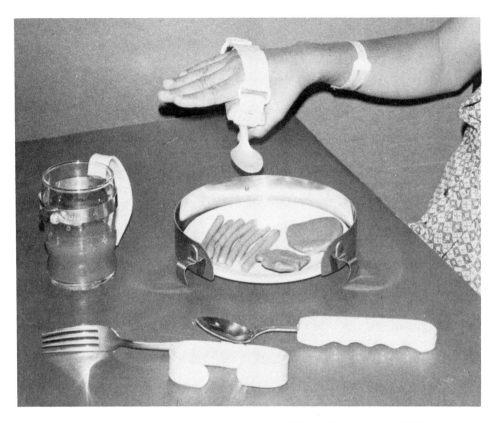

Fig. 8-15. Devices used in occupational therapy to make possible self-feeding for the disabled child. Note the metal frame to keep the plate from sliding.

parents is encouraged so that when the child returns home the therapy will continue.

Other specialties

Recreation, speech, and hearing specialists and bedside teachers provided by the public schools are among others who may be called on to meet the hospitalized child's needs. Although the services of these specialists must be approved by the doctor, the need for them may first be recognized by the bedside nurse who cares for the child from day to day. In recent years some hospitals serving children have created Child Life Departments that combine the services of psychological and occupational therapy, recreation, and other specialties.

Nursing observations

One of the important roles of pediatric nurses is to be a keen observer. Their observations provide valuable information about the child's condition that aid in diagnosis and treatment. To make meaningful observations, nurses must know about the common signs and symptoms of illness and how to accurately report and record them. These symptoms are sometimes treated separately from the disease that caused them. Nurses need to understand the basic physiological causes for these symptoms and the treatment usually given to relieve them. Table 8-3 is provided to assist the nurse in identifying and describing common signs and symptoms.

Nursing observations are reported and re-

Table 8-3. Common childhood signs and symptoms

Signs or symptoms	Descriptive terms	Definition and/or physiological cause
General conditions		
Pain	Intense Pounding Radiating Sharp, dull Localized	A defense mechanism of the body, caused by transmission of stimuli to cerebral cortex of brain; one of the cardinal symptoms of inflammation
Fever	High Moderate Low grade Afebrile Crisis	Elevation of body temperature above normal; it is increased heat production and decreased heat elimination No fever A high fever dropping suddenly to normal
Chills	Severe Moderate Slight Prolonged	A reaction of the body to toxins in it, similar to that produced by extreme cold, caused by an irritation of the hypothalamus, usually occurs at the onset of high fevers
Convulsions	Generalized Localized Clonic tremor Tonic tremor	Alternating contraction and relaxation of the voluntary muscles, caused by disturbance of normal central nervous system impulses, also called paroxysms Shaking, with intervals of rest Continuous shaking
Gastrointestinal conditions		
Anorexia	Mild Severe	Abnormal loss of appetite caused by a number of emotional and physical causes; often described in terms of appetite, as fair, poor
Nausea	Occasional Persistent Psychic Induced	Inclination or desire to vomit Occurs repeatedly Caused by emotions Produced purposefully, by emetic drug, etc.
Vomiting	Wretching Severe Blood tinged Projectile	Forceful ejection of gastric contents through mouth, caused by combination of nervous stimulation and muscle action; also called emesis Ejected a distance of several feet
Regurgitation	Occasional Persistent	Act of returning food to the mouth from stomach immediately after ingestion; often occurs when infants are overfed
Rumination	Occasional Habitual	Return of food to mouth from stomach for purposes of rechewing or retasting it
Constipation	Habitual Mild Severe	Sluggish action of bowels, resulting from megacolon, emotional anxiety, poor habits, inactivity; may lead to a fecal impaction
Diarrhea	Acute Chronic Blood tinged Frothy Mucous	Defecation of loose, watery, unformed stools, caused by diet, drugs, or irritation of mucosa of intestine

Table 8-3. Common childhood signs and symptoms—cont'd

Signs or symptoms	Descriptive terms	Definition and/or physiological cause
Gastrointestinal conditions—cont'd		
Diarrhea—cont'd	Clay colored	Black stool caused by old blood
	Tarry	
Nose		
Epistaxis	Frequent	Bleeding from nose caused by break in nasal vessel walls, may be caused by increased pressure as during a coughing spasm, by picking, or by fragile vessel walls as in some diseases
	Periodic	
Respiratory system		
Coughing	Continuous	A violent expiratory effort preceded by a preliminary inspiration, caused by irritation of nerves in bronchial tree
	Persistent	
	Painful	
	Hacking	
	Whooping	
	Crowing	
	Productive	
Croup	Mild	An inflammation of larynx causing a noisy stridulous breathing
	Severe	
Hiccoughing	Persistent	Spasmodic contractions of diaphragm causing short, noisy inspiratory coughs, caused by abnormal stimulation of phrenic nerve
	Intermittent	
	Continuous	
Dyspnea	Mild	Difficult breathing, effort of child to prevent anoxia
	Severe	
Anoxia	Chronic	Deficiency in oxygen caused by blood changes, cardiac malformation, metabolic rate increases, emotional upset, or lung impairment
	Temporary	
	Cyanosis	Dusky, blue color of skin resulting from anoxia
Skin		
Rash	Mottled	Any eruption of skin, usually temporary; also called erythema, or redness
	Dry, moist	
	Abraided	Scraped area of skin
	Petechia	Small hemorrhage spot in skin
	Macule	Discolored spot
	Papule	Pimple
	Vesicle	Blister
	Pustule	Pimple filled with pus
Jaundice	Mild	Yellow color of skin caused by increased amount of bilirubin in blood
	Severe	
Nevus (birthmark)	Elevated	Mark existing on the body from birth
	Circumscribed	Raised above surrounding skin
	Vascular	Well-defined edges
	Hair covered	Prominent blood vessels
	Wartlike	Hair growing from area
		Horny, like a wart

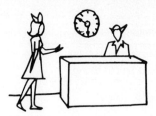

1. Arrive on time at the nursing station of the pediatric unit

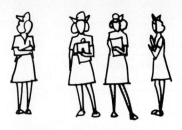

2. Receive report, medical orders, and nursing directives for each child assigned to your care

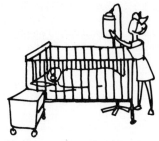

3. Take a tour to see your children during which you:
   a. Meet your patients
   b. Check for the safety of the children, including siderails, restraints, and toys
   c. Check the equipment around them, including that required for intravenous fluids, oxygen, humidity, and traction
   d. Evaluate need for supplies, such as linens, dressings, clothing, and special equipment
   e. Help with breakfast trays as needed

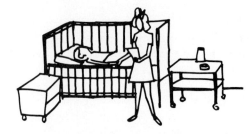

4. Evaluate the needs of your patients for priority and sequence of care, using the following criteria:
   a. Prior appointments that have been made for radiography, surgery, special therapists, and bedside teacher
   b. General condition of the child — caring for the least comfortable first, the quiet and nonacute cases last
   c. Types of treatment that the child is to have that day, such as blood transfusions, enemas, and shampoos; do sterile dressings after ward activity is at a minimum
   d. Hospital routines that come at regular hours such as meals and measurement of vital signs

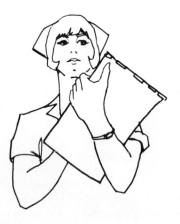

5. Plan your day's work with some degree of flexibility, knowing that change is a characteristic of children's illness

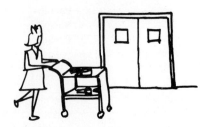

6. Go about your day's work, with neither an empty hand nor an empty head, but with enthusiasm, skill, and good humor

Fig. 8-16. The pediatric nurse begins the day.

corded so that they will be available to all who are responsible for treating the child. To reach the pediatrician, the nurse must make use of appropriate channels for communication. Information of an acute nature should be reported at once, orally, and then recorded on the child's chart. In pediatric units where team nursing is employed, information is reported to the team leader. When functional and individual nursing plans are employed, information is usually reported to the supervising or head nurse. In primary nursing, associates report to the primary nurse who takes appropriate action. (See the discussion on nursing care organization earlier in this chapter.)

Written records of nursing observations are an important part of care. A variety of forms have been developed on which to record information, such as graphs for vital signs, checklists for routine types of care or treatments, tally sheets for cumulative totals as for medications and for intake and output, and lined spaces for nurses' and doctors' comments. These forms vary from hospital to hospital. When nurses begin to work in any pediatric unit, they should acquaint themselves with the forms, practices, and policies used there.

The principles for recording nursing observations are as follows:

1. Records must be accurate. All information must be as precise and correct as humanly possible.
2. Records should be descriptive. Nurses describe what is observed and make nursing diagnoses; physicians make medical diagnoses.
3. Records should be appropriate and significant. Irrelevant information should be eliminated. The beginning nurse should ask the instructor or supervisor if in doubt about the importance of some observation.
4. Records should be complete and concise. Unnecessary words should be eliminated, but not at the expense of clarity or content.
5. Records should indicate the time. A date and hour should be a part of each notation.
6. Records must be legible. The unreadable notation is valueless; fancy frills are inappropriate. Special care should be taken in writing numbers clearly.

Planning daily care

Pediatric nurses carry great responsibility as they care for their small patients from day to day. To accomplish a seemingly impossible number of tasks, they must organize their work carefully. If they do this according to a system of priorities, deciding what is most important, their schedules will become flexible enough to cope with the ever-changing needs of children. A well-thought-through plan of daily care pays dividends in peace of mind and efficiency of effort (Fig. 8-16).

SURGERY AND THE CHILD
Psychological preparation

The psychological preparation of the child for hospital admission discussed earlier in this chapter is an integral part of preparation for surgery. Parents play an important part in that preparation. Nurses can help parents by their attitude of understanding and acceptance and by a calm optimism based on confidence in the medical staff. Such a cheerful expectancy helps combat fear and build hope.

Physical preparation

Before surgery the child's condition is evaluated for respiratory infections and nutritional deficiencies. If these are present, surgery may be delayed until the child's general condition improves.

Physical preparation for surgery usually begins the night before, emergencies excepted. If the child is to be admitted the morning of surgery, preliminary laboratory tests are done ahead of time and parents prepare the child according to instructions from the doctor. Most patients are admitted the afternoon before surgery to allow adequate time for completion of necessary procedures.

Preoperative hospital requirements include the signing of permission forms by a parent or guardian and routine laboratory analysis of blood and urine.

Specific doctor's orders vary according to the surgery to be performed, but they may be divided into the following three general areas of preparation: (1) skin, rectum, and bladder, (2) tests, supplies, x-ray examinations, and consultations, and (3) food, fluids, and drugs.

If orthopedic or plastic skin surgery is to be done, the child is given a tub bath with careful washing and inspection of the operative site. Fingernails and toenails of any extremity to be involved are trimmed. Shaving of the operative site may be done the night before surgery. Cleansing enemas are ordered in some cases. On rare occasions the child is catheterized just before surgery, but if not, the child should be encouraged to void. An infant should go to surgery with dry diapers.

In addition to routine urinalysis and blood count, a variety of x-ray films and tests may be ordered before surgery. Specialists may be called in to consult with the pediatrician. When extensive diagnostic workups are required, the child may be admitted to the hospital several days before surgery. If blood is ordered for surgery, it must first be cross-matched with the child's. After surgery is scheduled, the anesthetist examines the child and prescribes the preoperative medications to be given.

Food and oral fluids are usually withheld 6 to 12 hours before surgery, particularly when a general anesthesia is to be administered, because of the potential danger of aspired vomitus. A precautionary sign saying "nothing by mouth" is conspicuously posted by the bed, and in addition children should be told of the fact so that they do not think they have been forgotten when trays are passed. Teeth are also a potential danger if they are aspirated. Loose or missing ones should be noted on the child's chart.

Preoperative drugs are usually administered in two stages—the sedative, given about 2 hours before surgery, and the analgesic and atropine mixture, administered "on call," when surgery calls for the patient. After the sedative is given, every effort should be made to reduce noise and bright lights so that the child may rest.

After the child is taken to surgery, the parents should be directed to a waiting room or the cafeteria for food and relaxation. They will want to know when and where they will see their child again. Some means of giving parents this information is provided in each hospital. The nurse should know what it is so that anxious parents may be informed.

While the child is in surgery, the return unit is prepared, according to postoperative needs. Special equipment is collected, including an intravenous standard, suction machine, oxygen and humidifying equipment, and restraints. Orthopedic patients may need bed boards under the mattress, an overbed frame and trapeze, and extra waterproofed pillows. Frequently beds of orthopedic patients are taken to surgery, and the child is placed directly on the bed from the operating table and positioned by the surgeon.

Postoperative care

Immediate postoperative care is usually provided in the recovery room. When blood pressure is stable and the patient has roused sufficiently from general anesthesia, the patient is moved to the return unit. If it is a different location from his preoperative one, the child may become disoriented. Disorientation can be lessened if the child sees a familiar face or the move is explained ahead of time.

The following care should be given to the postoperative child by the nurse:

1. Note the child's general condition, state of consciousness and restfulness.
2. Check for signs of shock—rapid pulse; cold, clammy skin; pallor; and dilated pupils.
3. Take the pulse, respiration, and blood pressure periodically. If there is a sudden change, report it immediately.
4. Keep the child on the abdomen with the head

turned to the side and with no pillow, unless contraindicated by surgery. This position allows mucus and vomitus to flow out of the mouth instead of into the lungs.

5. Restrain as necessary to prevent disruption of needles, tubing, or sutures.
6. Check dressings, their location, condition, and drainage, if any. Record findings.
7. Connect urinary drainage and see that the flow is unobstructed. Measure and record the amount periodically. If no urinary catheter is in place, check for voiding. Report anuria of more than 4 to 6 hours.
8. Check intravenous infusions for correct rate of flow and any infiltration. Record amount received.

The decision as to when to introduce oral fluids and food to the postoperative child depends on the child's condition and is made by the doctor. Sometimes fluids and food are withheld for several days, during which time the child is fed intravenously. When oral feedings are introduced, they are changed gradually, according to the child's tolerance and age, beginning with clear liquids and progressing to full liquids and then soft and finally regular foods. Only nonspicy, easily digested foods are included in a surgical diet.

After surgery, toddlers and young children usually move about in their cribs without difficulty, and if allowed, ambulate with relative ease. Older children act more like adults postoperatively. They may be afraid of pain and reluctant to move or get up, and so they may need to be assisted and encouraged. Early postoperative ambulation is of great benefit to the functioning of each of the body systems. Except for special cases, most patients ambulate the day after surgery and even sooner in some cases. When it is impossible for a child to get out of bed, the child should be turned frequently, receive good skin care, and encouraged to take deep breaths at regular intervals. To aid lung expansion, the doctor may order a type of inhalation therapy called intermittent positive pressure breathing (IPPB).

Except for children who must undergo extensive plastic surgery, the hospital stay of most surgical patients is brief. They recover rapidly and go home to their families in a few days.

DISMISSAL

When the doctor decides that a child is ready to go home, an order to that effect is written in the child's chart. The doctor may also leave a variety of other instructions, an appointment for a return visit to the office, and prescriptions for medications that are to be taken home with the child. The doctor may recommend the services of a visiting nurse when there is a need for special teaching or complex treatments. In other circumstances parents may be encouraged to come to the hospital on several consecutive days in advance of dismissal for instruction on some phase of the child's care, such as colostomy irrigation. Whenever it is possible, the child is taught to assume responsibility for personal care with only a minimum of adult supervision. For example, they are taught to give their own insulin injections.

In addition to the preparations for home care of the child during convalescence, the parents must arrange for safe transportation from the hospital. An adolescent in a body cast will probably require an ambulance, but most children can go home in the family car or a taxicab.

The day and approximate hour of dismissal are agreed on in advance by the parents, the doctor, and the hospital staff. The morning hours are more convenient because the hospital must prepare for new admissions that arrive in the afternoon. In most hospitals the parents must first go to the business office to take care of the bill and sign a release for their child. They then proceed to the nursing station where they are given any medications, appointments, or instructions. These instructions should be written down so that the parents can read them later when they are less distracted.

Regulations of the Joint Commission on Accreditation of Hospitals require that hospitals show evidence that patients have received discharge instructions and that they understand those instructions.

If the nursing staff knows in advance of the approximate time the parents will come for their child, planning is greatly facilitated. When all is ready the nurse (1) gathers up the child's belongings, including clothing, toys, and treatment supplies, (2) dresses the child in the child's own clothing, (3) gives the parents last-minute information about what meals the child has had, treatments, and care, (4) places the child in a wheelchair or cart or on a gurney, (5) checks one last time with the supervising nurse, (6) sees that the child is accompanied to the hospital exit and into the waiting transportation, and (7) records the facts about the dismissal in the child's record.

The dismissal notations in the chart should include the following information:

1. Time of departure
2. How the child was transported, as "by gurney" or "by wheelchair"
3. To whom the child was dismissed, as "to the parents"
4. Any important descriptive notes, as "with casted left arm in a sling"
5. Notation about what prescription drugs or instructions were given to the parents

SUMMARY OUTLINE

  I. The pediatric unit
    A. The physical plant
      1. Psychological support
      2. Physical comfort and safety
      3. Medical treatment and care
    B. The pediatric team
    C. Nurse-child-parent relationship
    D. Nursing care organization
  II. The nursing process
    A. Assessment
    B. Planning
    C. Implementation
    D. Evaluation
    E. Responsibility for the nursing process
  III. Isolation technique
    A. Terminology
    B. Infection chain

      1. Infectious organisms
      2. Reservoirs of infection
      3. Portals of exit
      4. Transmission means
      5. Portals of entry
      6. Susceptible hosts
    C. Breaking the links of the infection chain
    D. Categories of isolation
      1. Strict isolation
      2. Respiratory isolation
      3. Protective (reverse) isolation
      4. Enteric isolation
      5. Wound and skin precautions
      6. Discharge precautions
      7. Blood precautions
    E. Nursing roles in controlling infection
    F. The principle of isolation technique
    G. The practice of isolation technique
      1. General precautions
      2. Personal precautions
      3. Isolation unit
      4. Isolation cart
      5. Masks and gloves
      6. Gowns
        a. Gowning and handwashing
        b. Donning the gown
        c. Removing the gown and handwashing
        d. Leaving the isolation area
      7. Technique papers and small plastic bags
      8. Meal service
      9. Linen and diaper care
     10. Waste disposal
     11. Toys, books, and religious articles
     12. Recording nursing observations
     13. Disinfection
     14. Organization of nursing care
    H. Effects of isolation on children and their parents
  IV. Admission
    A. Preparation of the child and the family
      1. General preparation
        a. Of parents
        b. Of children
        c. Methods
      2. Specific preparation
    B. Preparation of the hospital
    C. Procedure
      1. Hospital admission and identification
      2. Pediatric admission
        a. Undressing and dressing
        b. Establishing rapport
        c. Weighing and measuring
        d. Vital signs
        e. Restraints

f. Urine specimen
g. Settling the child
h. Orienting the parents
i. Hospital records
    (1) Bed card
    (2) Kardex cards
    (3) Chart
j. Nursing care plan
V. Basic needs and daily care
  A. Safety
    1. Restraints
        a. Waist restraints
        b. Sleeve restraints
        c. Elbow restraints
        d. Wrist and ankle restraints
        e. Mummy restraints
        f. Jacket restraints
        g. Positioning-holds used as restraints
        h. Wheelchair and gurney restraints
    2. Bassinets, cribs, and side rails
    3. Precautionary signs
    4. Toys and hazardous objects
        a. Plastic bags
        b. Sharp objects or toys with sharp parts
        c. Small objects
        d. Lead paint
        e. Toy stuffing
    5. Continuous observation
  B. Personal hygiene and weight measurement
    1. Oral hygiene
    2. Bathing
        a. Tub bathing
        b. Sponge or bed bathing
    3. Dressing
    4. Hair and scalp
  C. Vital signs
    1. Temperature
    2. Pulse
        a. Age or size
        b. Drugs
        c. Infections
        d. Emotions
        e. Activity
        f. Environment
    3. Respiration
    4. Blood pressure

  D. Food and fluids
    1. Hydration
    2. Mealtime management
  E. Rest and positioning
  F. Physical therapy
    1. Body temperature alteration
    2. Local application of heat
        a. Dry heat
        b. Moist heat
    3. Local application of cold
        a. Dry cold
        b. Moist cold
  G. Psychological therapy
  H. Occupational therapy
  I. Other specialties
  J. Nursing observations
  K. Planning daily care
VI. Surgery and the child
  A. Psychological preparation
  B. Physical preparation
  C. Postoperative care
VII. Dismissal

STUDY QUESTIONS

1. Describe a pediatric unit that meets the psychological and physical needs of the child.
2. Define the pediatric team and explain individual, functional, primary, and team nursing.
3. Who is responsible for the total nursing process?
4. Define asepsis, sepsis, disinfection, carrier. Explain the differences between strict, protective, and reverse isolation.
5. Describe the steps in admitting and dismissing a child in the pediatric unit in the hospital where you work.
6. State the average normal range of temperature, pulse, respiration, and blood pressure for a child 3 years of age. Beside age, what are the indications for taking the temperature rectally? orally? How much of the arms should be covered by the blood pressure cuff to ensure accuracy?
7. Describe the routine for beginning a typical day in the pediatric unit.

REFERENCE

Joint Commission on Accreditation of Hospitals: Accreditation manual for hospitals, Chicago, 1981, The Commission.

9
Diagnostic tests

VOCABULARY

Fractional urine specimen
Fasting
Parasites
Subarachnoid space
Ventriculogram
Lavage
Aspiration
Excision

Diagnostic tests play an important part in modern pediatric care. They enable nurses and physicians to more quickly and accurately identify the cause of illness and to institute prompt treatment. The variety, number, and complexity of these tests increase constantly, as do the consequences of their results. Although nurses seldom actually perform the tests, their role in the collection of specimens and preparation of the patient is of great importance.

All diagnostic tests can be grouped into two broad categories—tests of specimens taken from the child and tests, measurements, and x-ray examinations of the child's body as it functions. The principle behind all testing is the *comparison of standardized data*, that is, the comparison of the test results of the ill child with those of well children under similar circumstances. Unless the conditions are standardized, the test results cannot be compared accurately and so they become invalid. The responsibility for standardized conditions rests with the nurses. They must see that in both the collection of specimens and the preparation of the child the prescribed conditions for each test are met. To meet the conditions, they must have information about each test. Such information is usually supplied by the hospital laboratory on request or is available to the nurses on the pediatric unit. Information about some of the most common diagnostic tests is provided in the last section of this chapter.

COLLECTION OF SPECIMENS

The excretory products, blood, gastric juices, mucus, spinal fluid, and tissues of the body are all examined and tested in an effort to identify disease. The urine and blood are of such importance in this regard that they are routinely examined for every patient admitted to the hospital. Stool, sputum, and other materials are examined by special order of the physician.

Precautionary rules. To ensure the accuracy and validity of each test, the following general precautionary rules must be followed in the collection of specimens for any test:

1. The special conditions for the test must be met. For example, a fasting blood test requires that the patient fast for 8 to 12 hours before its collection.
2. The specimen must not be contaminated with any foreign material.
3. The container in which the specimen is placed must be appropriate, clean, and, in some cases, sterile.
4. In their zeal to collect a fresh, uncontaminated specimen according to prescribed directions, nurses must use great caution to see that the child's tender skin is not damaged by tight restraints, collection tubes, or adhesive tapes.
5. The specimen must be labeled correctly.
6. Specimens must be as fresh as possible and so should be delivered to the laboratory promptly, or in some cases they may be stored in a refrigerator temporarily.

Labeling of specimens. In some pediatric units, labels and order forms for routine laboratory examinations are completed at the time of admission and placed on the Kardex file or some other designated place until the specimen is collected (Fig. 9-1). If additional laboratory tests are requested by the doctor during the child's hospitalization, labels and forms are completed at the time of the order and these, too, are placed where the nurses can see if a specimen is needed. Although each hospital has its own forms, every label should include the child's name and hospital identification number; bed number and hospital unit; the nature and description of the specimen, such as "catheterized urine"; the date and hour of its collection; the type of test requested, such as "for culture"; and any special instructions, such as "phone results to Dr. Hart."

Collection of urine. The collection of a clean urine specimen from a child who is toilet trained is no particular problem. Whichever sex is involved, the perineal region or the penis is cleansed, and the child voids into the specimen container, a clean potty chair, bedpan, or urinal. As is necessary, the specimen is transferred to the clean container, correctly labeled, marked as a "voided" specimen, and sent to the laboratory. If urine is contaminated with fecal matter, it cannot be used.

The collection of a clean urine specimen from a child who is still in diapers is not as easy as for one who is toilet trained. A variety of devices have been invented to collect the urine, including the older method of strapping a test tube over a boy's penis or a bird-seed cup over the girl's perineum. Commercial products are now available to replace these methods. Most are made of plastic; some have adhesive surfaces to stick to the child's skin; some are of various shapes to be positioned inside the diaper (Fig. 9-2). It may also be helpful to prop the child with padding in a position that will facilitate collection of the urine. Special care must be taken to avoid injuring the child with any of these restraints.

Sterile catheterized urine specimens are collected directly from the indwelling catheter with a sterile syringe and needle or temporarily placed urethral catheter over a sterile container. The basic procedure for catheterizing an infant or young child is the same as for an adult. But because considerable skill is required (the urethra of a female infant curves posteriorly) and the consequences of urinary tract infection are so grave, catheterization of children is never done routinely. A doctor's order is required. The specimen is correctly labeled, marked "catheterized," and sent to the laboratory promptly.

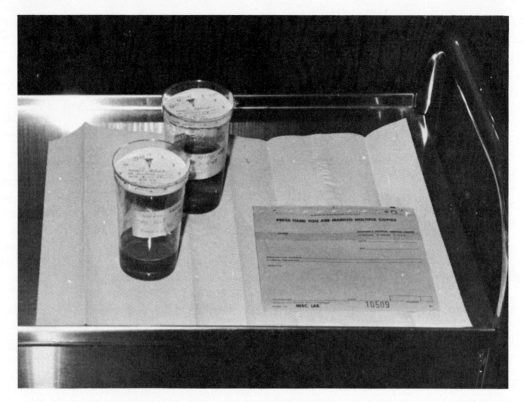

Fig. 9-1. Specimens ready for the laboratory. Note the label attached to each container to prevent mixups. In addition, laboratory forms accompany specimens.

Timed specimens are usually of voided urine, although they may involve drainage from a urinary catheter. To begin, the patient empties the bladder and the urine is discarded. The time is noted as the "opening" of the specimen. All subsequent voidings are added to a large collecting bottle that has been labeled properly. If a special preservative is not used, the bottle should be kept in a refrigerator. At the end of the period the patient voids again, and this is added to the container as the "closing" or final voiding. The entire collection is then sent to the laboratory. When a continuous sequence of timed specimens are taken so that the closing specimen of one initiates the opening of another at specific time intervals, the specimens are called "fractional."

Collection of blood. Blood specimens are not usually drawn by nurses, but nurses are the ones who prepare children and help restrain them while the specimen is drawn by the doctor or laboratory technician. Blood specimens may be obtained by a toe, finger, or heel prick or arterial or venous puncture in the neck, arm, or groin (Fig. 9-3). The sample should be properly labeled, stored temporarily in a refrigerator, or taken directly to the laboratory.

Collection of stool. Stool specimens may be obtained from a diaper, bedpan, or rectal swab. By the use of tongue blades, a representative sample is placed into a clean, nonporous container, which is tightly covered, labeled, and sent to the laboratory.

Stool is examined for the presence of blood,

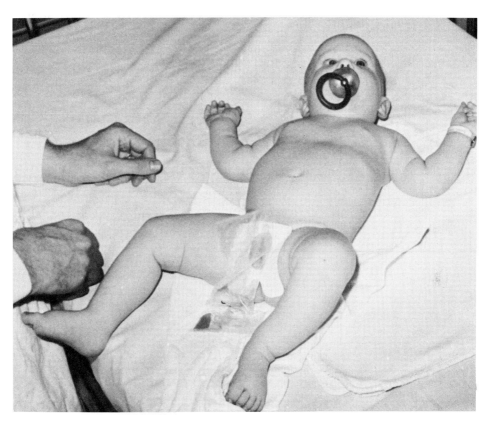

Fig. 9-2. Urine-specimen collection device.

parasites, bile, and undigested food. Some of these tests are distorted if the feces is contaminated by urine; others require that the specimen be kept warm until it is examined. The special instructions must be followed if the test is to be valid. To keep a stool specimen warm, the nonporous container should be placed into a warm-water bath as soon as it is obtained and taken directly to the laboratory.

Collection of cerebrospinal fluid. Cerebrospinal fluid is a lymphlike fluid formed primarily of blood plasma that filters from networks of capillaries known as choroid plexuses found in the ventricles (cavities) of the brain. It circulates through the spaces of the brain and spinal cord and is reabsorbed in the arachnoid layer of the membrane that covers them. At birth there is about 5 ml of this fluid. By adult life the constant level is about 135 ml, with approximately 550 ml secreted and reabsorbed each day. The spaces in which the fluid is contained are the subarachnoid space around the brain and cord, the ventricles and aqueducts inside the brain, and the central canal inside the spinal cord. Specimens of cerebrospinal fluid are taken from several locations in the central nervous system, depending on the tentative diagnosis.

The following procedures involving the cerebrospinal fluid are usually carried out by a physician using sterile techniques.

Lumbar puncture. A spinal needle is inserted into the subarachnoid space of the lumbar region of the cord. The pressure may be measured and a specimen of fluid removed for laboratory ex-

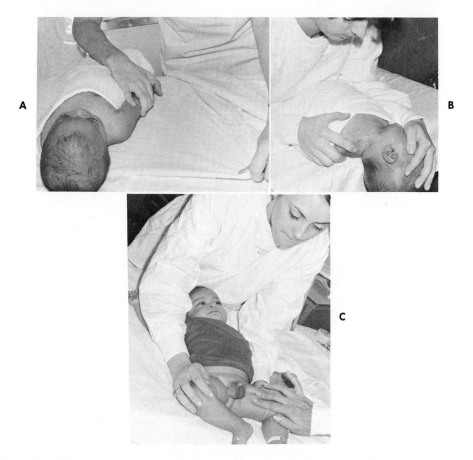

Fig. 9-3. A, Mummy restraint being applied in preparation for venipuncture. **B,** Venipuncture site in neck is exposed, as the infant's head is lowered over the edge of the table. Note position of the nurse's hands, arms, and body. **C,** Venipuncture site in groin is exposed and the child is safely restrained by nurse's arms and hands.

amination (Fig. 9-4). *Pneumoencephalograms* are x-ray films of the spinal cord and brain taken when fluid is removed through a lumbar puncture and replaced by air that is allowed to rise to the proper level for contrast visibility.

Cisternal puncture. A spinal needle is inserted into the fourth ventricle of the brain at the base of the skull. The pressure may be measured, and some fluid may be removed and replaced with air, which is visible in x-ray films called *ventriculograms.* A specimen of the fluid may also be sent to the laboratory for examination.

Ventricular tap. A large needle, attached to a syringe, is inserted into the spaces between the parietal and frontal bones of the infant's skull into the lateral ventricles to remove the excessive amounts of fluid that collect there when there is interference with normal circulation and reabsorption of fluid. (See discussion of hydrocephalus in Chapter 18.)

Subarachnoid tap. Fluid from the subarachnoid space around the brain is removed to relieve pressure caused by hemorrhage or tumor growth and for laboratory examination. The site depends on the location of the lesion.

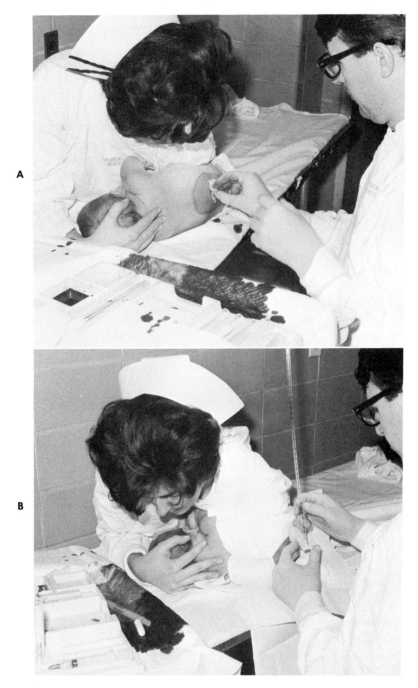

Fig. 9-4. A, Lumbar puncture. The nurse restrains the child without obstructing the airway. With sterile gloves the doctor cleans the injection site. **B,** Spinal fluid pressure is measured before specimens of the fluid are removed. Note the nurse's hand as she maintains the arched position of the infant's back.

These procedures are carried out in whatever is the most convenient and appropriate location in the hospital. Lumbar punctures are usually done in the treatment room of the pediatric unit. The nurse is responsible for preparing the room and the sterile equipment and for assisting the doctor. The nurse may need help in positioning and restraining the child so that movement will be minimal during the procedure. *Great care must be taken to see that the child's breathing is not hampered.* When the needle is in place in the prepared site, a series of three successive specimens of spinal fluid may be collected in test tubes. They are labeled as *1, 2,* and *3* and taken to the laboratory as soon as possible. The needle is removed and a small pressure dressing is placed over the site. After this procedure the child is returned to the unit to rest, preferably flat in bed. Pulse, respirations, and general reaction are assessed and recorded.

Collection of sputum. To be of value, a sputum specimen must be of the deep mucous secretions of the lungs and bronchial tree. A single specimen may be ordered, but the total sputum collection of a 24-hour period is more common. The patient is instructed to cough up secretions from deep in the chest and expectorate them into a container that is kept covered when not in use. Infants and young children are not able to cooperate, but older children and adolescents may be able to do so. When postural drainage is ordered, the resultant sputum may provide a representative sputum specimen. Preliminary aerosol vapor inhalation may be ordered to facilitate collection of a single specimen. Once the specimen is obtained, the container is placed in an outer cover such as a plastic bag, labeled, and taken to the laboratory.

Collection of stomach contents. Stomach contents are examined when poisoning is suspected, when there is a possibility of hemorrhage or intestinal obstruction, and when the degree of acidity must be known. Stomach contents are most commonly available for examination as vomitus but may also be obtained through a gastric tube. When it is possible, vomitus should be saved until the physician can examine it; if it is not possible, representative portions may be sent to the laboratory for examination.

A gastric tube may be passed for a specimen or lavage (washing) by an experienced nurse or physician. A nurse prepares the equipment, assists the physician or another nurse, and positions and restrains the child. A portion of the initial undiluted material aspirated through the gastric tube is placed in a clean container and sent to the laboratory. If poisoning is suspected, an analysis is performed immediately to identify it. The stomach is lavaged by the repeated introduction and removal of large quantities of water. When the poison is known, an antidote is administered. After the lavage, the exhausted child is allowed to rest. Intensive nursing care may be indicated if poisoning occurred.

Collection of sweat. Sweat is collected to detect the presence or carrier state of cystic fibrosis. An abnormally large amount of sodium chloride (salt) is present in the sweat of afflicted persons. The three common methods of sweat collection are the hand impression technique, the plastic bag technique, and the iontophoresis technique.

The hand impression technique is used for screening large numbers of children. Hands are washed, rinsed, dried, and then pressed against a test medium for color change. Children with positive results are then given more exact tests.

The plastic bag technique involves enclosing a clean extremity in a clean plastic bag. A heating pad may be applied to hasten the production of perspiration. When enough is collected in the bottom of the bag, it is removed carefully, closed, and taken to the laboratory.

The iontophoresis technique is usually carried out in the laboratory, where perspiration is stimulated by the injection of pilocarpine and the use of special electrodes. The special collecting pads are then weighed and chemically analyzed.

Collection of tissue for biopsy. Tissue is removed from the body for microscopic examination to determine a variety of diseases. It may be removed by excision (cutting out), by punch, scraping, rubbing with an absorbent sponge, and by aspiration through a needle. Excision and punch biopsies are used to obtain skin and muscle specimens; scraping is used for cervical and mucous membrane specimens; sponging is used for wounds and mucous membrane; and aspiration is used to obtain specimens for such tissue as bone marrow and liver. Any surgical procedure requires great caution. An operative permit is required for biopsies, except those obtained by scraping or sponging. The procedures are carried out in the treatment room or other appropriate location by a physician with the assistance of a nurse who prepares the child, the equipment, and the room. Depending on the procedure, a sedative may be given to the child 30 minutes ahead of time and food and fluids may also be withheld preoperatively.

When everything is ready, the child is brought into the treatment room, positioned, and restrained as necessary. The skin is draped and prepared. A local anesthetic may be infiltrated into the site if the procedure is painful. A variety of instruments and devices may be used to obtain tissue specimens. Bone marrow is obtained through a large hollow needle with a removable inner plug inserted into the sternum, femur, or crest of the ilium. A similar needle is used for liver biopsy. A delicate blade is used for excisions, a punch for punch biopsies, and scraping and sponging devices for other biopsies. The precious specimen is placed in prepared tubes or on slides; sometimes these tubes or slides contain special chemicals. The labeled specimens are sent to the laboratory for examination as soon as possible. The area is dressed, as needed, and the child is returned to bed. A pressure dressing and close observation are necessary after liver or bone marrow biopsy because of the danger of hemorrhage. The child's vital signs and reaction must be watched closely, reported, and recorded.

Collection of material for culture. "To culture" means "to care for" or "to cultivate in a medium." When microorganisms are grown in an artificial medium, they are said to be cultured. To determine the causative organism of various infectious diseases, a specimen of matter from the patient is placed in or on a culture medium where it grows under controlled conditions. Microscopic studies are then made to identify the organism and sensitivity tests may be done to determine the most effective antibiotic.

Cultures may be made of material from any part of the body but are most commonly taken from the mucous membrane of the nose, throat, or vagina and from wounds, urine, and spinal fluid. The nurse, physician, or trained technician may obtain culture matter, with swab technique, but great care must be taken to prevent the spread of pathogenic organisms. The one taking the specimen should wear a mask or not breathe near the sterile swab that is rubbed in the matter and placed into a sterile receptacle, stoppered aseptically, labeled, and taken to the laboratory promptly. The procedure is not painful nor time consuming, but the frightened child may resist if cooperation has not been gained.

When urine is to be cultured, a catheterized specimen is so labeled and sent to the laboratory promptly.

PREPARATION OF THE CHILD

A great many tests and studies are performed on the whole child, not just on specimens of the bodily processes. Some of these tests are determination of metabolic rate, electrical impulses in the brain and heart, psychological reactions and reasoning, and x-ray films. For these studies to be of value, the child must be prepared according to standardized conditions. These preparations fall into two categories—specific and general. The pediatric nurse must understand the importance of these preparations and know how to fulfill them.

Text continued on p. 224.

Table 9-1. Common diagnostic tests

Test material	Test	Purpose	Preparation of specimen and child	Special considerations or method of testing	Normal range
Urine	Routine urinalysis	To determine common deviations from normal	Clean, voided specimen	Ordered for all patients on admission and preoperatively	(See below)
	*Ketone (acetone, diacetic acid, beta hydroxybutyric acid)	To determine presence of ketones, a sign of acidosis	Clean, voided specimen	Place 1 drop of urine on Acetest tablet; color changes in 30 seconds; check color scale	No ketones present
	*Protein (globulins and albumins), qualitative	To detect loss of albumin through kidney tubules; may mean heart or kidney disease or poisoning	Clean, voided specimen or 24-hour collection for qualitative analysis	To urine, sulfosalicylic acid is added, which precipitates protein; degree of cloudiness indicates amount	No albumin present Small amount globulin present
	*Sugar (glucose, lactose, galactose)	To detect presence and amount; may indicate diabetes mellitus	Clean, voided specimen	Clinitest, Clinistix, and various commercial products; follow directions; color scale indicates amount of sugar; administration of cephalothin and ascorbic acid give false results	No glucose present
	*Gross appearance	To observe color and clarity and kidney's ability to concentrate urine	Clean, voided specimen	Color depends on hydration; some drugs color urine; sediment and cells cause cloudiness	Clean, straw color
	*pH	To determine the alkalinity or acidity	Clean, freshly voided specimen	Strip of Nitrazine paper moistened in urine becomes red in acid, blue in alkaline; if urine is allowed to stand, bacteria multiply; by their metabolism of urea render the urine alkaline	pH 4.5 to 8.0
	*Specific gravity	To measure kidney's ability to concentrate or dilute urine	Clean, voided specimen	Calibrated float (urinometer) placed in urine; distance it sinks is measured	1.1010 to 1.025

Test	Purpose	Procedure	Notes	Normal values
*Microscopic cells and casts	To determine kidney health; disease allows cells and casts (solid particles) to pass	Clean, voided specimen (urine of menstruating girl may show red cells)	Urine is placed in centrifuge; sediment, if any, is examined microscopically	No red cells Few white and epithelial cells No casts
Addis count	To aid in diagnosis of kidney disease (chronic, acute, latent, etc.); cells and casts are counted	24 hours of a dry diet (no fluids); after first 12-hour period, a 12-hour timed specimen is collected with care to prevent contamination; bottle and keep it in cool place	Used to follow progress of known kidney disease, especially acute glomerulonephritis; 12-hour specimen is mixed and sample centrifuged for sediment and cell count; total excreted number calculated as results	No red cells; few white cells; no casts
Phenolsulfon-phthalein (PSP)	To determine ability of kidney tubules to excrete a dye; in chronic nephritis and urinary tract obstruction dye excretion decreases; in some liver diseases it increases	Patient voids; specimen is discarded; patient drinks pint of water; doctor injects 1 ml of dye intravenously; then urine specimens are collected in separate containers at 15-, 30-, 60-, and 120-minute intervals (time varies with hospital)	Urine becomes red; patient should be warned to prevent anxiety; laboratory compares voidings with colorimeter to determine percent excreted	Elimination of 75% to 80% of dye in 120 minutes (2 hours)
Blood (venous) Total protein, albumin/globulin (A/G) ratio	To aid in diagnosis of kidney, liver, and other diseases; main function of albumin is to maintain osmotic pressure; A/G ratios are lower in chronic nephritis, nephrosis, malnutrition, and liver disease	Fasting patient; specimen is 6 ml. of venous blood into an unoxalated tube to allow clotting; serum is used for test	Serum is tested for total protein albumin and globulin, and A/G ratio is found	Albumin: 3.2 to 5.6 gm Globulin: 1.3 to 3.2 gm Total protein: 6.0 to 8.0 gm (all values per 100 ml of serum)
Antistreptolysin O (ASO) titer	To aid in diagnosis of possible rheumatic fever and glomerulonephritis; indicates presence of antibodies formed by body to combat group A streptococcus	Fasting patient; specimen is 5 ml of venous blood in unoxalated tube to allow clotting; serum used for test	Test is unreliable for 20% of cases; if test is negative, other antibody test can be used to aid in diagnosis	Ages 0 to 5 years: up to 300 Todd units; 5 to 12 years: up to 200 Todd units; 12 and over: up to 125 Todd units

*All part of routine urinalysis.

Continued.

Table 9-1. Common diagnostic tests—cont'd

Test material	Test	Purpose	Preparation of specimen and child	Special considerations or method of testing	Normal range
Blood— cont'd	Bilirubin	To determine amount of bilirubin in blood; amount increases when red blood cell destruction is excessive or liver's excretory function is impaired	Fasting patient; specimen; 5 ml of venous blood in unoxalated tube to allow clotting; serum used for test	Test reveals excessive bilirubin before jaundice appears	0.1 to 1.0 mg/100ml of serum; up to 12 mg/100ml in newborn infants
	Bleeding time	To measure time needed for a small cut to stop bleeding (not the same as clotting time since constriction of small vessels is also involved); bleeding time is prolonged in thrombocytopenic purpura and hemophilia	Nonfasting patient	Ivy bleeding time method: standardized stab wound is made on forearm while blood pressure cuff is maintained at 40 mm Hg; drops of blood are blotted at 30-second intervals; time when bleeding stops is recorded	2 to 6 minutes
	Clotting time	To determine time needed for blood to clot outside body; depends on complex coagulation mechanism	Nonfasting patient; specimen; freshly drawn venous or capillary blood	Several methods used, such as Lee-White	Normal values depend on standardized result of method used
	Platelets (thrombocytes)	To aid in diagnosis of bleeding tendencies such as aplastic anemia, purpura; platelets are necessary in clotting mechanism of blood	Nonfasting patient; specimen; drops of oxalated blood	Known dilution of blood is placed on slide in counting chamber; with microscope, platelets are counted and number per cubic millimeter is calculated	At birth: 350,000/mm^3 At 2 days: 400,000/mm^3 6 months to adult: 250,000/mm^3

Red blood cells (erythrocytes)	To aid in identifying effects of primary or secondary blood disease; elevated count may indicate polycythemia or hemoconcentration; low counts indicate inadequate cell formation, hemorrhage, or abnormal cell destruction	Nonfasting patient; specimen; drops of oxalated blood	Known dilution of blood is placed on slide in counting chamber; with microscope, cells are counted and number per cubic millimeter is calculated	At birth: 5.1 million/mm³ At 2 days: 5.3 million/mm³ At 3 months: 4.3 million/mm³ 8 to 12 years: 5.1 million/mm³ Adult: 4 to 6 million/mm³
Reticulocytes (immature red cells less than 1 day old)	To indicate bone marrow activity; elevation above normal numbers indicates increased hemopoiesis in response to hemorrhage, hemolysis, and bone marrow disease	See foregoing section of this chapter on collection of tissue for biopsy	Bone marrow sample is stained with dye and microscopic study made; number of reticulocytes per 1,000 mature red cells is determined	At birth: 2 per 100 RBC At 2 days: 3 per 100 RBC At 3 months: 0.5 per 100 RBC At 8 to 12 years: 1 per 100 RBC
White cells (leukocytes)	Leukocytes help defend body against invading organisms; in infections and certain diseases, such as leukemia, number is increased (leukocytosis); number is reduced by toxic chemicals, blood dyscrasias, and overwhelming infection, especially viral (leukopenia)	Nonfasting patient; specimen; drops of oxalated blood	Blood is mixed with a chemical that destroys red cells, then known dilution placed on slide in counting chamber; cells are counted under microscope	At birth: 15,000/mm³ At 2 days: 21,000/mm³ At 14 days: 11,000/mm³ 4 to 12 years: 8,000/mm³ 12 years and over: 5,000 to 10,000/mm³

Continued.

Table 9-1. Common diagnostic tests—cont'd

Test material	Test	Purpose	Preparation of specimen and child	Special considerations or method of testing	Normal range
Blood—cont'd	White cell differential	To aid in diagnosis of disease; various conditions cause changes in percentages of the five types of white blood cells Neutrophils: increase in bacterial infection Eosinophils: increase in allergic and parasitic conditions Basophils: increase in leukemia Lymphocytes: increase in leukemia and viral infections Monocytes: increase in chronic infections	Nonfasting patient; specimen; drops of fresh blood placed on slide	By use of another slide blood is spread evenly over glass; after it is dry, it is stained and examined under microscope; each type of white cell is counted separately; a total of 100 of all kinds is counted and percentage of each calculated	Birth to 12 years: Neutrophils: 45% to 60% (160–170) Eosinophils: 1% to 5% Basophils: 0% to 1% (0–5) Lymphocytes: 20% to 30% Monocytes: 5% to 8%
	Coombs'	To detect antired cell antibodies that become attached to red cells	Nonfasting patient; specimen; 2 to 5 ml clotted or oxalated blood (depends on type of test to be performed)	When Rh or ABO incompatibility is suspected, this test may be performed at frequent intervals during last 4 to 6 weeks of pregnancy	Negative
	Culture	To identify microorganisms in blood; drug sensitivity test usually performed after organism found and grown	Nonfasting patient; specimen; blood placed in container of culture media immediately	Specimen is placed in nutrient media to foster growth and facilitate identification of pathogens	No organisms (sterile)

Glucose tolerance	To discover disorders of glucose metabolism that have not become severe enough to show up in a fasting blood sugar determination	Patient to have adequate diet for 3 days before, then fasts for 12 hours; venous blood and urine specimens saved, followed by collection of blood and urine samples collected at hourly intervals	Time each specimen of urine and blood is taken must be noted on its label; amount of glucose in each sample is calculated	Intravenous glucose: Return to fasting in 1 hour. Oral glucose: Return to fasting in 2 hours. Peak of not more than 150 mg/100 ml of serum
Glucose (semiquantitative)	To determine blood glucose level	Nonfasting patient; obtain blood from heel or finger stick; place one drop on Chemstrip b6 or Dextrostix; follow manufacturer's directions	Not a substitute for quantitative studies, but more accurate than urine tests for glucose	65 to 105 mg/100 ml (read color values on commercial product)
Blood urea nitrogen (BUN)	To determine kidney disease or urinary tract obstruction; urea, the end product of protein metabolism, is normally excreted by kidneys; blood levels rise if urinary system fails	Fasting patient; specimen, 5 ml of venous blood in an oxalated tube	A rising blood urea nitrogen level may cause mental confusion, convulsions, or coma	7 to 20 mg/100 ml blood
Carbon dioxide combining power	A measure of the amount of carbon dioxide that can be absorbed by serum or plasma; increase occurs with alkalosis; decrease occurs with acidosis	Nonfasting patient; specimen; 8 ml of venous blood in an oxalated tube (avoid contact with air)	Plasma or serum is extracted and saturated with carbon dioxide; amount is then freed by adding acid, and volume is measured	22 to 30 mEq/liter

Continued.

Table 9-1. Common diagnostic tests—cont'd

Test material	Test	Purpose	Preparation of specimen and child	Special considerations or method of testing	Normal range
Blood—cont'd	Protein-bound iodine (PBI)	To test thyroid function; iodine is bound chemically to the hormone thyroxin; increased amounts indicate hyperthyroidism; decreased amounts indicate hypothyroidism	Fasting patient who has not had any iodine for 6 months preceding test or thyroid hormone for 14 days before test; specimen, 8 ml blood in unoxalated tube	Laboratory test results give amount of iodine per 100 ml or serum; many drugs, states, and conditions give falsely elevated results	After 1 month: 4 to 8 μg/100ml of serum
	Sedimentation rate	To aid in determination of inflammation and tissue breakdown; useful in following course of such diseases as rheumatic fever and arthritis	Nonfasting patient; specimen, 4 ml of oxalated blood	Blood sample is put in calibrated tube; rate formed elements settle is determined; corrections for anemia are sometimes reported as "corrected" sedimentation rate	Westergren method: 0 to 20 mm per hour
	Hematocrit	To measure the relative proportion of cells and plasma; reading is low in anemias and after hemorrhage, high in polycythemia and dehydration	Nonfasting patient; specimen, 4 ml venous blood in an oxalated tube	Measured amount of blood is placed in calibrated tube and spun in centrifuge; height of column of packed red cells is measured	35 to 50 vols % (mm of red blood cells per 100 mm of column height)
	Hemoglobin	To determine amount of hemoglobin available for oxygen transport, hemoglobin levels affect color and are not always parallel with red cell count; in iron-deficiency anemia, hemoglobin is reduced more than	Nonfasting patient; specimen, venous or capillary blood in oxalated tube.	Sahli method gives results in terms of grams per 100 ml of blood	At birth: 17.6 gm; At 2 days: 18.0 gm; At 1 year: 12.2 gm; 8 to 12 years: 14.1 gm; Adult: 12 to 16 gm

		red cell count; in pernicious anemia, red cell count is reduced more than hemoglobin		
Blood typing Major groups, Rh factor	To determine blood type for possible transfusion or maternal-infant blood studies	Nonfasting patient; specimen, both nonoxalated and oxalated blood used for transfusion cross matching tests	Agglutination tests: major types are A, B, AB, and O; the Rh factor is not present in 15% of population:	Found in general population: A 38% B 12% AB 5% O 45% Rh+ 85% Rh− 15%
Serology test for syphilis; Veneral Disease Research Laboratory (VDRL)	Screening test for syphilis; results are reported as reactive, weakly reactive, and nonreactive; reactive results are confirmed by specific *Treponema pallidum* tests; infants born to mothers with history of syphilis	Nonfasting patient; specimen, 5 ml of venous blood in unoxalated tube	False positives or negatives may occur because of other conditions in body; all positive results should be brought to doctor's attention, but kept confidential	Nonreactive
Blood (arterial) Blood gases (bG): pH, Po_2, Pco_2	To determine oxygenation, acidosis, alkalosis, base excess or deficit	Warm puncture site for 15 minutes unless obtained from arterial line; take to laboratory immediately	Be sure blood is arterial; irrigate arterial line before and after; place pressure on puncture site after withdrawal	pH 7.35 to 7.45 Po_2 80 to 100 mm Hg Pco_2 36 to 40 mm Hg Base: no excess or deficit
Stool Fat determination	To confirm diagnosis of steatorrhea, excessive fat in the stool, as seen in celiac syndrome	Patient on normal diet for 3 days before test; then timed specimen is ordered	Save all stools during the test period; unnecessary ones can be discarded, but lost ones are gone forever	15% to 25% of total weight of stool specimen

Continued.

Table 9-1. Common diagnostic tests—cont'd

Test material	Test	Purpose	Preparation of specimen and child	Special considerations or method of testing	Normal range
Stool—cont'd	Occult blood	To detect presence of fecal blood; blood from high in intestinal tract is changed chemically; blood from lower may appear bright red	Patient on normal diet; specimen collected; if positive, meat-free diet for 3 days, then another specimen	Until stool is collected, patient should not brush teeth so that blood from broken gum tissue will not give false results	No occult blood
	Parasites	To detect presence of parasites or their eggs in stool	Oily cathartics are never given; specimen preparation depends on parasite: cold stool is suitable for ova anal amebic cysts; and swabs for pinworms; warm stool for some mobile worms; proctoscopic scraping, aspiration, and biopsy may be necessary in some cases	Specimens are examined microscopically and identification made

Some antibiotic drugs kill normal inhabitants of bowel, causing a disruption of normal balance and allowing pathogenic organisms to grow; diarrhea may result | Large numbers of normal parasites like *Escherichia coli* and certain flagellates |
| Cerebrospinal fluid (CSF) | Cell count | To determine presence of infection within brain or spinal cord; cell count is moderately increased in poliomyelitis, neurosyphilis, and encephalitis; cell count is greatly increased in meningitis | Collection of CSF is discussed in a prior section in this chapter | A known dilution of CSF is placed in counting chamber; by use of microscope the number of cells per cubic millimeter of CSF is calculated | 0 to 5 cells/mm³ |
| | Chlorides | To measure chloride level of CSF as an aid in differential diagnosis; chlorides are reduced in tuberculous meningitis | Specimen: 2 ml CSF in special test tube | The laboratory procedure similar to that for blood serum; results expressed in milligrams per 100 ml; blood chlorides are reported as milliequivalents per liter | 720 to 750 mg/100 ml of CSF |

Test	Purpose	Procedure	Notes	Normal values
Colloidal gold curve (albumin/globulin ratio of CSF)	To aid in differential diagnosis of central nervous system disease such as neurosyphilis, poliomyelitis, in which the A/G ratio is changed from the normal 4/1	Specimen: 1 ml of CSF in small test tube	Bloody spinal fluid gives a false positive and so cannot be used; colloidal gold suspension is added to 10 dilution samples; pattern and amount of precipitation suggests particular diseases	No precipitation (negative) or small amount in a few tubes
Sputum Culture	To aid in differential diagnosis of respiratory diseases, particularly tuberculosis	Specimen: mucous secretions brought up from lungs and trachea; see prior section on collection of sputum	Treat all sputum as potentially infectious; sample is placed in culture medium, and resultant growth stained and examined microscopically; special attention given to identify acid-fast (tubercle) bacilli	No pathogenic organisms (a single negative test is not conclusive)
Sweat Pilocarpine iontophoresis for sodium and chloride ions	To identify cystic fibrosis victims	A dilute solution of pilocarpine is given intradermally on forearm; weak electric current then is used to stimulate sweating	The sweat is collected on a gauze pad and analyzed for sodium and chloride; results are expressed in milliequivalents per liter	Sodium: less than 70 mEq/liter Chloride: less than 50 mEq/liter
Child Basal metabolism rate (BMR)	To measure rate at which metabolic processes take place under standard conditions; BMR is elevated in hyperthyroidism and infection, lowered in hypothyroidism and sedation	Good night's sleep before test; fasting after 10 PM night before; may have water; on morning of test patient lies on comfortable bed and breathes through machine apparatus that records amount of oxygen used	Anxiety, fear, or activity before test give elevated results; basic metabolic rate calculated by using the child's age, weight, height (body surface), and amount of oxygen used during timed period	-20% to $+20\%$
Electrocardiogram (ECG, EKG)	To determine irregularities in electrical impulses controlling heart action; to diagnose heart disease or damage	No special preparation, except an adequate explanation to allay fear; painless procedure	Electrical leads are positioned at various points on body by technician; child must lie still for brief periods while electrical impulses are being recorded on special graph paper	A specialist reads tracings for abnormalities

Continued.

Table 9-1. Common diagnostic tests—cont'd

Test material	Test	Purpose	Preparation of specimen and child	Special considerations or method of testing	Normal range
Child—cont'd	Electroencephalogram (EEG)	To aid in determination of abnormal brain waves; used in diagnosing epilepsy and tumors	No special preparations except explanation; sedation may be given young children; special machine records electrical potentials	Electrodes are placed on scalp with adhesive and fastened to a sensitive machine that records tracings; test takes about 1 hour in a quiet atmosphere, free of electrical interference	A specialist in neurology reads tracings for abnormalities
	Barium swallow	To aid in diagnosis of obstructions or strictures of esophagus and stomach	Nothing by mouth for 8 to 12 hours before x-ray examination	Patient slowly swallows flavored barium under fluoroscopic examination; x-ray films are taken as directed	Specialist observes fluoroscopy and reads x-ray films
	Barium enema	To aid in diagnosis of lower bowel pathology by outlining colon with radiopaque material and taking x-ray film; may be used in treatment of intussusception	Day before x-ray examination, clear liquid diet and cathartic or cleansing enema	Barium enema given in x-ray department when child is under fluoroscope; many x-ray films taken during 1- to 2-hour procedure; cathartic or enema may be given after x-ray films taken	Specialist reads x-ray films for pathological conditions
	Gastrointestinal (GI) series	To aid in diagnosis of stomach and small bowel pathology by outlining these structures with radiopaque material	Night before test; light supper, then no food, fluid, or drugs after midnight until procedure is completed	Barium given in x-ray department under fluoroscope; child remains NPO until 6-hour studies are completed; food and fluids resumed after procedure	Specialist reads x-ray films for abnormal conditions
	Cystogram	To aid in diagnosis of urinary obstruction or abnormality by visualization of urethra, bladder, and ureters with radiopaque material	Indwelling catheter inserted prior to procedure	Radiopaque dye is injected into the bladder through a catheter; x-ray films are taken immediately and again during voiding	Specialist reads x-ray films for pathological conditions

Test	Purpose	Preparation	Description	
Intravenous pyelogram (IVP)	To detect urinary tract disease by intravenous dye injection followed by x-ray films	Day before x-ray examination, cathartic or enema to empty bowel; light supper with few fluids; food, fluids, and drugs withheld after midnight	X-ray films of abdomen are taken before and after intravenous injection of iodine-containing dye by physician; force fluids after procedure; allergy to iodine is a contraindication to routine procedure	Specialist in urology reads x-ray films for abnormalities
Capillary fragility (tourniquet test)	To detect platelet or vascular defects present in some hemorrhagic diseases	Blood pressure cuff is applied and inflated to a pressure between systolic and diastolic for 5 to 15 minutes	A circle 2.5 cm in diameter is drawn on the forearm before the test; the number of petechiae that appear during the test are counted	Less than 10 petechiae
Pneumoencephalogram	To detect abnormalities of brain by contrast x-ray films by use of injections of air into spinal canal; this procedure is extremely painful and not without risk	No food or fluid 6 hours before; preoperative sedation given; may be done under local or general anesthesia in x-ray department	Spinal puncture performed, fluid removed, and equal amount of air injected; this air is allowed to rise to ventricles of brain; x-ray films taken; postoperative care includes keeping child flat and observing for signs of increasing intracranial pressure	Specialist in neurology reads x-ray films for abnormalities
Ventriculogram	To detect abnormalities of brain by contrast x-ray films by use of injections of air directly into ventricles through burr holes in skull	Preoperative care, NPO after midnight the day before; sedation and analgesic administered just prior to surgery	Procedure is performed in operating room under general anesthesia; craniotomy patients require intensive postoperative observation and care	neurosurgeon performs surgery and reads x-ray films for abnormalities
Computerized tomography (CT scan or computerized axial tomography CAT scan)	To provide three-dimensional views of cranial contents; largely replaced pneumoencephalograms	NPO 4 to 6 hours before scan; no other preparation; ask if patient is allergic to iodine, the contrast medium given IV to enhance results	Noninvasive procedure with the patient lying on a table with the head placed in an opening of the scanner; small beam of x-ray is passed through brain; computer forms a picture based on x-ray absorbed	Specialist in neurology reads scan for abnormalities
Psychological tests	To determine emotional disturbance and intellectual ability	No preparation	Psychologist administers battery of tests as indicated	Varies with test

Specific preparations

Each test or study has a set of specific conditions in the form of directions to be followed. It is a nursing responsibility to see that these directions are followed. Some of the most common terms used for testing follow.

Fasting. The child is to receive no nourishment of any kind for the designated period. It does not necessarily mean that the child must be deprived of water or sugarless beverages.

Nothing by mouth (NPO). No food or fluids of any kind may be given to the child for a designated period of time. Special mouth care can be done to relieve discomfort from dryness unless specifically contraindicated.

Sedation. The child is given a sedative to quiet but not necessarily to cause unconsciousness. Sedation is especially useful when the procedure is frightening or mildly painful.

Enema. The type of enema ordered varies with the procedure to be done, but it is commonly a cleansing enema, given to evacuate the lower bowel. It should be given long enough in advance so that violent peristalsis has ceased by the time of the test or x-ray examination.

Activity. Physical activity such as walking, standing, or sitting increases the metabolism and affects the functioning of every organ of the body. The results of some tests are significantly altered by physical activity.

Voiding (urinating). Many procedures require that the patient void just before the test. Doing so assures that the bladder will occupy the minimum space in the pelvis. On the other hand, the first voiding in the morning is considered best for tests requiring more concentrated, representative specimens of urine.

Catheterization. When an indwelling catheter must be in place during tests and studies, often it is inserted beforehand by a staff nurse.

General preparations

Although many tests are not especially painful or exhausting, the child who is old enough to know they are planned may experience anxiety and fear. The three best ways to counteract fear are with information, physical rest, and emotional support. To the degree it is possible, the nurse should provide each child scheduled for tests with all these anxiety-relieving measures. The results will not only be evident in the child's personal reaction, but also in the child's ability to cooperate with the hospital staff during the procedures.

Children have vivid imaginations. If they hear only a few whispered words about what is "scheduled for tomorrow," they may suffer needless fear. To relieve such anxiety, the nurse should offer a simplified but truthful explanation of impending tests.

Physical rest is important to both the physical and psychological preparation of a child for tests and studies. The child should not be disturbed unnecessarily during the night before a test.

Emotional support is of great importance in the general preparation of a child for a test or study. Although it involves much more, one of the practical ways to provide this support is by the physical contact and presence of someone the child trusts. The nurse may remember this while taking the child to the x-ray department for a gastrointestinal series, or as the doctor approaches with rubber gloves and mask. By both actions and attitudes the nurse communicates warmth and genuine acceptance, thus fortifying the child for the coming procedure.

SUMMARY OUTLINE

I. **Collection of specimens**
   A. Precautionary rules
   B. Labeling of specimens
   C. Collection of urine
   D. Collection of blood
   E. Collection of stool
   F. Collection of cerebrospinal fluid
      1. Lumbar puncture
      2. Cisternal puncture
      3. Ventricular tap
      4. Subarachnoid tap

G. Collection of sputum
H. Collection of stomach contents
I. Collection of sweat
J. Collection of tissue for biopsy
K. Collection of material for culture
II. Preparation of the child
  A. Specific preparation
    1. Fasting
    2. Nothing by mouth (NPO)
    3. Sedation
    4. Enema
    5. Activity
    6. Voiding (Urinating)
    7. Catheterization
  B. General preparations

STUDY QUESTIONS

1. What is the principle behind all testing? What can the nurse do to make test results valid?
2. List the precautionary rules that must be followed in specimen collection.
3. Describe the procedure for collecting a 24-hour urine specimen.
4. Describe the procedure for collection of stool, sputum, and sweat.
5. Describe the purpose, the preparation of the specimen and the child, and the normal range of results for the following: glucose tolerance, ECG, EEG, and GI series.

10
Pediatric medications

with Louise Burkett Snead

Administration of medications to children carries great responsibility. Laws and regulations must be followed precisely. The effective dose of drugs varies from child to child according to body weight, surface area, and metabolic condition. The action of drugs, both intended and untoward, occurs more rapidly in children than in adults. Children's body structure and ability to cooperate are constantly changing as they grow and mature. All these variables impose the need for special skill and knowledge on the nurses who must be able to calculate drug dosages correctly, administer them safely, know their expected actions, and recognize untoward reactions.

LEGAL IMPLICATIONS AND RESPONSIBILITIES

Until about 5 years ago, consumers of hospital services were unaware of many of the measures used by medical science. They were hesitant and were sometimes discouraged from asking questions about alternate methods of treatment.

Then consumer groups began to challenge medicine. Consumer demands resulted in generic price listings and a rapid increase in successful lawsuits against medical personnel. Until that time, the nurse remained in the background. Nurses were protected by the physician, because they were only "following orders." The tables have now turned. Consumers now are recognizing nursing as a separate, somewhat independent and distinct entity from medicine and are holding nurses accountable for their actions. More and more lawsuits are being litigated successfully against nurses, particularly concerning medication administration. Successful lawsuits against nurses often result in the revocation of their licenses. For nurses to avoid such legal actions, and loss of license, they first must recognize and adhere to several groups of rules and regulations that govern their practice, particularly in regard to giving medications.

Federal regulations
Controlled substances

Though the prescribing, manufacturing, and dispensing of all drugs fall under its domain, the federal government has developed several regulations that govern nurses in the administration of medications. These regulations are concerned primarily with the administration of controlled substances. Controlled substances are drugs that are regulated or monitored because of their high abuse potential and their addictive properties. Originally, when the Harrison Narcotic Act was enacted in 1914, controlled substances were limited to opium and cocaine derivatives. Since that time other substances have been added. Now controlled substances are listed in five categories, called "Schedules" according to their potential for abuse. Schedule I drugs are considered to have the highest potential for abuse; Schedule V drugs have the least potential for abuse. Currently, the method of classification is as follows:

Schedule I	Narcotics and hallucinogenics not approved for medical use, such as heroin and PCP
Schedule II	Narcotics and stimulants used for medical treatment, such as meperidine hydrochloride (Demerol) and amphetamines
Schedule III	Analgesics and sedatives used for medical treatment, such as aspirin (Emprin #3) and pentabarbital (nembutal).
Schedule IV	Tranquilizers and analgesics such as diazepan (Valium) and propoxyphene hydrochloride (Darvon).
Schedule V	Antitussives and other groups with small amounts of narcotics such as paregoric and elixir of terpin hydrate with codeine

When nurses administer controlled substances they must account for every dose. If the controlled substance is used from stock supplies, they must record certain information on a special record that bears the hospital registry number. The form of this record may vary from institution to institution but the following information must be included: (1) the date of administration of the drug; (2) the patient's name; (3) the name and amount of drug administered (if part is not given, another nurse must witness its wasting and sign the record verifying that the drug was, in fact, discarded); (4) the name of the physician ordering the drug; and (5) the signature of the nurse administering it.

In an emergency, nurses may take verbal orders for controlled substances. When they do they must write the complete order on a physician's order form, state that it is a verbal order, and write the physician's name along with their own names. The order must be countersigned by the physician within 24 hours.

Experimental drugs and treatments

In addition to federal regulations that affect controlled substances, there are regulations that affect the use of experimental or investigational drugs. Informed consent must be obtained before such a drug or treatment may be given. The physician is expected to explain fully all aspects of the treatment, and the patient, parent, or legal guardian must sign a consent form. Nurses may witness such a signature, and they may wish to reinforce the information given by the physician. They must not, however, administer an experimental drug without consent.

State regulations: nurse practice acts

In addition to federal guidelines, each state has developed its own laws and regulations that govern nursing, called nurse practice acts. They have grown out of community needs for health services, availability of nurses and physicians, and standards of care. As a result, nurses in some areas are allowed to carry out functions reserved for physicians in other areas.

With the advent of two categories of nurses, registered nurses and practical-vocational nurses, the differences between states has been multiplied. For example, functions permitted for licensed practical nurses in Arizona are proscribed for registered nurses in California. Nurses must know the scope of the practice in the state for which they are licensed. Copies of nurse practice acts are available from the licensing body of each state.

Although there are differences between states, nurse practice acts have the following common characteristics:

1. They define licensing procedures including educational requirements, testing, and fees.
2. They define scope of practice, that is, what a nurse can and cannot do.
3. They identify some of the facts that may result in revocation of the license.

The effect nurse practice acts have on the administration of medications is that the acts may specify whether nurses can or cannot do the following:

1. Accept verbal prescriptions from doctors, and if so, under what circumstances.
2. Superimpose intravenous solutions and if so, what types are permitted.
3. Administer intravenous, intracardiac, or intraspinal (intrathecal) medications.
4. Perform venipunctures, and if so, under what circumstances.

5. Make decisions about patients' conditions relative to the administration of drugs.
6. Function in an "expanded role" if qualified by advanced education, in which nurses administer drugs without direct medical supervision.

Implicit in the nurse practice acts is the requirement that licensees (1) have knowledge of the purpose, course, and side effects of drugs they administer; (2) only administer what was prescribed by a physician; (3) know and only administer the safe dosages of a drug; (4) observe the patient for reactions to drugs; and (5) report or record that a drug was administered and the effects observed in the patient.

Hospital policies and procedures

Even though the federal and state governments define specific rules and regulations required for licensing, individual institutions have their own set of rules and regulations that govern nurses in their particular setting. The institutions' rules and regulations generally are in the form of policies and procedures. Similar to state regulations, institutional regulations vary from one institution to another. The institutional policy or procedure may be more strict than the state or federal regulation, but it cannot be more liberal. For example, a federal regulation may state that any licensed person trained to do so may give medications using any route. A state regulation may state that LPNs and LVNs may give medications using any route except intravenous. Institutional policy may state that LPNs and LVNs may give oral medications only. *The strictest rule always prevails.*

Institutional policies and procedures affecting the administration of medications include those that regulate (1) who may accept verbal and written medication orders, (2) who may administer medications, (3) the process for certification to administer medications, (4) the medication system to be used in the institution, and (5) the procedures for discharge prescriptions and instructions. The nurse must become thoroughly familiar with the institution's policies and procedures.

• • •

In summary, three sets of rules and regulations govern nurses' actions: federal, state, and institutional. It is important for nurses to know these rules and regulations for their own sake and for the safety of the patient. When nurses perform outside established regulations, willfully or not, they may be guilty of malpractice.

Individual responsibilities

Negligence is the omission of acts a reasonably prudent person would do, or the commission of acts a reasonably prudent person would not do.

Malpractice is the omission of acts a professional person with similar education and in similar circumstances *would do*, such as the failure of a license practical-vocational nurse to observe and report an adverse drug reaction, and the commission of acts a professional person with similar education and in similar circumstances *would not do*, such as administering an overdose of a medication.

When nurses commit acts of malpractice, they may be sued individually for their actions. If their acts of malpractice are also violations of laws, they may be convicted of those criminal offenses, and their licenses may be revoked. For example, if nurses divert controlled substances for self-administration, they could be sued by deprived patients for malpractice, and the state could prosecute them for breaking the law. If convicted, their license to practice nursing could be suspended or revoked.

PRINCIPLES

Five principles, or "rights," apply to the administration of medications in any situation and to any patient, young or old. These five rights are as follows:

1. The right patient
2. The right medication in the right amount and route

3. The right dosage
4. The right method of administration
5. The right time

PRACTICE

To apply the five principles of safe drug administration, hospitals have developed various processes and instruments. These include identification methods (right patient), medical prescriptions (doctor's orders), calculation of safe dosages, systems of drug administration, and times of administration.

Identification methods (the right patient)

Administering medicines to the right patient requires some form of identification, especially in a pediatric unit where the patients may not know their own names. Most common forms of patient identification are bed cards and wrist or ankle bands. Bed cards are certainly helpful, but they cannot substitute for identification actually attached to the child. Johnny sometimes gets put into Billie's bed, and sometimes playful hands switch bed cards! No matter how well nurses know their patients, before administering any medicine they must actually read the name on the identification band, compare it with the name on the medicine card, listen to such remarks as "I've never had that before," and double-check if they have any doubts. A moment of error-prevention is worth hours of remedial care.

Medical prescriptions (doctor's orders)

No medication should be given without a prescription. The following information must be included in all prescriptions: (1) patient's name, (2) date the prescription is written, (3) name of medication, (4) route of medication, (5) frequency with which the medication is to be administered, and (6) physician's signature. If one of these elements is missing, the prescription is incomplete. The nurse must not guess the missing part, but must ask the physician for it. Prescriptions for drugs to be taken at home by the patient also must state the total quantity to be dispensed by the pharmacy, the number of refills, and the address of the patient.

Forms

Prescription forms vary in design and name. They may be called "doctor's order forms," "medication order forms," or the like. They may be single or multiple sheets with carbon copies attached. The forms may serve more than one purpose. For example, there may be space provided on the form for charting the medication after it is administered. Carbon copies of the form may be sent to the pharmacy for ordering and billing purposes.

Some institutions have different forms to be used for discharge prescriptions. Many states require physicians to write prescriptions for controlled substances to be taken home on a special form with carbon copies. Nurses need to review both in-house and take-home prescriptions to be sure they are correctly written and on the right form. Nurses also have the responsibility for explaining prescriptions for drugs to be taken or treatments to be followed at home to the patient and family, and to note the degree of apparent understanding on the patient's record.

Procedures

Ideally, when a drug is needed the physician comes to the nursing care unit and writes (or places into the computer) a prescription in the patient's record. The physician then "flags" the record indicating that new orders have been written. The nurse should review the prescription with the physician and ask questions to be sure the prescription is understood. The nurse or unit clerk then transcribes the new prescription to all the appropriate places, dates them, and countersigns them.

Standing orders are prescriptions for care or drug administration that apply to groups of patients, classified by some criteria; for example, "All patients over 6 months of age are to be given a tuberculin test on the inner aspect of the right forearm on the day of admission." Because standing orders apply to groups of patients, they are not written individually in every patient's record by the physician. Instead, a preprinted copy is added to each patient's record. Before standing orders can be instituted they must be approved by the medical staff and a signed copy must be on file in the hospital. Standing orders are noted and implemented by nurses as meticulously as any other orders.

Verbal orders, which include telephone orders, are prescriptions given orally by a physician to a nurse. Usually, verbal orders are given when the physician is not readily available to write them or is in an emergency situation. Verbal orders must contain the same information as a written prescription. The only difference is that in place of the physician's signature, the nurse taking the verbal order writes the physician's name followed by the nurse's name. The physician must still sign the order, but may do it at a later time, usually before the end of 24 hours. Whenever a nurse takes a verbal order, it should be repeated to the physician immediately to ensure that the information has been understood and written correctly.

Drug dosages

The *therapeutic dose* of a drug is the amount that produces the desired effect. A *lethal dose* is one large enough to cause death. *Toxicity* is any degree of poisoning from a drug. *Untoward actions* of drugs are undesirable and atypical actions of drugs. The amount of a drug that might be effective for a large child could be lethal for an infant. Children's dosages are calculated as a part, or fraction, of therapeutic adult dosages. Because the consequences of administering an incorrect dose of medicine to a child are so grave, careful nurses check their calculations with one another or consult their pharmacist before they administer fractional dosages of drugs.

Verification of safe dosages

Nurses practice under their own license, not under the physician's license. They are responsible for their own actions. The physician may order a medication, but as the giver of the medication, the nurse must know that the prescribed dose is safe. If a medication is given to the patient as ordered by the physician and the order is not safe, then both the physician and the nurse are considered negligent. Because the gap between a therapeutic dose and an overdose in the pediatric age group is so narrow, great care must be taken to ensure accuracy.

Physicians do err. This may be particularly true in teaching institutions where physicians who have previously worked in adult settings rotate briefly through pediatrics and are unfamiliar with pediatric doses. Nurses must be alert to catch these errors and correct them.

Before the actual pouring up of medications, the nurse should ask the question, "Is the dose of medication I am administering a safe one?"

If a nurse should discover that a prescribed dosage is too large for a child, the nurse has the legal responsibility to withhold the medication and report the fact to the charge nurse or physician immediately. The nurse discusses the matter with the physician tactfully. Most physicians are appreciative of the nurses' efforts to be conscientious. Sometimes the physician has good reason for prescribing a larger dose than recommended. For example, the patient may have developed a tolerance to the drug or the disease process may be more severe than usual. With such information from the physician nurses will be able to make informed decisions about whether to administer the medication. They will gain in understanding and will enhance patient care.

Reference manuals

To determine the therapeutic dose for a pediatric patient one needs a drug reference manual that states the therapeutic range. The manual should also list side effects and contraindications. If such a book is not available, the nurse can obtain information about drugs from the manufacturer's printed insert or the hospital pharmacist. A list of drugs commonly used in pediatrics is given in Table 10-1. Note that the routes of administration are indicated as follows: oral (PO), subcutaneous (SC or SQ), intramuscular (IM), intraveneous (IV), and rectal (R).

Calculation methods

There are several methods for calculating drug dosages for children, including age, weight, surface area, and Fried's, Clark's, and Young's rules. These methods, together with some practice problems, follow.

Age. Age is the least accurate criterion for determining a safe dose because of the wide range in size of children within the same age group. For example, a 1-month-old premature infant may weigh 3 pounds; a 1-month-old full-term infant may weigh 12 pounds. Because of this variance, medication dosages determined by age are usually oral medications that are not especially potent, such as plain antitussives, decongestants, minerals, and vitamins. To verify that a doctor's order is safe, using age as the criterion, follow these steps:

Step 1. Determine the age of the child.
Step 2. Look up the medication and determine the safe dose for that age group.
Step 3. Compare the dosage recommended for that age group with the doctor's order.

Example: The physician orders Dimetapp, 1 tsp. PO, q.i.d. for a patient of 1 year of age. Is this a safe dose?
Step 1. Determine the age of the child.
The child in this instance is 1 year old.
Step 2. Look up the medication and determine the safe dose for the age group. (Refer to Table 10-1.) The safe dose of Dimetapp for a 1 year old is ½ tsp.
Step 3. Compare the recommended dosage for that age group with the doctor's order. The physician has ordered 1 tsp; the maximum safe dose is ½ tsp, so the doctor's order is *unsafe*.

Table 10-1. Safe dose chart of commonly used medications for children

Medication	General classification	Recommended maximum dosage by route for 24 hours unless specified otherwise	Forms available
Acetaminophen (Tylenol)	Antipyretic Analgesic	*PO, R:* 3-6 mo—30 mg q 4-6 hr 6-12 mo—60 mg q 4-6 hr 1-3 yr—60-120 mg q 4-6 hr 3-6 yr—120 mg q 4-6 hr 6-12 yr—240 mg q 4-6 hr	Elixir (drops), oral suspension, syrup, tablets, capsules, suppositories
Acetazolamide (Diamox)	Anticonvulsant	*PO, IV:* 8-30 mg/kg	Capsules, tablets, sterile powder for injection
Actifed (contains triprolidine hydrochloride and pseudoephedrine hydrochloride)	Antihistaminic Sympathomimetic	*PO only:* Syrup 4 mo-2 yr—¼ tsp 3-4 times a day 2-4 yr—½ tsp 3-4 times a day 4-6 yr—¾ tsp 3-4 times a day 6-12 yr—1 tsp 3-4 times a day Tablet 6-12 yr—½ tablet 3-4 times a day	Syrup, tablets*
Actinomycin D (Dactinomycin, Cosmegen)	Antineoplastic	*IV only:* 0.4-0.6 mg/m² for 5 days; maximum single dose, 0.5 mg	Sterile powder for injection
Amikacin (Amikin)	Antibiotic	*IM, IV:* 15 mg/kg divided into 2-3 doses	Sterile powder for injection
Aminophylline (Somophyllin Liquid, Somophyllin rectal solution—contains theophylline and ethylenediamine)	Bronchodilator	ACUTE ASTHMA—INITIAL DOSE†: *PO:* 7 mg/kg/dose *IV:* 6 mg/kg/dose *R:* 3-5 mg/kg/dose	Tablets, oral liquid, elixir, sterile solution for injection, rectal solution, suppositories
Amobarbital (Amytal)	Sedative/hypnotic	SEDATION: *PO:* 1-2 mg/kg *IM:* 1-2 mg/kg SLEEP: *PO:* 2-3 mg/kg/dose *IM:* 2-3 mg/kg/dose	Sterile powder, tablets, elixir, capsules, suppositories
Amoxicillin (Amoxil, Polymox)	Antibacterial	*PO:* Under 20 kg—20-40 mg/kg Over 20 kg—250-500 mg q 8 hr	Oral suspension, drops, capsules
Amphotericin B (Fungizone)	Antifungal	*IV:* 0.25-1 mg/kg *Topical:* 2-4 applications of 3% suspensions	Cream, lotion, ointment, sterile powder

Drug	Classification	Dosage	Forms
Ampicillin (Polycillin, Amcill)	Antibiotic	*PO, IM, IV:* Under 20 kg—50-100 mg/kg Over 20 kg—500-2000 mg	Capsules, oral suspension, drops, sterile powder for injection
Asbron G (In-Lay Tabs; contains theophylline and guaifenesin)	Bronchodilator Expectorant	*PO only:* 1-3 yr—75-200 mg theophylline 3-6 yr—150-300 mg theophylline 6-12 yr—300-600 mg theophylline	Elixir, tablets
Atropine sulfate	Anticholinergic	*PO, SC:* 0.01-0.02 mg/kg/dose *IV:* 0.01 mg/kg/dose	Tablets, sterile solution for injection
Bactrim (Septra; contains trimethoprim and sulfamethoxazole)	Antibacterial	*PO only:* 8 mg/kg of trimethoprim; 40 mg/kg of sulfamethoxazole	Tablets, oral suspension
Benzathine penicillin G (Bicillin)	Antibiotic	*IM only* (single dose): under 60 lb—0.05-0.90 million units/dose, adjusted for age	Sterile suspension for injection
Benylin (contains diphenhydramine hydrochloride‡ and alcohol)	Antihistamine Antitussive	*PO:* 2-6 yr—½ tsp 4 times 6-12 yr—1 tsp 4 times	Syrup
Bisacodyl (Dulcolax)	Cathartic	*PO:* 0.3 mg/kg/dose *R:* 5-10 mg/dose	Tablets, suppositories
Bleomycin (Blenoxane)	Antineoplastic	INITIAL DOSE: 1-2 units *IM, SC, IV:* 0.25-0.5 units/kg/3-7 days (total dose should not exceed 400 units)	Sterile powder for injection
Busulfan (Myleran)	Antineoplastic	*PO only:* 1.8 mg/M²	Tablets
Caffeine	Stimulant	*PO:* 10 mg/kg	Tablets, capsules
Calcium gluconate	Electrolyte	*PO:* 500 mg/kg *IV:* 0.2 ml/kg/dose of 10% solution, diluted, given slowly with cardiac monitoring	Tablets, sterile solution for injection
Calcium lactate	Electrolyte	*PO:* 500 mg/kg	Powder, capsules, syrup, wafers
Carbenicillin (Geopen, Pyopen)	Antibiotic	*IM, IV:* Infants under 2 kg—first 7 days, 100 mg/kg/12 hr; after 7 days, 100 mg/kg/8 hr Infants over 2 kg—first 7 days, 100 mg/kg/12 hr; after 7 days 100 mg/kg/6 hr Children—50-400 mg/kg depending on severity of infection	Sterile powder for injection

Continued.

*Each 5 ml tsp contains 1.25 mg triprolidine HCl and 30 mg pseudoephedrine HCl.
†This amount is given to attain therapeutic blood levels; maintenance doses are adjusted to maintain desired response.
‡Each 5 ml contains 12.5 mg of diphenhydramine.

Table 10-1. Safe dose chart of commonly used medications for children—cont'd

Medication	General classification	Recommended maximum dosage by route for 24 hours unless specified otherwise	Forms available
Cefaclor (Ceclor)	Antibiotic	*PO only:* 20-40 mg/kg	Powder for oral suspension
Cefamandole nafate (Mandol)	Antibiotic	*IM, IV:* 50-100 mg/kg	Sterile powder for injection
Cefazolin sodium (Ancef)	Antibiotic	*IM, IV:* 25-100 mg/kg	Sterile powder for injection
Cephalexin (Keflex)	Antibiotic	*PO only:* 25-50 mg/kg	Capsules, oral suspension
Cephalothin (Keflin)	Antibiotic	*IM, IV:* 60-150 mg/kg	Sterile powder for injection
Chloral hydrate (Noctec, Somnos)	Sedative	*PO, R:* 10-50 mg/kg	Syrup, capsules, elixir, suppositories
Chloramphenicol (Chloromycetin)	Antibiotic	*PO, IV:* Newborns—25 mg/kg; Infants and children—50-100 mg/kg	Capsules, oral suspension, sterile powder for injection, ophthalmic ointment
Chlorothiazide (Diuril)	Diuretic Antihypertensive	*PO:* 2-15 mg/kg/12 hr	Suspension, tablets, sterile powder for injection
Chlorpromazine (Thorazine)	Antipsychotic Antiemetic	*PO, IM, IV:* 2 mg/kg; *R:* 3-4 mg/kg; Dosages not established for children under 6 mo	Syrup, tablets, sterile solutions for injection, suppositories
Clindamycin hydrochloride (Cleocin)	Antibiotic	*PO:* 8-20 mg/kg; *IM, IV:* 15-25 mg/kg	Capsules, granules for reconstitution for oral use, sterile solution for injection
Clonazepam (Clonopin)	Anticonvulsant	INITIAL DOSE: *PO:* 0.01-0.05 mg/kg; MAINTENANCE DOSE: *PO:* up to 0.1-0.2 mg/kg	Tablets
Cloxacillin (Tegopen)	Antibiotic	*PO:* Under 20 kg—50-100 mg/kg; Over 20 kg—1000-2000 mg	Capsules, powder for oral solution
Codeine	Analgesic	*PO:* 3 mg/kg; *SC:* 3 mg/kg	Sterile solution for injection, syrup, tablets
Colistimethate (Coly-Mycin)	Antibiotic	*PO:* 5-15 mg/kg; *IM, IV:* 2.5-5 mg/kg	Oral suspension Sterile powder for injection
Corticotropin (Acthar)	Anterior pituitary hormone	*SC, IM:* 0.5-1.6 units/kg	Sterile powder for injection, sterile gel for injection
Cortisone	Corticosteroid	*PO:* 1-10 mg/kg; *IM:* 5-6 mg/kg	Sterile suspension, syrup, tablets

Drug	Classification	Dosage	How supplied
Cytarabine (Cytosar)	Antineoplastic	*IV continuous infusion:* 200 mg/m² for 5 days	Sterile powder for injection
Demeclocycline hydrochloride (Declomycin)	Antibiotic	*PO only:* 6-12 mg/kg; Not for use in children under 8 yr	Capsules, tablets, oral suspension
Dexamethasone (Decadron)	Corticosteroid	*PO, IM, IV:* 0.08-0.3 mg/kg	Elixir, tablets, aerosol, sterile solution for injection, oral suspension, ophthalmic solution
Diazepam (Valium)	Sedative, Antianxiety agent	SEDATIVE/MUSCLE RELAXANT: *PO:* 0.1-0.8 mg/kg; *IM, IV:* 0.04-0.2 mg/kg; ANTICONVULSANT: *IV:* 0.3-0.75 mg/kg; may repeat in 15 minutes	Tablets, sterile solution for injection
Dicloxacillin (Dynapen, Pathocil)	Antibiotic	*PO:* Under 40 kg—12-25 mg/kg; Over 40 kg—500-1000 mg/kg	Capsules, oral suspension
Digoxin (Lanoxin)	Cardiotonic	DIGITALIZING DOSE: *PO:* Newborns—0.04-0.06 mg/kg/dose; 1 mo-2 yr—0.06-0.08 mg/kg/dose; 2-10 yr—0.04-0.06 mg/kg/dose; Over 10 yr—0.125-0.5 mg/dose; *IM, IV:* Neonates—0.025-0.04 mg/kg/dose; 2 wk-2 yr—0.035-0.05 mg/kg/dose; 2-10 yr—0.025-0.04 mg/kg/dose; MAINTENANCE DOSE: $\frac{1}{5}$-$\frac{1}{3}$ of digitalizing dose	Tablets, elixir, sterile solution for injection
Dimercaprol (BAL)	Antidote	*IM:* 2.5-5 mg/kg	Sterile solution in oil for injection
Dimetapp (contains brompheniramine, phenylephrine hydrochloride, phenylpropanolamine hydrochloride)	Antihistaminic, Decongestant	*PO only*:* 1-6 mo—¼ tsp 3-4 times daily; 7-24 mo—½ tsp 3-4 times daily; 2-4 yr—¾ tsp 3-4 times daily; 4-12 yr—1 tsp 3-4 times daily	Syrup, elixir, tablets; tablets not recommended for children under 12 yr
Diphenhydramine hydrochloride (Benadryl)	Antihistamine	*PO, IV:* 5 mg/kg	Elixir, capsules, tablets, sterile solution for injection

Continued.

*Dosages are for the elixir containing 4 mg brompheniramine, 5 mg phenylephrine HCl, and 5 mg phenylpropanolamine per each 5 ml tsp.

Table 10-1. Safe dose chart of commonly used medications for children—cont'd

Medication	General classification	Recommended maximum dosage by route for 24 hours unless specified otherwise	Forms available
Diphenoxylate hydrochloride (Lomotil)	Antidiarrheal (with atropine)	*PO only:* 2-5 yr—6 mg; 5-8 yr—8 mg; 8-12 yr—10 mg	Liquid, tablets
Docusate sodium (Colace)	Stool softener	*PO only:* Under 3 yr—10-40 mg; 3-6 yr—20-60 mg; 6-12 yr—40-120 mg; Over 12 yr—50-200 mg	Liquid drops, capsules, tablets, syrup
Donnatal (contains phenobarbital, hyoscyamine sulfate, atropine, hyoscine)	Antidiarrheal	*PO only*: 22 kg—0.5 ml-0.75 ml q 4-6 hr; 45 kg—1.25-2 ml q 4-6 hr; 68 kg—2.5 ml q 4-6 hr; 110 kg—¾ tsp-1 tsp q 4-6 hr; 175 kg—1-1½ tsp q 4-6 hr	Elixir, tablets, capsules
Doxycycline (Vibramycin)	Antibiotic (tetracycline class)	INITIAL DOSE: *PO, IV:* Under 45 kg—4.5 mg/kg; Over 45 kg—200 mg. MAINTENANCE DOSE: *PO, IV:* Under 45 kg—1.1-2.2 mg/kg; Over 45 kg—100 mg	Oral suspension, capsules, tablets, sterile powder for injection
Ephedrine	Antiasthmatic	*SC, IM, PO:* 3 mg/kg	Capsules, tablets, syrup, sterile solution for injection
Epinephrine (Adrenaline, 1:1000; Susphrine, 1:200)	Bronchodilator	*SC:* 1:1000 solution: 0.01-0.025 ml/kg/dose; 1:200 solution: 0.005 ml/kg/dose	Sterile solution for injection
Erythromycin (Erythrocin, Pediamycin)	Antimicrobial	*PO:* 30-100 mg/kg; *IV:* 15-20 mg/kg	Tablets, drops, oral suspension
Ferrous sulfate (Ferosol, Fer-in-Sol)	Iron supplement	*PO:* 1-2 mg/kg	Elixir, tablets, spansule, drops, capsules
Flucytosine (Ancobon)	Antifungal	*PO only:* 50-150 mg/kg	Capsules
Furosemide (Lasix)	Diuretic	INITIAL DOSE: *PO:* 1-2 mg/kg/dose, not to exceed 6 mg/kg/dose; *IM, IV:* not to exceed 6 mg/kg/dose	Oral solution, tablets, sterile solution for injection

Gentamicin (Garamycin)	Antibiotic	*IM, IV:* Premature infants or neonates under 1 wk—5 mg/kg; 1 wk-1 yr—7.5 mg/kg; Over 1 yr—6-7 mg/kg	Sterile solution for injection
Glucagon	Hormone	HYPOGLYCEMIC REACTION: *SC, IM, IV:* 0.025 unit/kg/dose	Sterile powder for injection
Griseofulvin (Fulvicin-U/F, Grifulvin V)	Antifungal	*PO only:* 10 mg/kg	Tablets, oral suspension
Guaifenesin (Robitussin, Robitussin-CF)	Expectorant Antitussive	*PO only:* 2-6 yr—15 ml; 6-12 yr—30 ml; over 21 yr—60 ml	Syrup
Hydralazine hydrochloride (Apresoline)	Antihypertensive	*PO:* 0.75-3.5 mg/kg; *IM, IV:* 1.7-3.5 mg/kg	Tablets, sterile solution for injection
Hydrochlorothiazide (Hydrodiuril)	Diuretic Antihypertensive	*PO:* 0.5-2.0 mg/kg	Tablets
Hydrocortisone sodium (Solu-Cortef)	Antiinflammatory	ASTHMA: *IM, IV:* 10-20 mg/kg; ENDOTOXIC SHOCK—INITIAL DOSE: 50 mg/kg; MAINTENANCE: 50-75 mg/kg	Sterile powder for injection
Hydroxyzine hydrochloride (Atarax, Vistaril)	Antihistaminic, antiemetic, sedative	*PO:* 2 mg/kg; *IM:* 1 mg/kg/dose	Syrup, tablets, capsules, sterile solution for injection
Indomethacin (Indocin)	Analgesic	*PO only:* Under 14 yr—not recommended; Over 14 yr—75-150 mg	Capsules
Ipecac	Emetic	*PO only:* Infants—5-10 ml/dose; Children—15 ml/dose	Syrup
Iron dextran (Imferon)	Iron supplement	*Deep IM (Z-track only):* dose variable depending on extent of deficiency	Sterile solution for injection
Isoniazid (INH, Nydrazid)	Antitubercular	*PO:* 10-30 mg/kg; *IM:* 10-30 mg/kg	Tablets, syrup, sterile solution for injection
Kanamycin sulfate (Kantrex)	Antibiotic	*PO:* 25-50 mg/kg; *IM:* 15 mg/kg	Capsules, sterile solution for injection
Lidocaine (Xylocaine)	Antiarrhythmic	*IM:* 403 mg/kg/dose; *IV:* 1 mg/kg/dose	Sterile solution for injection

Continued.

*Dosages are for elixir containing 16.2 mg phenobarbital, 104 µg hyoscyamine, 19 µg atropine, and 6.5 µg hyoscine.

Table 10-1. Safe dose chart of commonly used medications for children—cont'd

Medication	General classification	Recommended maximum dosage by route for 24 hours unless specified otherwise	Forms available
Magnesium and aluminum hydroxide (Gelusil, Mylanta, Maalox)	Antacid	*PO only:* 0.5 ml/kg/dose	Tablets, oral suspension
Mannitol (Osmitrol)	Diuretic	OLIGURIA: *IV:* 200 mg/kg/dose CEREBRAL EDEMA: *IV:* 1-2.5 gm/kg/dose	Sterile solution for injection
Mechlorethamine (nitrogen mustard, mustargen)	Antineoplastic	*IV:* 0.1-0.2 mg/kg	Sterile powder for injection
Meperidine hydrochloride (Demerol)	Analgesic	*PO, IM, SC:* 6 mg/kg	Syrup, tablets, sterile solution for injection
Meprobamate (Equanil, Miltown)	Sedative/hypnotic	*PO only:* 6-12 yr—12.5-25 mg/kg	Syrup, capsules, tablets
Mercaptopurine (Purinethol)	Antineoplastic	INITIAL DOSE: *PO only:* 2.5 mg/kg MAINTENANCE DOSE: *PO only:* 1.5-2.5 mg/kg	Tablets
Methicillin (Staphcillin, Celbenin)	Antibiotic	*IM, IV:* Neonates under 7 days—50 mg/kg Neonates over 7 days—75 mg/kg	Sterile powder for injection
Methotrexate (Mexate)	Antineoplastic	DISEASE DEPENDENT: *PO, IM:* 6.6-60 mg/m²/wk *IV:* 2.5 mg/m² q 14 days	Tablets, sterile powder for injection
Methyldopa (Aldomet)	Antihypertensive	INITIAL DOSE: *PO, IV:* 10 mg/kg; may increase or decrease; not to exceed 65 mg/kg	Tablets, sterile solution for injection
Methylphenidate hydrochloride (Ritalin)	Stimulant	*PO:* start with 5 mg q 12 hr; increase as needed by 5 mg/dose/wk; not to exceed 60 mg/day; not recommended for children under 6 yr	Tablets
Methylprednisolone (Solu-Medrol, Medrol)	Antiinflammatory	*PO, IM, IV:* 0.4-2 mg/kg	Sterile powder for injection, tablets
Metronidazole (Flagyl)	Antibacterial	AMEBIASIS: *PO:* 35-50 mg/kg	Tablets
Minocycline hydrochloride (Minocin)	Antibiotic	*PO, IV:* 2-4 mg/kg; not for children under 8 yr	Oral suspension, sterile powder for injection
Morphine	Analgesic	*IM, SC:* 0.06-0.2 mg/kg/dose	Tablets, ampules

Drug	Classification	Dosage	Form
Nafcillin (Unipen)	Antibiotic	*PO:* Neonates—30-40 mg/kg, Children—25-50 mg/kg; *IM, IV:* Children—100-200 mg/kg	Capsules, tablets, powder
Naloxone hydrochloride (Narcan)	Narcotic antagonist	*SC, IM, IV:* 0.01 mg/kg/dose	Sterile solution for injection
Neomycin (Mycifradin)	Antibiotic	*PO only:* 50-100 mg/kg	Tablets, oral solution
Nitrofurantoin (Furadantin, Macrodantin)	Antibacterial	*PO:* 5-7 mg/kg; Contraindicated in infants under 1 mo	Tablets, oral suspension
Novahistine Elixir (chlorpheniramine maleate, phenylpropanolamine hydrochloride, alcohol)	Antitussive decongestant	*PO:* 7-11 kg—½ tsp, 11-16 kg—¾ tsp, 16-23 kg—1 tsp, 23-41 kg—2 tsp	Elixir
Nystatin (Mycostatin, Nilstat)	Antifungal	*PO only:* Infants—400,000-800,000 units, Children—1.6-2.4 million units	Tablets, oral suspension
Oxacillin (Prostaphlin, Bactocill)	Antibiotic	*PO, IM, IV:* Under 40 kg—50 mg/kg, Over 40 kg—2-3 gm	Capsules, oral solution, sterile powder for injection
Oxtriphylline (Choledyl)	Bronchodilator	*PO only:* 2-9 yr—24-37.5 mg/kg, 9-12 yr—20-31 mg/kg, 12-16 yr—18-28 mg/kg, Over 16 yr—13-20 mg/kg (or up to 1400 mg)	Syrup, elixir, tablets
Pancrelipase (Cotazym)	Pancreatic enzyme	*PO only:* 1-3 capsules or 1-2 packets of powder with each meal	Capsules, powder
Penicillin (Pentids 400, pfizerpen G, Sugracillin)	Antibiotic	*PO, IM, IV:* Children—25,000-400,000 units/kg; *IV, IM:* Neonates under 7 days—50,000-400,000 units/kg, Neonates over 7 days—100,000-200,000 units/kg; MENINGITIS: *IV, IM:* Neonates under 7 days—150,000-250,000 units/kg, Neonates over 7 days—150,000-250,000 units/kg	Tablets, oral suspension, sterile powder for injection

Continued.

Table 10-1. Safe dose chart of commonly used medications for children—cont'd

Medication	General classification	Recommended maximum dosage by route for 24 hours unless specified otherwise	Forms available
Pentobarbital (Nembutal)	Sedative/hypnotic	*PO, R, IM:* 6 mg/kg	Capsules, tablets, elixir, suppositories, sterile solution for injection
Phenobarbital (Luminal, Eskabarb)	Central nervous system depressant	SEDATION: *PO:* 6 mg/kg SLEEP: *PO:* 4-6 mg/kg/dose ANTICONVULSANT OR STATUS EPILEPTICUS—LOADING DOSE: *IV, IM:* 10-15 mg/kg MAINTENANCE: *PO:* 4-6 mg/kg	Elixir, tablets, capsules, suspensions, sterile solutions for injection
Phenoxymethyl penicillin (Penicillin V, Compocillin VK, Penn-Vee K, V-cillin K)	Antibiotic	*PO only:* 25,000-50,000 units/kg	Tablets, oral solutions, oral suspension
Phenylephrine hydrochloride (Neo-Synephrine)	Vasoconstrictor	*PO:* 1 mg/kg *SC, IM:* 0.1 mg/kg/dose	Syrup, elixir, sterile solution for injection
Phenytoin sodium (Dilantin)	Anticonvulsant	*PO, IV:* 5-7 mg/kg up to maximum of 300 mg	Tablets, capsules, sterile powder for injection
Phytonadione (Aquamephyton)	Vitamin K₁	PROPHYLAXIS IN NEWBORN: *IM, SC:* 0.5-1 mg/dose	Sterile solution for injection
Prednisone (Deltasone, Paracort, Meticorten)	Antiinflammatory	*PO only:* 2 mg/kg	Tablets
Procaine penicillin G (Crysticillin, Duracillin A.S., Wycillin, Bicillin C-R)	Antibiotic	*IM only:* 25,000-100,000 units/kg	Sterile suspension for injection
Prochlorperazine (Compazine)	Antiemetic	*PO, R:* 13-18 kg—up to 10 mg 18-39 kg—up to 15 mg *IM:* 0.132 mg/kg	Tablets, syrup, capsules, suppositories, sterile solution for injection
Promethazine hydrochloride (Phenergan)	Sedative, antiemetic	*PO, IM, R:* 0.25-0.5 mg/kg	Tablets, syrup, suppositories, sterile solution for injection
Propantheline bromide (Pro-Banthine)	Antispasmodic	*PO:* 1.5 mg/kg *IM:* 0.8 mg/kg	Tablets, sterile powder for injection

Drug	Classification	Dosage	Forms
Propranolol hydrochloride (Inderal)	Antihypertensive Antiarrhythmic	ANTIHYPERTENSIVE: *PO:* 1-5 mg/kg ANTIARRHYTHMIC: *PO:* 0.3-1.2 mg/kg *IV:* 0.01-0.02 mg/kg/dose	Tablets, sterile solution for injection
Prophylthiouracil (PTU, Tapazole)	Thyroid inhibitor	INITIAL DOSE: *PO only:* 6-10 yr—50-150 mg Over 10 yr—50-300 mg MAINTENANCE DOSE: 75-2000 mg/day	Tablets
Pseudoephedrine (Sudafed)	Nasal decongestant	*PO only:* Infants—15 mg q 4-6 hr not to exceed 60 mg/day Children—30 mg q 4-6 hr not to exceed 120 mg/day	Syrup, elixir, capsules, tablets
Reserpine (Eskaserp, Serpasil, Snadril, Raurine)	Antihypertensive	INITIAL DOSE: *PO, IM:* 0.02 mg/kg MAINTENANCE DOSE: *PO:* 0.005 mg/kg Not for use in young children	Elixir, tablets, sterile solution for injection
Rifampin (Rifadin, Rimactane)	Antitubercular	*PO only:* 1-20 mg/kg	Capsules
Secobarbital (Seconal)	Sedative/hypnotic	SLEEP: *PO, IM:* 2-3 mg/kg SEDATION: *PO, IM, R:* 1-2 mg/kg	Tablets, capsules, elixir, suppositories, sterile solution for injection
Streptomycin	Antibiotic	*IM only:* 20-40 mg/kg (maximum of 1 gm)	Sterile solution for injection
Sulfisoxazole (Gantrisin)	Antibacterial	INITIAL DOSE: *PO:* 75 mg/kg *SC, IM, IV:* 50 mg/kg MAINTENANCE DOSE: *PO:* 150 mg/kg *SC, IM, IV:* 100 mg/kg	Tablets, oral suspension, syrup, sterile solution for injection
Tetracycline (Achromycin)	Antibiotic	*PO, IM, IV:* 25-50 mg/kg Not recommended for children under 8 yr	Capsules, syrup, oral suspension, sterile powder for injection
Oxytetracycline (Terramycin)	Antibiotic	*PO:* 25-50 mg/kg *IM, IV:* 10-20 mg/kg Not recommended for children under 8 yr	Tablets, capsules, oral suspension, sterile solution for injection
Theophylline (Accurbron)	Bronchodilator	*PO only:* 16-24 mg/kg; highly toxic; serum levels not to exceed 20 µg/ml	Elixir, syrup, capsules
Tobramycin (Nebcin)	Antibiotic	*IV:* Neonates—4 mg/kg *IM, IV:* Children—3-5 mg/kg	Sterile solution for injection

Continued.

Table 10-1. Safe dose chart of commonly used medications for children—cont'd

Medication	General classification	Recommended maximum dosage by route for 24 hours unless specified otherwise	Forms available
Triiodothyronine (Cytomel)	Thyroid hormone	INITIAL DOSE: *PO only:* 2.5-5.0 μg MAINTENANCE DOSE: 15-20 μg	Tablets
Tripolidine (Actidil)	Antihistaminic	*PO only:* 4 mo-2 yr—1.24 mg 2-4 yr—2.5 mg 4-6 yr—3.75 mg 6-12 yr—5 mg	Tablets, syrup
Valproic acid (Depakene)	Anticonvulsant	*PO only:* INITIAL DOSE: 15 mg/kg MAINTENANCE DOSE: increase every week by 10 mg/kg up to 30 mg/kg	Capsules, syrup
Vancomycin hydrochloride (Vancocin)	Antibiotic	*PO, IV:* Children—45 mg/kg Neonates—10 mg/kg	Sterile powder for injection, oral solution
Vincristine (Oncovin)	Antineoplastic	IV: 0.05-0.15 mg/kg/wk	Sterile powder for injection
Viokase	Pancreatic enzymes	PO: 750 mg with each meal	Granules, tablets, capsules

Kilogram weight. The most frequently used criterion for determining a therapeutic dose of pediatric medication is by kilogram weight. To verify that the doctor's order is safe using weight as the criterion, follow these three steps:

Step 1. Determine the kilogram weight of the child. In some institutions, only kilogram scales are used, thereby making this step a simple one. In other institutions, however, pound scales are used; therefore, pounds must be converted to kilograms. To convert the weight in pounds to kilograms, divide the pounds by 2.2 (1 kilogram is equal to 2.2 pounds). In many neonatal nurseries, infants are weighed on gram scales. To convert gram weight to kilograms, divide the gram weight by 1,000 (1,000 grams equal one kilogram).

Step 2. Multiply the kilogram weight by the *safe dose factor* (SDF). The SDF is the recommended amount of medication determined through research to be appropriate for pediatric patients. It can be found by going to a reference book and looking under "recommended pediatric dosage." In many cases, the SDF is a single number; a dosage range is common, however, depending on the severity of disease. On Table 10-1 the SDF is listed in the column listing recommended maximum dosage by route. It is important to note whether the SDF in the reference is in *terms of dosage each time or dosage per 24 hours.* Usually, the SDF is written per 24 hours. The answer obtained when multiplying the kilogram weight by the SDF is the maximum amount a patient of that kilogram weight is to receive.

Step 3. Compare the doctor's order with the maximum recommended dosage. (Obtained in step 2.) Be sure the two comparisons are for the same time period. If the maximum amount is determined for 24 hours, the amount that the physician ordered for 24 hours must be used for comparison. If the doctor's order exceeds the recommended amount, the order is unsafe and the dosage should not be administered.

Practice problem 1: The physician orders amoxicillin, 135 mg PO q 6 hr. The child weighs 22 pounds. Is this a safe dose?

Step 1. Find the kilogram weight: Because the weight is in pounds, it must be converted to kilograms. To get the kilogram weight, divide the weight in pounds by 2.2.

$$\frac{22}{2.2} = 10 \text{ kg}$$

Step 2. Multiply the kilogram weight by the SDF. The SDF for amoxicillin on Table 10-1 is 20 to 40 mg/kg per 24 hours.

$$40 \text{ mg} \times 10 \text{ kg} = 400 \text{ mg}$$

The maximum amount of amoxicillin that a child who weighs 10 kg (or 22 pounds) should receive in 24 hours is 400 mg.

Step 3. Compare the doctor's order with maximum recommended dosage. The physician has ordered 135 mg per dose. It is ordered every 6 hours or 4 times a day. Therefore, to determine what the doctor has ordered for 24 hours, it is necessary to multiply the dose by the number of times a day it is given. In this case 135 mg × 4 a times = 540 mg per 24 hours. The maximum safe amount of amoxicillin for a child of kg is 400 mg per 24 hours. The physician has ordered 540 mg per 24 hours so the doctor's order is *unsafe*.

Practice problem 2: The physician orders meperidine hydrochloride (Demerol), 15 mg IM q 4 hr p.r.n. for a child who weighs 40 pounds. Is this a safe order?

Step 1. Find the kilogram weight (by dividing pounds by 2.2).

$$\frac{40}{2.2} = 18.18, \text{ or } 18.2, \text{ kg}$$

Step 2. Multiply the kilogram weight by the SDF. The SDF for meperidine hydrochloride is 6 mg/kg per 24 hours.

$$6 \text{ mg} \times 18.2 \text{ kg} = 109.2 \text{ mg}$$

The maximum amount of meperidine a child of 18.2 kg should receive is 109.2 mg.

Step 3. Compare the doctor's order with the recommended safe dosage. The physician has ordered 15 mg per dose to be given every 4 hours or 6 times a day.

$$15 \text{ mg} \times 6 \text{ times} = 90 \text{ mg}$$

The physician has ordered 90 mg per 24 hours. The maximum amount the child can receive is 109.2 mg per 24 hours so the doctor's order is *safe*.

Surface area or square meters (M²). A third criterion used for calculating the safe pediatric dosage is by surface area or square meter (M²). This method is probably the most accurate method, as it considers not only body weight and length, but also physiological processes that affect the utilization of medication such as heat loss and cardiac output. This method is used to determine dosage for medications that are unusually potent or have severe side effects, such as those of the antineoplastic group or steroids. Like the other methods for calculating dosage, there are three steps:

Step 1. Find the surface area in square meters. To do this, a nomogram such as the West nomogram (Fig. 10-1) is used.

Step 2. Multiply the surface area of the child by the recommended SDF. (Make sure that the SDF is per M², not kg.)

Step 3. Compare the doctor's order with the safe maximum dosage amount (obtained in step 2).

Practice problem 3: The physician orders cytarabine, 75 mg IV, b.i.d. for a patient of 60 pounds. Is the doctor's order safe? On consulting a reference, the nurse sees that the safe dose is determined according to surface area.

Step 1. Find the surface area. The West nomogram shows that the surface area of a child of 60 pounds is approximately 0.98 M².

Step 2. Multiply the surface area by the recommended maximum SDF as listed on Table 10-1. Thus,

$$0.98 \text{ M}^2 \times 200 \text{ mg} = 196 \text{ mg}$$

The maximum amount of cytarabine that a child of 60 pounds should receive is 196 mg per 24 hours.

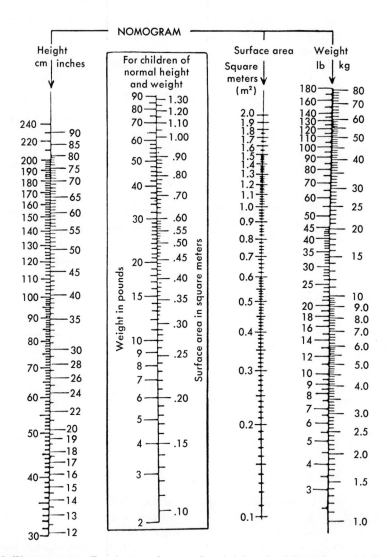

Fig. 10-1. West nomogram. To estimate surface area from height and weight: with a straight line connect the height and weight and read the square meters (m^2) in the surface area column. To establish the surface area for children of normal height and weight: use the enclosed column and read the square meters opposite their weight in pounds. (Modified from data of E. Boyd by C.D. West. From Shirkey, H.C.: Drug therapy. In Nelson, W.E., editor: Textbook of pediatrics, ed. 9, Philadelphia, 1969, W.B. Saunders Co.)

Step 3. Compare the doctor's order with the safe maximum dosage amount. The physician has ordered 75 mg per dose twice a day or 75 mg × 2 times = 150 mg per 24 hours. The safe maximum dose is 196 mg per 24 hours so the doctor's order is *safe*.

Practice problem 4: The physician orders busulfan, 1 mg PO, t.i.d. for a child of 35 pounds who is 25 inches tall. Is this a safe order?

Step 1. Find the surface area in square meters. Using the West nomogram, the point intersection of the surface area column from a height of 35 inches and a weight of 35 pounds is approximately 0.64 M².

Step 2. Multiply the surface area by the SDF. The maximum SDF for busulfan as listed in Table 10-1 is 1.8 mg/M² per 24 hours. Thus,

$$0.64 \text{ M}^2 \times 1.8 = 1.15 \text{ mg}$$

Step 3. Compare the doctor's order with the recommended maximum safe dose. The physician has ordered 1 mg 3 times per day or 1 mg × 3 times = 3 mg. The recommended safe maximum safe dose is 1.15 mg per 24 hours. Thus, the doctor's order is *unsafe*.

Other rules. There are several other rules that may be used in calculating a safe pediatric therapeutic dose. These rules are not very reliable because the bases on which they were developed are not reliable: age and adult weight. Because of their inaccuracies, the only time these formulas should be used is when there is no recommended pediatric dosage. Medications that are new, or for which pediatric ranges have not been determined may not have a recommended pediatric dosage.

Three of the pediatric formulas that will provide an infant's or child's fractional dose are as follows:

1. *Fried's rule* (used for patients less than 1 year old)

Approximate infant's dose =
$$\frac{\text{Infant's age in months} \times \text{Adult dose}}{150}$$

2. *Clark's rule* (for a child 2 years old or over)

Approximate child's dose =
$$\frac{\text{Weight in pounds} \times \text{Adult dose}}{150}$$

3. *Young's rule* (also used for children 2 years old or over)

Approximate child's dose =
$$\frac{\text{Age of child (in years)}}{\text{Age of child (in years)} + 12} \times \text{Adult dose}$$

The "150" that is used as the demoninator in Fried's rule and Clark's rule represents the average adult weight in pounds. This explains why these rules give inaccurate information, as the average adult weight varies from one population to another, and in the United States average adult weighs far exceeds 150 pounds.

Systems for the administration of medications

Several systems exist for the preparation and administration of medications. Systems vary from institution to institution. Nurses should become familiar with the systems and procedures utilized in the institution where they work.

Stock medications

With stock medications, medications are delivered to the nursing unit in bulk. This system requires that nurses be particularly knowledgeable about methods of calculating dosages and using various formulas. They must know how to mix drugs in the correct solution, how to maintain sterility when mixing medications for parenteral use, the life of drugs after mixing, labeling of the strength after reconstitution, and proper disposal of unused medications.

Unit dose systems

Many hospitals are using the unit dose system for administration of medications with a portable medication cart (Fig. 10-2). With this system, the pharmacy department assumes all responsi-

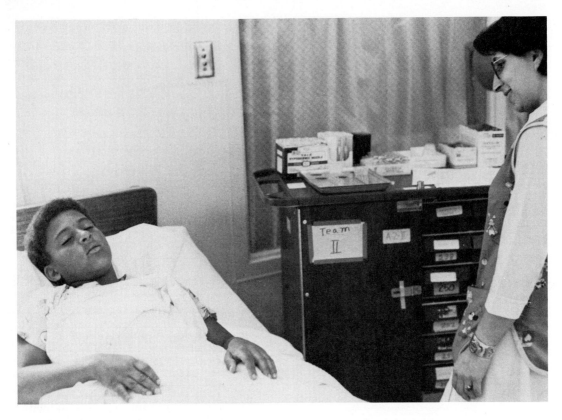

Fig. 10-2. With a unit dose system, medications of all patients are prepared in individual doses by the pharmacist and stored in a portable medication cart that can be moved near to the patient.

bility for calculating, mixing, and labeling the medications. When the medication arrives at the nursing unit, it is packaged and labeled in single individual doses. With this system, much of the work of calculating and measuring drug dosages is taken over by the pharmacist.

In the pediatric setting, it is extremely difficult to have a pure unit dose system. Many of the medications are unstable and must be administered within a few minutes after mixing. For this reason a combination system of medication administration may be used. Stable medications may be prepared by the pharmacy department using the unit dose system, whereas unstable medications may be sent to the nursing unit in bulk to be mixed by the nurse just before administration.

• • •

Regardless of the system used, the nurse must take appropriate measures to ensure that the "five rights" are followed.

Medication cards

Many hospitals use a medication card for administration of medications. With this system, a card is completed in ink for each medication to be administered. If the medication is to be discontinued after that particular administration, the card is destroyed.

The medication card contains all the information given in the doctor's order: the name of the child, the name of the medication, the amount of the medication, the route of administration, and

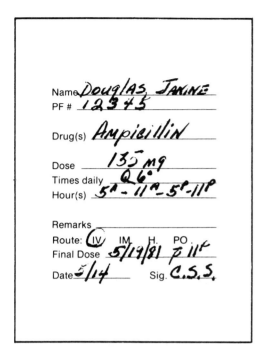

Name *Douglas, Janine*
PF # *12345*

Drug(s) *Ampicillin*

Dose *135 mg*
Times daily *Q 6°*
Hour(s) *5ᴬ - 11ᴬ - 5ᴾ - 11ᴾ*

Remarks _____
Route: (IV) IM H. PO
Final Dose *5/19/81 p̄ 11ᴾ*
Date *5/14* _____ Sig. *C.S.S.*

Fig. 10-3. Medication card.

the frequency of administration (Fig. 10-3). Additional information may also be placed on the medication card such as "mix with applesauce," or "give with meals." Start dates for the medications and stop dates or expiration dates may also be required on the medication card.

To use this system, the nurse gathers the medication cards for all the patients for whom she is to administer medications. At the beginning of the shift, the card is reviewed for completeness and checked for expiration dates, and the safety of the dose is verified.

Having done this, the nurse then places the cards in time sequence. At the time the medication is due, the nurse prepares the medication according to the instructions on the medication card. Immediately after administration, the nurse charts the medication, using the card as the source of information. The cards are then returned to their storage area until the next time the medication is due.

Some hospitals have moved away from this system because of the increased error factor associated with transcribing doctors' orders in many places and because of lost or misplaced cards.

Medication Kardex

In the Kardex system of medication administration, all medications are transcribed from doctor's order forms to individual medication Kardex cards, one for each patient. As with medication cards, all of the components of the doctor's prescription are included, but may be spelled out in more detail. For example, if the prescription reads, "b.i.d. (twice a day)," the Kardex card might specify "9 am and 6 pm," depending on the established custom on that nursing unit (Fig. 10-4).

As with the medication card, all the pertinent information is reviewed at the beginning of the shift. At the time of the preparation of the medication, the Kardex is taken to the area, and the medications are prepared according to the information on the Kardex.

After administration, the medications are charted in the patient record, using the Kardex card as the source of information. Should the medication be discontinued or changed, a line is drawn through it to indicate that the order is no longer valid. Variations of this system have been devised, such as using color-coded stickers with each drug on a separate sticker.

Because this system is fraught with problems, many hospitals have abandoned it in favor of unit dose systems.

Original prescription system

Because of the problems inherent in systems that require transcription of doctor's orders, some hospitals have instituted one in which medications are administered from the original doctor's order (Fig. 10-5). With this system, each patient's medication orders are listed on a single page. The order sheets are usually kept in a notebook or chart out of the patient's record. Because

Start Date	Exp. Date	MEDICATION	DOSAGE	MODE	FREQUENCY	AM		PM		RN Initial
5/14	5/19	Ampicillin	135 mg.	I.V.	Q 6°	5	11	5	11	C.S.S.
5/14		Aminophylline	100 mg.	I.V.	Q 8°	2	10	4		C.S.S.
5/14		Dimetapp Syrup	3/4 Tsp	P.O.	T.I.D	9		1	5	C.S.S.
5/14	5/17	Acetaminophen	gr ii	P.O.	Q 4° PRN For T > 101°	9		5		C.S.S.

DRUG ALLERGY: NONE

DIAGNOSIS PNEUMONIA   AGE 2 y/c BIRTH DATE 8/17/78 ADM. DATE 5/14/81 P.F.# 12345

NAME Douglas, Janine D.   ROOM 347 DOCTOR Celsa Clifford

Fig. 10-4. A medication Kardex is made for each patient.

MEDICATION PRESCRIPTION AND ADMINISTRATION RECORD

Patient's name_____

ID number_____

Date	Time	Order	Date: 5/14/81 AM	PM	Date: 5/15/81 AM	PM	Date: 5/16/81 AM	PM
5/14/81	10 PM	1) Ampicillin 135 mg, IV q 6° ———		11 ^{PM} - css	5 ^{AM} - D.J. 11 ^{AM} - mℒθ	5 ^{PM} - css		
5/14/81	10 PM	2) Aminophylline 100 mg IV q 8° ———			2 ^{AM} - D.J. 10 ^{AM} - mℒθ	4 ^{PM} - css		
5/14/81	10 PM	Dimetapp Syrup 3/4 Tsp P.O. T.I.D. ——			9 ^{AM} - mℒθ	1 ^{PM} - mℒβ 5 ^{PM} - css		
5/14/81	10 PM	Acetaminophen gr ii P.O. q 4° PRN for T > 101 ^{R} Dr. C. Clifford Noted C. Stanley, R.N.		10 ^{PM} - css	3 ^{AM} - D.J.			

Fig. 10-5. A medication order form that is also used to record the actual administration of medication.

the original order is used, transcription is not necessary. At the time of administration, nurses take the notebook to the medication area and prepare the medication from the original order. After administering the medication, they chart the time of administration and sign the original order form. If a medication is discontinued, the nurse draws a line through the remaining times. When the sheet is filled, it is placed in the patient's record as a permanent part of the chart.

Because of the structure of the form, the physician is required to reorder frequently. The advantage of this is that medication orders are not "lost" or forgotten. This system also eliminates additional forms for recording medications.

Computerized systems

The advent of computerized medical records has changed dramatically all methods for storing and retrieving information. In hospitals with such systems physicians type out prescriptions on a keyboard to put them into the computer. The pharmacy then knows instantly to supply medications to the nursing units. As the time comes to administer them, the display screen indicates to nurses what drugs and their dosages are due. As soon as they give a medication, nurses record the fact in the computer. This system appears to be the most accurate and efficient system yet devised.

• • •

Regardless of the system used, the nurse must be aware of the policies and procedures associated with the system of administration used in a particular facility. Information such as who is allowed to note orders, the expiration dates for medications, various places medications are noted, and charting procedure must be a part of the nurse's knowledge before administering medication.

Times of administration

Medications are given at various times throughout the day. Some are given only once,

such as preoperative analgesics; others are ordered to be given as needed (p.r.n.) every so many hours. Some drugs are to be given once a day (q.d.), some are given twice a day (b.i.d.), some three times a day (t.i.d.), some four times a day (q.i.d.). The times that drugs are to be given are usually standardized in each pediatric ward, such as at 8, 12, 4, and 8.

Some drugs are excreted from the body rapidly, and so they must be given at regular intervals throughout the day and night to maintain a constant blood level. The orders for these drugs indicate the intervals between doses rather than the number of times per day. For example, penicillin may be ordered every 12 hours rather than twice a day (q 12 hr). It should be administered exactly as ordered.

Measurement systems

There are three systems of measurement: household, apothecary, and metric. Nurses need to be able to make conversions between them. A full conversion table should be posted in the area where medicines are prepared, but nurses' work is greatly facilitated if they know the basic equivalents from memory. Table 10-2 is a list of basic equivalents, conversion rules, and a dose calculation formula.

Measuring containers commonly used for liquid medicines are 3 to 10 ml syringes and an ounce glass or cup. For quantities of less than 5 ml or for fractions of less than 10 ml, such as 7.5 ml, nurses should use syringes for measurement. All air bubbles should be removed to ensure an accurate amount. An ounce cup can be used for amounts between 10 and 32 ml. Remember that after liquid is placed in a container, it is drawn upward by capillary attraction where it contacts the glass. This attraction produces a *meniscus*, or a concave surface. Liquids should always be measured at the lowest point of meniscus (Fig. 10-6).

Droppers may be used for liquid medicines, such as nose drops, or for fluids being administered over a time period, such as intravenous

Table 10-2. Basic equivalents measurements, conversions, and calculation formula

A. Liquids

Metric	*Apothecary*	*Household*
0.06 milliliter*	1 minim	1 drop†
1 milliliter	15 or 16 minims	15 or 16 drops
4-5 milliliters	1 fluidram	1 tsp or 60 drops
16 milliliters	4 fluidrams	1 tablespoon
30 milliliters	1 fluid ounce	2 tablespoons
240 milliliters	8 fluid ounces	1 cup
500 milliliters	1 pint	2 cups
1000 milliliters (1 liter)	1 quart	4 cups

C. Conversion

To convert grains to grams, divide by 15.
To convert grams to grains, multiply by 15.

D. Dose calculation formula

To calculate the correct amount to administer (CATA) divide the dose desired (DD) by the dose on hand (DOH) times the amount of the dose on hand (ADOH):

$$CATA = \frac{DD}{DOH} \times ADOH$$

B. Weights

Metric	*Apothecary*
1 gram	15 grains
60 milligrams	1 grain
4 grams	1 dram
30 grams	1 ounce
1 kilogram	2.2 pounds

*The milliliter and the cubic centimeter are considered equal.
†This "drop" does not necessarily refer to the drop of an intravenous administration unit.

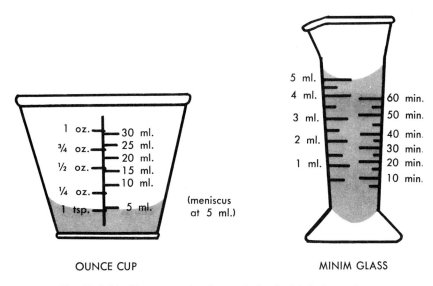

Fig. 10-6. Liquid measures showing menisci at 5 ml in both containers.

infusions. The size of the lumen of the dropper determines the size of its drops.

Routes of administering medications

Medications are administered enterally through the gastrointestinal tract and parenterally by other routes, such as topically into the eyes, ears, nose, or on the skin, or intradermally, subcutaneously, intramuscularly, or intrathecally. Because nurses assist with or administer medications by all of these routes, they need to learn about the special equipment and techniques required to do so.

Enteral routes

The enteral routes are oral, rectal, and directly into the stomach by means of gastric tubes.

Oral. As with adults, the oral route is the most common one for administering medications to children. Unlike adults, however, children often

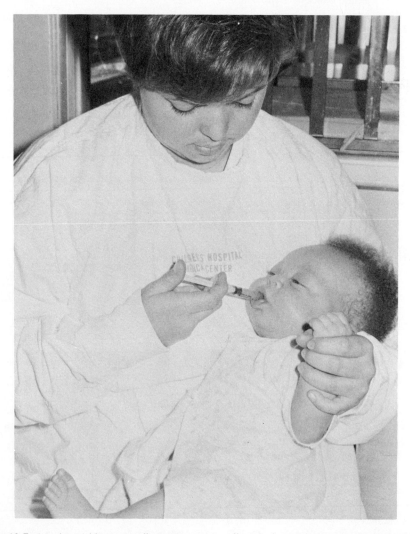

Fig. 10-7. A syringe without a needle serves as an excellent device to give oral liquid medications.

require creative approaches to make the medicine go down.

Oral medications are available in many forms—as dry powder, pressed tablets, capsules or coated tablets, syrups, tinctures, or suspensions. When the physician prescribes an oral medication, often it is the nurse who decides what form is most appropriate, considering the child's age and illness and the amount and taste of the medicine.

When drugs are dispensed in tablet form they may need to be crushed before they are administered. A mortar and pestle are useful for this purpose but the nurse should remember to clean them before and after use. Crushed tablets can be mixed with honey or jam to make them more palatable.

Once the form of medication is decided, further preparation by nurses may be required. If the form is to be liquid and the drug comes in a powdered form, the medication must be reconstituted. As a rule, the manufacturer recommends the amount and type of solution to use as a diluent. Though reconstituting an oral medication is not a sterile procedure, the nurse must use aseptic technique when mixing it. Recalculations and remeasuring are necessary if all the reconstituted medication is not to be given. All liquid oral medications, whether reconstituted at the time of administration or premixed by the pharmacy or pharmaceutical company, must be mixed thoroughly.

As a rule, capsules should not be crushed or taken apart. Capsules are gelatin-like containers used to delay the absorption of the medication. Because of the time it takes the capsules to dissolve, the medication is either timed release (a small amount utilized at a time) or immediately absorbed in the intestine, thus eliminating gastric irritation typical of some medications. If the medication is removed from the capsule, the medication may not be absorbed in the manner intended.

Nurses should select equipment that will facilitate the administration of medication. For infants and smaller children, a syringe without the needle is appropriate (Fig. 10-7). A nipple is not usually appropriate, as many medications adhere to the sides of the nipple. Toddlers and older children like the autonomy associated with taking a medication from a medication cup. Nurses should offer the child something to drink after taking the medication.

When approaching children with oral medications, nurses should use tender loving care but also establish themselves as authority figures. If children are able to understand, nurses should explain unequivocally that it is time to take the medicine. It should not be referred to as candy. Nurses should permit children to decide who holds the cup, which allows them to demonstrate their independence even in their dependent role. Nurses should praise children after they have taken their medications successfully. An extra hug confirms approval. If a parent is present, he or she may be able to hold the child while the nurse administers the medicine (Fig. 10-8).

When administering oral medications to infants, nurses must remember that it is a slower, messier process than for older children, and should allow extra time. Nurses should cover themselves with a protective gown and place protective bibs on the infants. They then should pick up the infants, restrain their arms, and administer small quantities at a time. To prevent aspiration, the medication should be administered just after inhalation. If infants resist swallowing, pinch the nose gently. This action causes them to swallow. Then continue to hold these babies for a time to calm and comfort them.

Rectal. Medications may be administered rectally in solutions as retention enemas or in a firm base such as cocoa butter as suppositories. Because the medication is absorbed slowly and sometimes incompletely, dosages may be higher than for other routes. Rectal medications may be given for their local effects or for their systemic effects. Those made to melt at body temperature are refrigerated until used.

When a retention enema or suppository is prescribed the nurse must explain the procedure at the level of understanding of the child. Children may have more questions about this route of administration than others because bowel control is a major childhood learning task.

The necessary supplies for inserting suppositories include the medicine, gloves, and lubricant. The child is turned to the Sims's position or onto the abdomen and asked to hold the breath at the time of insertion and to try to retain the medication. Then the medication is inserted slowly, past the rectal sphincter. When the finger is removed, the fold of the buttocks must be held

together for a few minutes until the medication begins to dissolve. As with other routes of administration, these children need tender loving care immediately afterward.

Gastric. Medications may be administered directly into the stomach by means of a nasogastric tube passed through the nose or mouth or by a gastrostomy tube inserted into the stomach through a surgical opening in the upper abdomen.

When medications or feedings are to be administered through a nasogastric tube, nurses first must be sure that the tube is in the stomach

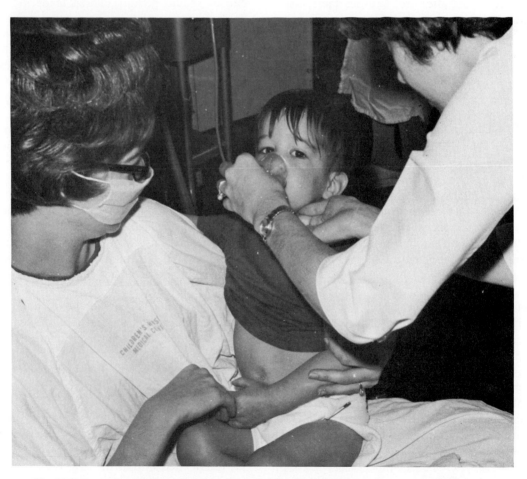

Fig. 10-8. Medicine goes down easily when mother is there. (Note the position of the mother's hands.)

and not in the lungs. Three tests can be made to determine this: (1) aspiration of stomach contents with a syringe indicating that the tube is in the stomach; (2) observation of bubbles when the end of the tube is submerged in water indicating that the tube is in the lungs; and (3) hearing a whoosh of air instilled in the tube by means of a stethoscope placed over the epigastric area indicating that the tube is in the stomach.

Having determined that the tube is in place, the nurse pours the medication into the tube and allows it to flow down the tube by gravity (Fig. 10-9). Following the administration of the med-

ication, the tube is usually rinsed with water to ensure that no medication is left in the tubing.

Frequently, patients who have nasogastric tubes are premature babies and infants. The nurse should remember that this age group needs to suck or they will lose their natural sucking reflex. A pacifier is a useful means to supply this sucking need.

Parenteral routes

Parenteral routes for the administration of medications include the eyes, ears, nose, skin, and blood vessels, cavities, and tissues. When

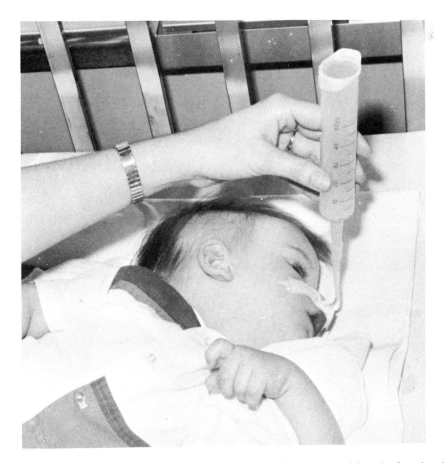

Fig. 10-9. When a nasogastric tube is in place, oral medications are poured into the funnel syringe followed by water.

administering medications by these routes, the nurse may need to restrain infants and young children. A mummy restraint can be used, or another staff member may hold the infant for that moment of stillness required for safety (Fig. 10-10).

Eyedrops. A variety of drugs are prescribed as eyedrops to produce such diverse local effects as anesthesia, dilation or constriction of the pupil, and antisepsis. The exact number of drops and whether the child's left (o.s.), right (o.d.), or both eyes (o.u.) are to be medicated are specified. Before instilling eyedrops the nurse's hands should be washed carefully and the medicine checked with the medicine card. The child is

then positioned on the back with the head turned toward the eye receiving the medication. The nurse takes a tissue in one hand and the medicine dropper in the other, places the palm of the hand against the child's forehead, and instructs the child to look away. The nurse then draws the lower lid down, and instills the correct number of drops into the space (Fig. 10-11). Eye medication should never be instilled directly onto the cornea. The eyes should then be allowed to close gently, permitting the drug to spread about under the lids with the excess absorbed by the tissue.

When bitter or painful drugs such as atropine are instilled, the nurse should put pressure on the inner canthus to prevent the medication from

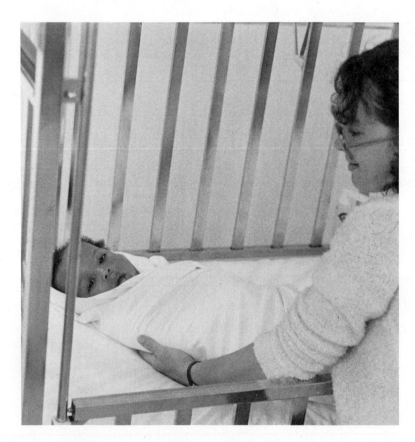

Fig. 10-10. A mummy wrap may prove useful to restrain an infant when medications are to be given into the eyes, nose, or ears, or into a scalp vessel.

going down into the nose through the nasolacrimal ducts. The child should lie still for several minutes after the instillation. The calming presence of one or both parents may be most helpful at this time.

Eardrops. Eardrops are instilled to relieve pain, to treat local inflammation of the canal, and to soften and lubricate collected matter. The medication should be warmed to at least body temperature to reduce pain. The child is positioned with the head turned first to one side and then to the other. In infants and young children the earlobe (pinna) should be pulled down and back to help straighten the canal for the medication to pass along more readily. For older children draw the pinna up and outward (Fig. 10-12). Cotton should not be placed in the ear immediately, because it absorbs the medication; instead, the head should be held in position for at least 1 minute before instilling drops in the opposite ear. Special care should be taken when a glass dropper is provided.

Nosedrops. Nosedrops, such as Neo-Synephrine 0.25%, may be ordered for children with nasal inflammation to shrink the tissue and reduce congestion. They are most effective if preceded by nasal suctioning and are often ordered just before feeding time to open the passages, because it is difficult for a child to eat and breathe through the mouth simultaneously.

Nosedrops are valueless if they merely go into the nose and down the throat. Ideally, nasal secretions are removed first and the drops instilled as the patient inhales them up into the nasal pas-

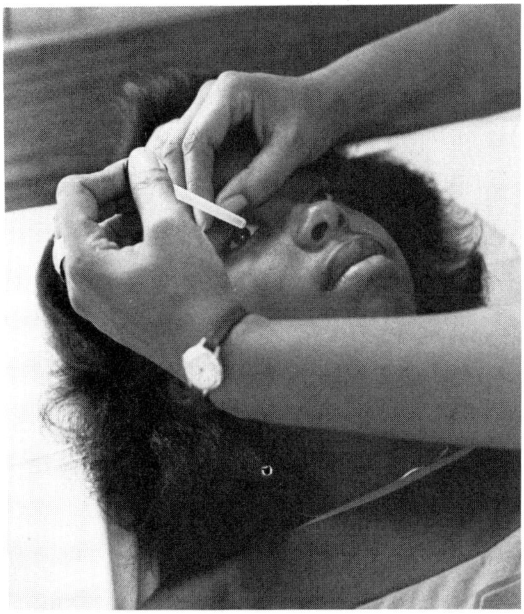

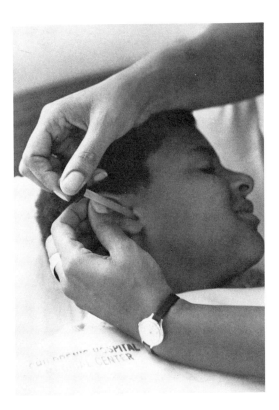

Fig. 10-11. Preparing to instill eye medications. The child is positioned on the back with the head turned toward the eye to be medicated. The lower lid is drawn down and the medicine is dropped into the space.

Fig. 10-12. Ear drops are instilled in the ears of children over 5 years of age by pulling the pinna upward and outward.

sages in a kind of self-vaporizing effect. Unfortunately, few children of any age understand this process, and so the child's head must be held lower than the body long enough for the drops to flow by gravity into the swollen passages. Care must be taken that the child does not aspirate the secretions in the process. To prevent aspiration, a pillow can be placed under the shoulders and the head tilted back, first to one side and then to the other, while the drops are instilled. Another method especially effective with infants and young children is to hold the child's head down on the gowned nurse's lap while sitting on a firm chair. The head is placed between the nurse's knees and held firmly in place as the drops are instilled and until they

have time to flow to the nasal passages (Fig. 10-13).

If individual bottles of nosedrops are not provided for each child, a clean dropper should be used for each instillation so that the stock bottle is not contaminated. Nosedrops are recorded as medications on the child's chart.

Skin applications. Ointments, creams, and lotions are applied to the skin for a variety of reasons. Depending on the conditions, they may be buttered on with a tongue blade, rubbed in with bare hands, or applied with gloved hands. If the child is especially susceptible to infection or is contagious, or if the medication (such as silver nitrate) causes stains, gloves should be used. All specifically ordered skin medications

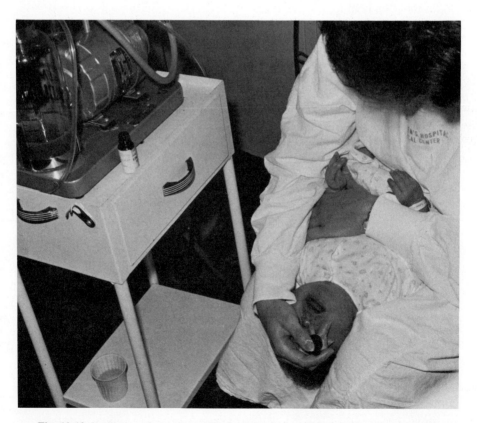

Fig. 10-13. Instillation of nose drops. Suction is ready for use to remove nasal secretions.

are recorded as are other medications on the child's chart. Routine back-rub lotions need not be recorded.

Injections and infusions. The administration of medications and fluids by injection and infusion requires great care and skill. When using these routes to administer drugs and fluids, nurses must adhere to the following principles:

1. All supplies and equipment must be sterile.
2. Drugs and fluids must be in perfect condition. Cloudy or discolored ones should be returned to the pharmacy or central supply.
3. Equipment must be correct for the task, and provide the most accurate measurement and the least discomfort for the patient. If the amount of medication to be given is less than 1 ml, a tuberculin syringe should be used because it is calibrated in millimeters on one side and minims on the other. The needle length and gauge are selected according to the task. At issue are the size of the child, the medication to be injected, and the tissue site. Some nurses carry several sizes of needles to the bedside so they can select the correct size after they have assessed the child.
4. A firm but kind approach is essential. The nurse must let the child know who is in control, but the child should have a non-frightening explanation, select the injection site, and "play nurse" whenever possible. Even though children may understand

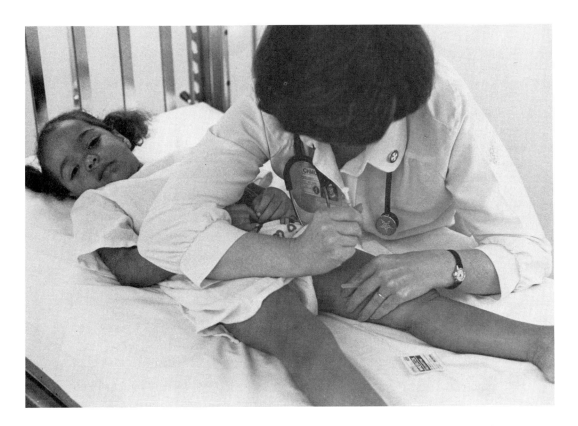

Fig. 10-14. A "hold" used to minimize movement of the patient during an intramuscular injection.

the procedure, they may resist an injection. For safety's sake, however, the nurse must have total control of the injection site. Various "holds" may be used to provide this control. Administer the medication as quickly as possible. Even the most compliant child will not stay still for long (Fig. 10-14).

5. With few exceptions the injection site should be massaged to promote absorption. Sites of injection should be recorded and rotated. Sites of former injections should be observed for signs of inflammation (redness, heat, pain, swelling). Never inject a medication into inflamed tissue.

6. Give an extra measure of tender loving care to the child receiving injections. Take extra time to soothe the tears and praise cooperation. Remember to apply the bandage! It is a badge of courage, a symbol of prestige.

Intradermal injections. Certain drugs are administered by fine-gauge needles into the layers of the skin, intradermally. This route is usually used for tuberculin or allergy testing. The amount of allergen or medication is usually less than 1 mm. A short, 26- or 27-gauge needle and a tuberculin syringe are used. A site is selected on the arms, thighs, back, or abdomen. After cleansing the skin the needle is inserted, bevel up, at a 15-degree angle with the tip just below the surface of the skin. A small bleb is formed by the injected solution. The needle is withdrawn quickly, and the site is not massaged. Many nurses mark or number multiple sites so that they can be "read" at a specified later time.

Subcutaneous injections. Subcutaneous injections are administered by relatively fine needles into the fatty tissue just below the skin. If children are premature there will be little adipose tissue. Consequently, the needle should be short (½ to ⅝ inch) and inserted at a 45-degree angle (Fig. 10-15). If there is little adipose tissue, the nurse can pinch the site as the needle is inserted to be sure it is not in a muscle. There

are different schools of thought about whether the needle should be aspirated. When heparin is injected the site should *not* be massaged. Because patients may have several injections per day, it is important to rotate the injection sites and keep a record of each one. Some nurses place a small round bandage over the latest site as a marker.

Intramuscular injections. Many medications are administered using the intramuscular route. This route is used when others are not available and when rapid absorption and distribution are

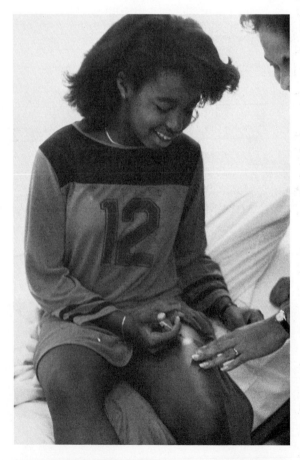

Fig. 10-15. The nurse supervises the adolescent giving her own subcutaneous injection. Note 45-degree angle of insertion.

desired. When a drug is prescribed to be injected intramuscularly, the tip of the needle must be in a muscle (Fig. 10-16). It is important to assess the amount of adipose tissue before giving an injection. If the needle is not long enough, the medication will be administered subcutaneously. If this occurs, not only will the absorption rate be slowed, but the fatty tissue may be damaged because some drugs are caustic to adipose tissue. Therefore, needle may be from ½ to 1½ inches long and should be inserted at a 90-degree angle to the skin. If the patient is obese, the fatty tissue is spread so that the needle will go into the muscle.

Not only should intramuscular injections be made into muscles, but the muscles should also be those which are exercised. This is important because when a muscle is exercised, foreign substances such as injected drugs are absorbed into the bloodstream more rapidly. Medications injected into seldom-used or paralyzed muscles will be absorbed more slowly. As a result, the following guidelines are recommended: (1) Neonates: *vastus lateralis* and *rectus femoris*; (2) nonwalking infants and children: *vastus lateralis, rectus femoris*, and *deltoid*; and (3) toddlers and older children who walk: *vastus lateralis, rectus femoris, deltoid*, and *gluteus* muscle group. Injection sites should be massaged to further promote absorption (Fig. 10-17).

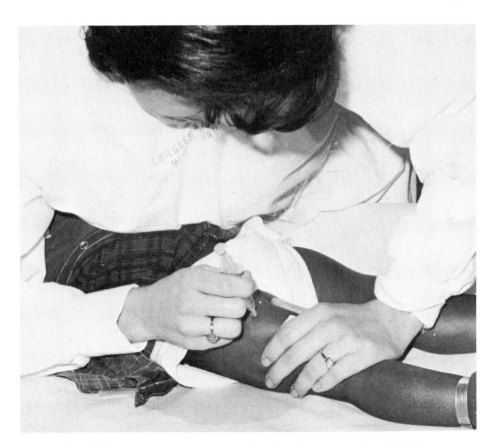

Fig. 10-16. Intramuscular injection given into the midanterior muscles of the thigh.

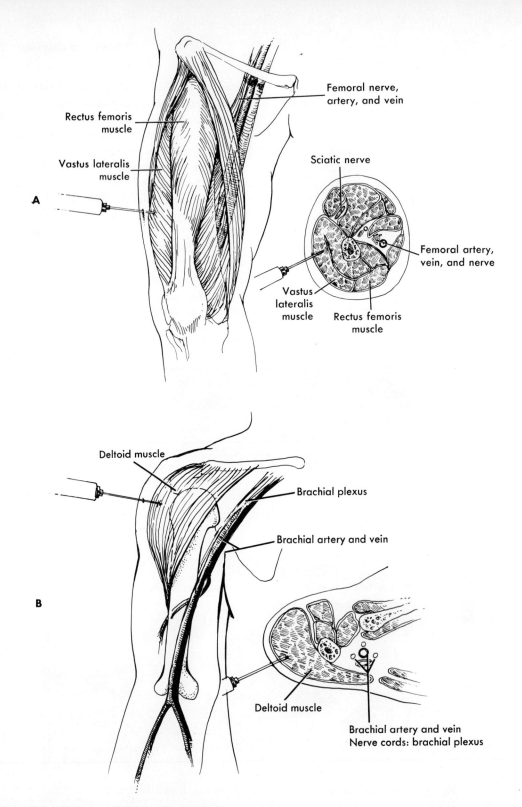

Fig. 10-17. Intramuscular injection sites for children. **A,** *Vastus lateralis* and *rectus femoris* muscles. **B,** *Deltoid* muscle.

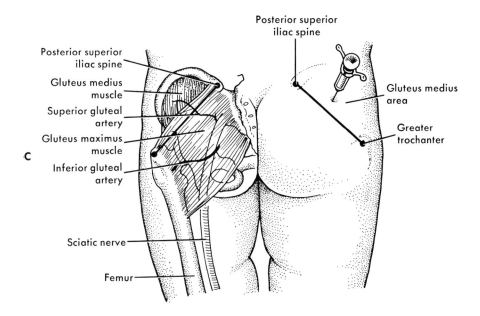

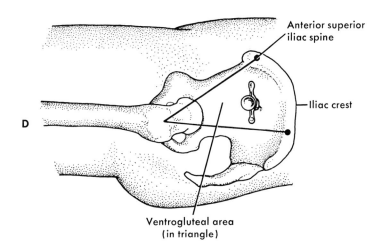

Fig. 10-17, cont'd. C, *Gluteus medius* area (above diagonal line). **D,** *Ventrogluteal* area (in triangle).

It is important not to overload the absorption capacity of a muscle. Authorities consider 2 ml the largest amount of fluid that should be injected in a site at one time. If more than 2 ml is prescribed, it should be divided between two sites.

The preparation of drugs for injection requires skill and concentration. Only sterile injectables may be used. Some must be stored in the refrigerator; others must be diluted with special solvent or be shaken before measurement. The correct dosage must be calculated. Antiseptic is used to clean the stoppered top or the breaking line of the glass vial, and the correct amount is drawn into the syringe. Intramuscular injections must be given as soon as they are prepared.

Most children learn during their first year of life that a needle and syringe mean pain. Thereafter they resist all injections with varying de-

grees of intensity. Because of this unfortunate fact, nurses may need assistance in restraining the child during the injection. When it is possible, nurses gain the cooperation of children by having them participate in the procedure. Older children may hold the side of the bed and count to 10 or be asked to stand on the opposite leg to help relax the muscles at the site of the injection. To reduce pain, nurses should allow the alcohol used to cleanse the skin to dry and then, using a sharp needle, insert quickly, pull back on the plunger to be sure that the needle is not in a blood vessel, inject the drug slowly, and remove the needle at the same angle as it was inserted. If signs of inflammation or allergy develop after an injection, they should be reported immediately and the injections withheld until the physician has been consulted. Signs of inflammation

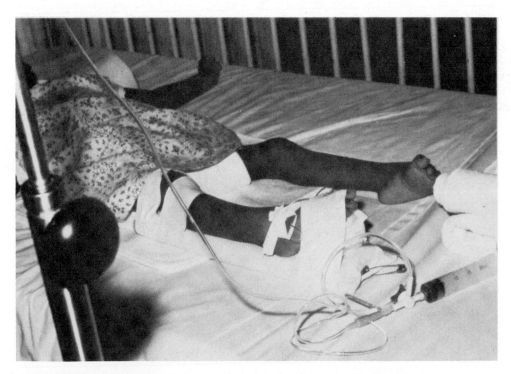

Fig. 10-18. A common site for a cutdown is the ankle. Leg is fastened securely to a padded board and the board fastened to the bedding.

and allergy are pain, redness, itching, heat, and skin rash. Injections should never made into old hemorrhage sites. After the injection, massage the area, check for bleeding, comfort the child, return the equipment to its proper place, and record the injection on the child's chart.

Intravenous injections. The intravenous route for administration of medications and fluids is the most direct, giving immediate access to the whole body. With the intravenous route a needle is inserted into a peripheral vein or a major central vein. Peripheral veins are those found on the arms, legs, or scalp. Major interior veins include the jugular and subclavian. Selection of the vein depends on type of therapy needed. In general, peripheral veins are used for dilute fluids and noncaustic medications. Major interior vessels are used for such concentrated solutions as those used in hyperalimentation therapy and diagnostic x-ray studies.

Various types of needles are inserted into the veins for intravenous therapy. They range from a simple short metal needle to multiple-post cannulated catheters. Needles may be inserted with or without anesthesia. Some are inserted into deeper peripheral veins through an incision into locally anesthetized tissue and sutured into place. Such a surgically positioned intravenous infusion is called a *cutdown* (Fig. 10-18).

Depending on institutional policy and state regulations, nurses may be authorized to insert any or all intravenous needles. The insertion of a needle is always an aseptic procedure. It may be long, tedious, and painful for the child. The nurse assembles the equipment and explains the procedure to the child, if possible. Two or more persons are required to insert an intravenous needle in a child; one to immobilize the limb, the other to insert the needle. The limb must be immobilized with restraints. The site, kind, rate of flow must be recorded.

Nursing responsibilities continue through the course of intravenous therapy. The insertion site must be monitored at least every hour for signs of infiltration into the tissue, reaction to the tape,

or impairment of circulation to the limb because of the restraint. Intravenous needles can be extremely "positional" because the veins of children are small and flexible. The infusion rate also must be monitored constantly. Many hospitals use infusion pumps to maintain an accurate rate of flow (Fig. 10-19). Nurses are responsible to be sure the pumps are functioning properly. Untoward reactions or infiltration should be reported to the physician immediately, and the intravenous infusion discontinued according to hospital policy.

When patients need intravenous medications but do not need fluids, a "heparin lock" may be inserted. A heparin lock is an intravenous needle connected to a short piece of tubing with a stopper and secured in place with tape. The tubing is irrigated with a solution of heparin every 3 to 4 hours to prevent blood from clotting in the tube. Medications or fluids are administered through the stopper tube followed by heparin solution to flush the tubing.

Two modes of administering medications intravenously are used: push and drip. The *push method* is used for immediate response. The medication is not diluted or diluted only minimally. It is drawn up into a syringe and introduced into the intravenous tubing slowly according to the correct length of time recommended in a drug reference. The nurse observes the patient closely for untoward reactions during and after the administration.

In the *drip method* of administering medications, the drug is diluted in various amounts of solute and is administered drop by drop over a period of time. The nurse should consult a drug reference to determine the amount and type of solute along with the least and most time in which to administer the medication. Drip-administered medications may be added to the total amount of solution, given "piggy-back" in smaller bottles, or placed in measured dispensers such as Volutrol or Metroset (Fig. 10-20). Whether the drip method or push method is used, the nurse should flush or irrigate the tubing be-

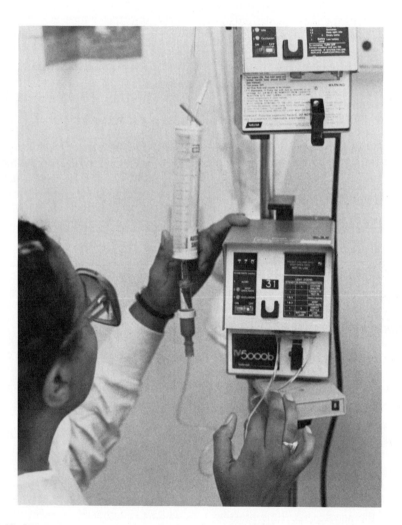

Fig. 10-19. Intravenous infusion pump maintains a constant rate of infusion and sounds an alarm if something goes wrong.

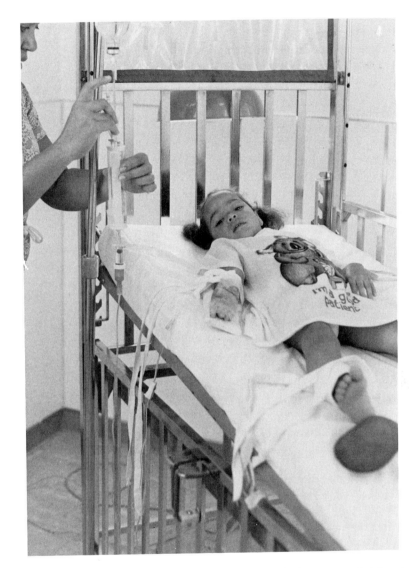

Fig. 10-20. The nurse puts the medication directly into the Volutrol for intravenous administration using the drip method. Note restraints of child's limbs.

fore and after the administration of the medication to prevent crystallizing or precipitation of one medication with another.

Fluid and electrolyte therapy
Principles and rationale

The cardinal principle of fluid balance is that intake must equal output, a matter of *quantity*. The body loses or uses up water through the kidney, skin, lungs, tissue metabolism, and intestine. To maintain health, the amount of water lost must be made up with intake. If the output increases, so too must the intake.

The second principle concerns the *quality* of the body fluids. They are not made up solely of water (H_2O) but contain numerous chemical components. These components are divided into three groups—protein molecules, electrolytes, and nonelectrolytes. In their various proportions these components are responsible for maintaining the amazing fluid balance found within blood vessels, cells, and spaces between cells.

Some chemicals, especially the salts, form electrically charged bodies called ions when they are dissolved in water. Because these ions can pass an electric current through the solution, they are called electrolytes. The body's chief ions are sodium (Na^+), potassium (K^+), calcium (Ca^{2+}), magnesium (Mg^{2+}), chloride (Cl^-), bicarbonate (HCO_3^-), phosphate (HPO_2^-), and sulfate (SO_4^-). Categories of fluid and electrolyte imbalance are as follows:

Categories of fluid and electrolyte imbalances*

I. Imbalances caused by a deficiency or excess of water and/or electrolytes
  A. Water-salt imbalances
    1. Water deficit: dehydration, hypernatremia, hypertonic dehydration
    2. Water excess: water intoxication, hyponatremia, hypertonic water excess
    3. Saline deficit: extracellular volume deficit, hypovolemia, salt deficit
    4. Saline excess: extracellular volume excess, hypervolemia, salt excess
  B. Potassium imbalances
    1. Potassium deficit: hypokalemia
    2. Potassium excess: hyperkalemia
  C. Calcium imbalances
    1. Calcium deficit: hypocalcemia
    2. Calcium excess: hypercalcemia
  D. Magnesium imbalances
    1. Magnesium deficit: hypomagnesemia
    2. Magnesium excess: hypermagnesemia
  E. Hydrogen ion (acid-base) imbalances
    1. Metabolic acidosis: primary base bicarbonate deficit of extracellular fluid
    2. Metabolic alkalosis: primary base bicarbonate excess of extracellular fluid
    3. Respiratory acidosis: primary carbonic acid excess
    4. Respiratory alkalosis: primary carbonic acid deficit
II. Imbalances caused by nutritional deficiencies
  A. Calorie deficiency: starvation
  B. Protein deficiency: hypoproteinemia, kwashiorkor
III. Imbalances caused by shifts in the position of the extracellular fluid
  A. Plasma shifts to the interstitial spaces
  B. Interstitial fluid shifts into plasma

When a child is unable to take sufficient fluids by mouth or has lost large amounts of vital electrolytes or proteins as a result of burns, diarrhea, defective kidneys, vomiting, or high fever, imbalances result and parenteral fluids must be given. The record of the child's daily fluid intake and output and the laboratory analysis of the blood chemistry tell the physician what proportion of electrolytes is needed to establish fluid balance.

Types of fluids

After evaluating the child's general condition, blood chemistry, daily intake and output, and diagnosis, the physician prescribes parenteral fluids from among three general types—whole blood, plasma, and solutions of water and

---

*Adapted from Sorenson, K.C., and Luckman, J.: *Basic nursing, a psychophysiological approach*, Philadelphia, 1979, W.B. Saunders Co.

chemicals. When the child is undergoing long-term parenteral therapy, vitamins, proteins, and fats are added to the minerals and carbohydrates in these solutions.

Whole blood is obtained from blood banks on special order. The child's blood is typed and cross-matched with the blood to be given. An intravenous infusion of normal saline solution is begun followed by the blood. Extraordinary caution and watchfulness must be maintained during the infusion because of the danger of reactions to the "foreign" blood. Chills, fever, skin rash, or any unusual symptoms should be reported immediately.

Plasma, the liquid noncellular part of blood, may be given, but it, too, may produce serious reactions.

Solutions of electrolytes, carbohydrates, and other chemicals are as varied as they are common. Some of the frequently used fluids are 5% and 10% dextrose in water, saline solution, and lactated Ringer's solution; there are many more, each one containing different proportions of chemicals.

SUMMARY OUTLINE

I. Legal implications and responsibilities
  A. Federal regulations
  1. Controlled substances
  2. Experimental drugs and treatments
  B. State regulations: nurse practice acts
  C. Hospital policies and procedures
  D. Individual responsibilities
II. Principles
III. Practice
  A. Identification methods (the right patient)
  B. Medical prescriptions (doctor's orders)
  1. Forms
  2. Procedures
  C. Drug dosages
  1. Verification of safe dosages
  2. Reference manuals
  3. Calculation methods
    a. Age
    b. Kilogram weight
    c. Surface area or square meters (M^2)
    d. Other rules
  D. Systems for the administration of medications
  1. Stock medications

  2. Unit dose systems
  3. Medication cards
  4. Medication Kardex
  5. Original prescription system
  6. Computerized systems
  E. Times of administration
  F. Measurement systems
  G. Routes of administering medications
  1. Enteral routes
    a. Oral
    b. Rectal
    c. Gastric
  2. Parenteral routes
    a. Eyedrops
    b. Eardrops
    c. Nosedrops
    d. Skin applications
    e. Injections and infusions
      (1) Intradermal injections
      (2) Subcutaneous injections
      (3) Intramuscular injections
      (4) Intravenous injections
  H. Fluid and electrolyte therapy
  1. Principles and rationale
  2. Types of fluids

STUDY QUESTIONS

1. Controlled substances are categorized into five schedules. By what criteria are they placed in these schedules? What classifications of drugs are in each schedule?
2. List the characteristics common to all nurse practice acts. What are the implicit requirements in these acts in regard to the administration of drugs?
3. Compare, contrast, and give examples of the meaning of the words *negligence* and *malpractice*.
4. Discuss the "five rights" of drug administration and the procedures used to implement them in the hospital where you practice.
5. What is the safe dose factor (SDF)? What should the nurse do if a physician orders an *unsafe* dose of medicine?
6. What is considered the most accurate method for calculating pediatric dosages? Demonstrate how to use the West nomogram to calculate drug doses.
7. Define the following symbols: q.d., q.i.d., t.i.d., b.i.d., p.o., q.4 h., p.r.n., o.s., o.u., o.d. What is a meniscus?
8. What special precautions should you take when you administer a medication per nasogastric tube; into the ear, eyes, or nose; topically; intramuscularly; and intradermally? What are the nursing responsibilities when a patient is receiving intravenous fluids and medications in your hospital?
9. Discuss the cardinal principle of fluid balance. List the three components of body fluids and describe each one.

REFERENCES

American Academy of Pediatrics, Committee on Infectious Diseases: Report, ed. 17, Evanston, Ill., 1974, The Academy.

Babson, S.C., and Benson, R.C.: Management of high-risk pregnancy and intensive care of the neonate, ed. 3, St. Louis, 1975, The C.V. Mosby Co.

Bergersen, B.S., and Goth, A.: Pharmacology in nursing, ed. 13, St. Louis, 1976, The C.V. Mosby Co.

Garb, S.: Laboratory tests in common use, ed. 6, New York, 1975, Springer Publishing Co., Inc.

Levison, H.: Textbook for dental nurses, ed. 4, Philadelphia, 1971, F.A. Davis Co.

Pagliaro, L.A., and Levin, R.H., eds.: Problems in pediatric drug therapy, Hamilton, Ill., 1979, Drug Intelligence Publications, Inc.

Physician's desk reference to pharmaceutical specialties and biologicals, Rutherford, N.J., printed annually, Medical Economics, Inc.

Ryan, S.A., and Clayton, B.D.: Handbook of practical pharmacology, ed. 2., St. Louis, 1980, The C.V. Mosby Co.

Schuberth, K.C., and Zitelli, B.J.: The Harriet Lane handbook, ed. 8, Chicago, 1978, Yearbook Medical Publishers, Inc.

Shirkey, H.C.: Pediatric drug handbook, Philadelphia, 1977, W.B. Saunders Co.

Spock, B.: Doctor Spock's baby and child care medical record, New York, 1971, Hawthorn Books, Inc.

Squire, J.E., and Clayton, B.D.: Basic pharmacology for nurses, ed. 7, St. Louis, 1981, The C.V. Mosby Co.

Squire, J.E., and Welch, J.M.: Basic pharmacology for nurses, ed. 6, St. Louis, 1977, The C.V. Mosby Co.

Vernon, D., and others: The psychological responses of children to hospitalization and illness, Springfield, Ill., 1965, Charles C Thomas, Publisher.

Williams, S.R.: Mowry's basic nutrition and diet therapy, ed. 6, St. Louis, 1980, The C.V. Mosby Co.

Wing, K.R.: The law and the public's health, St. Louis, 1976, The C.V. Mosby Co.

Disorders common to children and their care

11
The infant at risk

With the conquest of most infectious diseases and surgical emergencies, modern medicine has turned to the next most pressing medical problem—infant morbidity and mortality. Certain categories of infants are known to have a higher incidence of birth defects and death. These infants at risk have become the object of considerable study. As a result, prevention and care have been expanded and a new terminology has developed.

TERMINOLOGY

Once all underdeveloped babies were called *premature*. As the study and care of these infants expanded, the terminology used to describe them became more precise. More specific words describing weight, gestational age, and maturity are now used, as follows:

At risk; high risk	All categories of infants with a high incidence of mortality and morbidity
Low birth weight	2,500 gm or less at birth
Full size	2,500 gm or more at birth
Immature	Up to 27 weeks gestation
Premature	28 to 33 weeks gestation
Preterm	34 to 37 weeks gestation
Term	38 to 42 weeks gestation
Postterm	Over 43 weeks gestation
Dysmature	Poor development, fragile

Regardless of cause or description, all babies who are not robust at birth need special intensive nursing care.

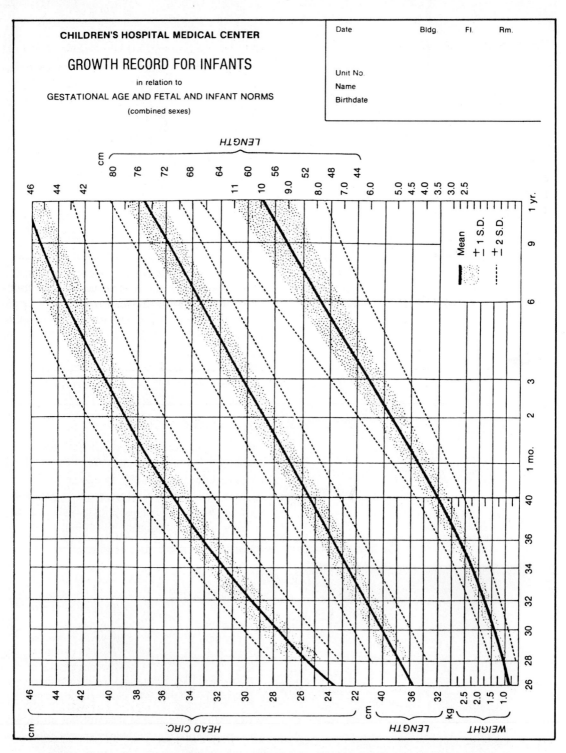

Fig. 11-1. Growth chart for early born infants. (Courtesy Children's Hospital Medical Center, Oakland, Calif.)

THE EARLY BORN INFANT
Description

Infants who are born before term are deprived of the benefits of intrauterine life for varying periods. They must breath and eat and carry on the functions of mature babies while they are still immature. As a result it takes them longer to "catch-up" with babies who remained in the ideal environment of the uterus until they were fully mature. A standardized growth chart has been developed for early born infants (Fig. 11-1).

The underdeveloped, early born infant resembles a little old man. The features are sharp, and bones are pronounced and unsoftened by subcutaneous fat. Through the transparent skin the exposed capillary beds give a dark red hue. The fontanels and suture lines of the too-large skull are prominent. Fine lanugo hair may cover the entire body in a downy coat, while the pasty, lubricating vernix caseosa, so conspicuous on a full-term baby, is absent. The infant's cry is weak and pitiful, matching the frail appearance (Fig. 11-2).

Handicaps

The underdeveloped infant has numerous special handicaps:

1. Reduced, respiratory function caused by the incomplete development of the air sacs, thoracic muscles, blood supply, and nerve reflexes of the respiratory system
2. Inadequate regulation of the body temperature caused by a lack of subcutaneous fat, feeble muscle activity, immature sweat glands, and a surface area that is too large in proportion to the infant's weight

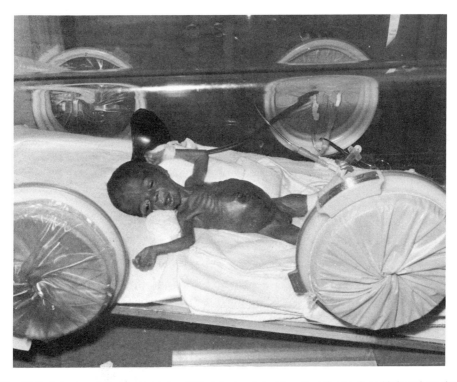

Fig. 11-2. Immature infant in incubator. This infant weighed less than 2 pounds at birth and required immediate surgery for a herniation of the abdominal contents at the umbilicus called an "omphalocele."

3. Inadequate development of the mouth, stomach, and reflexes of sucking and swallowing, making it difficult for nutritional needs to be supplied
4. Inefficient elimination of body wastes by immature kidneys and skin
5. Reduced resistance to disease caused by incomplete development of the enzyme system, body chemistry balance, antibody production and having not received immune substances, hormones, and nutrients from the mother
6. Reduced storage of body nutrients and production of blood-clotting elements resulting from immature liver function
7. Defective hemopoiesis (blood cell production) and increased capillary fragility, making even a small blood loss dangerous
8. Increased possibility of brain damage during the birth process caused by fragility of capillaries and a tendency to bleed
9. Lack of adequate amounts of surface-active material (surfactant) needed to reduce surface tension in the air sacs. The lungs are less compliant and fatigue occurs as a result of attempts to ventilate "stiff lungs"

Besides overcoming all of these handicaps of premature birth, the underdeveloped infant is threatened by two common complications associated with prematurity—hyaline membrane disease and retrolental fibroplasia. These complications are discussed among the diseases of the premature infant later in this chapter.

Special needs
At birth

Although every effort is made to prevent labor and delivery before term, when it becomes inevitable, preparations for the infant are made. The nursery is alerted and a person trained in resuscitation stands by at the delivery. Essential equipment includes a preheated incubator and ready-to-use resuscitation devices. At the birth the physician evaluates the baby's condition and emergency care is given as needed. The cord is clamped. The naked baby is placed in an incubator. After proper identification and eye care

the baby is transferred to the neonatal nursery. Weighing, measuring, and other care are secondary to life-maintaining measures. Sometimes it is several days before the baby is strong enough to be weighed.

The underdeveloped infant may be cared for in the regular newborn nursery or may be transferred to a neonatal intensive care unit, a designated facility where specially trained personnel care for babies at risk, using the most advanced equipment and techniques.

Environmental needs

Incubator. The incubator is designed to duplicate as closely as possible the environment of the uterus. Heat, humidity, and oxygen content are carefully controlled (Fig. 11-3). Because the defenses of infants at risk against infection are poor, every effort is made to keep the bacterial count low. Transparent sides and top allow for continuous observation of the infant. Nursing care is given through adjustable portholes, so that the infant need not be removed from the incubator or handled excessively. Regulating controls, air analyzers, and warning signals are added features of some models. A variety of incubators are manufactured; the nurse should become thoroughly familiar with those in the nursery.

Radiant heat cribs. These cribs provide a special advantage because the infant is more accessible for nursing care. They provide warmth from a heat source above the infant. Other specialized equipment such as positive pressure respiratory tubes, intravenous infusions, and hoods for oxygen administration can be supplemented as needed.

Temperature and humidity. The infant needs an environment of 85° to 95° F with the relative humidity at 60%. If the infant is in an incubator the temperature is noted and recorded on the infant's chart at regular intervals. Specific orders may be given by the physician for the exact temperature and humidity levels for each at risk infant, or the supervising nurse may be asked to

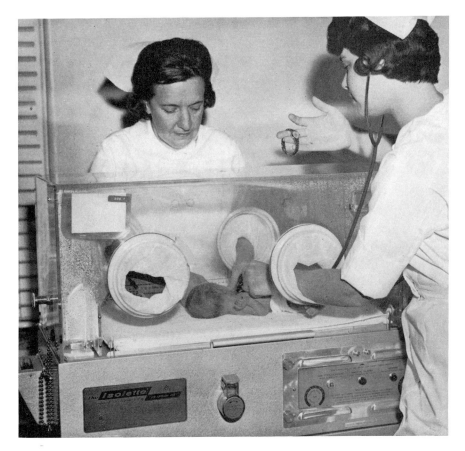

Fig. 11-3. The incubator provides a controlled environment for the infant. Control panel and warning lights are in lower right. Nursing care is given through portholes. (From Hamilton, P.M.: Basic maternity nursing, ed. 4, St. Louis, 1979, The C.V. Mosby Co.)

adjust them in an effort to stabilize the infant's body temperature.

Oxygen. The normal concentration of oxygen in the air is about 21%, which is sufficient for a healthy baby, but a sick infant may become cyanotic and die from anoxia unless given additional oxygen. Unlimited amounts of oxygen cannot be used, however. It has been found that prolonged administration of oxygen to premature infants in concentrations over 40% causes *retrolental fibroplasia*, a serious condition that produces partial or total blindness. This condition is discussed more fully later in this chapter.

To prevent such a tragic aftermath of prematurity, oxygen is never administered unless it is definitely needed, and then the concentration is rarely maintained over 40% for prolonged periods.

Nutrition

Nutrition plays an important part in the survival of infants at risk. Calories, water, electrolytes, and nutrients are no longer withheld for the first 1 to 3 days of life but are administered intravenously and orally within a few hours after birth. The infant's nutritional needs are calculated every 12 to 24 hours on the basis of intake, output, weight, and blood chemistry tests.

Intravenous feedings. Intravenous fluids may be given through the umbilical vessels, peripheral arteries, or jugular vein. A cutdown operation may be done by the physician to position an intravenous catheter (Fig. 10-12).

Hyperalimentation. When all of the nutritional needs are supplied by intravenous solution, the treatment is called *hyperalimentation*. The individually calculated, highly concentrated solution of dextrose, electrolytes, and vitamins is administered through a catheter into the superior vena cava. The child is monitored closely, including daily weight, urinary and blood glucose levels, urine output, and electrolyte balance. Although hyperalimentation provides total parenteral nutrition, it does not satisfy the infant's sucking and security needs. These needs can be met by giving the baby a pacifier to suck and by holding a hand against the baby's body when possible.

Oral feedings. The baby is not removed from the incubator for feeding until specifically permitted by the physician. The method of oral feeding and the amount given depend on the baby's development, size, and strength. A variety of methods are used, such as gavage or tube feeding; with a tiny rubber or polyethylene catheter that is passed down into the baby's stomach, using a medicine dropper with a rubber tip, and special nipples that are small and very soft. Only specially trained persons should attempt to insert a gavage tube, because of the serious consequences of improper placement.

Nasogastric feedings. Nasogastric feedings may be continuous, controlled by a pump, or intermittent with the tube clamped between feedings. Before a feeding the nurse should check the position of the tube by injecting air and listening with a stethoscope over the stomach.

General precautions. Underdeveloped infants should be fed small amounts, slowly, with frequent rest periods and burpings. Overfeeding is dangerous because it may cause regurgitation and, because the gag reflex is weak, the infant may suffer aspiration of formula into the lungs. To help prevent aspiration, the infant should be positioned with the head elevated for several minutes after each feeding.

Records. An accurate record of the exact amount of formula taken at each feeding and the infant's response is important to the physician in evaluating progress.

Observations

The physician provides medical supervision of the infant at risk. The physician examines, evaluates, writes orders, and directs, the medical care. The physican relies, however, on the team of nurses for information about any changes that might occur and for giving the infant continuous skilled care essential to survival. A specially trained professional nurse leads each team in caring for infants at risk. The professional nurse may delegate responsibility to assistants on the nursing team. Because the condition of these infants may change rapidly, constant observations of significant symptoms must be made by each team member. Important symptoms that should be noted, reported, and charted are the following:

1. Color: cyanosis (blueness) caused by anoxia, or jaundice (yellowness) from free bilirubin in the tissue
2. Respiration: regularity or cessation; sternal retraction (epigastrium caves in with each expiration)
3. Pulse: rate and regularity
4. Abdomen: distention (may occur suddenly)
5. Feeding: sucking ability, regurgitation, amount of satisfaction, and vomiting
6. Skin: excoriation, edema, rashes, and turgor
7. Cord and eyes: discharge
8. Skull: fontanels and sutures sunken or bulging
9. General responsiveness: degree of lethargy or hyperactivity; the cry as compared with former condition

10. Stools: frequency, color, consistency, and amount
11. Urine: time and frequency of voiding and amount
12. Mouth: dry lips or small white patches that do not wipe away

Handling, positioning, and care

The underdeveloped or sick infant should be handled as little as possible to conserve strength. The usual bath procedures are modified to do only that which is essential. There is no need for clothing, and so the extra handling required for dressing is avoided. The absence of clothing also makes close observation of the infant possible.

The baby is too weak to turn alone and is totally dependent on others for help. The baby should be turned from side to side at least every 2 hours. Air and water mattresses are used to promote circulation. If the airways are filled with mucus or fluid, they should be suctioned and the baby placed head down and to the side.

The delicate skin tends to become dry, and the buttocks excoriate easily. Gentle cleansing followed by exposure to the air or application of protective ointments may promote healing.

Prevention of infection

Because of an untimely birth, the early born baby has been deprived of the immune bodies normally obtained from the mother's blood. The baby's own body defenses are also underdeveloped. Therefore, the baby is easy prey to every variety of infectious disease. The nurse must maintain meticulous cleanliness in every aspect of care, including washing hands, sterilizing supplies and equipment, and maintaining protective isolation.

The parents

The mother of an underdeveloped or sick baby may have difficulty adjusting to her unnatural role. The baby may have been taken from her in the delivery room, placed in an incubator, and sometimes even transferred to a neonatal intensive care center many miles away. She and her husband may have difficulty identifying with the tiny stranger who bears their name but whom they have never held or even seen closely. They may develop feelings of inadequacy about their ability to care for the new baby, especially when they see their tiny infant cared for by highly trained persons using complex-looking equipment. As a result, the parent's insecurity mounts and they wonder whether they will ever be able to care for their infant.

The nurse can do much to overcome these problems. The parents should be encouraged to phone the nursery regularly for a progress report. The nurse should speak of the infant by name. Doing so helps the parents to think of the infant as a real child, their own child. As soon as possible the parents may be allowed to go to the nursery to hold and feed their baby. The nurse should use every opportunity to instruct the parents in infant care so that when the baby is finally ready to go home, they will feel competent to take over.

The decision of the physician regarding dismissal of the baby at risk is based on two factors—condition and home environment. When feeding well and gaining weight, weighing 5½ pounds, and in good condition, the baby is usually ready to leave the nursery. To evaluate the home situation, a community health nurse may be asked to make a home visit, during which not only the physical facilities are assessed but also the attitudes toward health teaching, cleanliness, and continued medical supervision. It would be folly to send a high-risk baby to a home where the baby would be neglected and exposed to disease. After receiving a favorable report, the physician writes the dismissal order.

Arrangements for dismissal include careful instructions to the parents, home visits by the public health nurse, and return appointments with the physician.

DISEASES OF THE EARLY BORN INFANT
Retrolental fibroplasia

Retrolental fibroplasia is the chief cause of blindness in newborn infants. It occurs only in immature and premature babies who are exposed to prolonged periods of high oxygen concentrations administered during the first 7 to 10 days of life. The immature blood vessels commence a period of excessive growth that continues for several days or weeks. The extent of growth that has occurred cannot be detected for 4 to 6 weeks but by the age of 3 months it is well defined.

The overgrown veins of the retina eventually regress and leave varying degrees of scar tissue. If the swollen veins rupture and a hemorrhage occurs, the blood may cause the retina to detach from the inner surface of the eye. Glaucoma and corneal opacity may then follow, with partial or complete blindness.

Prevention is the only way to reduce the incidence of this tragic disease. In the past, oxygen concentrations of 40% have been considered safe, but recent studies show that any concentration of oxygen above the normal 21% atmospheric level is *unsafe* for noncyanotic premature infants and that any concentration is *safe* for the cyanotic infant until the blood gas levels are within normal limits. These facts place great responsibility on the nursery staff, because the concentration of oxygen must be constantly adjusted to the infant's condition.

Such grave responsibility underlines the need for highly trained and unusually perceptive nurses to act as members of the nursery team. Not only must they be keen observers, but they must also be conscientious in recording the oxygen concentrations in relation to the child's condition, giving specific times and observations. This is necessary to protect the hospital and staff against malpractice liability judgments should a premature infant become sightless in months and years to come.

Hyaline membrane disease (respiratory distress syndrome, RDS)

Hyaline membrane disease is found in 50% of all early born infants and, until recently, killed 25,000 babies each year. It is seldom found in full-term infants but may develop in infants of diabetic and other high-risk mothers.

The disease occurs because the underdeveloped lungs of these infants fail to function properly. The failure largely stems from a lack of *surfactant*, which reduces surface tension within the tiny air sacs. The reduced surface tension helps the air sacs inflate with ease, preventing them from collapsing completely after each breath. Eventually, damaged lung cells, white blood cells, and serum combine to form fibrous material called *hyaline membrane*, which fills the air sacs and prevents oxygen from reaching the infant's bloodstream.

The typical victim is born without obvious respiratory distress; then, within minutes or hours a membrane forms in the lungs, closing off the oxygen supply. The respiratory rate zooms to 60 times a minute or more; the baby makes a desperate effort to obtain oxygen. The ribs retract; there is an expiratory grunt, a weak cry, oral bubbling, and deepening cyanosis. More than half of these infants die within 18 hours if untreated. Now, more than 85% of RDS babies can be saved, including many weighing less than 2 pounds.

When hyaline membrane disease is suspected the infant is transferred to a neonatal intensive care unit for continuous observation and specialized care. Ordinary respirators usually do not work because the lungs of RDS babies collapse with each breath. The problem has been overcome with the use of *continuous positive airway pressure* (CPAP). In CPAP, oxygen is given under pressure through an intubation airway or by a plastic hood. The pressure keeps the baby's lungs from collapsing until the body begins producing enough surfactant, usually in 3 to 5 days.

In addition to this successful treatment of RDS

babies, a number of preventive measures have helped reduce infant mortality from this disease. Prenatal monitoring has helped detect trouble before a baby is born. By taking samples of amniotic fluid and measuring the amounts of *lecithin*, a component of surfactant, the maturity of the baby's lungs can be determined. Administering steroid drugs, such as betamethasone, to the mother 1 to 2 days before expected delivery may prevent RDS. The drug enters the fetal bloodstream and stimulates the infant's lungs to produce surfactant. Planned cesarean section deliveries for high-risk babies with immediate intensive treatment has further reduced the death rate of infants from RDS.

Vomiting

The most common cause of vomiting in early born and full-term infants alike is overfeeding or too rapid feeding. The obvious way to prevent this is to feed smaller amounts more slowly. An early born infant who can be removed from the incubator should be held for feeding, burped several times during the course of it and at its conclusion, and then carefully returned to bed without excessive juggling. It may be helpful to elevate the head slightly immediately after feedings and to place the infant on the right side to enhance the flow of stomach contents toward the small intestine.

Some vomiting is caused by congenital deformities of the gastrointestinal tract or by increased intracranial pressure of the central nervous system. To help the physician evaluate the symptoms and diagnose the cause, the nurse should record the following information about any infant vomiting: (1) time in relation to the last feeding, (2) amount, (3) color and consistency of vomiting, (4) odor, (5) force of ejection (projectile or not), and (6) the infant's general response (for example, cyanosis or evidence of pain). Repeated vomiting of feedings can disrupt an infant's fluid balance very quickly and cause serious dehydration and electrolyte imbalance.

Parenteral fluids may then be necessary to correct this deficiency.

Whenever an infant vomits, regardless of the cause, there is immediate danger that the vomitus will block the airway. Every nursery worker should be prepared to give emergency care, as follows: quickly wipe the vomitus out of the infant's mouth, lowers the head, milk the trachea toward the mouth, and suction with a bulb syringe. More extensive suctioning can then be instituted if it is needed. As a precaution against such aspiration, an infant should never be left lying supine, but, instead, the head should be turned to one side.

Diarrhea

A newborn infant usually has four to five stools a day. More frequent or loose stools are called *diarrhea*. It is especially serious for an underdeveloped or sick infant because a loss of water and chemicals can produce fatal electrolyte imbalance.

Two common causes of diarrhea in underdeveloped infants that are not related to illness are overfeeding and a formula too rich in fat. These problems can be corrected easily by a simple adjustment of ingredients and the amount of feedings.

Diarrhea may be caused by infections anywhere in the infant's body, but the most dangerous is diarrhea caused by pathogenic organisms that invade the intestinal tract. They may be highly contagious, affecting a whole nursery of helpless infants. It is against such epidemics that many nursery practices are maintained, including routine handwashing, sterilization of the linen, and overhead antiseptic lights. When symptoms of diarrhea occur, the physician is immediately notified and the suspect infant isolated. Stool cultures and clinical signs are used to diagnose the cause. Treatment includes replacing lost water and chemicals to restore electrolyte balance and protecting the skin from excoriation.

Dehydration

Dehydration is especially serious in underdeveloped infants because their tolerance for variations in body fluid is so poor. It is caused by inadequate fluid intake or by excessive output. Vomiting and diarrhea are recognized easily as causes, but evaporation through the skin may also dehydrate infants. This is why the warmed air in incubators and nurseries always must be humidified.

Symptoms of dehydration are fever, sunken fontanels, tight, drawn skin without turgor, concentrated urine, or reduced urinary output. Careful records of all fluid intake and approximate output are important. If dehydration develops, parenteral fluids may be necessary to restore essential fluid balance.

Jaundice

Jaundice is caused by excessive amounts of bilirubin in the tissue. Bilirubin is the pigment found in hemoglobin and bile. It breaks down more quickly in the presence of light and is largely eliminated in urine. When bilirubin levels become elevated, the excess is deposited in various body tissues. In the skin these deposits cause a yellowness; in the brain they may cause permanent damage, mental retardation, and death.

Immediately after the birth of all infants free bilirubin level rises because of the normal destruction and reduction in numbers of red blood cells. This rise may cause a so-called *physiologic jaundice*. Jaundice may also stem from such abnormal conditions as erythroblastosis fetalis, bile duct defects, and septicemia. Because of an immature liver, the early born infant is less able to eliminate excess bilirubin than is the full-term infant, and so is more likely to become jaundiced. All jaundice should be reported at once, so that tests may be ordered for blood level of bilirubin. Treatment for jaundice includes the use of a blue-spectrum lamp to hasten bilirubin breakdown, intravenous fluids, and exchange

transfusions, depending on the infant's needs. It is important to cover the infant's eyes when exposed to these lamps to prevent retinal damage.

Convulsions

Convulsions in any newborn infant are serious. In a sick or underdeveloped infant they are especially so because the accompanying anoxia and stress threaten survival. An accurate description of a convulsion helps form the diagnosis. It should include: how long it lasted, where it started, if it was generalized or localized, and what parts of the body were involved. Convulsions may be caused by intracranial hemorrhage, a congenital cerebral defect, prolonged anoxia, hypoglycemia, hyperglycemia, fever, or an overwhelming bacteremia (bacteria in the blood) (Chapter 18).

THE POSTTERM INFANT

Most babies are born after 38 to 40 weeks of gestation. About one in 20, however, stays in the uterus beyond 42 weeks. Surprisingly, these babies are not better off for having remained in their watery prison. They seem to have lost weight and to have grown long fingernails and hair. Their skin has become waterlogged because it is no longer protected by vernix caseosa. Meconium from the bowel may have stained their nails and may be found in their lungs.

These babies are generally poor risks. Their mortality rate is two or three times higher than that of a full-term infant. The cause of their poor condition and apparent malnutrition is thought to be placental aging. As the weeks pass, the placenta becomes less and less efficient in providing the infant with needed nutrients and oxygen.

When a mother is quite sure of the date of conception so that the calculated length of the pregnancy seems accurate, the physician may elect to induce labor or perform a cesarean section to reduce risk to the life of a postterm infant.

SUMMARY OUTLINE

STUDY QUESTIONS

1. Define low birth weight, full-size, immature, premature, preterm, and postterm infant.
2. Describe an early born infant and list six special handicaps such an infant has.
3. How does retrolental fibroplasia cause blindness in children? How can it be prevented?
4. Describe the course of hyaline membrane disease. What is the prognosis?
5. What makes the skin yellow in jaundice? Is all newborn jaundice abnormal?

12

Respiratory aids and oxygen therapy

RESPIRATION
Definition

Respiration is the exchange of gases between the atmosphere and the cells of the body. It is divided into two parts—external and internal.

External respiration, or the act of breathing, is the exchange of gases between the air and the blood in the lungs. It is the primary function of the respiratory system.

Internal respiration is the transportation and exchange of gases between the blood and the cells of the body. It is one of the important functions of the circulatory system.

External respiration

Breathing. Normal breathing, called *eupnea*, is a two-part act—inspiration of air into the lungs and expiration of air out of the lungs. It occurs without conscious effort, although it can be temporarily controlled by "holding the breath" or increasing the rate for a time. The diaphragm and intercostal muscles contract and force air out and then relax as the atmospheric pressure pushes them back into the hollow, treelike spaces of the lungs. Diaphragmatic respirations are deeper and more relaxed. They are characterized by the abdomen bulging out first, followed by the thorax. In costal respiration, first the upper ribs move and then the abdomen. This type of respiration requires greater effort and usually indicates some degree of stress or oxygen hunger. The absence of breathing is called *apnea*.

Table 12-1. Differences in composition of inspired and expired air*

	Inspired air	Expired air	Difference
Nitrogen	79%	79%	0
Oxygen*	20%	16%	−4
Carbon dioxide	0.04%	4%	+3.96
Rare gases	Traces	Traces	
Water vapor	Variable	Almost saturated	
Temperature	Variable	Nearly body temperature	

*Note that the concentration of oxygen in expired air is still 16%, enough to help the victim who needs mouth-to-mouth resuscitation.

Gaseous exchange. As air is inspired and expired, gases are exchanged through the walls of the tiny capillaries that are situated in profusion about the air sacs of the lungs. Oxygen passes into the bloodstream and carbon dioxide passes out in a continual adjustment of internal and atmospheric pressures (Table 12-1).

Internal respiration

As the oxygen molecules pass into the bloodstream, most form relatively unstable chemical compounds with the hemoglobin of the red blood cells. These oxyhemoglobin cells, as they are then called, travel to the various parts of the body, where the oxygen separates and enters into the complex chemistry of metabolism. At the same time, waste carbon dioxide is carried in the blood and released through the capillaries of the air sacs, together with water vapor, into the expired air.

Necessary components

A number of components must be present and functioning if the respiratory process is to occur. Without adequate gaseous exchange, body cells die. If the necessary components are missing or are temporarily malfunctioning, artificial aids must be supplied until the body can take over independently. The six necessary components to respiration are discussed here.

Adequate oxygen. There must be an adequate supply of oxygen in the air at normal atmospheric pressures. If not enough is present or if atmospheric pressure is lower than normal (as occurs at high altitudes), additional oxygen must be supplied.

Open airways. The passages that would normally allow gaseous exchanges must be open. If they are blocked at any point from the nose to the air sacs in the lungs, the exchange of gases is hampered.

Nervous stimulation. Respiratory effort occurs as a result of the triggering of certain nervous pathways in response to air pressure in the lungs, to carbon dioxide levels in the blood, and to psychic factors. The respiratory center in the medulla of the brain and the phrenic and intercostal nerves are chiefly responsible for respiratory stimulation and regulation.

Muscle action. The muscles of respiration, the diaphragm and intercostals, respond to nerve impulses sent to them. As they contract, air is forced out of the lungs in expiration. As they relax, air rushes into the lungs under atmospheric pressure in inspiration. Without this action, respiration could not occur.

Rigid frame. The bony structure that creates the rib cage is essential for establishment of the volume of air in the lungs. Without this rigid frame, movement of air in and out would be impossible.

Functioning circulatory system. The blood cells must be sufficient in both numbers and maturity to carry the gases to the capillary beds in the lungs. The pumping action of the heart and the ability of the vessels to carry blood must be adequate for this transfer to take place. A test called tidal volume is an indicator of the adequacy of ventilatory effort. In it the amount of air in a single expiration is measured.

Hypoxia

A deficiency in any one or all of the necessary components of respiration is called hypoxia. Hypoxia is a condition caused by an inadequate supply of oxygen to meet one's needs. These needs vary with age, size, activity, and state of health. The nurse must be able to recognize the symptoms and signs of hypoxia so that corrective measures can be instituted. Some of the most important ones are as follows:

1. Labored breathing (dyspnea)
2. Restlessness, apprehension, and disorientation
3. Flared nostrils and the use of neck and facial muscles in attempts to aid respiration
4. Squatting or sitting position in an effort to improve aeration (orthopnea)
5. Paleness (pallor) or gray-purple skin color (cyanosis) may be generalized or may be more noticeable around the mouth (circumoral cyanosis) or in the fingers and toes (achracyanosis)
6. Sternal or costal retraction as the muscles of respiration contract with special effort, causing a "falling in" of the chest on inspiration
7. Increased tachypnea or decreased bradypnea rate of respiration, depending on the state of hypoxia
8. Clubbing of the fingers and toes, caused by the overgrowth of capillary beds in response to prolonged hypoxia
9. Mouth breathing or gasping mouthfuls of air

Relief of hypoxia

Regardless of the cause, treatment of hypoxia usually consists of the administration of additional oxygen above the normal 21% of atmospheric air. This is a general measure to increase the available oxygen for respiration. Specific measures are then taken to relieve the basic cause

for the individual's hypoxia, such as opening blocked air passages, improving nerve stimulation and muscle action, and correcting skeletal and cardiovascular defects.

PROVIDING AN OXYGEN-RICH ENVIRONMENT

The administration of oxygen to treat hypoxia is accomplished in a variety of ways. Nurses must have an understanding of these methods and the nursing care associated with each one. They must also recognize the potential dangers of oxygen therapy, understand the reasons for certain safety precautions, and be able to interpret them to ill children and anxious parents.

Safety precautions

Oxygen therapy can suffer risks caused by the hazards of fire and explosion, faulty equipment, excessive concentrations of oxygen, and overuse. Oxygen therapy is also expensive and requires special equipment and continuous nursing care. For these reasons it is used only when necessary.

Fire and explosions. Oxygen does not cause fire, but does support combustion and will explode under certain circumstances. Without oxygen, no fuel will burn. With increased concentrations of oxygen, all fuels burn more readily. This means that although a spark might die if it fell on a bed sheet in normal atmospheric air, in the presence of higher oxygen levels the sheet might be ignited and consumed in moments. Because of this danger, open flames, smoking materials, spark-producing electrical appliances and toys, or cloth (such as wool blankets or nylon uniforms) should not be used in the same area with oxygen therapy. Ungrounded electrical equipment is prohibited, including television sets, vaporizers, and electrical call bells. Nurses may be required to wear cotton clothing and conductive shoes that ground static electricity.

Grease, oil, and alcohol should not be used on or near oxygen equipment. If they seep into the oxygen container, they might diffuse into the oxygen and cause an explosive mixture of gases. Thus, at no time should administering apparatus or regulators be oiled or greased, nor should alcohol backrubs be given to patients receiving oxygen.

Equipment. All oxygen equipment should be in perfect running order. It should be carefully inspected by persons knowledgeable about its care and be assembled and used according to the manufacturer's instructions. Gauges and controls must be protected from falls to avoid damage. Tubing must be open and free of kinks so that the flow of oxygen will be continuous.

In most hospitals, oxygen is piped to the bedside from a central source. The administering devices are then connected to the oxygen outlet. The oxygen is turned on or off through a flow-meter that tells the amount of oxygen being released in liters per minute (Fig. 12-1).

Oxygen is also supplied in heavy metal cylinders or tanks in various sizes. They must be transported and positioned with care because of their great weight and because they contain compressed gas. If a cylinder falls, it might cause serious injury from its weight or from the sudden release of oxygen if the controls are damaged. For prevention of these dangers, oxygen tanks should be strapped to the bed or positioned to a tank carrier or baseplate (Fig. 12-2). Full tanks of oxygen should be so labeled and partially used ones should be labeled with the amount remaining. Nurses, or in some hospitals, respiratory therapists, are responsible for seeing that an adequate supply of oxygen is on hand at all times.

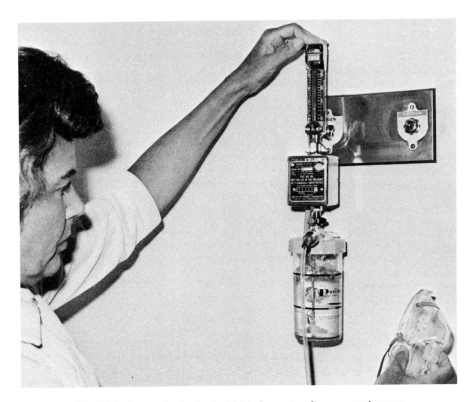

Fig. 12-1. Oxygen is piped to bedside's flowmeters from a central source.

They must never go off duty leaving a nearly empty tank. To avoid tragic errors, empty tanks should be plainly labeled "empty" and removed from the bedside.

When oxygen is supplied in tanks, regulators must be used to reduce the pressure to safe levels before it reaches the patient. The regulator has a dial that measures the amount of oxygen remaining in the tank and a flowmeter that tells the amount of oxygen to be administered (Fig. 12-3). A number of different types of regulators are manufactured; the particular type employed must be thoroughly understood before it is used. The following principles, however, apply to all types.

1. All oxygen tanks should be momentarily opened, or "cracked," before the regulator is attached to blow out dust from the aperture. This causes a loud cracking sound and so should be done outside the patient's room. The nurse stands on the side as the tank is "cracked."
2. The regulator is attached with a hand wrench or key to assure a tight connection.
3. With the flowmeter closed and the operator standing on the side, the main tank valve is opened slowly. When it is open and the needle registering the contents of the tank comes to rest, the flowmeter may be opened according to the amount needed. The "full" sign should be removed after the tank is in use.
4. When discontinuing tank oxygen for periods of 30 minutes or less, only the flowmeter need be closed. When longer periods without oxygen are desired or when a tank is to be replaced, the main valve is closed first, and when the dial of the regulator registers zero and all the oxygen is exhausted in the flowmeter, the flowmeter is closed. If the cylinder is to be changed, a wrench is used to detach the regulator. An "empty" sign is then attached and the tank removed.

Concentrations and overuse. The amount of oxygen being administered to a patient can be determined by analyzing the oxygen concentration of an enclosed space or by reading the flowmeter when oxygen is being administered through

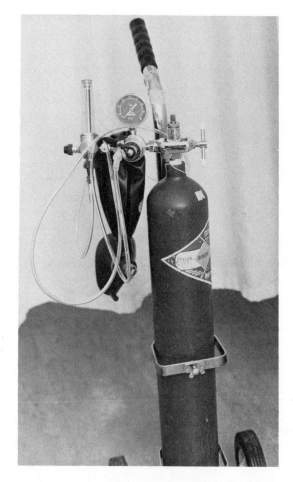

Fig. 12-2. Small, portable oxygen cylinder, equipped with a regulator (small dial), a pressure-compensated flowmeter, and a mask and bag for emergency use.

tubing from the oxygen source. In either method, the minimum concentration that will relieve hypoxia should be used. Immature and premature infants are especially vulnerable to excessive levels of oxygen, sometimes developing retrolental fibroplasia with subsequent blindness (p. 280). In older infants and children, excessive concentrations of oxygen serve no purpose and are wasteful. The physician usually indicates the amount of flow or concentration of oxygen in the order. The physician may set limits, depending

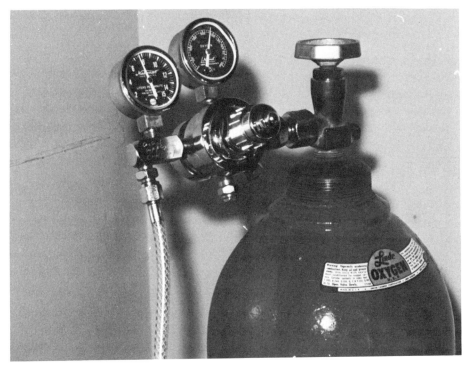

Fig. 12-3. Oxygen regulator and flowmeter attached to tank that is wheeled to the bedside in a metal carrier.

on the patient's symptoms, and rely on the nurse's judgment regarding the exact amount of oxygen to be administered.

Whenever oxygen is administered, no matter what the method, it must be humidified to prevent drying of and damage of the mucous membrane.

Oxygen therapy is discontinued as soon as possible to reduce the psychological dependency that may develop in some children and also to reduce the expense it incurs for their families. It is usually discontinued gradually, both in amounts of oxygen administered and in the duration of treatment periods.

Nursing observations. Continuous nursing observation must be made of all patients receiving oxygen, of the amounts being administered, and of the equipment being used. These obser-

vations should be recorded at regular intervals on the patient's chart. Any changes should be reported verbally to the supervising nurse for immediate action.

Methods of oxygen therapy and nursing care

There are two basic methods of administering oxygen: (1) placing the patient in an oxygen-rich chamber such as an incubator or tent and (2) allowing oxygen to flow directly into the respiratory passages by means of tubes or masks. Various modifications of these methods are made by adding humidifiers and employing various sizes and shapes of catheters, cannulas, masks, hoods, and tents. The method is selected to provide the patient maximum comfort, relief from hypoxia, and ease of nursing care. Emergency oxygen is usually administered by means of a mask or bag with relatively high oxygen flow. As soon as possible, other methods are instituted according to the physician's orders. The physician also indicates any modifications to be used, the amount of oxygen to be administered, and the duration of the therapy.

In some hospitals the services of individuals specially trained in various methods of oxygen therapy are available when oxygen is ordered for a patient. The *respiratory therapist*, as this person is called, sets up all types of oxygen equipment, administers the various types of inhalation therapy, instructs the staff on their continued operation if this is required, and terminates the treatment when it is discontinued by the physician. In hospitals where a respiratory therapist is not employed, the nurse assumes these responsibilities.

In addition to knowledge of oxygen therapy, the nurse must be able to explain its functions to the parents, who may share the common misconception that oxygen is only administered to the dying. The nurse can help allay fears by comparing oxygen with other therapeutic measures, such as drug or physical therapy, and by showing the parents how the equipment works, such as how the portholes of a tent open to provide access to the child. Fire safety should be stressed to the parents as a normal precaution observed wherever oxygen is used and not as an unusual, additional hazard to their child. The parents should be encouraged to ask questions and these should be answered with respect and understanding. Confident, assured parents are better able to reassure an ill child.

Oxygen chambers. When it is desirable to control the humidity, oxygen content, or temperature of a patient's environment, the patient is placed in a chamber appropriate to size and needs. For this purpose environmental control rooms, incubators, and large- and small-sized tents are used. Environmental control rooms are relatively rare and used only in unusual circumstances. Incubators and tents, however, are common in pediatric units everywhere.

Incubators. Incubators are small cabinets equipped to provide oxygen, humidity, warmth, and easy observation of infants. They are sometimes used only to provide additional heat by means of a preset, thermostatically controlled heating unit. Sometimes the temperature of the incubator is regulated by the baby's own body heat as determined by a temperature probe taped to the body. Temperatures between 80° and 85° F are usually maintained, but higher levels may be ordered, depending on the infant's condition.

When oxygen is added to the incubator, its source is either the central source through the wall flowmeter or a tank through an attached regulator. The flow is adjusted to maintain various oxygen concentrations as determined by an oxygen analyzer. The concentration is never allowed to remain above 40%, unless ordered specifically by the physician.

Humidity in the incubator is provided from a reservoir of distilled water and controlled by a preset dial. The degree of humidity ordered for each infant may vary considerably. High humidity may be supplied by jet humidifiers, together with aerosol medications.

Some incubators are made with lift-up lids that open for nursing care. Others are made with side portholes that allow for nursing care without major oxygen loss if it is being administered. This kind may also have a removable lid for special procedures and various innovations inside such as a rocking device to assist the infant with regular diaphragm motion. The small mattress is usually covered with a pillowcase and a pad is placed under the infant.

Tents. Large oxygen tents may be ordered for older children or adolescents (Fig. 12-4). These tents usually consist of a plastic canopy suspended from an overhead rod and attached to a cabinet containing a machine. When the machine is properly adjusted, it regulates the tent's ventilation and temperature and may also provide for increased humidity in connection with the oxygen flow. Manufacturer's instructions should be followed for each individual unit, but the following general recommendations may prove helpful:

1. A bath blanket should be placed between the bed mattress and bedsprings to prevent the plastic canopy from catching in the springs and tearing. Oxygen loss can be reduced if a plastic or rubberized sheet is placed over the mattress and under the bottom bed sheet.
2. The tent canopy and control cabinet are brought to the bedside. The overbed bar is extended and the tent folded out along the bar.
3. The electric cord leading to the control cabinet is plugged in and the motor turned on. Ventilation is provided by a fan that is initially set at medium speed. If deflectors are provided, they should be arranged to prevent the cold air from blowing directly on the patient.
4. The temperature-controlling thermostat is usually set at about 70° F, except in hot weather when the temperature inside the tent should not be more than 15° F below room temperature to reduce shock to the patient if the canopy is lifted and to increase the efficiency of the tent.
5. The oxygen inlet tube is connected to the wall flowmeter or the oxygen tank regulator. Desired concentrations of oxygen can be obtained by holding the flush valve open for about 2 minutes or by allowing the oxygen to flow at 15 liters per minute for about 30 minutes. At that time analysis of the concentrations in the tent should be made and the flow reduced to 10 to 12 liters per minute.
6. When all is in readiness, the patient is placed under the canopy or the canopy is placed over the patient. Care should be taken to see that the canopy sides do not touch the patient's face. The tent skirts are tucked under the mattress between bath blankets or sheets in such a way that leakage is minimized. Special care should be taken in raising or lowering the head of the bed to prevent tearing of the plastic canopy.

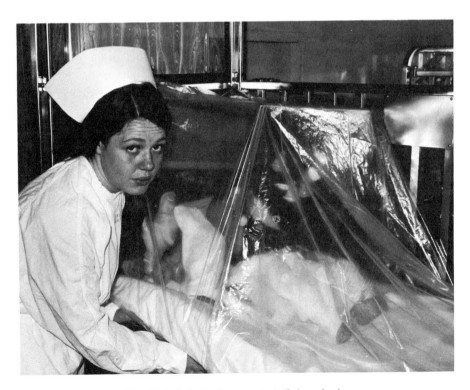

Fig. 12-4. Crib-sized oxygen tent of clear plastic.

7. Nursing care is planned to provide maximum rest for the patient and minimum loss of oxygen. The ventilator fan should be turned off before opening the tent to reduce oxygen loss. Hypoxic patients usually are more comfortable if the head of the bed is raised somewhat, orders permitting. Because the constant circulation of cold air inside the tent promotes evaporation, many patients feel cold and are more comfortable if they wear hooded sweat shirts or head covers of some kind. If linen becomes wet from the humidifier, they should be changed.

8. When high humidity is desired, jet humidifiers containing distilled water or special medications may be added to the standard oxygen tent as ordered by the physician.

Often small-sized, bed-top chambers of a variety of models are used for small children. They are particularly useful for high-humidity environments. This type of chamber usually does not include an electric ventilating fan or a refrigeration unit, as does the large-sized tent. To prevent overheating and to keep the temperature in the interior about 70° F, ice or a mixture of ice and water is added to a container located inside the tent. As the ice melts, it is drained off into a collection container and emptied periodically. The nurse is responsible for seeing that the ice container is full and the collection container empty. In the Hudson tent, the air or oxygen passes through tubing bathed in ice water. In the Mistogen tent, ice is simply placed in its perforated metal chest inside the chamber.

The chief function of these units is to act as a humidifying unit. Distilled water or medicated solution is placed in a container and oxygen or air bubbled through, producing a fine mist. When oxygen is used, the flow rate is usually set between 4 and 10 liters per minute, depending on the physician's orders. If the apparatus does not produce a mist when it is turned on, the nurse should check to see if (1) the oxygen tubing is connected and the flow rate sufficient, (2) the fluid level is high enough in the solution container, and (3) the mist-making apparatus is

clogged with lint or other matter. Thorough, periodic cleaning of all the apparatus parts should eliminate most of these difficulties.

Oxygen masks, cannulas, hoods, and catheters. Masks are an ideal means for emergency use, because high concentrations of oxygen can be administered by them very quickly. The oxygen passes through a tube leading to the light plastic mask. A wide variety of masks are made in various sizes, many of disposable material (Fig. 12-5). Some kinds allow for the rebreathing of the first one-third of the expired air along with fresh oxygen from the supply. The BLB mask (named for its inventors—Boothby, Lovelace, and Bulbulian) is one of the rebreathing types. Rebreathing masks must fit the face tightly, but simple face masks should not be applied tightly unless an escape valve for carbon dioxide is provided (Fig. 12-6).

Nasal cannulas are short, paired, open tubes made of plastic that are attached to the larger tube leading to the oxygen supply. The tubes are placed just inside the nostrils. Because of the drying effect the steady flow of oxygen has on the nasal mucosa, oxygen administered by cannula should pass through a humidifier. This method of administering oxygen is particularly useful when concentrations less than 35% are desired. The apparatus is light, disposable, and relatively easy to set up.

Clear plastic hoods are small chambers that fit over the infant's head. They are an efficient means of administering oxygen to infants. They permit unobstructed observation and care of small infants (Fig. 12-7).

Oxygen administered by nasal catheter is only rarely used with children because it is unnecessarily irritating and confining (the child must be restrained to prevent pulling out the catheter). A nasal catheter is made of soft plastic or rubber tubing attached to the oxygen supply. The catheter is passed into one nostril until the tip is located just behind the uvula. It must be securely taped to the face to prevent movement in or out. The nostril must be cleansed and lubricated fre-

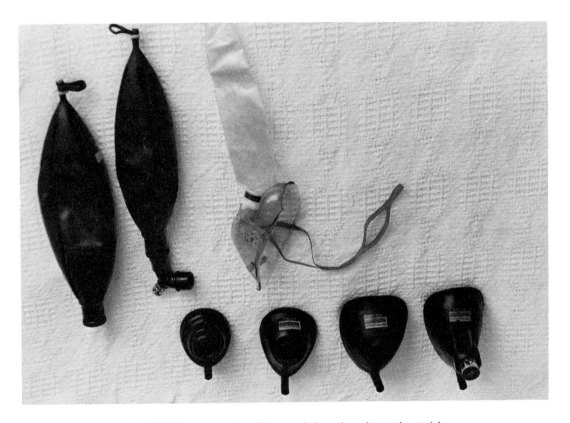

Fig. 12-5. Oxygen masks and bags made in various sizes and materials.

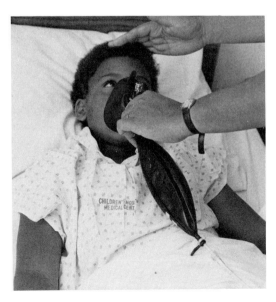

Fig. 12-6. The BLB mask, a rebreathing mask, must fit the face tightly.

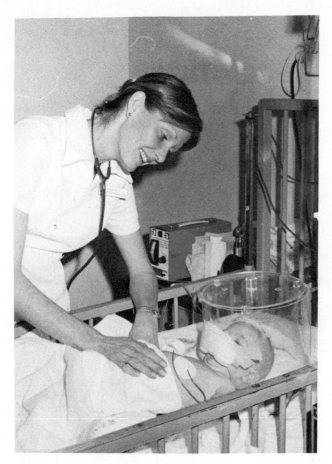

Fig. 12-7. Clear plastic hoods such as this Olympic Oxyhood provide an efficient means of administering oxygen to small infants while permitting unobstructed access for care and observation. (Note heart monitor attached to infant's chest.)

quently to remove crusts and reduce irritation to the skin. Eating and drinking are greatly complicated by this method of oxygen administration because the catheter passes down into the back of the throat. Oxygen flow is generally discontinued temporarily during meals to prevent swallowing oxygen.

OPENING AIR PASSAGES

For external respiration to occur, the air passages must be open. Mucous membrane secretions, foreign objects, the tongue, and swollen tissue may obstruct the airway and hamper the child's breathing. Various measures can be used to open closed passages and help maintain open

ones; such measures are positioning, artificial cough maneuvers, suctioning and liquefying mucus, shrinking mucous membranes, and tracheostomy. The nurse may be called on to assist with or perform all of these life-saving measures.

Positioning

Correct positioning can prevent many problems of blocked airways in infants, postoperative and unconscious children, and those with disorders such as Down's syndrome. These helpless persons should never be left on their backs because of the danger that regurgitated matter might be aspirated or the tongue might obstruct

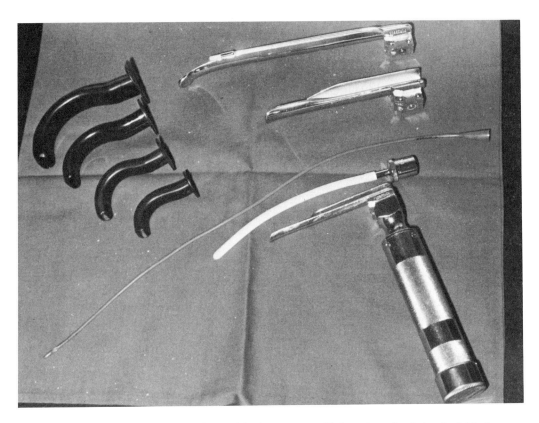

Fig. 12-8. Airways of various sizes; lower right, laryngoscope. Various sizes of catheters for intubation are shown in metal pan at top.

the airway. Instead, they should be maintained on the side or abdomen with the head to the side. If positioning is impossible because of special conditions such as the administration of anesthesia, the head should be lowered and turned to the side during episodes of vomiting. An airway may be left in place after anesthesia to ensure an unobstructed air passage until consciousness is regained (Fig. 12-8).

Artificial cough maneuvers

Three basic maneuvers produce an artificial cough and clear the airway. They all carry some risk to victims, such as broken ribs, lacerated livers, or ruptured stomachs, but they may be life-saving. They are abdominal compression (Heimlich maneuver), low chest compression, and back blows.

Abdominal compression is especially useful for adults and larger children. A fist is pressed from behind against the victim's stomach with a quick upward thrust.

Chest compression is especially useful for small children. A rescuer picks up and bends the child over an arm while giving a quick blow between the shoulder blades.

Back blows are delivered between the shoulder blades, preferably with the victim's head below the body. This maneuver may be used for any age, but especially for infants and small children.

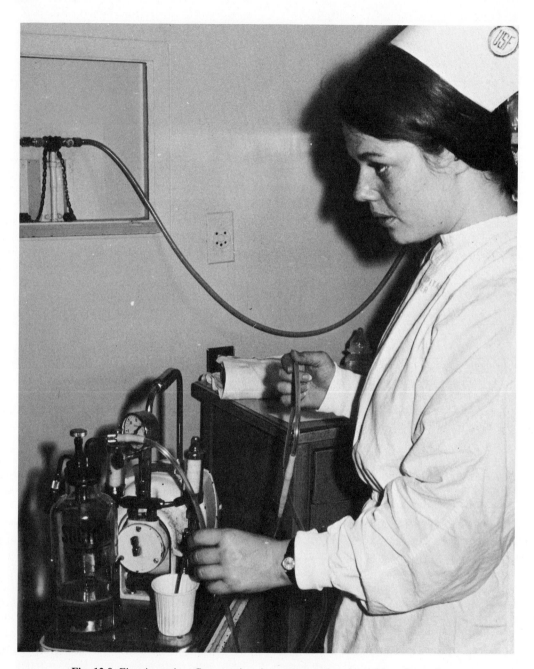

Fig. 12-9. Electric suction. Cup contains clean water used to clear tubing after each use.

Suctioning

Suctioning can be accomplished by using a bulb syringe, a manual suction catheter (DeLee trap), or a catheter setup attached to electric suction. A suction bulb is usually provided for each newborn infant to remove matter from the nose and mouth. The DeLee trap has been largely replaced by electric suction but is still seen in emergency kits. Regardless of the type, some form of suction apparatus should be available at all times for all infants and other persons who might develop respiratory difficulties, including those patients with respiratory or nervous system diseases, those patients undergoing an operation, and postoperative and unconscious patients (Fig. 12-9).

The following recommendations are made for the use of all suction apparatus:

1. The apparatus should be personal for each patient and kept free from contamination. In some hospitals catheters are not reused; a fresh one is employed for each suctioning.
2. The catheters should be lubricated with water before use to ensure greater ease of insertion. Oil should never be used because it might go down into the lungs.
3. During the insertion of a catheter the suction should be temporarily interrupted by pinching the catheter or uncovering the Y-tube control to keep it from clinging to the wall of the air passage and damaging the delicate tissue.
4. Suctioning should not be prolonged (no longer than 9 seconds) nor should unnecessarily high amounts be used because these practices may aggravate the congestion instead of relieve it.
5. For dilution of the collected secretions, the drainage bottle should contain about an inch of water at the onset. The bottle should be covered or shielded from view for esthetic reasons.

Humidifying the atmosphere and liquefying and shrinking tissue

By increasing the water content of inspired air, breathing is made easier. Two common methods of increasing the humidity of air are by boiling water to produce steam and by forcing oxygen or air through a solution of fluid to produce a fine mist. To add to the efficiency, various drugs are used to liquefy thick secretions and shrink the tissue, thus further assisting respiratory effort.

Steam. A steam or croup tent is one of the oldest means of treating croup, bronchitis, and sinusitis. But both steam and the boiling water that creates it are very dangerous, especially near a small child who does not understand their dangers. Many tragic burns have been caused by vaporizers or tea kettles that have overturned. For prevention of such tragedy, vaporizers should be stable, preferably kept at floor level with a long nozzle that is shielded so that the live steam cannot contact the child. For greatest efficiency the steam should be trapped in a relatively small space where the child will gain maximum benefit from it while breathing. For infants and small children a tent or sheeting can be formed over the crib and the nozzle of the vaporizer placed into it, shielded by a wooden frame to protect the child from the incoming steam. For larger children and adolescents a whole room may be filled with steam.

When assigned to care for a child receiving steam, the nurse should check the vaporizer regularly to see that it is functioning correctly and that there is sufficient water in the storage reservoir. In the home, oil of eucalyptus or tincture of benzoin may be added to the water, but in the hospital distilled water is used to prevent the deposit of hard water salts in the appliance.

Humidifying devices. By forcing air or oxygen through distilled water or some special solution, a fine, nonheated mist can be produced (Fig. 12-10). There are various names for these devices, such as aerosol, nebulizer, humidifier, and many trade names created by the manufacturers. The Hydrojet is one such device. It is useful in treating a relatively calm child who will remain in the humid steam. The Mistogen detergent solution, aerosol, and tent are usually used together with oxygen passing through the solution to produce a fine mist. Whatever the unit,

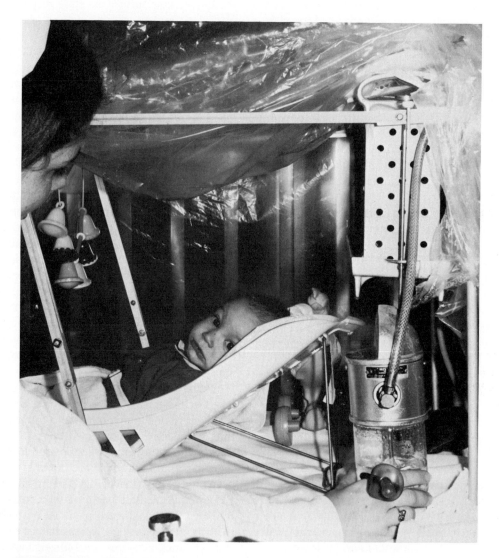

Fig. 12-10. Mist-producing device serves to humidify the small plastic tent (drawn up in photo to show icebox used to cool the enclosed air). This infant has been placed in semi-Fowler's position to facilitate breathing.

manufacturer's instructions should be followed and the nurse should see that the level of solution in the aerosol bottle is sufficient to produce the desired effects.

Medications

In addition to the therapeutic gases used in the treatment of respiratory conditions, a number of drugs have also proved useful, including the bronchodilators, mucolytic agents, antitussives, expectorants, and decongestants.

Bronchodilators. When the bronchial passages become constricted, the exchange of gases is disrupted. The bronchodilator drugs are used to relax the smooth muscles of the bronchial tree, resulting in an increased lumen size. Some of the most commonly used bronchodilators are epinephrine, isoproterenol hydrochloride (Isuprel), terbutaline sulfate (Brethine), and aminophylline.

Mucolytic agents. These drugs reduce thickness and stickiness of pulmonary secretions. They are usually administered by aerosol inhalation. Acetylcysteine (Mucomyst, Respaire) is an amino acid derivative that is administered in a 10% to 20% solution of water or saline. Desoxyribonuclease (Dornavac) is an enzyme that degrades DNA in cells. It is administered in a saline solution by aerosol.

Antitussants. These drugs act to supress the cough reflex. Codeine and methadone are narcotic antitussants. Benzonatate (Tessalon) and dextromethorphan hydrobromide (Romilar) are nonnarcotic antitussants.

Expectorants. Drugs that increase mucus secretions and thereby reduce their thickness and facilitate expulsion are called expectorants. Ammonium chloride and sodium iodide increase secretion by irritating the gastric mucosa.

Nasal decongestants. These drugs are administered as nasal sprays and shrink the engorged nasal mucous membranes. When overused they may result in "rebound" engorgement, or swelling of the mucous membranes. Some of the most common are phenylephrine hydrochloride (Neo-

Synephrine), ephedrine sulfate, and naphazoline hydrochloride (Privine).

Artificial airways

When the airway is obstructed, it may be necessary to place a tube into the trachea to create an opening to the lungs. The trachea may be intubated in two ways: (1) by passing a tube through the nose or mouth, a procedure called endotracheal intubation, or (2) by making a surgical incision through the throat into the trachea, a procedure called a tracheotomy. The resulting opening is called a tracheostomy. It may be temporary or permanent.

Endotrachael intubation

Endotracheal intubation may be done to prevent aspiration of secretions and stomach contents, to provide an avenue of access, and to administer intermittent positive pressure and gases for anesthesia or treatment. In an emergency it is preferred to tracheotomy. Later, if prolonged support of the airway is needed, a tracheotomy is performed as a nonemergency procedure with the endotracheal tube left in until the tracheostomy tube is in place. Endotracheal tubes are made of rubber or synthetics with an inflatable cuff so that a closed system with a ventilator can be maintained if necessary.

Tracheotomy

A tracheotomy is needed when an endotracheal tube cannot be inserted, when it is contraindicated as in severe burns or in obstructions such as tumors, or when the patient is conscious and cannot tolerate an endotracheal tube. Tracheostomy tubes are made of silver, steel, or synthetics. They may be single lumen or double lumen and both types may be cuffed (Fig. 12-11). The newer plastic tubes come with a high-volume, low-pressure cuff that is less likely to cause damage to the trachea. Single lumen tubes must be changed every 72 hours. Double lumen tubes have an advantage because the inner tube can be removed for cleaning without disturbing the airway. They are secured in place with twill tapes tied around the patient's neck. If they are coughed out, however, a tracheal dilator or a curved hemostat kept at the bedside is used to hold the opening open until the tube can be replaced.

Using a cuffed tracheostomy tube or endotracheal tube has several implications for nursing care. Although the low-pressure cuff reduces the incidence of tracheal erosion from pressure on the wall of the trachea, some hazards inherent in their use remain. Therefore, the cuff is not inflated unless it is necessary to provide positive pressure ventilation, to prevent aspiration of secretions by the unconscious person, or to exert pressure on bleeding sites in patients who have had neck surgery. If the older kind of cuff is used, it must be deflated for several minutes every hour to prevent tracheal damage.

All persons with tubes require suctioning of the airway. The airway should be suctioned as often as necessary to remove obstructing mucus. The following guidelines are recommended:

1. Use sterile technique and equipment, including gloves or forceps, suction catheter, and water or saline solution.
2. Before suctioning, administer a few breaths of oxygen to reduce hypoxia.
3. Do not suction for longer than 10 seconds at a time, with 3-minute rests between aspirations, unless the airway is obstructed with mucus.
4. Use a fenestrated (windowed) catheter or a non-windowed catheter with a Y-tube connected to the suction machine so that the catheter can be

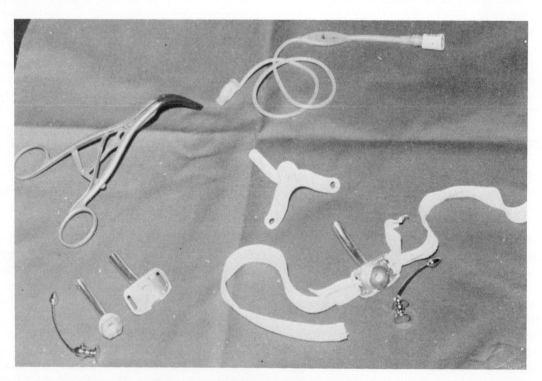

Fig. 12-11. Tracheostomy tubes of silver (lower left and right) and plastic (center) with inflatable rubber tube and clamp used to maintain airway in certain circumstances.

inserted without suction. Once the catheter is inserted, place the thumb over the window to institute suction as the catheter is withdrawn.

5. Insert the catheter deeply enough to stimulate coughing. Then begin suctioning.
6. If mucus is tenacious, 5 to 10 ml of sterile saline solution may be instilled into the tube just before suctioning if ordered by the physician.
7. To aspirate the left bronchus, turn the child's head to the right and tilt the chest to the left. Reverse the process for the right bronchus.
8. When double lumen tubes are in place, clean the inner tube at least every 2 to 8 hours using hydrogen peroxide, sterile water, detergent, and friction. Some hospitals use commercially packaged trachostomy care kits and some assemble their own.

Inserting an endotracheal and tracheostomy tube bypasses the natural secretions of the nose and mouth. Therefore, artificial humidification and warming of the air are necessary, through the use of mist-making devices. The nurse and respiratory therapist are responsible to see that these devices are working properly.

Nourishment of the child with an endotracheal tube is provided by intravenous or nasogastric tube feedings. The child with a tracheostomy may be able to swallow and take normal oral feedings, although they, too, may be fed by nasogastric tube or intravenous line. To prevent aspiration during oral or tube feedings, some experts recommend inflating the cuff of the tracheostomy tube. Others believe that such inflation bulges into the esophagus and makes swallowing more difficult; they therefore prefer that the cuff be deflated during feedings. The decision of what is best should be determined by nursing assessment.

Because the tracheal opening is made below the voice box (larynx), the tracheotomy patient cannot speak or make any vocal noises unless the opening is temporarily closed to allow air to pass up through the vocal cords. This situation can be frightening to children who have hitherto been able to communicate their wants by speaking or by crying. If children are old enough they can be given a bell to ring when they need help. (An electric bell call is allowed if oxygen is not in use.) Older children appreciate a pencil and paper or Magic Slate on which to write messages. As soon as permissible, children can learn to place a finger over the tracheostomy opening during expiration to divert the air up through their vocal cords so they can speak.

Because infants and children have shorter necks than adults, special care must be given to the skin around the outer tube and the folds of the child's neck to guard against excoriation. Moist ties should be changed periodically and the child's neck washed and carefully dried. A small towel placed under the shoulders of the infant will allow better positioning and prevent some excoriation under the chin. Lint-free gauze dressings placed under the flange of the outer tubes should be changed as they become moist.

When it is time to wean the child from a temporary tracheostomy, the physician may order a gradual, increasing occlusion of the opening each day until it is completely closed. When the child can tolerate a completely closed tube, the tracheostomy tubes are removed by the physician and the opening allowed to heal. A tracheostomy set should be kept available for emergency use for some time thereafter in case it is needed again.

STIMULATING OR SUBSTITUTING RESPIRATORY EFFORT

No matter how much oxygen is in the air or how open the air passages may be, if air does not move in and out of the lungs with alternating internal pressure, necessary gaseous exchange cannot take place, causing death. In other words, respiratory action is necessary to life. Sometimes newborn infants do not begin to breathe spontaneously, some have episodes of apnea, and sometimes disease or drug effects cause respirations to slow or cease. In these cases respirations must be stimulated and/or substituted until the child is able to take over.

Stimulation

Physical stimulation. Respirations can be stimulated by various physical shocks such as when the physician slaps the newborn infant's feet or buttocks or dips the body in a bath of cool water. The irritating effect of a suction catheter in the nasal passages may also stimulate the infant to take a first breath and cry out in protest.

Chemical stimulation. Drugs are frequently used to stimulate respirations, not only to initiate them but also to increase their rate and depth. The most common of these drugs administered to children are as follows.

Carbon dioxide. It may come as a surprise to learn that the gas carbon dioxide is an important, natural respiratory stimulant. As it builds up in the blood, it stimulates the respiratory center in the medulla of the brain to cause the individual to take a breath. The person who exercises produces more carbon dioxide, which stimulates the respiratory center to produce greater respiratory effort, thus supplying additional oxygen needs. For a sleeping person, the level of blood carbon dioxide is reduced, and respiratory stimulation and oxygen need are reduced. One of the effective means used artificially to stimulate respiration is to administer carbon dioxide together with oxygen. This principle is demonstrated in the effective use of rebreathing oxygen masks and mouth-to-mouth resuscitation.

Bemegride. The drug bemegride acts on the respiratory center of the brain to increase the respiratory rate. It is especially effective for the treatment of barbiturate poisoning when respirations are depressed. It is given intravenously in doses of 1 mg per kilogram of body weight and repeated in 3 to 5 minutes if necessary. Because of the danger of convulsions from an overdose, pentobarbital should be kept available.

Caffeine. Well known for its presence in coffee and tea, caffeine causes the respiratory center of the brain to be more sensitive to carbon dioxide and so works to stimulate both the rate and depth of respirations. It is administered for depression intramuscularly, intravenously, or subcutaneously, in amounts of 8 mg per kilogram of body weight per dose (maximum of 500 mg) repeated every 4 hours as needed.

Ephedrine sulfate. Ephedrine sulfate is a chemical cousin of epinephrine (Adrenalin) but is weaker and more prolonged in its action. It stimulates the respiratory center and relaxes hypertonic muscles in the bronchioles, thus making respiratory effort more efficient, and so it is especially useful in the treatment of asthma. It is administered orally, subcutaneously, or intravenously in amounts of 3 mg per kilogram of body weight per 24-hour period divided into four to six doses.

Nikethamide (Coramine). Frequently seen in emergency kits, nikethamide acts on the respiratory center in the brain to increase the rate and depth of respirations. It is used as a stimulant for respiratory, depression from poisoning by alcohol, barbiturates, and anesthesia. It is administered orally, intramuscularly, or intravenously in amounts of 25 mg (0.1 ml) per kilogram of body weight per dose, with a maximum dose of 10 ml, to be repeated as needed.

Pentylenetetrazol (Metrazol). Pentylenetetrazol is a potent stimulant for all parts of the brain and spinal cord. It is frequently used for barbiturate poisoning. It is administered intravenously in amounts of 0.2 ml (100 mg/ml) per kilogram of body weight per dose, with a maximum dose of 10 ml, to be repeated every 15 minutes as needed for marked barbiturate depression.

Picrotoxin. Picrotoxin stimulates the entire central nervous system and is used as an antidote for barbiturate poisoning and as a combatant for depression caused by tribromoethanol (Avertin) and paraldehyde. It is administered intravenously or intramuscularly in amounts of 0.2 mg per kilogram of body weight per dose. It may be repeated in 15 minutes as necessary, but the child must be watched closely for convulsions.

1. Place victim on back.
   Wipe foreign matter from victim's mouth.

2. Tilt victim's head back as far as possible.
   Lift the jaw forward to open air passageway.

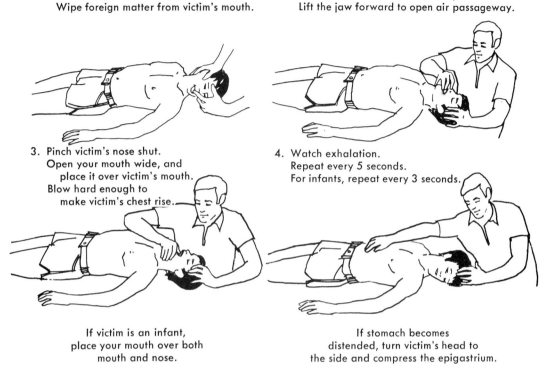

3. Pinch victim's nose shut.
   Open your mouth wide, and
      place it over victim's mouth.
   Blow hard enough to
      make victim's chest rise.

4. Watch exhalation.
   Repeat every 5 seconds.
   For infants, repeat every 3 seconds.

If victim is an infant,
place your mouth over both
mouth and nose.

If stomach becomes
distended, turn victim's head to
the side and compress the epigastrium.

Fig. 12-12. Mouth-to-mouth resuscitation.

Artificial respiration

When respirations cease, emergency resuscitation measures must be instituted promptly. This means that alternating positive and negative pressure must be provided in the lungs to cause the gaseous exchange to take place. If the heart continues to beat but the victim cannot take over the breathing effort, mechanical respirators may be employed to keep up the respiratory action. Some of the most common respirators in current use are the tank and chest respirators, the rocking bed, and the intermittent positive pressure apparatus.

Emergency measures

Mouth-to-mouth resuscitation. When there is no evidence of respiratory movement, emer-

gency resuscitation should begin at once. The most effective method is mouth-to-mouth resuscitation, in which the rescuer breathes air by mouth into the victim's lungs (Fig. 12-12). The following method is recommended by the American Heart Association:

1. Place the victim face up immediately. Do not waste time moving to a better place, loosening clothing, or draining water from lungs.
2. Quickly clear the mouth and throat if it is evident the victim has vomited. Remove mucus, food, and other obstructions.
3. Tilt the head back as far as possible. The head should be in a "chin-up" or "sniff" position and the neck stretched.
4. Lift the lower jaw forward. Grasp the jaw by placing the thumb into the corner of the mouth. Do not hold or depress the tongue.

5. For an adult, pinch the nose shut, or seal with the cheek. For an infant, cover both nose and mouth at the same time.

6. Open your mouth wide and cover the victim's mouth and blow until you see the victim's chest rise. (For infants, cover both nose and mouth and blow with small puffs of air from your cheeks.)

7. Listen for exhalation. Quickly remove your mouth when chest rises. Lift jaw higher if victim makes snoring or gurgling sounds.

8. Repeat every 5 seconds for adults, every 3 seconds for infants. Continue until victim begins to breathe normally, another means of resuscitation is provided, or the patient is pronounced dead by a physician.

9. NOTE: Children's stomachs tend to become distended with air during rescue breathing. If this becomes excessive, turn the head to one side and compress the epigastrium.

If the heartbeat cannot be felt, external heart massage may be attempted at the same time that resuscitation measures are begun.

External heart massage. Heart massage is an emergency method of stimulating the heart muscle to contract. It is sometimes called *artificial circulation*. Internal heart massage requires an incision into the chest cavity and direct massage of the heart by the surgeon's hand. Obviously, this method is unsuitable for most emergency conditions. External heart massage, however, involves the depression of the sternal bone down onto the heart, thus stimulating it to contract. This method is more suitable for a variety of emergency conditions. It is not without danger, however, because of possible broken ribs or traumatized liver, but it is worth the risk if death is the alternative. Emergency heart massage is not

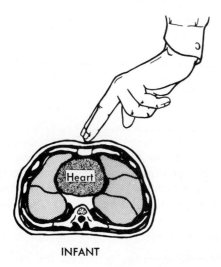

INFANT

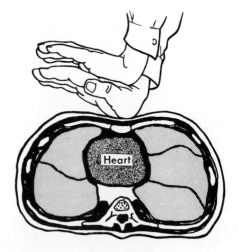

OLDER CHILD

Place victim on a firm surface.

For infant:

1. Place two fingers firmly on the midsternum.

2. Firmly depress ¾ inch at rate of 80 to 100 depressions per minute.

The ratio for both adults and children is 5 compressions to 1 ventilation.

Begin mouth-to-mouth resuscitation.

For older child or adult:

1. Place the heel of one hand on the sternum. Use the other hand to add strength.

2. Firmly depress at rate of 60 depressions per minute.

Fig. 12-13. External heart massage for infants and older children.

attempted for patients dying of debilitating or incurable diseases (Fig. 12-13).

The procedure for administering external heart massage is as follows:

1. Place the victim face up on a firm surface or slip a firm board under the thorax.
2. Mouth-to-mouth resuscitation is begun before external heart massage. The absence of a pulse is determined by feeling the brachial artery. In the case of infants, two fingers on the midsternum and firmly depress the bone ¾ inch at a rate of 80 to 100 compressions per minute and at a ratio of one ventilation to five compressions. In the case of an older child or adult, place the heel of one hand on the sternum and use the other hand depressing the bone 1 to 2 inches at a rate of 60 to 80 compressions per minute and at a ratio of one ventilation to five compressions. Because it is difficult for one person simultaneously to do both heart massage and mouth-to-mouth resuscitation, especially on an older child or adult, a second person should help in the rescue.
3. The effectiveness of the heart massage can be judged by the pupils of the eyes. Dilated pupils indicate that the brain is not receiving sufficient oxygen; nondilated pupils indicate adequate circulation and oxygenation of the brain tissue. Emergency heart massage can be discontinued when the victim's heart begins to beat spontaneously or when the victim is pronounced dead by a physician.

Portable emergency respiration. To avoid direct mouth contact, a number of mechanical devices have been manufactured; however, the principle and basic method of mouth-to-mouth resuscitation remains the same. Whatever the device used, valuable time must not be lost in obtaining it.

The simplest and most easily available protection against direct contact is a clean handkerchief or other type of porous cloth. Other devices fall into three categories—the simple face mask, the double airway, and the bag or bellows with mask.

Continuing measures

If the muscles of respiration are paralyzed or the nervous control of them is damaged, the patient cannot breathe unaided. Some conditions that cause these effects are polio-myelitis, muscular dystrophy, myasthenia gravis, and poisoning from various drugs and chemicals. For provision of the long-term needs of these patients for total or partial respiratory assistance, a number of mechanical respiratory devices have been devised, such as the tank and chest respirators, the rocking bed, and intermittent positive pressure machines. The nurse may be called on to assist in the care of patients using these devices. If the basic principle underlying their use is understood, the nurse will be better able to learn the particular details associated with the operations of each machine and the special nursing care required for patients using them.

Tank respirators. The tank respirator or iron lung was well known in the tragic days of the poliomyelitis epidemics before the Salk and Sabin vaccines were perfected. Tanks are still used for selected cases in which other respirators will not meet the need.

Tank respirators work by creating a pressure outside the body that is greater than that inside the air sacs of the lungs and then by reversing the pressures. This action creates respirations just as the normal respiratory effort alternately increases and decreases the pressure inside the lungs. The patient's body is completely enclosed in a metal tank, except for the head. A large bellowlike, flexible end to the tank is moved in and out mechanically, producing the preset amount of negative and positive pressure and the rate per minute. An emergency hand lever is provided so that if there were an electric power failure the alternating pressures could be maintained. The patient breathes through the nose and mouth in a normal manner.

Complete care is provided through the portholes in the side of the respirator. They must be open only when the pressure gauge registers zero and should be closed by the nurse's arms or attached lids within 2 seconds so as not to interfere with the respiratory pattern. The patient is taught to speak and swallow only during expiration. Suctioning, too, must be accomplished during expiration to avoid aspiration. The care of patients in tank respirators requires special knowledge of the particular tank and great patience and skill.

Chest respirators. Chest respirators work on the same principle as the larger, more efficient tank respirators. They are devices that fit over the chest and provide alternating pressure. They give greater flexibility of patient care and mobility for the patient and are used for limited periods of time as the patient's condition becomes less acute.

Rocking beds. Rocking beds provide respiratory assistance by alternately forcing the abdominal organs against the diaphragm, as the head is tipped back and down, and then reversing the action as the diaphragm is drawn down and the head is raised. The degree of seesaw action can be preset on the electric controls of the bed. The patient must learn to talk and swallow on expiration in time with the ups and downs of the bed. The nurse must also learn to feed the patient, bathe, and care for elimination needs in time with the bed. Patients with weak respiratory action may use more than one of the respiratory devices; for example, they may use the rocking bed during the day, a chest respirator with a portable power supply for travel, and a tank respirator at night during sleep.

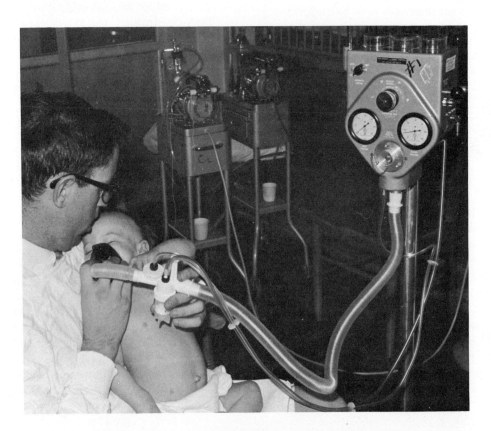

Fig. 12-14. Intermittent positive pressure breathing (IPPB) administered by an inhalation therapist.

Intermittent positive pressure. Intermittent positive pressure breathing (IPPB) is accomplished by a valve that alternately allows air or oxygen to be forced deep into the lungs during inhalation (Fig. 12-14). The device can be used for a variety of respiratory needs, from the patient who cannot breathe at all to the one who triggers the device by respiration. Various attachments provide further flexibility so that drugs can be nebulized and oxygen or air can be administered by means of a mask, mouthpiece, or tracheostomy dome (Fig. 12-15). The physician orders the amount of pressure to be exerted, the medication, and the duration and number of treatments per 24-hour period. The Bennett and Bird respirators are well-known IPPB devices. Although many hospitals employ respiratory

therapists, nurses may need to administer these treatments. If so, they should have special instructions and supervision in the use of such machines.

SUMMARY OUTLINE

I. Respiration
   A. Definition
   B. External respiration
      1. Breathing
      2. Gaseous exchange
   C. Internal respiration
   D. Necessary components
      1. Adequate oxygen
      2. Open airways
      3. Nervous stimulation
      4. Muscle action
      5. Rigid frame
      6. Functioning circulatory system
   E. Hypoxia
   F. Relief of hypoxia
II. Providing an oxygen-rich environment
   A. Safety precautions
      1. Fire and explosions
      2. Equipment
      3. Concentrations and overuse
      4. Nursing observations
   B. Methods of oxygen therapy and nursing care
      1. Oxygen chambers
         a. Incubators
         b. Tents
      2. Oxygen masks, cannulas, hoods, and catheters
III. Opening air passages
   A. Positioning
   B. Artificial cough maneuvers
   C. Suctioning
   D. Humidifying the atmosphere and liquefying and shrinking tissue
      1. Steam
      2. Humidifying devices
   E. Medications
      1. Bronchodilators
      2. Mucolytic agents
      3. Antitussants
      4. Expectorants
      5. Nasal decongestants
   F. Artificial airways
      1. Endotracheal intubation
      2. Tracheostomy
IV. Stimulating or substituting respiratory effort
   A. Stimulation
      1. Physical stimulation
      2. Chemical stimulation

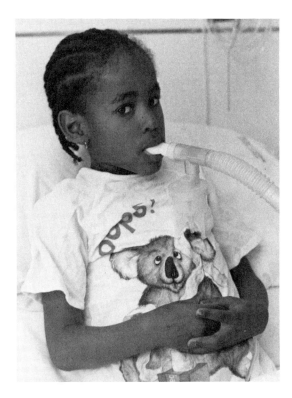

Fig. 12-15. Intermittent positive pressure breathing administered by a mouthpiece through a flexible hose. The child may need a nose pincher to ensure a closed system.

    a. Carbon dioxide
    b. Bernegride
    c. Caffeine
    d. Ephedrine sulfate
    e. Nikethamide (Coramine)
    f. Pentylenetetrazol (Metrazol)
    g. Picrotoxin

B. Artificial respiration
  1. Emergency measures
    a. Mouth-to-mouth resuscitation
    b. External heart massage
    c. Portable emergency respiration
  2. Continuing measures
    a. Tank respirators
    b. Chest respirators
    c. Rocking beds
    d. Intermittent positive pressure

STUDY QUESTIONS

1. Define external respiration, internal respiration eupnea.
2. What are the components essential for the respiratory process?
3. Describe the symptoms of hypoxia.
4. Describe in detail how to set up an oxygen tent. What are the objectives of nursing care? What special precautions need to be taken to meet these objectives?
5. What is a tracheostomy? When is it made? Discuss the nursing care of a child with a tracheostomy, including suctioning, communication, and weaning.
6. List three common respiratory stimulant drugs.
7. Demonstrate external cardiac massage and mouth-to-mouth resuscitation on a life-sized manikin.

13
Respiratory and cardiovascular conditions

The body is made up of many systems, all interdependent, all necessary to health, and all working together for the body's survival. Some of these systems, however, are more closely related in function than others and so are studied together. Two such systems, the respiratory and circulatory, are linked inseparably by the body's need for gaseous exchange. The structure, function, and childhood disorders common to these systems are discussed in this chapter. For the definition of respiration and the various aids to respiration, refer to Chapter 12.

RESPIRATORY SYSTEM

The respiratory system consists of all the organs that make it possible for blood to exchange gases with air: nose, pharnyx, larynx, trachea, bronchi, and lungs. Together these organs carry out external respiration (Fig. 13-1).

Structure and function

Nose and sinuses. The nose consists of external and internal portions. The external portion that protrudes from the face is formed by the *nasal bone* and its cartilage tip. The interior nose is hollow and is separated by a partition, the *septum*, into right and left cavities. The paired *palatine bones* form the hard palate, which serves as both the floor of the nose and the roof of the mouth. They separate the nasal cavities from the mouth cavity. Sometimes these bones

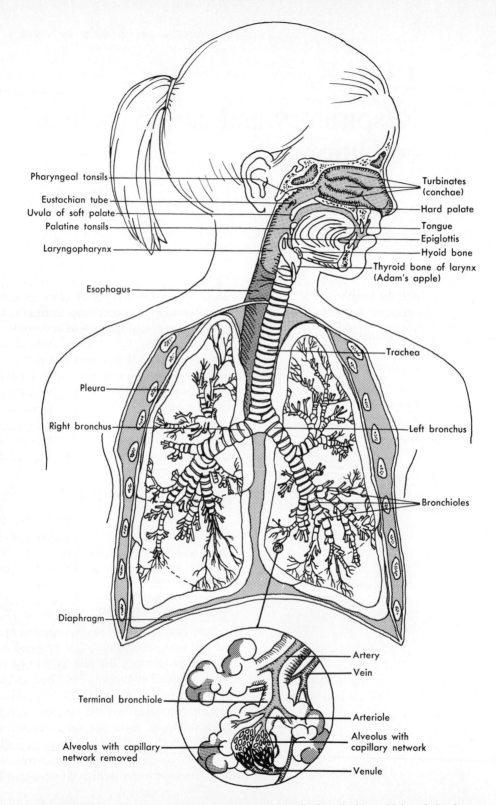

Fig. 13-1. The respiratory system, with a microscopic detail of terminal bronchiole and alveolus.

fail to unite completely, producing a condition known as a cleft palate.

Each nasal cavity is divided into three passageways by the projection of the *turbinate bones* from the walls of the internal nose. Closely associated with the nasal cavities are the *paranasal sinuses*, which are air-filled cavities in the frontal, ethmoid, sphenoid, and maxillary bones. These sinuses are connected to the nasal cavities by small ducts.

The external openings into the nasal cavities or nostrils are called *nares*. Hair grows just inside the nostrils for the purpose of straining larger particles of dust out of the air so that the particles will not go into the lungs.

The entire system of nasal cavities, sinuses, and ducts is lined with mucous membrane that is rich in blood vessels and cells that secrete mucus. The mucus aids in cleaning the air because particles of dust stick to it and so are not carried to the lungs. The surface is covered with hairlike projections, called *cilia*, that beat toward the larger channels and serve to carry the mucus and dust out of the body. Embedded in the mucous membrane of the nasal passages are tiny *olfactory nerve endings* important to the sense of smell. When a person has a head cold or an allergic condition, the mucous membrane swells, blocking off these nerve endings. As a result, the delicate food flavors that are largely perceived by smell cannot be enjoyed and the person complains that food is tasteless. Swollen mucous membrane may also block the movement of air between the nasal cavities and the sinuses, producing pain and chronic sinusitis.

Pharynx. The pharynx or throat is a muscular hallway serving both the respiratory and circulatory tracts because both air and food must pass through it before reaching the appropriate tubes. It is lined with mucous membrane and has three parts, the *nasopharynx* located behind the nose, the *oropharynx* located behind the mouth, and the *laryngopharynx* located behind the larynx. The following seven openings are found in the pharynx: two paired openings from the nasal cavities called *posterior nares*, two paired openings from the *eustachian tubes* coming from the ear, one opening from the mouth, one opening into the larynx, and one opening into the esophagus.

On the back wall of the nasopharynx, just opposite the posterior nares, are lymph nodes making up the *pharyngeal tonsils*. In children these frequently become enlarged to form *adenoids*. If they fill the space, they may block the passage of air from the nose. Other lymphoid tissue is found in the oropharynx—the paired *palatine tonsils* and the paired *lingual tonsils*. The palatine tonsils are the ones most commonly removed by tonsillectomy, together with the adenoids. Normally, tonsillar tissue shrinks to small tags by adulthood but may be stimulated to grow again from these tags or those left after surgery.

Larnyx and trachea. The *larynx*, or voice box, lies just below the pharynx and at the upper end of the trachea. The U-shaped *hyoid bone* is suspended just in front of it. The larynx is made up of nine pieces of cartilage held in place by a series of ligaments that allow a limited degree of movement. The *epiglottis* is the uppermost of these cartilages. It is leaf shaped, extends up into the pharynx, and is attached to the thyroid cartilage just below it in such a way as to form a lid that closes off the lower respiratory tract while food is being swallowed into the esophagus. The second and largest cartilage of the larynx is called the *thyroid*, or Adam's apple. It is shaped like a shield and forms the front and side walls of the larynx. It is more prominent in men than in women, especially after puberty. The other pieces of cartilage complete the larynx, with the *cricoid* attached to the trachea.

The larynx is lined with mucous membrane containing many glands that constantly secrete mucus to keep the surface moist. In the side walls of the larynx are two paired horizontal folds, the false (upper) and the true (lower) vocal folds. When the small muscles of the larynx contract, they produce tension on the true vocal folds, moving them together. Air from the lungs is forced between the folds, causing them to vibrate and produce sound waves. The tongue, lips, nose, bony sinuses, and teeth then form these sounds into meaningful expressions of thought under the direction of the brain. One can have normal vocal cords and still not be able to talk intelligently if there are defects in the brain or mouth, or if there is deafness, which prevents a person from hearing word sounds that can be imitated.

The *trachea*, or windpipe, extends from the larynx into the chest where it ends by dividing into the bronchi. Its walls are supported by a series of C-shaped rings of cartilage at regular intervals. The space between the cartilages is filled with smooth muscle and fibrous membrane. The inner surface is lined by secretory mucous membrane, as are the other respiratory passages. It serves as a passageway through which air can reach the lungs from the outside. Tracheotomy, the incision of which is made just below the first tracheal ring, is sometimes performed for obstructions.

Lower respiratory tract. The internal air passages of the lower respiratory tract resemble an upside-down tree, with the *trachea* likened to the main trunk, having two major branches, the *left* and *right primary bronchi*. The right bronchus is somewhat larger and more vertical than the left because it serves the three lobes of the right lung. This helps explain why aspirated foreign objects often lodge in the right bronchus. Each primary bronchus enters the lung on its respective side and soon divides into smaller branches called *secondary bronchi*. These branches divide to form smaller *bronchioles*, which subdivide into smaller and smaller tubes, eventually terminating in microscopic branches that divide into *alveolar sacs*, the walls of which form many outpouching alveoli, or air sacs. The structure of the alveolar duct and its branching alveolar sacs is like a cluster of grapes, the stem representing the duct, each cluster representing an alveolar sac, and each grape representing an alveolus.

The alveoli are enveloped in a network of cap-

illaries with a single layer of cells separating the blood from the air. It is in this maze of microscopic passages that gaseous exchange takes place. The oxygen enters the bloodstream and the carbon dioxide leaves, going out from alveolus to alveolar sac, to alveolar duct, to bronchiole, to secondary bronchus, to primary bronchus, to trachea, to pharynx, to nasal passage, and finally out into the atmosphere.

The structures in which all this takes place are the *lungs*, located one on each side of the *mediastinum*, the partition that separates them in the *thoracic cavity*. Each lung is cone shaped, with the *base* resting on the diaphragm and the rounded *apex* extending up to the level of the clavicle bone. The outer surface lies against the curving ribs. The medial surface of each lung is concave to allow room for the heart and the lung-communicating structures. These structures include the bronchi, the pulmonary and bronchial blood vessels, lymphatics, and nerves that pass through a central, inner opening called the *hilum*.

The right lung has three lobes, the left has two, leaving room for the heart within the thoracic cavity. Deep grooves mark the boundaries of the lobes. Elastic connective tissue holds the blood vessels and air passages together within the *visceral pleura*, the membrane that covers each lung. The *parietal pleural membrane* lines the entire thoracic cavity, leaving only a potential space that contains just enough fluid for lubrication so that when the lungs inflate with air the smooth, moist visceral pleura slips against the equally smooth, moist parietal pleura, thus avoiding friction. Pleurisy is an inflammation of the pleural membranes, usually causing pressure and pain. If pus develops in the pleural space, the condition is called *empyema*.

General nursing assessment of respiratory function

Regardless of whether a respiratory disorder has been diagnosed medically or not, nurses need to assess the respiratory function of all children as follows:

1. Check for air exchange. Is the chest rising and falling? Do you feel breath?
2. Count the respiratory rate. Is it normal for the child's age? (See Chapter 8.)
3. Identify abnormal respiration. Are there signs such as sternal retraction, wheezing, and grunting? (See Chapter 8.)
4. Report and record assessments.

Disorders

Epistaxis. Hemorrhage from the nose is a common emergency that results from a local disturbance or from a more serious systemic disorder. Some children seem to have an especially fragile network of capillaries in the mucous membrane of the nasal cavities, so that a slight fall, nose-picking, or physical activity causes bleeding. Infections, nasal allergy, and intranasal tumors are also local conditions that may cause epistaxis. Many systemic diseases cause nasal hemorrhage, such as measles, scarlet fever, rheumatic fever, pertussis, typhoid fever, hypertension, congestive heart failure, and chronic glomerulonephritis. In hemorrhagic disorders such as scurvy, leukemia, thrombocytopenia, and hemophilia, epistaxis is a typical symptom.

Emergency treatment consists of placing the child in a comfortable sitting position with the head bent forward and applying pressure by pinching the nostrils as if there were a bad odor. Cold applications to the neck and bridge of the nose may also be effective. The child should not blow or pick the nose. If bleeding persists, the child should be taken to the physician, who may apply a solution of epinephrine 1:1,000 to constrict the vessels, cauterize the bleeding vessels, or pack the nose with gauze for a 24-hour period. If the blood loss is excessive, transfusions may be indicated. Repeated nosebleeds should be investigated for their cause. A systemic disease may be responsible.

Foreign body in the nose. Children frequently push objects other than their fingers into the nasal cavities. Insects, too, may enter the nose. If the foreign body does not drop out or is not sneezed out immediately, it may become lodged in the tissue and cause pain, sneezing, foul discharge, and eventually a serious irritation. If these symptoms appear, especially unilaterally, one should suspect a foreign body and take the child to a physician promptly. The physician anesthetizes the suspected nares, may apply epinephrine solution to shrink the tissue, and then, with suction, irrigation, and instruments, removes the offending object. For prevention of such problems, small children should be discouraged from poking anything into *any* orifice in their bodies. They should not be allowed to play with beans, peas, or small buttons.

Nasal trauma. Injury to the nose is common, especially among school-aged boys. External lacerations should be treated as they are anywhere on the body. Compound fracture is suspected if there is also serious hemorrhage. Fractures are diagnosed by x-ray evidence. Simple fractures are corrected simply by molding the nose manually before edema develops. Antibiotics are administered for compound fractures. Old or serious fractures must be corrected with elaborate surgical procedures. In the treatment of any nasal fracture, however, maintenance of an airway is of utmost importance, as well as the creation of good cosmetic results. The widespread use of face guards for school athletes has helped reduce the incidence of fractured nose.

Deviated septum. When the central cartilaginous wall, or septum, that divides the nose into two parts is not straight down the midline, the condition is called a deviated septum. It may occur naturally or may be caused by a blow to the nose. Such a crooked nose may not only be disfiguring, it may also obstruct the airway so that the individual has difficulty breathing. The condition can be corrected by a surgical procedured called a submucous resection (SMR). It is usually deferred until adolescence or young adulthood unless breathing is obstructed.

Choanal atresia. Choanal atresia is a congenital obstruction of the posterior nares at the entrance into the nasopharynx. The obstruction may be caused by a membrane or, more rarely, by bone. It may close one or both nares. If both are closed, the infant is forced to breathe through the mouth, a most unnatural condition for an infant. The infant has great difficulty feeding and there is grave danger of aspiration of milk into the lungs as the infant tries to both eat and breathe through the mouth. The physician makes the diagnosis by inserting a soft rubber catheter into each nostril as far as it will go. If the obstruction is a membrane, it can be pierced readily by means of a nasoscope. If it is bone, more extensive surgery is required. Postoperative bleeding and maintenance of an airway are watched carefully until healing occurs.

Tonsillitis and adenoiditis. Part of the body's defense system against disease, tonsils and adenoids are lymphoid tissues that enlarge as they attempt to fight infections of the nose and throat. If they become so large as to obstruct the airway or so filled with infectious matter that they no longer serve to prevent but instead harbor infection, then they must be removed. Not all children need this surgery; those who do are ones with recurrent ear infections, sore throats, and rheumatic fever or ones who must breathe through the mouth because the airway is blocked. Infants and toddlers seldom need tonsillectomies. This surgery is more common among preschool- and school-aged children, although it may be necessary at any age.

Tonsillectomy and adenoidectomy (T & A). When physicians decide that surgical removal of the offending tonsils is necessary, the child is carefully prepared to be in maximum health, when the chances for recovery will be optimum. When it is possible, a season of the year is chosen that is relatively free of epidemic childhood diseases. Acute infections are treated with antibiotic drugs. Laboratory tests for clotting and bleeding time are done; a tendency to hemorrhage may be treated with vitamin K. Blood for possible transfusion during or after surgery is made ready. Fever is a contraindication to surgery. If fever develops, the surgery is rescheduled for a later date.

Preoperative nursing care for these children is similar to that for all surgical patients, as discussed in Chapter 8. The child may be admitted the morning of surgery if all preparations are made ahead of time. General anesthesia is usually used with children. Postoperative vomiting has been greatly lessened since the advent of anesthetic agents other than ether.

Postoperative care is primarily concerned with observing the child for hemorrhage, keeping the child quiet, and maintaining an open airway. To these ends nurses make frequent checks of the pulse and respiration, skin color, amount and nature of the discharge, and degree of restlessness. An ice collar may be prescribed to reduce pain and bleeding. There is always some blood-tinged mucus, but a steady flow or vomiting bright red blood indicates an abnormal amount of bleeding. Such discharge should be saved for examination by the supervising nurse or physician. If excessive bleeding occurs, the child may have to return to surgery where the bleeding vessels are tied off. Blood transfusions may also be administered.

Oral fluids should be given as soon as the nausea is over because an adequate fluid intake is important to recovery. The child progresses from clear to full liquid to soft diet at individual pace. Aspirin and antibiotics may be prescribed in gum preparations to encourage chewing, which relieves pain caused by muscle splinting. Most cases of uncomplicated tonsillectomy are dismissed from the hospital the day after surgery. As soon as the operative site has healed, the child may return to normal activities.

Common cold (upper respiratory infection or URI). The common cold has been known for centuries, yet there is still no specific treatment or cure. The nasal sinuses and nasopharynx are primarily involved, but the seriousness of the condition lies in its quick spread and the complications that develop. Children manifest different symptoms from those of adults.

The cause of the common cold is an invasion of one or more of a group of viruses. The secondary infections or suprainfections that so often follow are caused by various bacteria, such as staphylococci, hemolytic streptococci, and pneumococci. Everyone is susceptible, and children seem to have almost no resistance. They are particularly vulnerable when in a poor nutritional state, fatigued, chilled, or emotionally upset.

When catching a cold, the child first becomes irritable and restless and begins to sneeze. A clear nasal discharge appears, soon excoriating the nostril edges and upper lip. After a few hours the discharge turns yellowish green as bacteria invade the inflamed mucous membrane. The throat may be sore and the swollen tissues block the air passages, making breathing and eating difficult. The body temperature of infants and young children rises quickly to 102° to 104° F. The fevers of children over 3 years of age are usually not above 102° F. Because these beginning symptoms are similar to those of many childhood diseases such as measles and chicken pox, differential diagnosis is difficult. Allergic rhinitis (hay fever) presents similar initial symptoms, except for the high fever.

Complications of the common cold are caused by the rapid extension of secondary infection to nearby tissues. Serious conditions such as otitis media, mastoiditis, brain abscess, retropharyngeal abscess, trachobronchitis, sinusitis, pneumonia, pleurisy, and empyema may develop. These diseases are discussed later in the text.

Treatment of the cold consists of relieving the immediate symptoms and preventing complications. The child needs adequate rest, fluids, tissue-shrinking medications such as nosedrops, high humidity environment, and when secondary infection appears, antibiotics may be necessary. Children are not usually admitted to the hospital for a common cold, but they may present the first symptoms after admission. If so, isolation is required. They are more frequently hospitalized for complications that develop in the wake of a cold.

Retropharyngeal abscess. Retropharyngeal abscess may occur as a complication of an upper respiratory infection or by perforation of the pharynx by a foreign object such as a sharp toy. Most patients are 2 years of age or younger. The resultant abscess is dangerous because it may rupture and cause aspiration pneumonia or asphyxia, or the large blood vessels there may erode and cause fatal hemorrhage. Typically, the child has had or has an upper respiratory infection and develops difficulty in swallowing and breathing because of the bulging forward of the abscess. The child lies on one side with their heads drawn backward to displace the larynx forward. Saliva drools from the mouth because of inability to swallow. The cry is husky; the child is dyspneic, prostrate, and feverish, and the neck (cervical) lymph glands are enlarged.

Treatment consists of incising the abscess. The child should be placed in a head-low position to reduce the possibility of aspiration of pus both before and after the abscess is incised. Suction is kept ready for use. Large doses of antibiotics are administered and parenteral fluids given until the child can take fluids by mouth.

Streptococcal pharyngitis ("strep throat"). An inflamed sore throat is not always caused by the cold virus but may result from an invasion by a great many other pathogens. Among the pathogens of greatest concern are the various strains of group A beta-streptococci. This organism causes serious acute infections that often produce later complications. Acute infections include tonsillitis, pharyngitis, scarlet fever (pharyngitis with a toxic rash), and pneumonia. Later complications are probably caused by sensitization of the patient to streptococcal proteins and include rheumatic fever and glomerulonephritis. Because of the serious nature of both the acute diseases and late complications of streptococcal infection, it is important that children with severe sore throats, fever, enlarged lymph nodes, and a rash be seen promptly by a physician. Positive diagnosis is made on the results of throat cultures (see the diagnostic tests in Chapter 9).

Treatment is aimed at control of the acute infection and prevention of late complications that may produce crippling disease. The child needs bed rest with a period of protected convalescence. Diet should be liquid or soft, depending on the soreness of the throat, but nutrition must be maintained. High fevers in young children are controlled with sponge baths and aspirin. Penicillin is very effective when administered promptly and in large enough dosages to combat the infection. Children with a history of rheumatic fever or glomerulonephritis may be placed on a regimen of prophylactic antibiotics to reduce the possibility of streptococcal reinfection and a reactivation of their conditions. Their urine may be checked periodically for albumin, an early sign of kidney involvement.

Acute laryngitis. Acute laryngitis is a common infectious condition producing hoarseness, a brassy cough, and, at times, laryngeal obstruction. It is caused by both viruses and bacteria. Acute laryngitis is treated by placing the child in an atmosphere of high humidity, administering antibiotic drugs, if necessary, and observing the child closely for symptoms of respiratory obstruction.

Acute epiglottiditis. Acute epiglottiditis is an inflammation of the epiglottis and neighboring structures that comes with sudden, severe intensity, described as *fulminating*. It is described as "midnight croup." It occurs chiefly in children who are 1½ to 5 years of age and may cause death if a tracheostomy is delayed. After the tracheostomy is made, the child is placed in a mist tent with oxygen. Blood and throat cultures are taken with sensitivity tests to determine the most effective antibiotic for treatment. Intravenous fluids are administered to ensure adequate fluid intake, and the child is observed closely.

Spasmodic croup. Spasmodic croup is a common condition of children 2 to 4 years of age in which attacks of laryngeal obstruction occur chiefly at night. Although some attacks seem to be brought on by a mild upper respiratory infection or sleeping in a cold room, many occur for no apparent reason. Some children seem to be predisposed by familial tendency or by hy-

peractive dispositions. The condition seems to be caused by a spasm of the muscles of the larynx, causing partial obstruction of the airway.

In a typical attack the child wakens with dyspnea and a tight, barking, metallic cough, frightened and struggling for breath. A high-pitched rasp (stridor) occurs with each inspiration. The nostrils flare and there is sternal retraction. Body temperature is seldom elevated about 101° F. After 1 to 3 hours the attack subsides and the next day the child appears as on the previous day. Attacks may be repeated more than once in a night or on several succeeding nights.

Treatment consists of placing the child in a high-humidity atmosphere and giving reassurance. In some cases, the physician may prescribe an emetic drug to induce vomiting, which acts to relieve the laryngeal spasm by reflex stimulation. Hospitalization may be recommended to rule out other possible causes such as diphtheria or streptococcal infection. If hospitalized, the child should be placed in a quiet room having an even temperature and observed closely by a calm, even-tempered nurse. These children seldom require tracheostomy.

Perinatal hypoxia (anoxia). Chronic hypoxia during intrauterine development may cause mental retardation, low birth weight, and a variety of developmental defects. Studies show a much higher incidence of these defects in infants of mothers who smoked during the pregnancy.

Acute hypoxia may occur as a result of placental separation or oversedation of the mother during labor. It produces typical signs described as *fetal distress* in which there is an increase in activity of the heart, followed by irregularity, slowing, and finally cessation, indicating death. Immediate cesarean section is performed when possible to save the infant's life.

If these infants are alive at birth they may be cyanotic, lack muscle tone, and have irregular heart rates. See Chapter 4 for a discussion of the immediate care of the newborn infant.

Treatment depends on the cause and severity of the hypoxia. If hypoxia results from a depressed respiratory center in the brain from sedation of the mother, stimulants are administered. If hypoxia is caused by a blocked airway, suction and intubation may be used; if caused by anemia, transfusions are given; and if caused by a congenital malformation, corrective surgery is performed as soon as possible. Standard treatment of all hypoxia includes clearing the airway, providing additional oxygen, and initiating respiratory movement either by mouth-to-mouth resuscitation or by mechanical positive pressure.

Sudden infant death syndrome (SIDS). SIDS is a baffling disease that claims the lives of 10,000 babies each year in the United States. The typical victim is a low-birth-weight boy who has had a mild cold. He dies in his sleep and is found with blood-tinged froth about his nose and mouth. This occurs most often in the winter.

More is known about what does *not* cause SIDS than what does. The old notion that these babies suffocated in their blankets has been put to rest. Severe allergic reaction to milk, infections, deficiencies of hormones, and immune bodies have also been ruled out. The most promising research so far indicates that SIDS is the result of a genetic defect affecting the nerves that control reflex breathing movement, possibly exaggerated by a respiratory infection. This theory suggests that in sleep the respirations are slow; when the nasal airway becomes blocked the infant does not gasp for breath. As oxygen blood levels fall, the infant goes into a seizure and dies. If this theory is correct, many deaths could be prevented by pretesting low-birth-weight infants for respiratory reflexes. Those who scored poorly could be watched closely, especially when they caught colds. If breathing stopped, they could be resuscitated.

To accomplish this goal an apnea monitor has been invented. It is attached to susceptible infants when they are put down for sleep. If respirations stop, the monitor sounds a loud alarm alerting the parents, who institute resuscitation immediately. Episodes of apnea decrease with maturity.

Atelectasis. During fetal life the fetus receives all oxygen from the maternal circulation. After birth the normal infant takes a first breath and the lungs fill with air. Atelectasis is an airless state of all or part of the lung and may be acute or chronic. Fetal atelectasis is the failure of the lungs to expand adequately after birth. It may be caused by excessive central nervous depression from maternal drugs, prematurity, or excessive secretions in the respiratory tract. Acute atelectasis may be seen whenever there is a sudden obstruction of the airways from such things as foreign bodies, thick bronchial secretions, tumors, or enlarged lymph nodes that compress the bronchi, cutting off air.

Treatment of atelectasis is aimed at getting air into the lung tissue as rapidly as possible. If it is caused by lack of respiratory effort, stimulants, oxygen-rich environment, and positive pressure may be used. If it results from obstruction, measures must be taken to remove the obstruction.

Laryngotracheobronchitis. Laryngotracheobronchitis is a serious, acute inflammation of the larynx, trachea, and bronchi of infants and young children; it has deadly proportions. It is typically preceded by a common cold that prepares the way for hemolytic streptococci, staphylococci, or influenza pathogens to invade the irritated mucous membrane.

Typically, the child has had a mild upper respiratory infection, then rapid changes occur as the infection descends. A high fever and prostration ensue, together with grave dyspnea caused by severe edema of the mucous membrane and copious thick mucus that blocks the airways. The child becomes restless as the dyspnea increases; respirations are stridorous (noisy, strained, and shrill); the cough is brassy; the child does not cry or speak but uses all energy to breathe. Pallor and cyanosis indicate a losing battle for enough oxygen. Treatment must be instituted at once or death occurs in a few hours.

Treatment consists of placing the child in a warm atmosphere of high humidity and oxygen concentrations. Intravenous fluids and large doses of antibiotics are administered. Tracheostomy operations are frequently necessary. Intensive medical and nursing assessment and interventions are necessary. Even with prompt treatment the outlook is grave because of such complications as sepsis, pneumonia, and circulatory collapse. Prevention of this serious disease is best accomplished by limiting the exposure of infants and small children to persons with upper respiratory infections and by protecting those with colds from further infections.

Bronchiolitis. Bronchiolitis is an acute infectious disease that produces generalized emphysema, a condition in which air can pass into the alveolar ducts and sacs on inspiration but is trapped there by swollen bronchioles so that it cannot pass out on expiration. As a result the lungs become progressively overinflated with air (emphysematous). This leads to inadequate oxygenation of the blood and insufficient release of carbon dioxide, causing respiratory acidosis. In addition, the overinflated air sacs cause circulatory back pressure and an increased strain on the right heart that may lead to a condition in which the heart is not able to meet the needs of the body (cardiac decompensation).

Bronchiolitis usually affects infants younger than 6 months of age. It is believed to be caused by a virus because it is resistant to the usual antibiotic drugs. Typically, the disease begins as a simple cold with no fever and only a slight cough. The cough then worsens, coming in paroxysms similar to whooping cough; vomiting and fever may or may not be present. The baby must spend more and more energy in breathing and so is unable to suck. As the dyspnea increases, the child becomes restless, pale, and cyanotic. The chest may appear barrel shaped from overinflation. There is little respiratory movement, and because of the inflated lungs it is difficult to hear heart sounds through a stethoscope.

Treatment consists of placing the infant in an atmosphere of high humidity; if the infant is cyanotic, oxygen is added to the atmosphere. Intra-venous fluids are administered, as needed, with added electrolytes to relieve acidosis. Broad-spectrum antibiotic drugs (ones that destroy a variety of organisms) may be ordered to combat the bacteria that commonly invade inflamed mucous membrane. When infantile bronchial asthma is suspected, epinephrine may be prescribed in small amounts to avoid excessive heart strain. If there is evidence of cardiac decompensation, digitalis may be ordered to strengthen the failing heart.

Close nursing observation is of great importance, as are rest and fluid intake. As the child's condition improves, the combined use of oxygen and mist is changed to mist alone. With continued improvement the child is removed from the mist for brief periods and observed for pallor and dyspnea. These times are gradually lengthened until the child is able to do without the mist entirely and can breathe normally.

Bronchiectasis. Bronchiectasis is a chronic, inflammatory process that progressively destroys the mucous lining, leaving saclike dilations of the bronchi. It usually results from bronchial obstructions or severe infections during infancy or early childhood. Often the obstruction is the thick, tenacious exudate of whooping cough; sometimes it is blood from a tonsillectomy, aspirated vomitus, milk, or foreign body. Whatever the cause, atelectasis results from complete bronchial obstruction. Sooner or later infection ensues in the airless area, producing destructive changes in the mucous membrane and the formation of cystic pockets of pus. When these pockets drain, as they do occasionally, they cause paroxysms of coughing, spitting up of blood (hemoptysis) and copious amounts of foul, purulent matter. During childhood, hemoptysis is more often caused by bronchiectasis than by tuberculosis. Areas of bronchiectasis usually occur in the lower lobes of the lung, but they may involve an entire lung.

The diagnosis of bronchiectasis is made after the physician has taken a careful medical history; made a physical examination; tested and ruled out allergies, cystic fibrosis of the pancreas, chronic sinusitis, and tonsillitis; performed a bronchoscopy; and made bronchograms. These bronchograms not only help to identify areas of bronchiectasis but also tell the extent and degree of involvement. Treatment is planned accordingly. Because surgical excision of the diseased area is the only cure for well-advanced bronchiectasis, medical management may be employed for early, potentially reversible cases, for children who are too ill to tolerate surgery, and as a preparation for surgery.

The medical management of bronchiectasis is based on the following care:

1. Deep-cough sputum cultures to determine what organisms are causing the infection and sensitivity tests to determine what antibiotics will be effective against them
2. Administration of effective antibiotics by mouth, injection, or inhalation through a nebulizer directly in the bronchi
3. Postural drainage with mechanical vibration or hand clapping over the affected area to loosen mucus
4. Bronchoscopic aspiration weekly or bi-weekly
5. Diet high in calories, vitamins, and proteins
6. Treatment of anemia, if present

Nursing care includes skilled observations of the child's respiratory status and direct care to provide for skin and mouth cleanliness, postural drainage with chest clapping, suctioning, administration of antibiotics, taking vital signs, and providing adequate rest and much tender loving care. These children are often debilitated and frightened; they need quiet reassurance as they undergo painful treatments and long periods of care.

Bronchoscopy and bronchograms. Bronchograms are x-ray films taken of the bronchi by use of iodized oil as the radiopaque material. They show the shape and size of the bronchi and help the physician identify abnormal conditions. Bronchograms are considered most useful if the oil is placed in the exact area of concern by means of a bronchoscope.

A bronchoscope is a metal, periscope-like instrument used to visualize the bronchi. A child is prepared for bronchoscopy much as for surgery. Food is withheld preoperatively and sedation is administered. If bronchograms are to be made, bronchoscopy is done in or near the x-ray department. The child is restrained and positioned with the head hyperextended. The operator anesthetizes the child's larynx and trachea and slowly passes the approximately sized bronchoscope down to the level desired. The blunt-end obturator is then removed, and the bronchi can be visualized by means of a tiny light and mirror. Mucus can be aspirated, foreign objects lodged there can be removed, tissue samples can be taken (biopsy), and when bronchograms are desired, radiopaque oil can be injected into the exact area to be x-rayed. Gravity is also used to aid in the distribution of the oil. When the bronchoscope is to be removed, the obturator is replaced and the instrument slowly withdrawn.

Postbronchoscopy care includes close observation for dyspnea caused by edema, nebulized mist to aid respiratory effort, and soft foods.

Cystic fibrosis (mucoviscidosis). The symptoms of cystic fibrosis are caused by changes in the endocrine glands throughout the body, so the disease, including the respiratory involvement, is discussed as a whole in Chapter 14.

The pneumonias. Pneumonia is one of the most common childhood diseases, occurring by itself or as a complication of other infectious or weakening conditions. Any inflammation of the lung tissue may be termed pneumonia. Many descriptive words are used with it, however, to give added information, including those that describe how the disease was acquired, what anatomy is involved, certain special symptoms, what caused it (etiology), and the age group involved. Examples of these groups of adjectives are as follows:

How acquired: aspiration (said of such things as turpentine), hypostatic (inadequate or incomplete aeration).

Anatomy involved: lobar (confined to a lobe), double (both lungs), disseminated (not confined to a single area), broncho- (bronchi inflamed, too).

Symptoms: fulminating (coming on rapidly with intense severity), walking (so free of symptoms that the victim goes about daily activities), atypical (as compared with the symptoms of pneumococcal pneumonia).

Etiology: pneumococcal, staphylococcal, streptococcal, viral, lipoid (aspirated oil), fungal. Pneumonias are more often classified medically according to their etiology rather than by any other characteristic.

Age group: neonatal, childhood, adolescent.

Diagnosis of pneumonia is made on the basis of physical findings, history, x-ray examination, and laboratory tests. When the air sacs of the lungs are filled with fluid and white blood cells and when capillary beds are engorged with blood, the tissue is said to be *consolidated*, or solid with substances other than air. Airless areas in the lung show on the x-ray film and allow the physician to identify the region involved and the degree of consolidation, that is, the extent of the pneumonia.

Identification of the causative organism is made by cultures—of the blood, of nasopharyngeal mucus, or of sputum (see Chapter 9).

Prevention of pneumonia has been greatly assisted by the availability of antibiotics and sulfonamides, which physicians now freely give to children with upper respiratory infections as a prophylactic (preventive) measure against the development of pneumonia as a complication. Likewise, the prognosis of pneumonia has improved since the advent of antibacterial drugs. Where once the death rate for infants was more than 80%, it is now less than 5% for those treated promptly.

Pneumococcal pneumonia. Pneumococcal pneumonia is also called "lobar" pneumonia because the infection usually involves one or more lobes. It is caused by *Diplococcus pneumoniae*, a bacteria transmitted by droplets from the nasopharynx of carriers. Infants and young children are particularly susceptible.

The onset in symptoms is sudden. Older children may experience a chill; younger ones may convulse. Nausea and vomiting are common. The temperature rises rapidly to a range of 101° to 105° F, the pulse to 130 per minute. There is sharp chest pain and blood-streaked sputum that becomes rust colored. Hypoxia is profound, with rapid, shallow respirations and an expiratory grunt. A slow pulse is a serious sign. The child may lie on the affected side to reduce pain, perspires profusely, and is acutely ill.

Treatment consists of antibacterial therapy and supportive care. Oxygen, together with a high-humidity atmosphere, is administered if there is cyanosis or severe dyspnea. Fever is controlled with cooling sponge baths and antipyretic drugs. The diet advances from liquid to soft, bland, and regular as the child improves. Fluid intake is very important to replace that lost by evaporation during the fever or by vomiting or diarrhea. The nurse should offer the child small sips of liquid frequently. Urinary output should be measured carefully, especially for those children receiving sulfonamides. Intravenous fluids may be administered if the oral intake is inadequate. Rest and relief from pain are important.

Most children respond rapidly to antibiotic therapy with no complications. A small amount of effusion, or leakage, of clear serous fluid into the pleural space may produce a mild pleurisy, but empyema (pus in the pleural space) is rare with modern treatment.

Staphylococcal pneumonia. When the lungs are invaded by large numbers of antibiotic-resistant staphylococci, a serious pneumonia develops. It is characterized by widespread microscopic abscess formation in the lung tissue that may spread into the pleural space and even involve the lining of the heart and spread throughout the body in the blood. Intensive medical and nursing care is necessary to effect a cure and prevent more serious complications.

Resistant staphylococci are commonly present

in hospitals but may be present in the community at large. Staphylococcal pneumonia is usually a primary infection, but it may follow other infections such as impetigo. Newborn infants and young infants are easily susceptible. In the typical case the child develops a fever, is listless and irritable, and has a nasal discharge and cough. The child becomes progressively dyspneic with rapid respirations; cyanosis may ensue.

The child should be hospitalized immediately, isolated, and given supportive care, including oxygen in a high-humidity atmosphere, intravenous fluids, control of fever, and even blood transfusions if necessary. Cultures are taken of the blood and nasopharynx to determine the organism and what antibiotics will be effective. Large doses of penicillin G may be given intravenously until the most effective antibiotic is identified. Other drugs are substituted if a child cannot take penicillin. Treatment with antibiotic drugs is continued long after the obvious symptoms subside because of the tendency for staphylococci to hide in minute abscesses and then later recur.

Streptococcal pneumonia. Streptococcal pneumonia occurs more often as a complication of measles and other viral infections than as a primary infection. Young children are particularly susceptible. Unlike the other pneumonias, after entering the lungs, the streptococci swiftly invade the lymph glands and produce empyema.

The disease begins with a high fever. The infected child is prostrate, respirations become shallow and rapid, and the child may become cyanotic. Diagnosis is made by the history of recent communicable disease such as measles and by cultures of the blood, nasopharynx, and the pleural fluid. Penicillin is usually effective. The physician may instill penicillin directly into the pleural space.

Viral pneumonia (primary atypical pneumonia). Many viruses, including those of measles and influenza, may cause pneumonia. A slight upper respiratory infection is often present. Symptoms vary from mild fever and slight cough to high fever, prostration, and cough. Although there is sometimes a secondary infection of bacteria, viral pneumonia does not usually respond to ordinary antibiotics and so must be treated symptomatically.

Allergic conditions. The two most common allergic conditions of the respiratory system are allergic rhinitis and asthma. A discussion of allergic conditions in general is provided in Chapter 19.

Allergic rhinitis. The well-known malady of allergic rhinitis is characterized by sneezing, a running nose, burning eyes, and an itching throat. The seasonal form, called "hay fever," is caused by pollen and other seasonal allergens. The perennial form may be caused by any allergen, particularly inhalants such as smoke and dust. Allergic rhinitis affects 5% to 10% of the population and usually begins in childhood. Of those children who are not treated, 30% to 50% develop asthma later. Other complications may result from chronic inflammation or secondary infections of the mucous membrane, including overgrowth of the membrane (polyps) causing nasal obstruction and recurrent otitis media, leading to hearing loss.

Treatment consists of removing the offending allergens, reducing sensitivity by injection (hyposensitization) of those allergens that cannot be removed, and symptomatic relief of symptoms with antihistamines, soothing eye drops, and nasal decongestants. Overuse of nose drops such as Neo-Synephrine may produce a "rebound effect" that increases nasal swelling; they should be used sparingly.

Asthma. Bronchial asthma is the most serious allergic disease of childhood. It affects 1% to 2% of all children; onset may come at any age, although it is less frequent in infancy. The organs involved are the bronchioles, their mucous linings, and the associated smooth muscles. It is characterized by a wheezing type of dyspnea produced by a spasm of the bronchi and bronchioles and thick, tenacious secretions that tend to close the airways. Foods, inhalants, bacteria, and almost any allergen may cause asthma, but there also seem to be definite emotional factors that trigger attacks. It is frequently complicated by respiratory infections. Although few children die from asthma, many become semi-invalids from recurrent attacks. Parents need sound medical and psychological counseling in the home management of these children.

The typical attack is usually preceded by several days of increased nasal discharge and a dry, hacking cough. As the bronchial edema and spasm increase, the child develops an audible wheeze, both on inspiration and on expiration. The child uses accessory respiratory muscles to breathe; the older child may sit upright. As the attack progresses, the child sweats profusely, appears anxious, may be cyanotic, and cough up thick mucus. After a few hours, the symptoms gradually subside. If they continue for days or weeks, the condition is called *status asthmaticus* and requires intensive treatment. The inhalation of foreign substances into the lungs may produce symptoms similar to an asthmatic attack.

Treatment consists of identifying the causal allergen and removing it or hyposensitizing against it. Symptomatic treatment is the following:

1. Bronchodilator drugs such as epinephrine, ephedrine, and aminophylline, administered by injection or by nebulizer for children mature enough to inhale deeply (antihistamines are of little value in asthma)
2. Expectorants such as potassium iodide, ammonium chloride, and glyceryl guaiacolate that help reduce the viscosity of mucus
3. Maintenance of adequate fluids
4. Sedation for extreme anxiety
5. Oxygen for cyanosis administered with mist tent
6. Antibiotics for coexistent bacterial infections
7. Antiinflammatory drugs such as the adrenocorticol steroids

Treatment of chronic asthma in older children includes the use of aerosol drugs to liquefy the mucus and dilate the bronchi, followed by postural drainage. These children seem to benefit from pursed-lip expiration and diaphragmatic breathing exercises. Steroid therapy may be used for status asthmaticus because it often gives dramatic relief, but the dose is reduced to the lowest effective level as soon as possible to avoid side effects.

Tuberculosis

Description and cause. Tuberculosis is an ancient communicable disease once called "consumption." It is caused by *Mycobacterium tuberculosis*, a rod-shaped, acid-fast organism that can survive for long periods in a dried state. It usually affects the respiratory system but may involve the other body systems. Three types affect humans: human, cow (bovine), and bird (avian). In the United States the human type is responsible for practically all cases because the bovine type has been largely eradicated by strict enforcement of milk production standards and pasteurization. The avian type is very rare.

Public health factors. Tubercle bacilli enter the body through the respiratory tract, chiefly by droplet infection or direct contact with infected humans. Children, teenaged girls, and debilitated and malnourished elderly persons are particularly susceptible. It is not surprising to find a high incidence among the poor who live in crowded quarters. Young children are usually infected from family members, whereas older children may be infected from outside sources. Preventive measures are the isolation of known, active cases; regular testing of health workers and food handlers; mass screening by skin tests, prophylactic drugs for persons whose skin test has recently converted from negative to positive, and immunization of high-incidence communities.

Skin tests and diagnostic studies. The most common tuberculin skin tests are the old tuberculin (OT) and the precipitate of the protein of the tubercle bacillus (PPD). The three testing methods employing the PPD are the intracutaneous (Mantoux), the patch test (Vollmer), and the multiple puncture tests (Heaf and Tine). PPD is usually measured in international tuberculin units (ITU). It has been found that in mass screening approximately 99% of the cases can be detected by using 5 ITU of PPD. A positive test means that the individual has been infected with the tubercle bacilli and has become sensitive to tuberculoprotein. It does not tell anything about the infection, which must be determined by further testing. The results of the skin test are not 100% accurate; there are both false positives and false negatives. It does provide some method of screening and is particularly useful when employed annually to detect "converters" or those who have been exposed.

Positive diagnosis of tuberculosis is made if the tubercle bacillus is found in the sputum or gastric contents. If a child's skin test becomes positive, a sputum sample or gastric wash must be obtained for culture. The test must be repeated three times before the result is considered negative. If it is positive, x-ray examinations help the physician evaluate the extent of the infection.

Immunization. Immunization against tuberculosis is considered useful for children living where contact with tuberculosis cannot be avoided. It produces an allergic sensitization against the tubercle bacillus. The bacillus Calmette-Guérin (BCG) vaccine, made from a weakened bovine strain, is used for this purpose. Once the child has been sensitized, the skin test becomes positive and can then no longer be used to determine recent exposure.

Primary tuberculosis. The initial or primary infection of tuberculosis affects the body tissue quite differently than it does if reinfection occurs later. Fortunately, the great majority of children who have had a primary infection never are reinfected, but for those who are, the disease progresses much like the adult type. For this reason the primary and reinfection phases are discussed separately.

Primary tuberculosis occurs when the tubercle bacillus first enters the lungs and establishes a site of initial implantation called the "primary focus." The body then summons its defenses and builds a wall (tubercle) around the invaders. As the battle proceeds, some of the bacilli escape to the lymphatics of the hilum causing inflammation and an enlargement of the glands (lymphadenopathy). Some bacilli may also escape into the bloodstream and hide in the liver, spleen, kidneys, bones, or brain to await a time when they can renew their attack. The child may have a slight fever during this time but no other symptoms. The name "primary complex" refers to the primary focus and the inflamed lymph glands of the hilum. Occasionally the primary focus is the tonsils when the same response by the body occurs. The primary focus finally heals by itself, first forming a cheeselike mass (caseation) and then becoming calcified by the deposit of calcium. These primary lesions are usually located near the pleura in the lower lobe or in the lower part of the upper lobe of the lung. Their calcified remains can be seen in x-ray films for years afterward.

Miliary tuberculosis. Infants and young children are less capable of containing the initial tuberculosis infection. Instead of the lesion healing, it sometimes extends throughout the lungs, breaks into the blood, and spreads throughout the body with development of millet seed–like lesions, hence the term *miliary tuberculosis.* The child becomes irritable, has a fever that is higher in the afternoons, is increasingly toxic, loses weight, and may cough and become dyspneic. In untreated cases death may occur in 4 to 8 weeks.

Other complications. Tuberculous meningitis is one of the tragic and frequent complications of childhood tuberculosis. It usually begins within a year after the primary infection but may occur much later, or it may be a complication of miliary tuberculosis. The child becomes irritable, drowsy, and has a low-grade fever. Typical symptoms of an irritation in the meninges of the brain such as vomiting, stiff neck, headaches, and abnormal neurological signs develop; coma and death follow.

Tuberculosis of the lymph nodes of the neck, the peritoneum, and the bones may also occur as complications of primary tuberculosis. (See osteomyelitis).

Reinfection. The child who has had a primary infection and has become sensitive to the tubercle bacillus may be reinfected years later. The child is usually without any symptoms in the interval. The reinfections may be from an extension of prior well-controlled lesion, from lowered resistance, or from a new invasion from the outside. The child develops a low-grade fever and fatigue. As the disease progresses, the child loses an appetite and then weight, a cough develops, and chest pain may occur. The cough becomes productive as the lesion enlarges. The child may spit up blood (hemoptysis), have night sweats, and become anemic and wasted. A cavity of the necrotic tissue may form. Progressive destruction of the lung continues until death comes from hemorrhage or complicating disease.

Treatment. Although no single "miracle" drug has been found to eradicate tuberculosis, modern chemotherapy, together with supportive measures, prevention of reinfections, and surgical procedures have greatly improved the prognosis of the child with the disease. The tuberculostatic drugs most frequently used are isoniazid (INH), paraaminosalicylic acid (PAS), ethambutol, rifampin, and streptomycin. When a child's skin test changes from negative to positive, or when a disease such as diabetes is diagnosed or the child is living near a person with active tuberculosis, a course of prophylactic isoniazid may be prescribed to protect against an active infection.

Supportive measures are adequate rest in bed balanced with some activity, attention to the emotional needs of the child and the family, carefully planned nutritional diet and protection of the child from reinfection from outside sources. Nursing care is planned around these measures in consultation with the physician and cooperation with the child's family.

Communicable disease nursing is discussed more fully in Chapter 19.

CARDIOVASCULAR SYSTEM

The cardiovascular system includes the heart, blood vessels, blood, and lymphatics in an intradependent system of circulation. Working together, these organs and their fluids transport substances to and from the body cells, protect the body against invading organisms, and help regulate the body's heat. Disorders of this system commonly found in children result from birth injuries, structural defects, and diseases from a variety of causes. A knowledge of the structure and function of this system is vital to an understanding of the disorders.

Structure and function

Heart. The heart is a hollow muscular organ located slightly to the left in the midchest between the lungs, with its apex toward the diaphragm. It has three layers of tissue—the outer covering called the *pericardium*, the middle and thicker muscular layer called the *myocardium*, and the inner thin membranous lining that also forms the valves, called the *endocardium*. The heart is divided into four chambers, with a septum dividing the right from the left side. The right chamber (atrium) receives venous blood returning from the body; the left atrium receives oxygenated blood from the lungs. The lower right chamber (ventricle) pumps the venous blood through the pulmonary artery to the lungs where it receives oxygen and discharges carbon dioxide. The left ventricle pumps the oxygenated blood out through the aorta to all parts of the body. Four valves located in the inlet and outlet of each ventricle keep the blood flowing in one direction. The cuspid valves, *mitral* and *tricuspid*, guard between the atria and ventricles. The *semilunar valves* guard the exits inside the pulmonary artery and aorta. When the valves do not close completely, the condition is called valvular insufficiency. Disease sometimes causes scarring and narrowing (stenosis) of the valves.

The heart contracts as a result of nerve impulses going from the cardiac center in the medulla of the brain through the *vagus nerve* to the *sinoauricular node* (the pacemaker) and the *atrioventricular node* (the coordinator) and onward to the heart muscle by special neuromuscular fibers that are part of the heart's own electrical system. These impulses can be picked up on the body surface through leads and viewed on a cardiac monitor or recorded by an electrocardiograph machine.

The function of the heart is to pump the blood in sufficient amounts to meet the varying needs of the cells of the body for substances it transports.

Blood vessels. The blood vessels are the network of tubes that carry the blood to and from the heart. As the left ventricle contracts, blood leaves the heart by way of the aorta, which sends off branches that divide and subdivide into arterioles and finally become tiny capillary vessels. These capillaries then unite to form venules, which unite to form larger and larger veins that finally empty into the right atrium of the heart. The arteries have smooth muscle in their walls, which allows them to contract or to dilate and thus increase or decrease blood pressure. The veins are membranous tubes equipped with valves located at intervals to prevent backflow. The capillaries have thin walls, some only a single cell thick, which makes possible the essential exchange of gases, nutrients, and wastes (Fig. 13-2).

Lymphatic system. In addition to the system of tubes that carry blood, there is another system that carries lymph, the clear interstitial fluid that

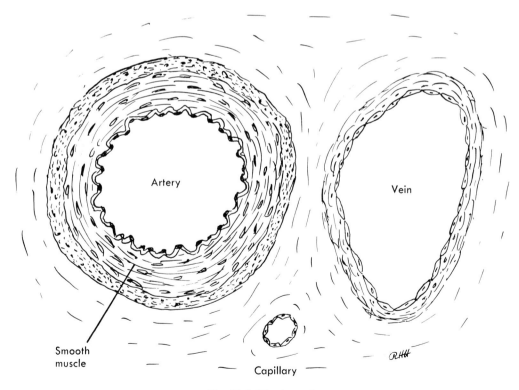

Fig. 13-2. Blood vessels.

bathes the cells. The lymphatic system is similar to the blood system without the heart or arteries. It is a system allowing for drainage of the excess fluid and protein that accumulates between the cells, thus playing a key role in fluid balance. Lymph is picked up in tiny capillaries similar to blood capillaries. These capillaries unite to form progressively larger ducts that unite to form two main channels—the *right lymphatic duct* and the *thoracic duct*. These ducts extend up to the subclavian vein of the neck, where the lymph is emptied into the venous blood.

Distributed along the lymph vessels at strategic points throughout the body are round bodies called *lymph nodes*, which act as filters to remove dead cells, bacteria, and intracellular waste. Special cells within the lymph nodes called *reticuloendothelial cells* digest the debris and convert it into harmless breakdown products. Lymph nodes also manufacture two kinds of white blood cells—*lymphocytes* and *monocytes*. When there is an inflammation in the body tissue, interstitial fluid from the area drains to the nearby lymph node. If a large defensive battle is waged there, the node becomes enlarged and sometimes tender. Swollen superficial lymph nodes can be felt in the groin, neck, and armpits. Sometimes the nodes themselves become the foci of the disease, as in tonsillitis.

Blood. "For the life of the flesh is in the blood' (Leviticus 17:11). The importance of blood in maintaining life was recognized in ancient times. It is indeed a marvelous substance, actually a circulating fluid tissue that accounts for about 7% of the body weight. Blood serves several functions in the body. It provides a vast transportation system that moves oxygen and carbon dioxide to meet respiratory needs, food and nitrogen wastes for nutritional and excretory needs, disease-fighting cells for protective needs, and heat for the regulation of body temperature. Blood also serves to maintain the proper acid-base balance that keeps the body in a state of chemical equilibrium. Blood also has its own built-in mechanism for self-preservation—clotting.

Plasma. Blood is composed of 55% plasma and 45% formed elements. Plasma is the clear liquid part of blood. It is a complex mixture of water, electrolytes, proteins, lipids, glucose, vitamins, gases, enzymes, hormones, and antibodies. Except for certain proteins, plasma is identical to the interstitial fluid that bathes the cells. Its proteins, *albumin*, *globulin*, and *fibrinogen*, play an important role in the regulation of the body. Albumin is responsible for holding the water in the blood vessels so that it will not seep out into the tissue and cause edema. Globulin is associated with immunity (almost all antibodies are gamma globulins). Fibrinogen is essential to the clotting process. When blood clots, the clear fluid that remains is called *serum*, which differs from plasma in only one way—its fibrinogen has been largely used up in clot formation.

Formed elements. Formed elements of the blood are of three types—red blood cells (erythrocytes), white blood cells (leukocytes), and platelets (thrombocytes) (Fig. 13-3).

Erythrocytes are characterized by the absence of a nucleus and the presence of an iron-bearing red protein called *hemoglobin*. Hemoglobin makes up about one third of the cell and averages 14 to 16 gm per 100 ml of whole blood. The chief function of the red cell is to transport oxygen from the lungs to the tissue. Erythrocytes are formed in the bone marrow and go through several stages before they emerge as flat, uniform disks without a nucleus. In some abnormal conditions, immature forms containing nuclei enter the bloodstream. Iron, folic acid, and vitamin B_{12} are needed for the proper development of red cells. The normal erythrocyte lives for 120 days and then disintegrates and is replaced by new cells from the bone marrow.

Leukocytes are colorless cells that average about 8,000 per cubic millimeter of blood. The leukocytes with granules in the cytoplasm are formed in the bone marrow and are the *neutrophils*, *eosinophils*, and *basophils*. Those without granules are formed in the lymph nodes and are the *lymphocytes* and *monocytes*. Unlike the red cells, the white cells have nuclei and can squeeze through the capillary walls, infiltrate the tissue, and aid in fighting infection. For this reason they seldom stay in the bloodstream more than 3 or 4 days.

The *platelets*, or thrombocytes, are not cells at all but are fragments of larger cells found in the bone marrow called *megakaryocytes*. Thrombocytes are essential to the clotting mechanism.

Blood products. Whole blood and various components of blood may be administered to patients to meet their specific needs. The nurse should have some understanding of these special products and the conditions and circumstances for which they are given. These products are whole blood, packed cells, plasma, fibrinogen, serum albumin, and gamma globulin.

Whole blood is seldom administered by direct transfusion from one person to another at the present time. Instead, it is collected from donors, processed, classified, and stored in blood banks in 500 ml (1 pint) containers, the amount that has become the standardized unit of whole blood.

Packed red blood cells are administered to patients whose blood volume should not be increased but who need additional blood cells. The unit of packed cells is a pint of fresh whole blood with the plasma drawn off, leaving 250 ml of concentrated fresh blood cells and a small amount of plasma. Typing and cross matching

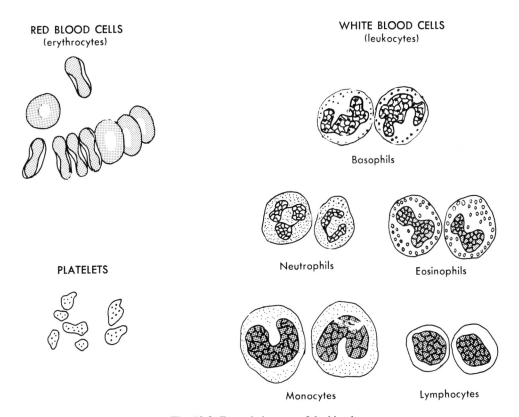

RED BLOOD CELLS
(erythrocytes)

WHITE BLOOD CELLS
(leukocytes)

Basophils

Neutrophils

Eosinophils

PLATELETS

Monocytes

Lymphocytes

Fig. 13-3. Formed elements of the blood.

are as necessary for packed cell administration as they are for whole blood.

Fresh-frozen and *liquid-stored plasma* are valuable aids in the treatment of patients who need the protein of plasma and additional blood volume. Fresh-frozen plasma is prepared by spinning whole fresh blood in a centrifuge and freezing the resultant plasma within 4 hours. It is thawed just before administration by placing its container in a bath of warm water. (Hot water would make the protein coagulate.) Liquid-stored plasma has been widely used as a life-saving measure to restore blood volume quickly. It does not have to be prepared from fresh blood and does not have to be frozen.

Fibrinogen is the protein substance in plasma that is essential for clotting. It is prepared in a concentrated form. Just before it is to be administered it is mixed with sterile distilled water. Then it is given intravenously by means of a blood filter infusion set.

Serum albumin is taken from plasma and is given to patients suffering from deficiencies of protein in certain diseases of the liver and kidneys.

Gamma globulins are the protein antibodies of the plasma responsible for immunity. They are extracted from the blood of persons with known immunity to specific diseases, such as measles and mumps, to give a recipient an immediate but temporary immunity to that disease.

Circulation. During fetal life the fetus does not need its liver to synthesize nutritional elements or lungs for gaseous exchange but instead uses the mother's. Three special shunts route most of the blood past these organs. They are the *ductus venosus*, which carry the blood through the liver, the *foramen ovale*, an opening in the septum of the heart, and the *ductus arteriosus*, which bypasses the lungs. As blood, rich with oxygen and food, leaves the placenta through the umbilical vein, it is diverted through the liver to the inferior vena cava via the ductus venosus. On reaching the heart, the blood next bypasses the nonfunctioning lungs by flowing

through the foramen ovale, from the right to the left atria of the heart. The third shunt is a short vessel called the ductus arteriosus, which diverts most of the blood from the pulmonary artery directly into the aorta. The blood then travels throughout the body and returns to the placenta via two unbilical arteries (Fig. 13-4).

At birth a dramatic change in blood circulation takes place. As soon as the lungs expand with the first breath, blood rushes past the bypass ductus arteriosus into the lung tissue, where it finds oxygen for the first time. Because the ductus arteriosus is an elastic muscular tube, it collapses when there is no longer pressure within it and shrinks from disuse. It normally closes a few hours after birth.

When the umbilical cord is clamped, the umbilical arteries and vein cease to function. These vessels, too, shrink and close, as does the ductus venosus. The one-way valve of the foramen ovale in the septum of the heart closes immediately from the increase in pressure on the left side and eventually grows shut from disuse.

Thus in a very short time fetal circulation converts to independent circulation. When the infant is born too soon, normal changes are delayed. When any of these changes fail to take place, congenital heart disease results.

Clotting. Clotting is the body's way of preventing blood loss. Although the process involves a series of complex biochemical reactions, the basic steps are as follows: A vessel is damaged and the platelets (thrombocytes) at the site of the injury disintegrate, thereby releasing an enzyme called *thromboplastin*. To speed up the disintegration of the platelets, normal blood contains an *antihemophilic factor*, the absence of which causes hemophilia. Thromboplastin now starts to work on a plasma protein called *prothrombin* (made in the liver from *vitamin K*), converting it into the enzyme *thrombin*. For conversion to thrombin to take place, however, *calcium* and a number of *other factors* must be present. Once thrombin is formed it works on the soluble *fibrinogen* in the blood to form inter-

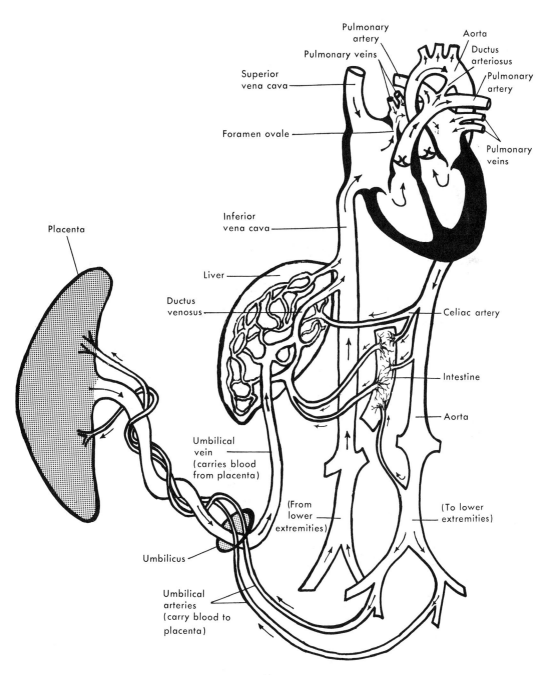

Fig. 13-4. Fetal circulation.

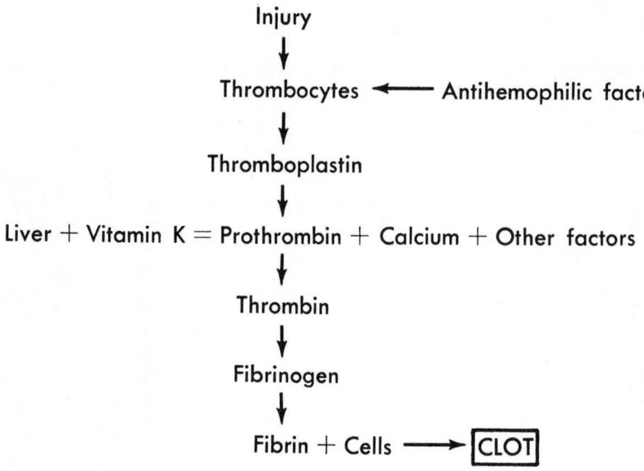

Injury

↓

Thrombocytes ←——— Antihemophilic factor

↓

Thromboplastin

↓

Liver + Vitamin K = Prothrombin + Calcium + Other factors

↓

Thrombin

↓

Fibrinogen

↓

Fibrin + Cells ——→ CLOT

Fig. 13-5. Formation of a clot.

lacing threads of insoluble protein called *fibrin*. These threads trap blood cells and form a *clot* (Fig. 13-5).Clotting may be affected at any step of the process by deficiencies or excesses of the necessary components.

Disorders

Congenital heart disease

A great many developmental defects may occur in the heart and associated vessels during the first 8 weeks of intrauterine life while these organs are being formed. These defects are caused by inherited traits or teratogenic agents. (See the discussion of influences on growth in Chapter 2.) Additional defects may result from a failure of the special structures of fetal circulation to close at birth. All such defects lead to congenital heart disease (Fig. 13-6).

Diagnosis. The diagnosis of heart disease is made by the physician on the basis of information gained by the following:

1. Health history of the child, including inherited traits and intrauterine stressors, noting growth and development, number of respiratory infections, and episodes of dyspnea or cyanosis
2. Observable symptoms of cardiac disease such as cyanosis, a characteristic squatting posture, and clubbing of the fingers and toes (Fig. 13-7)

3. Physical examination in which the physician inspects the child's general appearance, feels (palpates), taps (percusses), and listen (auscultates)
4. Laboratory tests of the blood, angiocardiography and other x-ray studies, electrocardiography, and cardiac catherization

Blood tests of special significance are the complete blood count and the hematocrit, whereby whole blood is centrifuged to determine the relative amounts of plasma and cells. Patients with heart diseases may have anemia (too few cells) or polycythemia (too many). Polycythemia occurs because the body manufactures large numbers of erythrocytes in an attempt to deliver more oxygen to its deprived cells. This abnormally high cell count thickens and slows the circulating blood and may result in clots in the bloodstream. It may also cause pooling of the blood in the capillary beds of the fingers and toes, with resultant widening called *clubbing*, a characteristic symptom of congenital heart disease.

Fluoroscopic and *x-ray examination* of the structure and function of the heart and vessels is done by a variety of techniques using radiopaque material. Barium swallowed by mouth may show an abnormal indentation of the esophagus

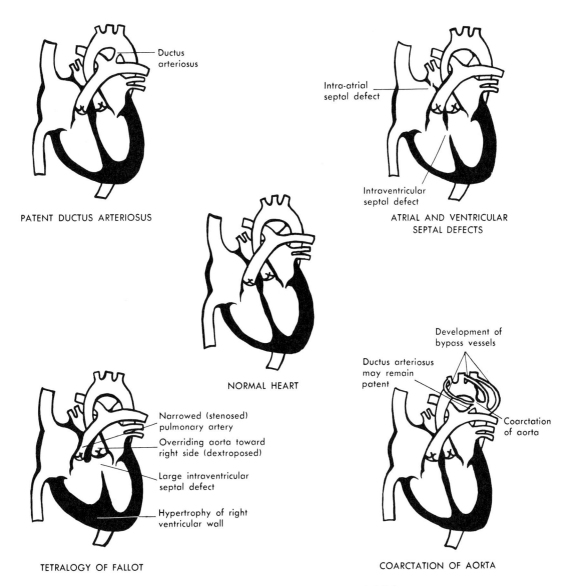

Ductus
arteriosus

PATENT DUCTUS ARTERIOSUS

Intra-atrial
septal defect

Intraventricular
septal defect

ATRIAL AND VENTRICULAR
SEPTAL DEFECTS

NORMAL HEART

Narrowed (stenosed)
pulmonary artery

Overriding aorta toward
right side (dextroposed)

Large intraventricular
septal defect

Hypertrophy of right
ventricular wall

TETRALOGY OF FALLOT

Development of
bypass vessels

Ductus arteriosus
may remain
patent

Coarctation
of aorta

COARCTATION OF AORTA

Fig. 13-6. Normal heart and common congenital defects.

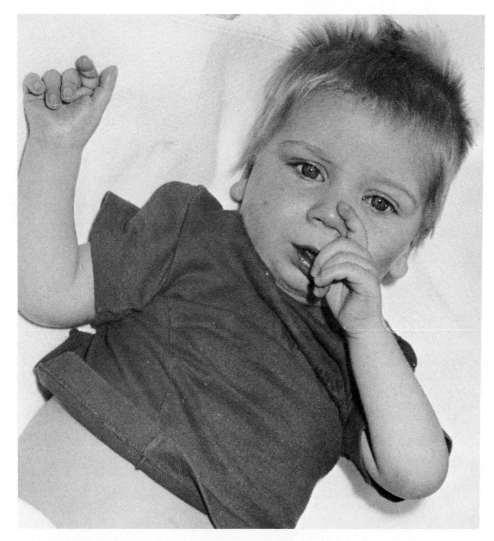

Fig. 13-7. Chronic hypoxia from an inoperable combination of heart defects gives this child a dusky purple color. His fingertips are especially dark and clubbed from an overgrowth of capillaries.

by the aorta and other nearby vessels. *Angiocardiography*, the procedure of injecting radiopaque dye into the circulating blood of certain vessels, during which x-ray films are taken, may reveal abnormal openings or structures of the heart and associated vessels.

Electrocardiography (ECG) provides valuable information about the electrical activity of the heart (Fig. 13-8).

Cardiac catheterization is an ingenious method that has been devised to examine the inside of the heart to determine possible defects. The child is anesthetized, and a small radiopaque catheter is inserted into a large vein of the arm or leg and pushed into the right atrium of the heart. With

the tip of the catheter the physician can examine the heart minutely for defects in the structure. The blood pressure in each chamber of the heart and samples of blood can be taken to determine the degree of oxygenation. After the procedure the child is cared for as if having undergone surgery. The insertion site is examined frequently for hemorrhage, and vital signs are checked often. Oxygen is kept available for immediate use.

Classifications. Congenital heart diseases are classified as acyanotic and cyanotic. *Acyanotic diseases* are those in which the defects do not cause a connection between pulmonary and systemic circulation, or if there is a connection, the

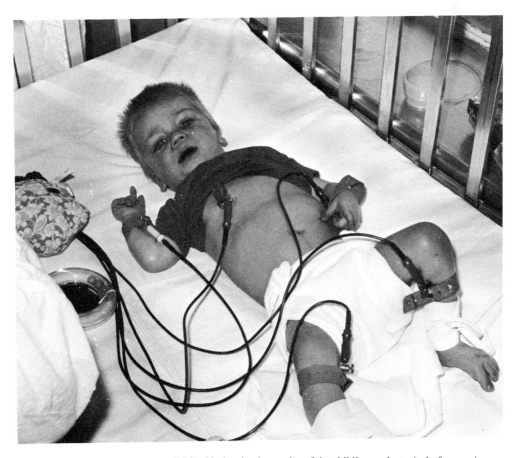

Fig. 13-8. Electrocardiogram (ECG). Notice the deep color of the child's mouth, typical of cyanosis.

pressure is higher in the left side of the heart than in the right side of the heart, and the baby does not appear to be "blue." Acyanotic diseases include patent ductus arteriosus, ventricular and atrial septal defects, coarctation of the aorta, and pulmonary and aortic stenosis.

Cyanotic diseases are those in which the defects permit the unoxygenated venous blood of the right side to mix with the oxygenated blood of the left side of the heart or in which there is severe pulmonary congestion and the baby appears to be "blue." Cyanotic diseases include tetralogy of Fallot, transposition of the great vessels, truncus arteriosus, total anomalous venous return, and tricuspid atresia.

Patent ductus arteriosus. The ductus arteriosus is one of the special structures of fetal circulation (Fig. 13-4). At birth it normally collapses and shrinks from a normal drop in *prostaglandin* (a fatty acid) blood levels. If it remains open (patent), blood under pressure from the aorta is shunted into the pulmonary artery, with the result that oxygenated blood recirculates through the pulmonary circulation (Fig. 13-6). This causes the heart to work much harder than necessary to supply the body with its oxygen. Patent ductus arteriosus, an acyanotic heart disease, is the most common cardiac defect, occurring by itself and with other defects, especially among early born infants whose production of prostaglandin remains high.

The symptoms of patent ductus arteriosus in infants are often so slight that they go unnoticed for some time. As the child grows older, however, characteristic symptoms develop. The child is likely to show more and more dyspnea on exertion. The radial pulse is full and bounding, and pulse pressure is wide, that is, the systolic and diastolic pressures are further apart than normal. The left ventricle becomes enlarged from overwork, and is still not able to meet the body's circulatory needs. Congestive heart failure gradually appears.

Diagnosis is made on the basis of physical signs of a machinery murmur (a continuous

rough sound) of the heart and increased pulse pressure, x-ray films showing an enlarged pulmonary artery, and angiocardiograms showing the ductus arteriosus. Treatment consists of administering oral indomethacin, which inhibits prostaglandin synthesis, causing the ductus to close. If this fails, the ductus is surgically tied off, after which the heart becomes normal in size, the murmurs disappear, and the child's general condition improves.

Septal defects. After birth, any opening in the septum that divides the right and left sides of the heart is abnormal (Fig. 13-6). Such openings may occur anywhere from high in the atrial septum to low in the ventricular septum. One of the more common sites is between the atria caused by a failure of the foramen ovale of fetal life to close. Septal defects occur more often and in greater severity in girls than in boys.

Interatrial septal defects usually do not cause cyanosis because the blood pressure is higher in the left heart than in the right and unoxygenated blood does not enter general circulation. If other defects are present, particularly of the pulmonary valve, right-to-left flow may occur and cyanosis may result. Children with atrial septal defects usually have an overworked right heart and congestive pulmonary circulation because of the backflow through the defect to the right atrium. They are more susceptible to respiratory infections and may be physically underdeveloped. Without treatment, gradual heart failure occurs and few of those children reach adult life. Diagnosis is made on the basis of x-ray findings of an enlarged heart and pulmonary artery, electrocardiograms, and typical murmurs. Surgical repair is attempted according to the condition of the individual child.

Ventricular septal openings are never normal, yet recent studies have shown that this type is one of the most common heart defects in infants. Most involve only the membranous, not the muscular, tissue, and at least 18% close spontaneously. The more serious ventricular septal defects involve the muscular tissue. The severity of symptoms depends on the size of the left-to-right shunt and degree of pulmonary congestion. Fortunately, only 3% of children with large ventricular defects go on to develop the inoperable and fatal *Eisenmenger syndrome* in which the blood flow is largely reversed. Symptoms of a large interventricular septal defect consist of a rapid pulse, typical heart murmurs, abnormal electrocardiogram readings, enlargement of the heart from overwork, and pulmonary congestion. Treatment depends on the age of the child and a severity of symptoms. Infants often respond to medical management of their pulmonary congestion. Those who fail to respond to it are sometimes treated surgically by pulmonary artery banding that narrows the opening (lumen) and reduces the backflow into the lungs. Surgical repair of a ventricular septal defect is indicated if the pulmonary blood flow is twice as great as the systemic blood flow and the child's condition warrants the risk.

For repair of septal defect, open heart surgery is necessary. The abnormal openings are closed by sutures or by incorporating a plastic patch into the repair. The patch is eventually penetrated by growing tissue and becomes part of the septum. Cardiac surgery is discussed later in this chapter.

Coarctation of the aorta (Fig. 13-6). Coarctation means "a narrowing together." After the aorta leaves the heart, it normally arches to the left and three major vessels rise out of it before it descends into the thorax. These arteries supply the head and upper extremities with oxygenated blood. During fetal life the ductus arteriosus also joins the aorta in the same general area. When the aorta is coarctated, the ductus usually remains patent for the first year of life. Although the condition does not produce cyanosis, the combination of defects imposes an extra load on the left ventricle of the heart as it attempts to meet the needs of the body for blood. Closure of the ductus, either spontaneously or surgically, helps reduce the heart's work.

Surprisingly, only 50% of infants with coarctation of the aorta show symptoms (dyspnea, poor weight gain, and congestive heart failure). As the child grows older, however, heart murmurs develop and electrocardiograms become increasingly abnormal. Smaller vessels develop to bypass the obstruction in the aorta. By the prepuberty years, the outstanding symptom of coarctation of the aorta has appeared—that of hypertension in the upper extremities and hypotension in the lower extremities. The heart becomes noticeably enlarged, and the aorta dilates in the portion above the coarctation.

Surgical repair, the only permanent treatment, is usually deferred until the child is at least 3 years of age to allow for increased size. The narrowed portion of the aorta is removed, and the ends are either sewn together (end-to-end anastomosis) or a section of another artery is used as a graft. Before surgery the child with symptoms of congestive heart failure is treated with digitalis.

Pulmonic and aortic stenosis. Both the pulmonary artery and the aorta leave the heart guarded by semilunar valves. A variety of defects may occur in these vessels, including their valves causing both cyanotic and acyanotic heart disease. They narrow the opening and reduce their capacity to carry blood. When such stenosis occurs by itself without other serious defects, the child may not show any symptoms. The physician usually discovers the defect during routine examinations by the telltale murmurs that are heard. The diagnosis is confirmed by electrocardiograms, x-ray films, and angiocardiograms. If the defect is severe and it appears likely that the child's condition will progressively worsen, surgical repair is undertaken. In children under 2 years of age with pulmonary valvular stenosis, a closed valvulotomy can be performed with little risk and some degree of relief. For all other cases requiring valvuloplasty, open heart surgery is necessary.

Tetralogy (foursome) of Fallot. Louis A. Fallot was a French physician (1850-1911) who described four heart defects that characteristically occur together, namely, (1) a large inter-ventricular septal defect, (2) a narrowing of the opening of the pulmonary artery, (3) an overriding aorta that is positioned very near the septal defect, and (4) an enlarged, thickened right ventricular wall (Fig. 13-6). Often called "blue babies," infants with these defects are usually quite cyanotic. Many die soon after birth. Of those who survive, growth is stunted, the fingers and toes become clubbed, the nail beds appear dusky blue, and the child tires easily and may have dyspneic "spells." The young child may squat in a characteristic position to improve cardiac output. Diagnosis is made on the basis of physical and x-ray examinations, electrocardiograms, angiocardiograms, and cardiac catheterization. Medical and surgical treatment depends on the condition of the child. Two types of surgical therapy are used—a palliative shunt operation such as a Blalock-Taussig or a Potts and total corrective operation requiring the heart-lung machine for open heart repair. Because the mortality is relatively low and the relief of symptoms is high for the palliative shunts, many cardiology centers prefer to perform the shunt first and then the corrective surgery later after the child has grown larger and the risk lessened. Without surgical intervention of some kind, the infant with tetralogy of Fallot usually dies from metabolic acidosis and severe hypoxia in a short time.

Transposition of the great vessels. Transposition of the great vessels is one of the serious cyanotic heart diseases. In this condition the aorta arises entirely from the right ventricle and the pulmonary artery entirely from the left ventricle. If there are no other defects, the child will die immediately after birth because no oxygenated blood is able to reach the systemic circulation. Most, however, have a septal defect that allows for some mixing of blood and permits the infant to live for a few weeks. There are often other defects associated with transposition that further complicate the total correction of the disorder. A variety of surgical procedures may be attempted, such as performing the Blalock-Taus-

sig shunt operation, making a large atrial septal defect, creating a new atrial septum to redirect the flow of blood inside the heart, and giving the child a new heart by transplant. In any case, the infant's chances for survival are very poor.

Truncus arteriosus. Truncus arteriosus results from the failure of the embryonic structures to divide into the aorta and pulmonary artery. As a result, a single vessel overrides both ventricles, ejecting blood into the lungs and systemic circulation. Cyanosis increases as congestion increases in the lungs. Congestive heart failure, dyspnea, retarded growth, and early death result. Success of palliative and corrective surgery depend on the severity of the pulmonary disease.

Total anomalous venous return. In this rare defect there is no direct communication between the pulmonary vein and the left atrium. There is no palliative surgical treatment, but if the child survives to the age of 2 years, corrective surgery offers a good prognosis.

Tricuspid atresia. Tricuspid atresia is the absence of the tricuspid valve, resulting in no opening between the right atrium and right ventricle. It is usually associated with other defects that allow some shunting of blood into the lungs. Severe cyanosis, dyspnea, and signs of right-sided heart failure are evident soon after birth. Palliative treatment is the same as for tetralogy of Fallot and corrective surgery is now possible in older children who survive.

Cardiac surgery

In 1945 Doctors Alfred Blalock and Helen Brooke Taussig introduced the shunt operation known around the world as the "blue baby operation." Since that time enormous strides have been made in the field of cardiac surgery. The heart-lung machine was introduced in 1955, making possible total cardiopulmonary bypass and open heart procedures; then hypothermia and high-oxygen tension (hyperbaric) chambers were introduced. With each advance a larger group of malformations has been made correctable, including the removal of the severely damaged heart and its replacement with a transplanted one, first done successfully in 1968.

At the present time cardiac malformations are classified surgically into the following four groups: (1) those that can be corrected without opening the heart, (2) those that can be corrected by use of the heart-lung machine and total bypass, (3) those that can be corrected only partially with or without the bypass, and (4) those that are inoperable except to be totally replaced with a transplanted heart.

Heart-lung machine and cardiopulmonary bypass. Open heart surgery has been made possible by the development of machines that temporarily take the place of the heart and the lungs. These pump-oxygenators, as they are aptly described, permit total bypass for as much as 3 hours. Three types are currently in use—the bubble, membrane, and disk oxygenators. Regardless of their design, all must perform the following functions successfully: (1) the blood must be taken from the patient and pumped back into circulation at an ideal flow rate about equal to cardiac output at rest, (2) the normal oxygen–carbon dioxide exchange must be accomplished in the oxygenator, (3) the temperature of the blood must be controllable so that it can be raised or lowered, and (4) the components of the blood must not be destroyed by the machine (Fig. 13-9).

Before the cardiopulmonary bypass is instituted, the heart-lung machine is primed with blood carefully cross matched with the patient's. When all is ready, plastic cannulas are inserted

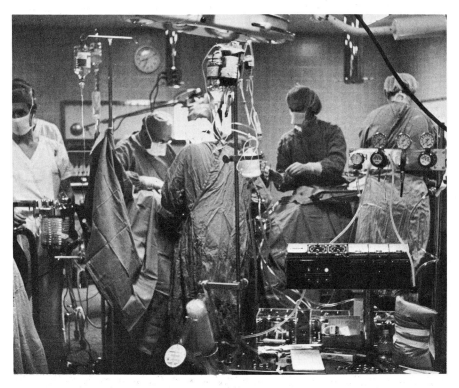

Fig. 13-9. Open heart surgery showing the pump-oxygenator (heart-lung machine) in foreground. (Courtesy Children's Hospital of the East Bay, Oakland, Calif.)

into the inferior and superior venae cavae and all the blood returning to the heart is diverted to the heart-lung machine where it passes through the oxygenator, in which the oxygen and carbon dioxide exchange takes place. The blood is then propelled back to the child by a pump at a flow rate equal to the child's own cardiac output. It enters the general circulation by a cannula placed in the aortic arch, the subclavian artery, or the femoral artery. Complete cardiac arrest with a dry operative field can be achieved by means of the bypass, by hypothermia, and by clamping off the coronary arteries.

The use of such complex equipment requires a team of highly skilled and specially trained surgeons, nurses, and technicians.

Preparation of the patient. Before heart surgery is scheduled, a tremendous amount of preparation takes place. The child's condition is carefully evaluated. Various diagnostic procedures may be performed during preliminary hospitalizations. With the findings of these studies in hand, the cardiologists and surgeons formulate a course of treatment that may involve several weeks or months of drug or diet therapy before surgery. The surgical repair of some defects may even be delayed for years to allow for increased size from growth.

As discussed in Chapter 8, the child should be prepared emotionally and physically for hospitalization and surgery. A prepared child presupposes prepared parents and therefore better adjustment. Although the physician usually discusses the actual surgery with the parents, the responsibility for general preparation is shared by members of the hospital staff.

Usually the child is admitted to the hospital several days before surgery for adjustment to the hospital and to provide a time for close observation and further tests. The child's weight is recorded each morning and vital signs checked at regular intervals. Appetite, degree of activity, posture, color, and responses are carefully recorded. Signs that might indicate infection such

as nasal discharge, skin rash, and cough should be reported promptly. They may necessitate a postponement of surgery.

This preliminary time is ideal for the nurse to help the child feel "at home," not only with the general surroundings but also with specific activities that will be undertaken after surgery, such as how to cough when the nurse holds the child's chest and how to use the intermittent positive pressure breathing device. Explanations should be geared to the child's ability to understand. Because several days may be spent in the special cardiac intensive-care unit after surgery, a brief visit there may benefit the older child.

Postoperative nursing care. Postoperative nursing care of the cardiac surgical patient is a specialty all its own. The child's heart action is monitored continuously. The child's color, respirations, and degree of consciousness are evaluated. Samples of blood are taken periodically through an arterial line to evaluate blood gas levels. Intravenous infusions and blood transfusions are calculated and maintained. Analgesic drugs for pain and cardiotonic drugs such as digoxin are administered. Humidified oxygen may be administered. Wound drainage and dressings must be checked. Chest tubes may be employed to prevent lung collapse from increasing fluid accumulation in the thorax. An indwelling catheter is checked to determine urine output. Tracheal and nasopharyngeal suction and temporary tracheostomies may be necessary, and the child may be placed on a respirator. The child's temperature may be subnormal at first, but later, fever reduction measures may be required. Continuous, complete, and accurate records must be maintained.

Such constant and expert nursing care requires special preparation that is not within the usual scope of practical-vocational nurses. They may, however, be called on to assist in turning the child during the critcal postoperative period. They should know that *any tube leading to or from the body must never be kinked or pulled.*

Of particular concern are the chest tubes connected by sealed drainage to a collection bottle that must be kept lower than the child's chest. If the tubing becomes disconnected or the bottle breaks, the tubes should be immediately clamped off near the chest wall to prevent air from entering the pleural cavity and collapsing the lung.

As the child's condition improves, chest suction is discontinued and the tubes removed. One by one the other life-supporting measures are suspended as the child's body takes over its normal functions. During this convalescent period care of the child includes weighing every morning before breakfast to determine fluid retention, carefully spacing a certain maximum oral fluid intake, encouraging the child to eat the low-sodium diet, taking the pulse before and after activities, observing for signs of fatigue, providing rest periods as needed, and taking the blood pressure and apical pulse at intervals as ordered. Cardiac surgical patients often recover from the most critical surgery in a surprisingly short time, soon returning to their homes for a period of continued convalescence and to a new life of health and development.

Medical treatment of cardiac conditions

Sometimes a child's cardiac condition cannot be helped with surgery or has to wait until the child is older or in better condition before surgery is attempted. In these cases the child is treated medically, that is, treated by medicines, special diet, and planned health supervision. The child may be in and out of the hospital frequently during such treatment. The nurse should be aware of the medicines the child is receiving, their side effects, and toxic reactions that may occur. A low-salt diet is often prescribed. Daily weight and accurate intake and output records are maintained. Limited activity may be necessary, although children with heart defects often limit themselves to what they can best tolerate. Quiet play is often more restful than an enforced "complete bed rest." Close and continuous ob-

servation of the vital signs, of dyspnea, and of respiratory infection must be maintained. Children receiving oxygen therapy should be disturbed as little as possible to reduce their exertion. Proper positioning contributes to rest and reduces the likelihood of contractures and skin breakdown. These children and their families often come to consider the hospital as kind of a second home because they spend so much of their time there.

Complications of congenital heart defects

Certain complications occur so commonly as a result of heart defects and their repair that preventive measures against them are included in the treatment of the defects. The most common of these complications are congestive heart failure, endocarditis, myocarditis, and pericarditis, all of which may occur aside from cardiac defects.

Congestive heart failure. Approximately 20% of all children with congenital heart defects develop congestive heart failure sometime during their illness. This condition develops when the heart cannot meet the needs of the body and cannot prevent abnormal congestion of the blood in various areas of the body. Sometimes the heart can maintain an adequate blood flow by gradually increasing its size and rate. By so doing the heart is said to be "in compensation." If the heart still cannot maintain the needed blood flow, it is said to be "in decompensation," or failure.

When the left ventricle fails to pump blood effectively, blood backs up in the lungs; the capillaries become engorged; fluid leaks out into the tissue and air spaces; the air is poorly oxygenated; breathing becomes increasingly labored; a cough, orthopnea, and cyanosis may develop. When acute pulmonary edema occurs, measures to reduce the heart's work load are ordered, such as the prescription of cardiogenic drugs. Emergency measures such as rotating tourniquets, whereby three of the four extremities are wrapped with elastic bandage in rotation every hour, and phlebotomy, where blood volume is reduced by bleeding, may also be necessary.

Right heart failure often occurs after left heart failure. If the condition develops gradually, the muscle of the right ventricle may become enlarged, the kidneys become congested and less efficient, the liver enlarges, congestion of the gastrointestinal tract causes distention and reduced function, and edema occurs in the tissue spaces and in the abdominal cavity (ascites). Infants may develop edema about the eyes.

Treatment of congestive heart failure in children is highly individualized. Assessment data used to form the medical and nursing plans include blood studies of the electrolyte and drug levels, electrocardiograms, liver and heart size, rate and rhythm of the pulse and respirations, and degree of edema. Nurses are involved in making or assisting with the collection of these data.

Edema is assessed as follows:

1+ = barely detectable swelling
2+ = indentation less than 0.5 cm
3+ = indentation less than 1.0 cm
4+ = indentation more than 1.0 cm

The principal drug used for the treatment of cardiac decompensation is a cardiotonic drug, digitalis, or one of its derivatives. It slows and strengthens the heartbeat and improves the excretion of sodium by the kidneys. Its toxic effects are nausea, vomiting, irregular heart rate, and cardiac standstill. *Digitalization* is the process whereby the dosage of digitalis is adjusted to just below the amount that will produce toxic symptoms. Parents' and nurses' observations are vital to the determination of the optimal dose.

Other important treatments include low-sodium diet, oxygen to relieve dyspnea, daily weight measurement, and rest. The sitting (orthopneic) position may provide some relief of respiratory distress.

It is important to involve the parents in carrying out the treatment plans. They need to know the what, when, where, and why of them and how they can assist the physicians and nurses in carrying out these plans.

Carditis. Any damage to the heart tissue or slowing of the blood flowing through it may make the heart vulnerable to inflammation. When the lining of the heart and its valves are inflamed, the condition is called *endocarditis*. When the heart muscle is involved, the condition is called *myocarditis*. When the membranous sac that encloses the heart is inflamed, the condition is called *pericarditis*. These inflammations usually result from bloodborne infections coming from other parts of the body or following surgical procedures such as dental extractions and tonsillectomy. Endocarditis and pericarditis frequently follow rheumatic fever.

Endocarditis. In endocarditis the main lesion is a vegetation composed of white and red blood cells, fibrin, and bacteria. It usually occurs on the valves but may also affect other areas of the endocardium. The most common causative agents are bacteria, fungi, and rickettsiae.

The most common portals of entry are the mouth from dental work, urinary tract from catheterization, and blood from intravenous infusions. Congenitally deformed heart valves or those damaged by rheumatic fever are predisposed to this infection. Symptoms are fever, increased white blood cell count, anemia, anorexia, spiderlike hemorrhages of skin capillaries (petechiae), and hemorrhages in the joints, eyes, and kidneys. Nephritis may develop, and death results from kidney or heart failure, malnutrition, and cerebral or pulmonary embolism. Prognosis of untreated cases is poor and those who survive often sustain valvular deformities from scarring. Prophylactic penicillin is administered to patients with congenital heart disease to prevent endocarditis when operations such as tooth extraction and tonsillectomy are necessary. Treatment includes bed rest, a highly nutritive diet, blood transfusions as required, and large doses of penicillin, the drug found to be most effective. Penicillin is continued for several weeks, the child checked regularly for many months for symptoms of recurrence, and penicillin treatment instituted again if necessary.

Myocarditis. When myocarditis occurs without a known cause, it is called *primary myocarditis.* When it is associated with a variety of systemic disorders such as infectious, metabolic, or nutritional disorders, carbon monoxide poisoning, and heat stroke, it is called *secondary myocarditis.*

Endocardial fibroelastosis is a primary myocarditis that affects infants. The tissue is changed, and the child develops congestive heart failure. Most patients die before 12 years of age. Viral myocarditis is quite common in the preschool child. Symptoms are air hunger, rapid pulse, and typical heart sounds and electrocardiograms. These patients are critically ill and are cared for in intensive care units. Digitalis, intravenous administration of epinephrine and steroids, oxygen, and complete bed rest are ordered. Rest must be continued until all evidence of inflammation has disappeared. Recovery depends on the severity of the involvement and expertness of care.

Pericarditis. Inflammation of the pericardium may be acute or chronic and may develop as a primary disorder or a secondary disorder to a variety of systemic diseases. When fluid accumulates in the space between the layers of the pericardial sac, the condition is called *effusion.* An audible friction rub may be heard with a stethescope as the layers move with each heartbeat. Acute pericarditis may cause excruciating pain. Chronic pericarditis may cause thickening and fusion of the tissue layers so that it interferes with normal filling and emptying of the heart. Diagnosis of pericarditis is made from the symptoms, the presence of systemic disease, electrocardiograms, heart sounds, x-ray and fluoroscopic findings, and blood count.

Treatment depends on the nature of the inflammation and its cause. If it occurs secondary to a systemic disease, that condition is treated. In acute, primary pericarditis, treatment is rest and sedation, medication for pain, ice to the chest, fever control, oxygen, and antibiotics. When a pericardial friction rub occurs in acute rheumatic fever, it always indicates severe cardiac involvement with myocarditis or an inflammation of the entire heart (pancarditis). Pericardial effusion may then develop. In severe, acute pericardial effusion, paracentesis of the fluid may be lifesaving. In chronic inflammation, when heart function is impaired by the constrictive fibrous tissues, the pericardium may be resected surgically.

The anemias

The primary function of the red blood cells is the transport of oxygen and carbon dioxide. The essential component that makes this possible is *hemoglobin.* Hemoglobin consists of an iron-containing pigment called *heme* and a simple protein called *globin.* Anemia results when the total hemoglobin content of the blood is below normal, either because of insufficient hemoglobin in the red blood cells or because of a lack of red blood cells. Anemia develops if there is (1) excessive blood loss from hemorrhage, (2) abnormal blood destruction as in hemolytic diseases, (3) decreased blood formation from lack of necessary building materials caused by dietary deficiency or faulty absorption, and (4) impaired hemoglobin or red blood cell formation, usually caused by bone marrow disorders.

Blood loss. Anemia from sudden, massive blood loss is most often caused by a traumatic accident injury. It causes dizziness, weakness, thirst, pallor, and weak rapid pulse and respirations. Blood pressure falls to shock levels and death ensues. Immediate treatment consists of stopping the bleeding, restoring the blood volume with intravenous blood and fluids, and combating shock with stimulants and external heat. Later a high-protein diet with supplementary vitamins and iron helps replenish the body's stores.

Chronic blood loss from such conditions as teenage ulcerative colitis or excessive menstrual flow may cause anemia. Together with specific treatment of the primary disease, the secondary anemia is treated with supplementary iron and vitamins.

Blood destruction. Hemolytic disorders cause abnormal destruction of the red blood cells. The most common ones in children are hemolytic disease of the newborn (erythroblastosis fetalis), sickle cell disease, and thalassemia.

Hemolytic disease of the newborn (erythroblastosis fetalis). Hemolytic disease of the newborn is caused by the development of antibodies in the mother's blood against antigens from the infant. The antigens pass into the mother through the placenta where the mother produces antibodies against them, a process called *isoimmunization*. These antibodies then pass back into the infant and destroy (hemolyze) the erythrocytes. The blood of the mother and her baby is then called *incompatible*. The baby's body attempts to make up for this destruction by producing an increased number of immature red cells called erythroblasts, hence the name "erythroblastosis" (Fig. 13-10). The two most important antigens that cause this reaction are the Rh factor and the A or B blood group substances.

Rh factor incompatibility. The Rh factor was discovered in 1941 to be inherited through an Rh-positive dominant gene. It is present in 85% of white women, 93% of black women, and nearly 100% of oriental women. Those who carry Rh genes are called Rh-positive; those who do not are called Rh-negative. Both conditions are normal.

The problem presents itself only when there is an Rh-negative mother, an Rh-positive father, and an Rh-positive fetus. While the Rh-negative mother is carrying the Rh-positive baby, some of its blood enters the mother's bloodstream. The mother's body reacts and produces antibodies against the Rh antigens from the baby and in so doing becomes sensitized. This sensitization usually happens just before or during delivery so that the antibodies do not affect the baby who sensitized her. If a baby of a subsequent pregnancy is Rh-positive, however, its antigens stimulate the already sensitized mother to produce large amounts of Rh antibodies. These hostile antibodies then cross the placenta and attack the unborn infant's red blood cells. Some infants of sensitized mothers are only mildly affected, but most are moderately affected, and some die before or soon after birth. Symptoms are caused by the destruction of red blood cells and the efforts of the fetus to make more red cells rapidly. The liver and spleen become enlarged; there is anemia and deep jaundice (icterus gravis); generalized edema may be present (hydrops fe-

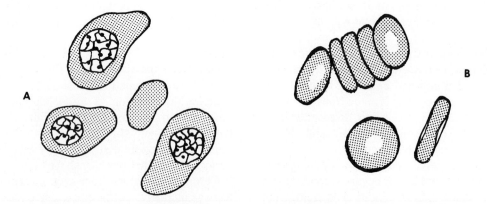

Fig. 13-10. Red blood cells (erythrocytes) and those of erythroblastosis fetalis. **A,** Immature erythroblasts of erythroblastosis. **B,** Normal mature erythrocytes.

talis); and pathological changes may occur in the nerve tissue from deposits of bilirubin (kernicterus), which results in brain damage, mental retardation, or death. An early sign of kernicterus is spasms of various muscle groups affected by the bilirubin deposits.

In 1968, a new weapon against Rh-hemolytic disease was introduced, called $Rh_o(D)$ immune globulin (human), or Rh_oGAM (Fig. 13-11). It is an injectable solution containing antibodies against Rh factor that have been manufactured by others. It is only effective when the Rh-nega-

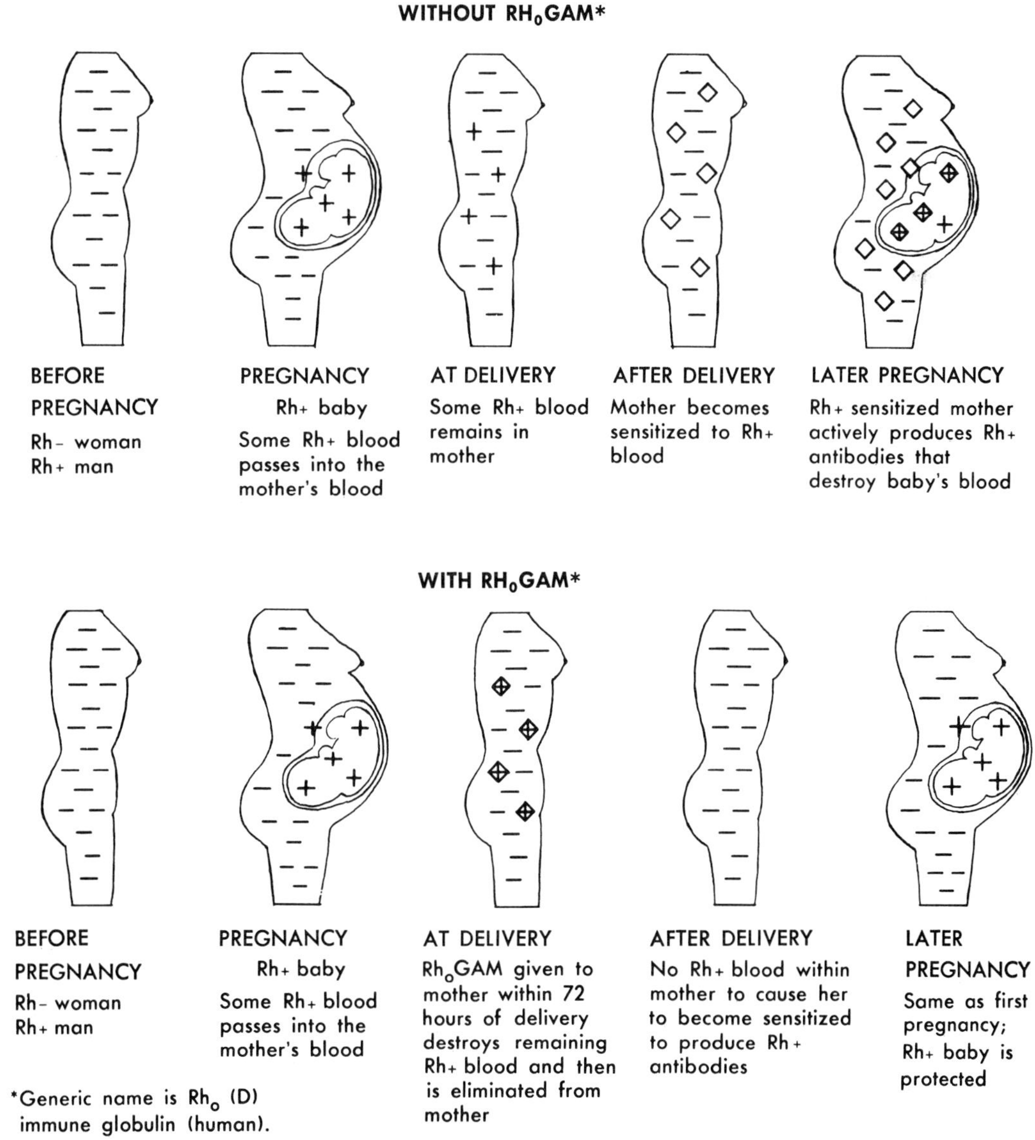

WITHOUT RH$_o$GAM*

BEFORE PREGNANCY	PREGNANCY	AT DELIVERY	AFTER DELIVERY	LATER PREGNANCY
Rh− woman Rh+ man	Rh+ baby Some Rh+ blood passes into the mother's blood	Some Rh+ blood remains in mother	Mother becomes sensitized to Rh+ blood	Rh+ sensitized mother actively produces Rh+ antibodies that destroy baby's blood

WITH RH$_o$GAM*

BEFORE PREGNANCY	PREGNANCY	AT DELIVERY	AFTER DELIVERY	LATER PREGNANCY
Rh− woman Rh+ man	Rh+ baby Some Rh+ blood passes into the mother's blood	Rh_oGAM given to mother within 72 hours of delivery destroys remaining Rh+ blood and then is eliminated from mother	No Rh+ blood within mother to cause her to become sensitized to produce Rh+ antibodies	Same as first pregnancy; Rh+ baby is protected

*Generic name is Rh_o (D) immune globulin (human).

Fig. 13-11. How Rh_oGAM prevents disease.

tive mother has not yet been sensitized to Rh factor. It is used in the following way. Immediately after an abortion or the birth of each baby of an Rh-negative mother, a sample of the baby's blood is taken to determine if the baby is Rh-positive. If so, Rh_oGAM is administered intramuscularly to the mother within 72 hours. It works immediately and provides temporary passive immunity to the mother against the baby's Rh-positive factor. The mother's body does not become sensitized to the red blood cells of the *next* Rh-positive baby, thus protecting that baby in advance against erythroblastosis fetalis.

Once the Rh-negative mother has been sensitized to Rh factor, that sensitivity is permanent. Rh_oGAM cannot help her. Fortunately, only 10% of Rh-negative women become sensitized, even with multiple pregnancies and without the help of Rh_oGAM. This low percentage may result because in some cases the infant is also Rh-negative or has an ABO incompatibility with the mother that somehow seems to prevent Rh sensitization. Fortunately, many sophisticated treatments have been devised to protect the infant of a sensitized mother. These treatments include periodic blood testing of the mother to ascertain the presence of Rh antibodies, amniocentesis, and intrauterine fetal blood transfusions until the baby is old enough to be born by induction at about 35 weeks' gestation.

Amniocentesis is done to determine the degree of anemia in the baby. This procedure may be carried out in the physician's office under local anesthesia. The mother's abdomen is cleansed and anesthesized. The amniotic cavity is entered on the side away from the fetal back and head. About 10 ml of amniotic fluid is removed and checked for the presence of bilirubin, a product of blood destruction. If there is an excessive amount of bilirubin, an intrauterine blood transfusion may be recommended.

Intrauterine blood transfusions are given in hospitals, where sonography or radiopaque dye and x-ray facilities are available. The mother is sedated; the amniotic cavity is entered by means of a special needle; then the peritoneal cavity of the fetus is entered and a catheter threaded into it. Between 50 and 100 ml of type O, Rh-negative packed cells are instilled, the catheter and needle are removed, and the wound is covered. The vital signs of both mother and fetus are observed for several hours. If satisfactory, the patient may leave the hospital that same day. Intrauterine transfusions are administered about 2 weeks apart so that the fetus will have enough blood until delivery. An exchange transfusion of Rh-negative blood is given the baby after birth.

ABO incompatibility. The importance of antigens A and B in the blood has been known since the advent of modern blood transfusion therapy. Only in recent years, however, have these antigens been recognized as a cause of erythroblastosis fetalis by the same isoimmune mechanism that operates in Rh incompatibility.

In the ABO system are two kinds of antigens—A and B. Those people who have neither are said to be type O. The rest of the population is of types A, B, or AB (both). When a fetus inherits a blood type from its father different from that of its mother, fetal blood may cross through the placenta and cause her to become sensitized to antigens of the foreign blood type. During a subsequent pregnancy, another baby with the same type as the first one might be affected by the hostile antibodies of the mother's blood and erythroblastosis fetalis might develop. Fortunately, ABO incompatibility is less common than Rh incompatibility because of a greater number of variables and a smaller percentage of persons in the population with A or B antigens. ABO incompatibility is less predictable, however, than Rh incompatibility, and to date there is no immune globulin to counter the antibody buildup.

Symptoms are a mild jaundice appearing during the first 36 hours of life, an enlarged liver and spleen, and usually no edema or nerve damage. The majority of affected infants need no treatment, but if the hemolysis of red blood cells is sufficient to cause jaundice and a rise in serum bilirubin; an exchange transfusion may be administered.

Nursing care. When there is a possibility that a baby will be born with erythroblastosis fetalis, preparations are made for an exchange transfusion. The umbilical stump is left longer than usual and wrapped in a saline-saturated gauze. The infant is watched closely for such symptoms of hemolysis as jaundice, pigmented urine, edema, and cyanosis. The blood is tested frequently for an abnormal rise in serum bilirubin levels. If these symptoms develop, an exchange transfusion is given. A plastic catheter is inserted into the umbilical vein or some other large vein, and small amounts of the infant's blood (10 to 20 ml) are withdrawn and equal amounts of Rh-negative blood injected. This process is continued until most of the infant's blood has been replaced—about 500 ml. Antibiotics may be given to prevent infection. After the transfusion, the infant is watched closely for changes in vital signs, increased lethargy, jaundice, edema, cyanosis, and convulsions. The infant is kept in an incubator and cared for by skilled, experienced nurses.

Sickle cell disease. Sickle cell disease is an inherited defect in the formation of hemoglobin that causes the outside of the red blood cells to become extremely fragile and rigid. Cells lose their usual concave form, no longer carry oxygen, clump together and clog blood vessels. They lose their cellular content, disrupt potassium levels, and create electrolyte imbalance. The red blood cells become holly-leafed in shape, or "sickled" (Fig. 13-12). Persons who inherit one of the parental genes for hemoglobin S (about 13% of black Americans) are said to have sicklemia, or a sickling trait. They do not develop symptoms. Those who inherit hemoglobin S genes from both parents (1.5% to 3% of black Americans) may exhibit symptoms as early as 2 months of age. The symptoms are caused by a clumping together of the malformed cells, which pile up in the capillaries, causing destruction of the red blood cells, and obstruction of the vessels. When this occurs it is called a "thrombocytic crisis" or "sickle-cell crisis."

Areas of dead tissue (infarcts) may result from the disturbed blood supply and may occur in the spleen, heart, kidneys, lungs, gastrointestinal tract, joints, and brain. The disease is characterized by crisis periods in which blood destruction with capillary obstruction is accelerated. The child has severe pain that may be generalized or

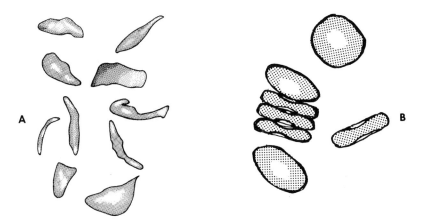

Fig. 13-12. In sickle cell anemia the membranes of the sickled cells are fragile and easily destroyed. **A,** Distorted erythrocytes of sickle cell anemia. **B,** Normal erythrocytes.

may occur in affected parts, depending on what vessels may be occluded; the child is pale, develops a fever, and may vomit. Convulsions, a stiff neck, coma, or paralysis may occur. Two or 3 days after the crisis, jaundice appears and may continue for some time. Growth may not be slowed, but the child may have long, thin arms and legs, a short trunk, a barrel-shaped chest, protruding abdomen, and an enlarged spleen and heart. Treatment consists of supportive measures such as blood transfusions and protection from infections. During crises, relief of pain, measures to control fever, and adequate fluid should be given. Patients with sicklemia (sickle-cell trait) should avoid high altitudes and air travel in unpressurized planes, because low-oxygen tension increases the sickling tendency of their blood, as does cold weather, cold water, and stress.

Thalassemia (Mediterranean anemia, Cooley's anemia). Thalassemia is an inherited defect of hemoglobin formation that causes severe anemia from excessive red blood cell destruction. It was first recognized in persons from countries that border the Mediterranean Sea but has also been found in Africa and the Orient. Persons who inherit the defective gene from both parents manifest the symptoms and are said to have "major thalassemia." Symptoms usually appear during the first year of life. The skin is jaundiced and bronze colored (hemochromatotic), cheek bones thicken (Mongolian facies) and fracture spontaneously, the spleen enlarges, and large numbers of immature red blood cells are found in the circulating blood. These persons are especially susceptible to infection. Treatment consists of regular blood transfusions, but even then, these children seldom live beyond puberty. Life expectancy is normal for those with "minor thalassemia," those who inherit only one defective gene.

Deficiency anemias. The normal manufacture of hemoglobin and red blood cells in the body depends on certain nutrients. When not enough of these nutrients are taken in the diet or when

they are not absorbed properly, deficiency anemias result. The most important of these nutrients are iron, folic acid, vitamin C, vitamin B_{12}, and vitamin B_6 (pyridoxine).

Iron-deficiency hypochromic anemia (milk anemia). The most common anemia in normal birth weight infants, called "milk babies," is caused by an inadequate intake of iron. It occurs when milk is almost the only source of the baby's nutrition. The skin looks like porcelain china; the child becomes weak and irritable. Treatment consists of giving iron by oral preparations and by revising the diet to include iron-rich foods such as liver, fortified cereal, and egg yolks. Intramuscular injections of iron may be ordered, but blood transfusions are seldom necessary. Health supervision of the infant during the first year of life is particularly important in preventing this condition.

Teenaged girls sometimes suffer from hypochromic anemia from a combination of iron-poor diet and heavy menstrual flow. Treatment includes supplementary iron preparations, protein- and iron-rich foods, and treatment of the menstrual difficulty.

Folic acid and vitamin C anemia (megaloblastic anemia). Vitamin C is essential to the absorption of folic acid, and folic acid is necessary for normal red blood cell formation. If either are inadequate, megaloblastic anemia results. This type of anemia is common in infants who do not receive supplementary vitamin C. It may also occur when barbiturates and methotrexate are given for other disorders because drugs interfere with the body's use of folic acid. Some diseases such as intestinal parasitism and hypothyroidism interfere with the absorption of folic acid. Treatment consists of withdrawing the harmful drug, treating underlying diseases, and supplying the needed nutrient.

Vitamin B_{12} anemia (pernicious anemia). Juvenile pernicious anemia is rare but occurs when there is an inadequate intake of vitamin B_{12} or the absence of an essential enzyme of the stomach, called the "intrinsic factor," which allows vitamin B_{12} to be absorbed by the body. Treatment consists of administering vitamin B_{12} by injection for the lifetime of the individual.

Vitamin B_6 anemia (sideroblastic anemia). Vitamin B_6 (pyridoxine) is necessary to the manufacture of hemoglobin. In some individuals severe anemia results because this vitamin is not absorbed by the intestinal tract. Treatment consists of administering it intramuscularly.

Bone marrow impairment. Because most of the red blood cells are manufactured in the bone marrow, disorders that disrupt its normal function cause anemia. The most common disturbances are as follows: (1) disturbance of the delivery of otherwise normal red blood cells to the general circulation from the bone marrow—associated with a variety of chronic conditions such as endocarditis and osteomyelitis; (2) replacement of the bone marrow with neoplastic (tumerous) or fibrous tissue; and (3) "aplastic anemia," or failure of the bone marrow to manufacture red cells caused by radiation or ingestion of toxic drugs such as the insecticide DDT, chloromycetin, benzene, and the sulfonamides. In all cases of bone marrow failure, the underlying disease is treated when possible and whole blood transfusions are given until the bone marrow can take over its normal function; a bone marrow transplant can be made.

Leukemia

Acute leukemia in children is a primary disorder of the bone marrow in which normal marrow elements are replaced by primitive white blood cells called "stem" or "blast" cells. When bone marrow is replaced, normal red blood cell and platelet production is seriously hampered, causing severe anemia and a marked tendency to bleed. The leukemic cells invade many areas of the body such as the liver, spleen, and lymph nodes and cause local symptoms. Diagnosis is made on the basis of discovery of immature forms of white blood cells in the bone marrow, circulating blood, and lymph nodes. At times the white blood count is extremely elevated; at other times it may be depressed. During periods of high count with large percentages of abnormal blast cells the blood picture is described as being "leukemic." During periods when the count is low and there are fewer immature forms, it is said to be "aleukemic."

Types. There are two basic types of the disease classified according to the kind of white blood cell principally involved: acute lymphoblastic leukemia (ALL) and acute myelogenous leukemia (AML). The cause for the abnormal cell growth of leukemia has not been found, even though extensive research has been going on for many years. In children leukemia is rapidly fatal. The average untreated child dies within 4 to 6 months from onset; some die in a few days. Death is usually caused by massive hemorrhage or secondary infection. Childhood leukemias seem to respond to drugs more readily than do adult types, but even with intensive drug therapy only 45% survive for 5 years after treatment.

Symptoms. The symptoms of leukemia may be very rapid in onset or may be slow and insidious. The child may appear to have a "cold" and develop a high fever and a secondary infection of the throat or lungs. The child may become progressively weak, appear pale, bruise easily, and lose weight. Because of the multiplying leukemia cells the child may have vague muscle and joint pains, swollen lymph nodes, and an enlarged liver and spleen. Laboratory tests confirm the tragic diagnosis. The course of the disease depends on the treatment attempted and the child's response and usually involves several hospitalization periods.

Treatment. At present no cure has been found for leukemia; however, a number of drugs have been developed that forestall death for varying periods. The principal action of the drugs is to destroy cells; therefore, the children who receive them are made very sick by their toxic effects. These drugs act independently, and when one is no longer effective, another may be for a while. There is always hope that by keeping the child alive for just a few more days a true cure will be discovered.

Adrenocortical therapy is often used initially for an acutely ill child. This therapy employs such steroids as ACTH, cortisone, and the synthetic hormone prednisone. These drugs often produce short-lived but dramatic remission of symptoms. But because they also make the patient easy prey to infection and cause bone deterioration, personality changes, and a moon-shaped face, other drugs are begun as soon as relapse appears.

Vincristine is another drug that may produce a temporary remission, but it causes loss of nervous control and muscle weakness and so cannot be continued indefinitely.

Administration of the antimetabolite group of drugs is begun during a period when the child is in good general condition or during the remission produced by adrenocortical or vincristine therapy. There are two kinds of antimetabolites: (1) the folic acid antagonists such as *aminopterin* and *methotrexate* and (2) a purine analog named *mercaptopurine*. This last drug produces remissions in 50% of the cases but must be stopped when the bone marrow is too severely depressed. Of the folic acid antagonists, methotrexate is far less toxic than aminopterin, but both cause hemorrhage, ulceration of the mouth and gastrointestinal tract, and depression of the bone marrow.

A nitrogen mustard derivative, called *cyclophosphamide* may be effective in combinations with other drugs. It produces remission of the disease in some children but also causes loss of hair and hemorrhagic inflammations of the urinary bladder and the mucous membrane of the mouth and so cannot be administered for long periods.

Daunorubicin is used for both types of lukeumia, producing remission in 50% of children treated. *L-Asparaginase* produces remission in 40% to 70% of children with ALL, but is rarely effective for AML.

Nursing care. Nursing care of the leukemic child and the parents is difficult. It requires a high degree of emotional stability, skill, and patience, and a philosophy of life that gives purpose to the present. See Chapter 7 for a discussion of children with terminal illness.

Physical nursing care is directed toward making the leukemic child more comfortable; observing and reporting significant changes in the child's condition, and carrying out specific therapy prescribed by the physician. The child is usually very uncomfortable and irritable. The body is sore and movement is painful, yet positions must be changed frequently to prevent skin breakdown and respiratory infections. The child bleeds easily from the mouth and rectum, and bruises seem to appear spontaneously. Gentleness should characterize all care, including oral hygiene and bathing. Soft toothbrushes, gauze applicators, and mouthwashes provide comfort without further tissue damage. Because fever is often present, measures to reduce temperature must be used often. Axillary temperatures may be necessary when there is rectal bleeding. Protective isolation may be required to protect the child from infection. The child is subjected to repeated, painful bone marrow aspirations and venipunctures for blood tests, intravenous feedings, and blood transfusions. Nurses must do everything possible to reduce the trauma and pain of these experiences. They must also support the parents, assuring them of their importance to their child at this time and encouraging them to do some of the special things that bring comfort to the child.

Hemorrhagic diseases

A number of diseases afflict children in which the outstanding characteristic is an abnormal tendency to bleed. This tendency may result from especially fragile blood vessels, defective platelets, or defects in the plasma coagulation of clotting (Fig. 13-5). Some of these defects are inherited or result from vitamin deficiency, some resemble an allergic reaction, and others simply occur with no known cause. To diagnose accurately what is causing the bleeding and then to identify the specific disorder behind it, the physician takes careful medical histories of these children and their families and orders laboratory tests. Among the most common tests are bleeding time, clotting time, prothrombin time, capillary fragility, platelet (thrombocyte) count, and fibrinogen measurement. (See the diagnostic tests in Chapter 9.)

The terminology used to describe hemorrhagic diseases is rather specialized, but the nurse is expected to understand and use it correctly. Some of the more common terms are:

capillary fragility easy breakage or damage to capillary vessel walls

ecchymoses irregularly formed hemorrhages into the tissue, bruises

epistaxis bleeding from the nose

hematuria blood in the urine

hemoptysis spitting up blood

melena darkening of feces by blood pigments

petechiae small purplish hemorrhagic spots

purpura a condition characterized by hemorrhages into the skin and other body tissue

telangiectases small red lesions usually found in the skin or mucous membrane caused by the dilation of capillaries, arterioles, and venules

Hemophilia. Classic hemophilia is an inherited, sex-linked, recessive disorder that occurs almost exclusively in males and is transmitted by females. It has become well known in history because it was carried for generations in the royal families of Europe. It is characterized by a deficiency of antihemophilic globulin (AHG), or factor VIII, involving a defect in the clotting mechanism of the blood so that even a minor wound may cause a life-threatening hemorrhage. Dental extraction, surgical procedures, and even the normal play of active children are hazardous for the hemophiliac patient. Bleeding into the soft tissue and joints may occur spontaneously. Repeated hemorrhages into the joints may cause permanent deformity. Treatment depends on the degree of blood loss and the area involved. Efforts to control bleeding by use of local measures such as pressure, cold, and applications of thrombin are attempted when possible. Whole blood, fresh frozen plasma, or antihemophilic

globulin may be administered. Some communities have hemophilia centers that are prepared to provide emergency care and intravenous therapy to hemophiliacs on an outpatient basis.

There are a number of hemophilias other than classic hemophilia. They are also inherited and may affect both boys and girls. They are caused by deficiencies of one or more clotting factors. The care of these children is the same as for those with classic hemophilia, except for the specific antihemophilic factor given during hemorrhages.

Supervision and care of hemophiliac patients must emphasize prevention. Parents need help in planning and managing their child to afford maximum protection and minimum restriction of normal activities. The slats of the infant's crib should be padded. The child learning to crawl and walk should be protected from falls. Knee pads may help. Sharp objects must be kept out of reach. Constant observation is needed, not only to protect the child from injury but also to detect bleeding as soon as it appears so that treatment can begin immediately. Such constant child care is exhausting to conscientious parents who want to protect their child from physical injury but do not want to make their child an emotional cripple. In some communities homemaker services and hospital day care are available to the parents to allow them an occasional "day off" for personal relaxation. Parents of hemophiliac children sometimes form local groups for mutual encouragement and education.

In spite of conscientious home care, hemophiliac patients are hospitalized frequently for intravenous therapy and uncontrolled bleeding. If the bleeding is into a joint, the child may be suffering severe pain. The child should be moved with gentleness and positioned with pillows. Ice packs may be applied to the affected part. The older child may be irritable, depressed, and angry because of a restricted life and repeated bouts of pain. The nurses should demonstrate that they accept and understand this despair and that they sincerely want to help. As the child begins to trust the nurses, they may be able to help the child come to terms with the disability and make the most of other abilities.

Scurvy. Scurvy is a hemorrhagic disease in which the capillaries become fragile and allow blood to escape into the tissue. It is caused by a vitamin C (ascorbic acid) deficiency. Scurvy is seen in infants fed with cow's milk who are not given supplementary vitamins in the diet or as oral preparations. Breast-fed infants usually receive enough vitamin C through the mother's supply. The disease usually develops between the fifth and fifteenth months, causing abnormal formation of the bones, connective tissue, and capillary cells. Hemorrhages occur in the bones and particularly in the knee joints, causing pain and a typical frog-like position. The gums swell and bleed and there are hemorrhages in the skin, bowel, bladder, and even eyes. The bones become porous and the ribs beaded. Treatment consists of administering vitamin C daily. Healing occurs rapidly and normal growth continues.

In severely malnourished older children, scurvy may exist along with the effects of other nutritional deficiencies. Mental and physical growth may be stunted in cases of long-term deprivation. Treatment consists of intensive nutritional therapy and educational opportunity to make full use of the intellectual capacities remaining.

Purpura. Purpura is a general name given to a great many conditions in which blood seeps out into the body tissues from damaged vessels and walls or because of a decrease in the number of thrombocytes (thrombocytopenia), which hampers clotting. Anaphylactoid purpura, the purpura of infections, and primary and secondary thrombocytopenic purpura are among the more common of these conditions seen in children.

Anaphylactoid Schönlein-Henoch purpura is a disease of unknown cause in which the small blood vessels throughout the body become inflammed. It is most often associated with upper respiratory infections and so is considered to be of allergic origin. This condition is relatively common, especially in children between 3 and 7 years of age. Boys are more susceptible than girls. Symptoms are skin rash, especially over the legs and face, petechiae, abdominal and joint pain, edema of the hands and feet, melena, hematemesis, telescoping of the bowel (intussusception), hematuria, and acute nephritis. Symptoms may disappear in a few days or may continue as long as 2 years. Recurrence is common. There is no specific treatment. Steroids seem to relieve some of the more severe symptoms, and, of course, surgery is required for such emergencies as intussusception.

The purpura of infections such as meningococcemia and subacute bacterial endocarditis is caused by injury of the vessel walls as a result of emboli and sometimes by thrombopenia. Large blotchy areas appear on the skin and there may be bleeding into other body tissues. When the underlying disease is cured, the purpura gradually disappears.

Primary thrombocytopenic purpura is also known as idiopathic thrombocytopenic purpura because the cause for such low thrombocyte production is unknown. The onset may be sudden, with showers of petechiae and bleeding mucous membranes, or it may follow months of easy bruising. Diagnosis is made after other conditions are ruled out and blood tests confirm the decreased thrombocyte count. Treatment is by transfusions of concentrated thrombocytes, platelets, or whole blood and steroids. Splenectomy may be required to reduce the destruction of thrombocytes because the formed elements of the blood are normally destroyed in the spleen.

Secondary thrombocytopenic purpura is associated with conditions in which the normal production of thrombocytes is disturbed, such as diseases of the connective tissue and bone marrow and exposure to radiation and toxic drugs. It may also appear in premature or full-term infants born to mothers with thrombocytopenia. The purpura is treated with whole blood and concentrated thrombocyte transfusions, together with such treatment as is available for the primary disorders.

Nursing care of the purpuric child is directed toward reducing further trauma and carrying out the specific treatment ordered. Intravenous therapy is administered under the watchful eye of the nurse to prevent infiltration into the tissue or disruption of the intended flow. The child should be cared for gently to prevent further hemorrhage into tissue. Tight band restraints should be well padded or avoided entirely. It may be comforting to the child to hold a soft cuddly toy or for the mother or the nurse to read aloud quietly. The child whose condition is improving is able to increase activities but should still be protected from trauma as much as possible.

SUMMARY OUTLINE

I. Respiratory system
  A. Structure and function
    1. Nose and sinuses
    2. Pharynx
    3. Larynx and trachea
    4. Lower respiratory tract
    5. General nursing assessment of respiratory function
  B. Disorders
    1. Epistaxis
    2. Foreign body in the nose
    3. Nasal trauma
    4. Deviated septum
    5. Choanal atresia
    6. Tonsillitis and adenoiditis
    7. Tonsillectomy and adenoidectomy (T & A)
    8. Common cold (upper respiratory infection or URI)
    9. Retropharyngeal abscess
    10. Streptococcal pharyngitis ("strep throat")
    11. Acute laryngitis
    12. Acute epiglottiditis
    13. Spasmodic croup
    14. Perinatahypoxia (anoxia)
    15. Sudden infant death syndrome (SIDS)
    16. Atelectasis
    17. Laryngotracheobronchitis
    18. Bronchiolitis
    19. Bronchiectasis
    20. Bronchoscopy and bronchograms
    21. Cystic fibrosis (mucoviscidosis)
    22. The pneumonias
      a. Pneumococcal pneumonia
      b. Staphlococcal pneumonia
      c. Streptococcal pneumonia
      d. Viral pneumonia (primary atypical pneumonia)
    23. Allergic conditions
      a. Allergic rhinitis
      b. Asthma
    24. Tuberculosis
      a. Description and cause
      b. Public health factors
      c. Skin tests and diagnostic studies
      d. Immunization
      e. Primary tuberculosis
      f. Miliary tuberculosis
      g. Other complications
      h. Reinfection
      i. Treatment

II. Cardiovascular system
  A. Structure and function
    1. Heart
    2. Blood vessels
    3. Lymphatic system
    4. Blood
      a. Plasma
      b. Formed elements
      c. Blood products
    5. Circulation
    6. Clotting
  B. Disorders
    1. Congenital heart disease
      a. Diagnosis
      b. Classifications
      c. Patent ductus arteriosus
      d. Septal defects
      e. Coarctation of the aorta
      f. Pulmonic and aortic stenosis
      g. Tetralogy (foursome) of Fallot
      h. Transposition of the great vessels
      i. Truncus arteriosus
      j. Total anomalous venous return
      k. Tricuspid atresia
    2. Cardiac surgery
      a. Heart-lung machine and cardiopulmonary bypass
      b. Preparation of the patient
      c. Postoperative nursing care
    3. Medical treatment of cardiac conditions
    4. Complications of congenital heart defects
      a. Congestive heart failure
      b. Carditis

   (1) Endocarditis
   (2) Myocarditis
   (3) Pericarditis
 5. The anemias
  a. Blood loss
  b. Blood destruction
   (1) Hemolytic disease of the newborn (erythroblastosis fetalis)
    (a) Rh factor incompatibility
    (b) ABO incompatibility
    (c) Nursing care
   (2) Sickle cell disease
   (3) Thalassemia (Mediterranean anemia, Cooley's anemia)
  c. Deficiency anemias
   (1) Iron-deficiency hypochromic anemia (milk anemia)
   (2) Folic acid and vitamin C anemia (megaloblastic anemia)
   (3) Vitamin B_{12} anemia (pernicious anemia)
   (4) Vitamin B_6 anemia, (sideroblastic anemia)
   (5) Bone marrow impairment
 6. Leukemia
  a. Types
  b. Symptoms
  c. Treatment
  d. Nursing care
 7. Hemorrhagic diseases
  a. Hemophilia
  b. Scurvy
  c. Purpura

STUDY QUESTIONS

1. Name the parts of the respiratory system through which air travels from the nose to an air sac.
2. Discuss the postoperative care of a tonsillectomy patient. What is the prime concern?
3. Compare bronchiolitis and bronchiectasis. Describe the symptoms and nursing care.
4. Describe the disease process of primary pulmonary tuberculosis from the time the bacteria enter the lung until the condition is "arrested."
5. Trace the path of a red blood cell as it circulates from a venous capillary back to an arterial capillary.
6. Define plasma, serum, platelets, leukocytes, erythrocytes. What is the function of each of the formed elements of blood?
7. Describe the defect in the following conditions: patent ductus arteriosus, ventricular septal defect, coarctation of the aorta, tetralogy of Fallot.
8. Describe the process that causes hemolytic disease of the newborn from Rh factor. How does Rh_oGAM protect future babies?
9. Describe the first symptoms of leukemia. What is the goal of nursing care as the disease progresses?
10. Discuss the nursing care of children with hemophilia and purpura.

14
Digestive and metabolic conditions

VOCABULARY

Peristalsis
Gastrostomy
Celiac
Exocrine glands
Enterobiasis
Incarcerated hernia
Eschar
Postprandial

For the body to maintain good health and to grow and develop normally it must have an adequate supply of the necessary nutrients found in foods, which are carbohydrates, proteins, fats, vitamins, minerals, and water. A discussion of how to provide these nutrients by means of a well-balanced diet is found in Chapter 3. But eating the right food is only the first step. The body must then be able to digest the foods and absorb and metabolize the nutrients they supply. This requires healthy, normal digestive and endocrine systems, a knowledge of which is necessary if the nurse is to understand the abnormal digestive and metabolic conditions that commonly afflict children.

THE DIGESTIVE SYSTEM

Function. The chief function of the digestive system is to prepare foods for absorption. Most food, when eaten, is in a form that cannot reach the cells because it cannot pass through the intestinal wall into the bloodstream, nor can it be used by the cells even if it could reach them. Food must therefore be broken up mechanically (by chewing and churning) and changed chemically (by enzyme action) so that it can be absorbed and used by body cells. These processes are carried out in the digestive tract, then the wastes are eliminated from the body.

Structure. The alimentary canal, or gastrointestinal tract, is a muscular tube extending through the body from the lips to the anus (Fig. 14-1). It consists of the mouth, pharynx, esopha-

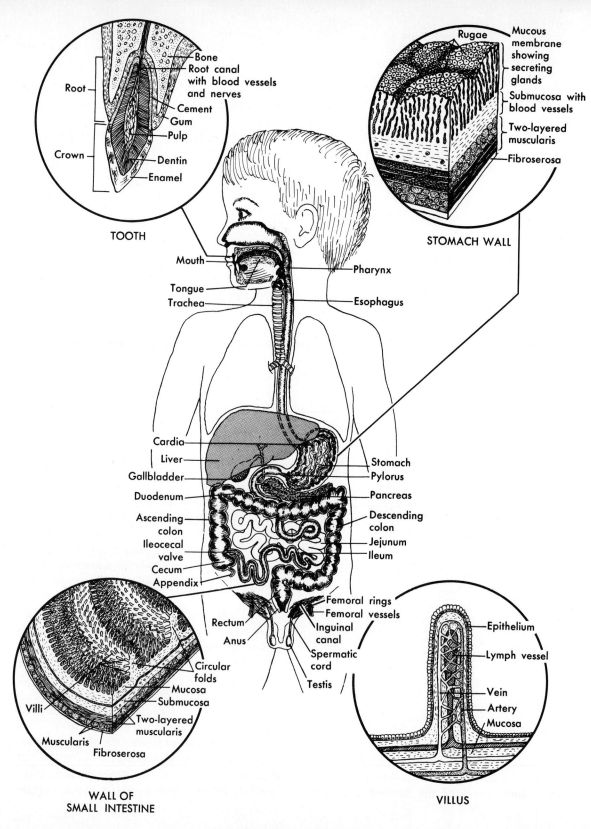

TOOTH

Bone
Root canal with blood vessels and nerves
Cement
Gum
Pulp
Dentin
Enamel
Root
Crown

STOMACH WALL

Rugae
Mucous membrane showing secreting glands
Submucosa with blood vessels
Two-layered muscularis
Fibroserosa

Mouth
Tongue
Trachea
Pharynx
Esophagus

Cardia
Liver
Gallbladder
Duodenum
Ascending colon
Ileocecal valve
Cecum
Appendix
Stomach
Pylorus
Pancreas
Descending colon
Jejunum
Ileum

Rectum
Anus
Femoral rings
Femoral vessels
Inguinal canal
Spermatic cord
Testis

WALL OF SMALL INTESTINE

Circular folds
Mucosa
Submucosa
Two-layered muscularis
Villi
Muscularis
Fibroserosa

VILLUS

Epithelium
Lymph vessel
Vein
Artery
Mucosa

Fig. 14-1. Gastrointestinal system.

gus, stomach, small intestine, and large intestine. After the food is swallowed, it is moved along by rhythmic waves of muscular contraction called *peristalsis*. Groups of nerve cells (ganglia) embedded in the muscle layer stimulate this action. The lining tissues secrete digestive fluids that mix with the food. They also absorb the digested food products. The accessory organs of digestion assist in the digestive process. They are the teeth, tongue, salivary glands, pancreas, liver, gallbladder, and appendix.

The *mouth* is especially made to receive food, to produce speech, and to accomplish the first steps of digestion. In the mouth the food is savored by the taste buds, chewed by the teeth, and softened and moistened by the secretions of the cheeks and tongue. The first chemical process of digestion takes place in the mouth as ptyalin, an enzyme found in saliva, changes starches into soluble sugars.

The *pharynx* is the muscular vestibule that serves as a passageway for both the digestive and respiratory systems. It receives the swallowed food and acts as a funnel through which food passes into the esophagus and then to the stomach without undergoing change.

The *stomach* is an enlarged part of the alimentary canal between the esophagus and the small intestine. It has two openings, the *cardia*, through which the food enters, and the *pylorus*, which leads into the small intestine. The pyloric sphincter is a thickening of the muscular layers of the stomach. It regulates the time food remains in the stomach. When the stomach is filled, the pyloric sphincter normally is closed until the food is churned and mixed with gastric secretions to form *chyme*. When the mixing is complete, the sphincter opens and some of the stomach content is discharged into the duodenum by peristalsis. In some newborn infants the pylorus is stenosed, or too tight. This stenosis prevents liquids from passing and the stomach becomes distended with milk. This distention causes reverse peristalsis and vomiting.

The lining tissues of the stomach are quite irregular, because of the presence of numerous folds called *rugae*. These rugae create a rough washboard surface that serves to enhance the mixing process. Gastric glands embedded in the stomach lining pour their secretions into the stomach chamber in response to complex hormonal and nervous stimuli. (See the discussion on the endocrine system in the following section.) The gastric secretions are the enzymes pepsin, rennin, and gastric lipase and hydrochloric acid. This strong acid provides the acid medium essential for gastric digestion of proteins and carbohydrates. It also destroys many organisms that enter the stomach with food. Excessive amounts of acid sometimes erode the stomach wall, producing ulcers.

The *small intestine* is composed of three regions—the *duodenum, jejunum*, and *ileum*. The duodenum is the part connected to the stomach. Secretions from the liver and pancreas are emptied into the duodenum. They are bile, emptied from the common bile duct, and pancreatic juice, emptied from the pancreatic duct. Bile is a greenish liquid containing bile salts and pigment that breaks up fat into a fine emulsion ready to be acted on by enzymes. Pancreatic juice supplies three important enzymes—amylopsin, trypsin, and steapsin. The jejunum and ileum make up the remainder of the small intestine and are similar in appearance and structure to the duodenum. Embedded in their walls are glands that secrete several more important digestive enzymes, such as enterokinase, erepsin, maltase, sucrase, lactase, and lipase. All these chemicals act on chyme in its final stages of digestion in the small intestines. Each one contains blood vessels, nerves, and minute lymphatic vessels that transport fats. Through these villi, food products are absorbed and carried to the liver.

The *liver* is the largest and one of the most important glands of the body, serving as its food-processing plant. It secretes bile, the emulsifier of fats, and stores carbohydrates in the form of glycogen. Then, as the body needs them, it reconverts the glycogen back into simple sugars and discharges them into the blood. The liver also regulates the protein levels in the blood, converting any excesses into usable sugar and urea. The liver also protects the body by aiding in the removal of poisons from foods that have entered the bloodstream.

The *gallbladder* is a storage place for bile. Bile is manufactured in the liver, collected in bile capillaries, moved through the bile ducts to the hepatic ducts and then to the cystic duct, which transports it to the gallbladder where it is concentrated and retained until needed in the intestine. When fat is present in the small intestine, complex chemical and nervous stimuli trigger the gallbladder to contract, thereby emptying bile into the duodenum just when it is needed.

The *pancreas* is a glandular organ made up of two types of tissues, those which secrete pancreatic juice to be transported by ducts into the small intestine to aid digestion and those which secrete hormones into the bloodstream. The latter are small masses of cells called pancreatic islets or islets of Langerhans. These masses of cells are made up of two kinds of cells, alpha and beta. The alpha cells secrete the hormone *glucagon*, which causes the liver to release glucose during emergency needs. The beta cells secrete *insulin*, which accelerates the transfer of glucose through cell membranes where it can be metabolized.

The *large intestine* is that part of the alimentary canal that lies between the ileum of the small intestine and the anus. The first part is a pouch-like structure called the *cecum*, which is connected to the ileum by the *ileocecal valve*. Coming from the cecum is a small blind tube, the *appendix*, which lies in the right lower quadrant of the abdomen. The appendix sometimes becomes obstructed with fecal matter and inflamed so that appendicitis results. Following the cecum are the *ascending*, *transverse*, and *descending colons*. They form an inverted U within the abdomen and connect to the *sigmoid colon*, the S-shaped part of the large intestine that joins the *rectum* and ends in the *anus*, the external open-

ing. The anal sphincter controls the passage of feces during defecation. The walls of the large intestine have no villi or circular folds, but as the rather liquid matter from the ileum passes through the colon, water is absorbed through its walls and the feces gradually become concentrated. Inflammation of the intestinal mucosa results in increased peristalsis, which propels the contents too rapidly toward the rectum, a condition called diarrhea. As a result, the feces are discharged in liquid form. Decreased peristalsis causes retention of feces, excessive removal of water, and constipation.

The *abdominal wall* consists of three muscle layers that run in several directions, thus providing strength and control. On each side of the groin the abdominal wall is pierced by an obliquely placed channel, the *inguinal canal*. In the male, the spermatic cord passes through the canal on its way to the testes. In the female, the round ligament of the uterus is anchored there. Nearby are the *femoral rings*, openings in the groin through which the main artery and veins of the legs pass out of the abdominal cavity.

The abdominal cavity is bounded by the diaphragm above and the pelvis below and is lined by a membrane called the *peritoneum*, which also serves to cover all or part of the abdominal organs. In certain places, the peritoneum folds back on itself. The peritoneal fold from the intestine is called a *mesentery*, and those from the stomach are called *omenta*. Of these omenta, the *lesser omentum* extends between the stomach and the liver and the *greater omentum* extends from the greater curvature of the stomach to form an apronlike fold in front of the intestine.

THE ENDOCRINE SYSTEM

Just as the nervous system provides the body with physical control of its functions, so too the endocrine system provides chemical control. These controls affect every other body system and are of particular importance because they affect the digestion of foods and the complex chemical process called *metabolism*, such that nutrients entering the bloodstream are utilized in cells to produce heat and energy, build and repair body tissue, and regulate body processes.

A summary of the more important hormones as they are currently known is provided in Table 14-1. The student is reminded that no matter where an endocrine gland is located, its secretions of hormones are discharged into the bloodstream and circulated throughout the body, affecting every cell.

Table 14-1. Endocrine glands, their hormones and action

Endocrine gland	Portion involved	Hormone	Action of hormone
Pituitary	Anterior	Somatotrophic (STH)	Stimulates growth and development of all tissue
		Thyrotrophic	Acts on thyroid gland to produce thyroxin
		Adrenocortico-trophic (ACTH)	Acts on adrenal cortex to release adrenocortical hormones
		Gonadotrophic:	
		Follicle-stimu-lating (FSH)	Acts on ovaries and testes to produce ova and sperm
		Luteinizing (LH)	Causes rupture and release of ovum
		Luteotrophic (LTH) or pro-lactin	Stimulates release of progesterone by corpus lu-teum; stimulates milk glands of breasts
		Interstitial cell-stimulating (ICSH)	Acts on testes to produce androgens
	Posterior	Vasopressin or an-tidiuretic (ADH)	Contracts smooth muscle causing increased blood pressure; stimulates reabsorption of water by kidneys
		Oxytocin	Acts on uterine muscle to cause forceful contrac-tions
Thyroid	Whole	Thyroxin	Increases metabolic rate and so enhances activities of all body tissues
Parathyroid	Four glands embedded in thyroid	Parathyroid hor-mone	Stimulates the release of calcium from bone, inhib-its phosphate reabsorption by kidneys
Adrenal	Cortex	Adrenocortical:	
		Mineralocorti-coids	Control extracellular concentration of sodium and potassium
		Glucocorticoids	Assist in metabolism of protein, fat, and carbohy-drates
		Androgens	Produce male characteristics
	Medulla	Epinephrine	Elevates blood pressure; dilates eye pupils; dilates bronchioles; decreases peristalsis; stimulates gly-cogenolysis; constricts all blood vessels except those of heart and muscles
		Norepinephrine	Elevates blood pressure by vigorous vasoconstric-tion

Continued.

Table 14-1. Endocrine glands, their hormones and actions—cont'd

Endocrine gland	Portion involved	Hormone	Action of hormone
Ovaries	Graafian follicle (when stimulated by FSH)	Estrogens: Theelin and estrin	Produce and maintain secondary sex characteristics; regulate menstrual cycle; stimulate breast growth
	Corpus luteum (when stimulated by LTH)	Progesterone	Inhibits uterine muscle contraction; prepares and maintains lining of uterus; stimulates breast development; suppresses ovulation in latter half of menstrual cycle
Testes	Interstitial tissue (when stimulated by ICSH)	Androgens: Testosterone is chief one	Related to progesterone, stimulates sex organs at puberty; produces and maintains secondary sex characteristics and sperm; inhibits pituitary gland; stimulates protein synthesis; causes retention of potassium and phosphate
Islets of Langerhans within pancreas	Alpha cells	Glucagon	Causes liver to release glucose into blood for emergencies
	Beta cells	Insulin	Accelerates transfer of glucose through cell membrane where it is metabolized
Hormone-secreting cells of gastrointestinal mucosa	Gastric cells stimulated by protein in stomach	Gastrin (may be histamine)	Stimulates release of gastric juices
	Intestinal cells stimulated by acid	Secretin	Stimulates pancreas to form pancreatic juice and liver to form bile
		Pancreozymin	Stimulates pancreas to produce digestive enzymes
	Intestinal cells stimulated by fatty foods	Cholecystokinin	Initiates contraction of gallbladder so that bile enters duodenum
		Enterogastrone	Decreases gastric secretions and movement
	Intestinal cells stimulated by chyme	Enterocrinin group of several hormones	Stimulates production of enzymes in intestine to digest proteins and carbohydrates

DISORDERS OF THE DIGESTIVE SYSTEM
Mouth

Abnormalities of the teeth. The development and eruption of first the primary and then the secondary teeth is a complex process, one in which abnormalities commonly occur. There may be an absence of all or some of the teeth (anodontia), or there may be too many teeth, or those that erupt may come together incorrectly (malocclusion). Because teeth are important to the child's nutrition, speech development, appearance, and emotional well-being, abnormalities should be corrected as soon as they appear and the child referred to an orthodontist, a person specializing in orthodontia, that branch of dentistry devoted to the correction of dental irregularities.

Dental caries and stains. Dental caries are areas of erosion in the enamel and dentin of teeth that result from a combination of acid-forming organisms and fermenting sugars and starches. If these areas are not treated, they gradually involve more and more of the tooth, eventually destroying the pulp, thereby causing inflammation and sometimes abscess formation. Treatment is given by a dentist, who cleans the decayed matter from the cavity and fills it with plastic or metal. More complex treatment may be necessary for deep cavities. Sometimes a diseased tooth must be extracted because of irreparable damage.

The enamel of teeth may be damaged or stained by the ingestion of acids, certain herbs, and such medications as tetracycline. To prevent these effects any such chemicals should be avoided if possible, and if not, they should be sucked in through a straw and followed immediately with water.

Positive measures for dental health are good nutrition, regular cleansing, flouridation, and regular dental examination. These are discussed in detail in Chapter 3.

Trauma. Active children often fall and cause severe trauma to their teeth, particularly to the front incisors. Even though the teeth involved may be primary teeth, every effort is made to preserve them until the permanent ones appear. For this reason the damaged teeth should be examined by a dentist immediately after the accident and periodically thereafter. Frequently abscesses develop at the roots of such teeth, causing damage to the permanent teeth beneath. Chipped or broken teeth should be treated by the dentist to prevent decay.

Stomatitis. Any inflammation of an opening of the body may be called stomatitis. The most common types involve the mucous membrane of the mouth. Some are the result of generalized disease conditions such as leukemia; some result from allergies or caustic chemicals; and some result from a local invasion of bacteria or fungus. *Thrush* is the name given to an infection by the fungus *Candida (Monilia) albicans*. It is characterized by slightly raised patches that resemble milk curds and can be removed only with difficulty, leaving raw, exposed tissue. This fungus is a normal inhabitant of the vaginal canal, and newborn infants are sometimes infected by it as a result of improper hygiene and feeding techniques after delivery. Thrush is also fairly common among children receiving long-term antibiotic therapy. The antibiotics destroy the normal flora of the alimentary canal and allow the fungus to multiply without competition. To combat this, a bacterial culture such as found in Lactinex granules may be given at meal time. Nystatin, or even the old standby gentian violet 1%, may be applied locally. All objects that have entered the infant's mouth should be sterilized until the condition responds to treatment.

Cleft lip and palate. Cleft lip and palate are fairly common congenital deformities. They appear alone or together about once in every 800 births. The cause is a failure of the union of the embryonic structures of the face, frequently the result of heredity.

The cleft lip, or harelip, is more common in boys and may vary from a single notching of the lip to a deep split extending through the lip into

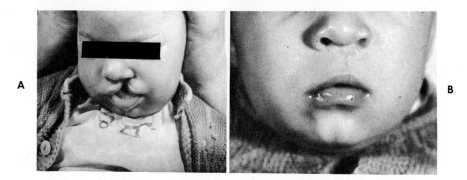

Fig. 14-2. A, Unilateral cleft lip. **B,** Same child after repair. (Courtesy Dr. Henry S. Patton, Oakland, Calif.)

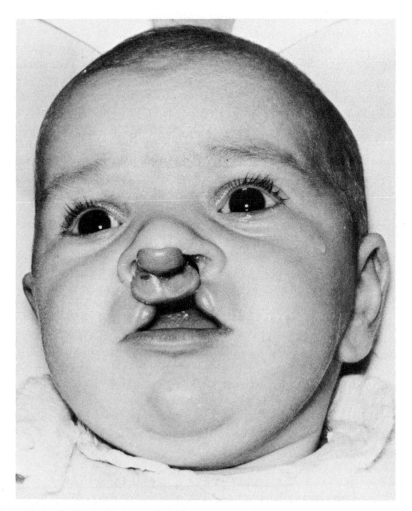

Fig. 14-3. Bilateral cleft lip and palate before repair. (Courtesy Children's Hospital of the East Bay, Oakland, Calif.)

the nose. It may be one sided (unilateral) (Fig. 14-2) or two sided (bilateral) (Fig. 14-3). A more severe cleft interferes with sucking, causes mouth breathing, and is psychologically distressing to parents, who may not give the infant the normal face-to-face cuddling. For maximum cosmetic results, plastic repair of a cleft lip is made within the first 2 months of life.

The cleft palate is more common in girls and may involve lack of fusion of only part of the hard or soft palate or may extend along the entire roof of the mouth. Its repair is usually delayed until the facial structures have grown somewhat and may involve a number of successive operations, depending on the severity of the defect.

Before taking their baby home to await surgery for cleft lip or palate, parents need to receive detailed instructions regarding care. They should have a number of opportunities to feed the infant under supervision. These babies usually have difficulty sucking because of an inability to create a vacuum in the mouth. They may be fed with a rubber-tipped medicine dropper, Asepto syringe, Brecht feeder, a very soft nipple such as a Lamb's nipple, or a spoon. Gavage is avoided if possible. The method of choice is the one most like a normal infant. The baby should be held in an upright position during feedings to prevent aspiration of milk into the lungs or regurgitation through the nose in the case of a cleft palate. Burping should be done frequently because of the increased tendency to swallow air. Some children with cleft palate are fitted early in life with a prosthesis to cover the open palate and guard against regurgitation and to aid in the formation of speech patterns until corrective surgery can be done.

After surgery for a cleft lip, the infant's arms must be restrained to prevent damage to the suture line. Both elbow and wrist restraints are used. Periodically, these should be removed, one at a time, to allow for circulation and exercise. A nasally inserted gastric tube is used for feedings for several days to reduce lip motion and protect the suture line. A soft nasal packing may

be positioned in the opposite nostril to balance the tissue stretching. It is removed after about 2 days. The suture line is protected by means of a Logan bow or bandage. The Logan bow is a metal loop placed over the suture line and attached to the cheeks by adhesive. The gavage tube may be taped to the Logan bow to prevent tension on the nose and eliminate the use of more adhesive on the skin. The suture line is kept scrupulously clean to prevent scarring crusts from forming. Various solutions such as hydrogen peroxide, warm, sterile water, or physiologic saline solution may be used with gentle persistence. After cleansing, the lip should be gently dried and a protective covering applied. This covering may be a ribbon of antibiotic ointment or a small piece of petrolatum gauze left on the lip.

Babies who have had a cleft lip repair need to be cuddled and held, not only because crying endangers their surgery but also because they are very young, cannot suck, and need the psychological support cuddling affords. Parents should be encouraged to hold their child and, as soon as possible, participate in feeding and giving other care. The gavage tube is usually removed about the third day after surgery. The infant is first fed with a rubber-tipped medicine dropper to the corner of the mouth, then graduated to other devices, and finally, when sucking is allowed, to a soft nipple.

The cleft palate repair is more complex than that of the cleft lip. It may involve a series of successive operations. After surgery the child may be gavaged for several days, or fed from a cup or side of a spoon. Nothing should be introduced into the mouth that might endanger the suture line. Unless a child is old enough to understand and cooperate, the arms must be restrained. The diet progresses from clear liquid to full liquid to soft foods over a period of about 1 week. The mouth should be rinsed with water after each feeding.

The problems of the child with a cleft lip or palate, or both, are so complex that they often

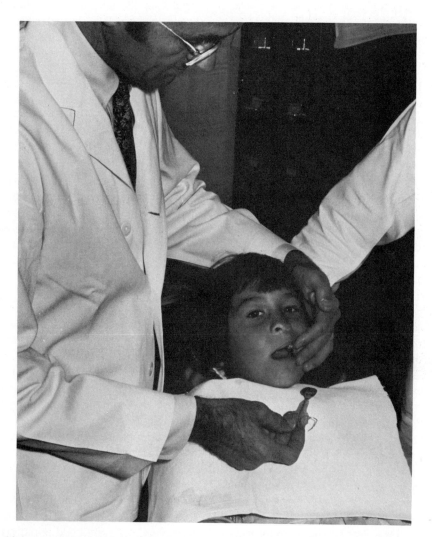

Fig. 14-4. An orthodontist fits this girl with a dental prosthesis to cover her palate and replace the missing front teeth.

require the combined services of the pediatrician, plastic surgeon, orthodontist (Fig. 14-4), speech therapist, child psychiatrist, and medical social worker. Parents play an important role in the child's care. They may need help to overcome their feelings about the child's defect and to be able to help the child develop to maximum potential.

Esophagus, stomach, and small intestine

Esophageal atresia and tracheoesophageal fistula. One of the more common abnormalities of the gastrointestinal tract is a condition in which the upper segment of the esophagus ends in a blind pouch and the lower portion is connected to the trachea by a tube (fistula). Obviously, such a gross defect must be discovered early before formula is fed in large amounts, because it would go directly into the lungs instead of the stomach. Any unusual choking, sputtering, or cyanosis at the time of the first water feeding should be reported at once.

When an esophageal atresia is suspected, all feedings are stopped. The child is suctioned and oxygen is administered for cyanosis. If the physician makes a positive diagnosis, surgery is performed as soon as possible. Where there is sufficient tissue, the two segments of the esophagus are sewn together in what is called *end-to-end anastomosis*. If there is insufficient tissue, a section of the colon may be transplanted to connect the esophageal stump to the stomach. A *gastrostomy* may then be performed, in which a tube is inserted through an opening in the abdominal wall to the stomach through which the child can be fed until the repair heals. A tracheostomy may also be performed.

After surgery, the infant is placed in an incubator with high humidity. Intravenous fluids, blood, and antibiotics are administered. After the immediate postoperative period, gastrostomy feedings are begun. The infant may be given a pacifier to suck during the feeding as an aid to relaxation and experiencing normal sensations.

The formula is allowed to run slowly into the stomach. When possible, the infant should be held quietly for a time after feedings. Special care should be given the skin around the gastrostomy opening, including cleansing and application of a thick ointment. As soon as possible, oral feedings are begun to reduce the degree of stricture at the operative site. When they prove successful, the gastrostomy tube is removed and the wound is allowed to heal. The tracheostomy tube is also removed when no longer needed. Dilation of the operative site may be necessary at a later time if strictures develop.

Esophageal stenosis. Esophageal stenosis is a narrowing of the lumen of the esophagus caused by a congenital defect or as a result of scars from ingestion of caustic poisons or postoperative tightening after corrective surgery. The child must undergo periodic dilation by catheters, or the narrowed area may have to be removed surgically (resected) and the ends joined together or a colon transplant inserted.

Foreign body ingestion. Children, particularly toddlers, are insatiably curious. Because their experience in life to that age has been centered about their mouths, it is only natural that curious items are placed there for testing, including such things as coins, small rocks, bits of dirt, bugs, pieces of glass, and safety pins. Most of these objects make the journey through the child's alimentary canal without incident. Sharp or irregular shaped ones, however, may not fare as well and may cut through (perforate) the canal wall. If there is a possibility that a child has swallowed such an object, feeding large amounts of bread or potatoes is of doubtful value and administering laxatives is dangerous. The abdomen should *not* be palpated. Most physicians take a conservative approach to such situations. If the object is metal, it can be followed from day to day with x-ray films. Surgery is performed only when the object appears to have become lodged in one place and when other symptoms indicating perforation develop. All stool should be saved, placed in a sieve, and run through with forced water. When the object is retrieved, the child is no longer in danger.

Congenital pyloric stenosis. Congenital pyloric stenosis is a rather common condition consisting of an abnormal narrowing of the pyloric sphincter, which forms the exit of the stomach, causing progressive vomiting and nutritional disorders in the infant. The narrowing is caused by spasm of the pyloric sphincter and overgrowth (hypertrophy) of the circular muscle fibers of the pylorus. The symptoms usually appear after the infant is 2 weeks old and before 2 months of age. It occurs more commonly in some family lines and in first-born males.

At first the vomiting is mild, but it becomes progressively more forceful until it is projectile. The vomitus does not contain bile but may contain mucus and streaks of blood. As the situation persists, the child loses weight and begins to show signs of dehydration, electrolyte imbalance, and malnutrition. Because little of the feeding is retained, the infant is always hungry and will take formula immediately after vomiting, only to vomit again. The physician makes the diagnosis on the basis of the history, x-ray studies with barium, and physical examination. A hard, olive-shaped mass can be felt (the hypertrophied pylorus) in the upper abdomen, and left-to-right peristalsis can be seen as the stomach tries to force its contents into the duodenum. When this proves ineffective, the peristaltic waves are reversed and emesis results. Without treatment the infant may go into convulsions from alkalosis and reduced blood calcium and eventually die from starvation.

Treatment for pyloric spasm alone consists of administering antispasmodic drugs such as atropine 15 minutes before specially prepared feedings. Phenobarbital may also be given. Feedings consist of precooked cereal added to formula to make it very thick and more difficult to vomit. These feedings are offered at frequent intervals. Vomited feedings are refed to preserve lost electrolytes and enzymes. A constant watch must be kept over the child's electrolytes, general well-being, and weight gain until the child has outgrown the condition.

Although the medical treatment as just described may be used for pyloric spasm, few physicians recommend it for pyloric stenosis because as the infant's condition worsens, the danger from operation increases. If an operation is performed early, the prognosis is excellent.

The surgical procedure most often used for pyloric stenosis is called the Fredet-Ramstedt operation, or a *pyloromyotomy*. The surgeon cuts down through the enlarged muscle of the pylorus to, but not into, the mucous membrane. Doing so relieves the constriction and enlarges the lumen.

Postoperative care consists of observing the surgical dressing for drainage and keeping it dry from urine. Oral feedings of dilute formula are introduced in small amounts, with the infant held in a nearly upright position. Gradually the amount and concentration of formula are increased. If too much is given too fast, it may lead to vomiting and strain on the suture line. Any postoperative vomiting should be reported at once. Intravenous fluids are discontinued as soon as the oral intake is sufficient and the child's condition warrants it. Complete relief of symptoms and dramatic improvement follow successful surgical repair.

Hiatal (diaphragmatic) hernia. During the eighth to tenth week of fetal life the diaphragm forms between the thoracic and abdominal cavities. The esophagus and great vessels pass through openings in the diaphragm. If these openings are too large, they may allow the stomach and other abdominal organs to protrude through them into the chest. When the infant is born, severe respiratory impairment may be present, necessitating immediate repair of the defect. If the defect is small, it may not be immediately evident. The upper, cardiac end of the stomach may slide back and forth through the opening, producing a backward flow (reflux) of stomach contents, a condition called *chalasia*.

The infant then may regurgitate the contents. Until surgical repair is scheduled, after feedings the infant should be held upright or placed in an infant seat.

Immediate postoperative care includes intravenous fluids and gastric suction to prevent abdominal distention. By the second or third day, feedings are begun by gavage and continued until the infant is less likely to swallow air while sucking and thus cause abdominal distention. The surgical dressing should be kept dry and the infant held whenever possible. With modern surgical techniques, the prognosis is excellent.

Meckel's diverticulum. During the embryonic development of a baby, a duct joins the intestine with the umbilicus, leading to the yolk sac, which temporarily provides nourishment for the developing child. In the normal course of events, the duct closes long before birth. In a small percentage of persons, however, the duct remains open or partially so, causing a variety of difficulties. Sometimes a fistula remains between the ileum and the umbilicus. More often, a blind pouch similar to an appendix remains. It may be ½ to 3 inches in length and may be lined with secreting gastric mucosa. If these secretions become blocked from the ileum, ulceration may result, with perforation, massive hemorrhage, and peritonitis. Diagnosis of a Meckel's diverticulum is usually not made unless emergency surgery is performed for perforation and hemorrhage. Then the defect is discovered. Treatment during and after surgery consists of blood transfusions, gastric suction, and comprehensive care, just as for other abdominal surgery.

Malabsorption (celiac) syndrome. There are a number of quite different conditions related to the poor absorption of foodstuffs in the body that produce similar symptoms. Because the outstanding symptom is a large protruding abdomen, or celiac distention, the group of symptoms is called *celiac syndrome*. Other typical symptoms in the syndrome include wasted extremities and buttocks, large foul-smelling stool, anorexia, pallor, and an irritable disposition. The

two most common pediatric disorders that manifest the celiac syndrome are gluten-induced enteropathy (also called sprue or idiopathic celiac disease) and cystic fibrosis of the pancreas.

Celiac disease (gluten-induced enteropathy). Celiac disease is believed to be caused by an inborn error of metabolism, an allergic-like reaction, or an enzyme defect. The child cannot ingest the gluten or protein portions of wheat or rye flour and sometimes cannot tolerate a protein in cow's milk. The child appears normal at birth but by late infancy begins to exhibit the celiac syndrome, which may last to the fifth year of life. There are characteristic episodes of diarrhea with anorexia, severe abdominal distention, loss of weight, and increased irritability. A "celiac crisis" may be precipitated by a mild upper respiratory infection or emotional upset during which the child vomits and has severe diarrhea. The resultant dehydration and acidosis may cause death if treatment with parenteral fluids and electrolytes is not administered promptly. The child's stools reflect the condition. When the child is acutely ill, the stools are foul-smelling, frothy, bulky, pale colored, and have a high fat content. Between acute episodes the stools become formed and normal in color.

Treatment consists of control of the diet, prevention of intercurrent infection, and psychological support. The diet must exclude all wheat and rye gluten and must limit fats. If the child cannot tolerate cow's milk, this too must be excluded from the diet. The child's caloric needs must be met, however, as well as the need for proteins, carbohydrates, vitamins, and minerals. Simple sugars are permitted, but starches are not. In the hospital, the nurse must work very closely with the dietitian and physician in observing and recording the child's reaction to different foods and the amount taken. With each new food added to the diet, the nurse should note the nature of the stool, the child's behavior, and the degree of abdominal distention that follows.

Skilled nursing care is needed for the child during the diagnostic period and subsequent acute episodes. Not only must the nurses make important observations about the child's food intake, they must also pay special attention to good hygiene because the child is anemic, malnourished, and easily susceptible to infections. The child perspires freely and must be kept dry. Because of an ungainly shape the child may not be able to move about freely and so must be turned periodically and given special skin care. While caring for the child, the nurse should take the opportunity to teach the parents.

The home care of the child with celiac disease is difficult. The parents may need special help in coping with their frustrations as well as understanding those of the child. The child is uncomfortable and hungry, yet cannot eat. The child is weak, unable to participate in normal activities, and, quite naturally, irritable. Normal development is impaired. During periods of acute illness the child may regress to younger emotional responses. The child's diet is a major concern. The parents should be given a list of permitted foods and warned to read the small print on the labels of prepared foods to avoid giving the child any of the forbidden proteins. The good services of a dietitian should be available to help the parents plan the child's diet. The physician may recommend regular visits by a community health nurse to provide general supervision and encouragement for the family.

The mortality from celiac disease is low, because of better understanding of electrolyte imbalance, use of parenteral fluids, dietary management, and control of infections by antibiotics. Although there is no cure for the disease, the symptoms decrease as the child grows older with fewer and fewer periods of worsenings (exacerbations) and longer periods of improvement (remissions).

Cystic fibrosis (mucoviscidosis). Cystic fibrosis (CF) is a congenital disease inherited as a recessive trait that follows Mendel's law of inheritance (see Chapter 2). Only infants who receive a CF gene from both parents manifest symptoms. Their parents may not know they are carriers of the disease. According to statistical averages, one fourth of the children of such parents will have cystic fibrosis. Only a few years ago the disease was considered rare and fatal but is now recognized as occurring once in every 1,000 live births. A variety of respiratory and digestive symptoms that were once thought to be caused by other conditions are now recognized as cystic fibrosis. More and more of these children are surviving to adulthood as a result of improved diagnostic methods and treatment. Symptoms of the disease vary from mild to severe. Respiratory involvement is present in almost all cases and digestive and nutritional problems in 80% of the cases.

The disease is caused by widespread dysfunction of the outward-secreting (exocrine) glands of the body, causing the sweat glands to produce unusually salty sweat and the mucous glands to secrete thick, gluey mucus that clogs the tiny bronchioles of the lungs and stops up the ducts of the pancreas and other organs of the body. The new name for the disease, mucoviscidosis, is derived from this characteristic. The older name, "cystic fibrosis of the pancreas," described the fibrous scarring that occurs in the pancreas when the tiny ducts are blocked. The disease continues to be called cystic fibrosis in common usage.

Digestive and nutritional involvement. In the child with cystic fibrosis, thick secretions block the ducts of the pancreas, intestinal glands, intrahepatic bile ducts, gallbladder, prostate, and sublingual salivary glands so that material from these glands cannot be released. In 5% to 10% of the cases, a serious complication occurs soon after birth called *meconium ileus*. In this condition, the already sticky meconium is even more thick and gluelike because of the absence of normal pancreatic digestive enzymes. The abnormal stool sticks to the walls of the ileum like paste and obstructs the lower digestive tract. The infant's abdomen becomes distended and no stool is passed. Vomiting and dehydration may follow. Emergency surgery must be performed to relieve the obstruction. Any newborn infant who does not pass stool within 24 hours after birth should be reported and evaluated for possible obstruction.

Whether or not the child who has cystic fibrosis develops meconium ileus, the blocked digestive juices soon cause a typical celiac syndrome. The stools become bulky, foul, and fatty, and a falling-out of the rectum (rectal prolapse) frequently occurs. The child develops a potbelly caused by putrefaction of non-absorbed protein and, despite a voracious appetite, fails to gain weight or to grow normally. Symptoms of vitamin deficiency and malnutrition appear. Without intensive nutritional help, prognosis is very poor.

The aim of therapy is to improve and maintain the nutrition status, to improve eletrolyte balance, and to prevent and control pulmonary infections. The cooperation and understanding of treatment by parents is essential.

The treatment of children with digestive involvement is tailored to the individual age and condition as follows: (1) high-protein, high-calorie, low-to-moderate-fat diet to compensate for poor food absorption; (2) supplementary vitamins, particularly the fat-soluble ones, A, D, E, and K, because of impaired fat digestion; and (3) pancreatic enzymes including lipase, protease, and amylose, given whenever food is eaten, at meals or snacks, because the child cannot supply them and they are necessary for the digestion of foods.

Respiratory involvement. The mucous glands of the tracheobronchial tree and upper respiratory tract secrete an excessive amount of mucus that is five to six times as thick as that of a person without cystic fibrosis (Fig. 14-5). This mucus is not eliminated in the normal way but accumulates in the air passages. A condition called *emphysema* develops, in which air can enter during inspiration but is trapped when the diameters of the bronchioles decrease during expiration. When air cannot move in or out, atelectasis (collapsed air sacs) develops. This lung involvement may progress through larger and larger channels of the tracheobronchial tree until whole segments of bronchi are impacted with mucus. Infection then invades the tissue. The capacity of the lungs to remove carbon dioxide from the body is reduced and respiratory acidosis results. Damage to the bronchial lining may occur, causing bronchiectasis, which may then progress to a serious congestion of the lung, right heart failure, and death. Pulmonary involvement is the cause of death in 90% of patients having cystic fibrosis.

Treatment of the patient with pulmonary involvement is highly individualized and is directed toward thinning the thick secretions, preventing infections, and strengthening heart action when it is failing. The child sleeps in a mist tent in which a solution of various mucus-thinning and tissue-shrinking medications is nebulized. As the child breathes, the mist enters the respiratory tract and does its work. "Clapping" is an important part of therapy. It is performed by placing the child in 16 different positions, and in each position the chest is clapped, then vibrated, and then the child coughs up the loosened mucus (Fig. 14-6). A child under 3 years of age may not be able to cough up the mucus. Tracheal suctioning with a catheter is then necessary after each position. Older patients may be able to give their own physical therapy by using a vibrating machine equipped with a rheostat to control the strength and frequency of vibrations. Whenever possible a family member, and eventually the patient, is taught to operate the inhalation equipment and to give the physical therapy so that the patient may be cared for at home.

Sweat, salivary, and lacrimal gland involvement. Although there are no pathological changes in the cells of the sweat, salivary, and lacrimal glands, all cystic fibrosis patients produce secretions abnormally high in salts (electrolytes). Because of this secretion, additional salt should be added to the diet each day. Excessive salt loss without replacement causes vomiting, vascular collapse, high fever, coma, and death. The characteristic of patients having cystic fibrosis to pro-

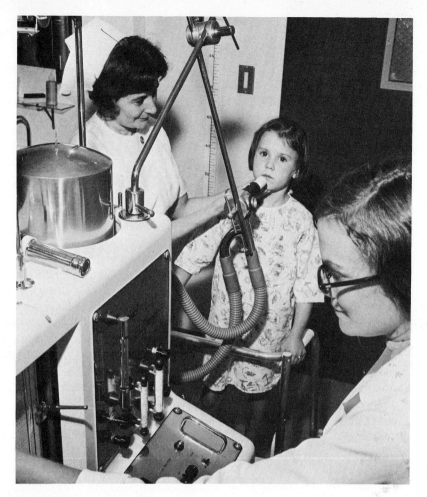

Fig. 14-5. Pulmonary function testing of a child with cystic fibrosis helps the doctors evaluate the degree of respiratory involvement. (Courtesy Children's Hospital Medical Center, Oakland, Calif.)

A

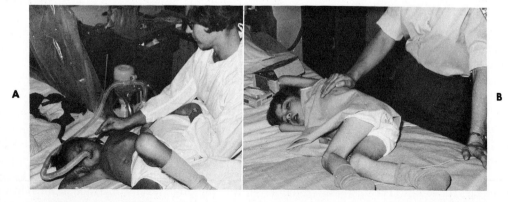

B

Fig. 14-6. Physical therapy of the child with cystic fibrosis consists of clapping the child's chest (note cupped hand in **A**) and vibration (**B**) in two of sixteen positions, after which the child coughs up the loosened mucus.

duce excessively salty sweat provides a valuable diagnostic test for cystic fibrosis. Of several methods in use to stimulate and collect sweat for chemical analysis, the pilocarpine iontophoresis technique is the most reliable and safest and can be used during the first few days of life. (See the diagnostic tests in Chapter 9.)

Prognosis. Outlook differs for each patient because of the degree of response to treatment. Most deaths result from severe pulmonary complications and lack of adequate treatment. Recent experience has shown that with early diagnosis and immediate, intensive care, prognosis can be greatly improved. Although there is no cure for the disease, more and more of these children are going to school, living relatively normal lives, and looking forward to adulthood.

Nursing care. Nursing care of the child with cystic fibrosis is vital to survival, both in the hospital and at home. It is adjusted to individual needs.

When there is digestive involvement, skin care is important. The rectal area must be kept clean and ointment applied to reduce irritation from the bulky stools. The size, color, consistency, and odor of the stools are recorded. Rectal prolapse, of course, requires special care. Soiled linens should be removed from the room. Air deodorants may be helpful. Nutrition should be maintained by a high-calorie, high-vitamin diet with supplemental enzymes and extra fluids.

Children with respiratory involvement are maintained in a mist tent with regular inhalation therapy and tracheal suctioning. They must be encouraged to eat and protected from exposure to infections. Every effort should be made to meet their emotional and social needs.

Few chronic diseases impose greater burdens on families, emotionally, socially, and financially. To add to the burden, cystic fibrosis often strikes more than one child in a family. The nurse and social worker can help the family by teaching, understanding, encouragement, and referral to various public agencies. Genetic counseling is especially important for parents of a child with the disease if they plan to have additional children.

A number of community resources are available to help these families. particularly the National Cystic Fibrosis Research Foundation, which provides a great variety of services to both parents and health workers.

Large intestine

Intussusception. Intussusception is the telescoping of one part of the bowel into another. This abnormal condition obstructs the lumen of the bowel, disturbs circulation, and results in gangrene and perforation. Although there may be a lead point such as Meckel's diverticulum or an outgrowth of tissue (polyp), intussusception usually occurs for no known reason. The most common site is at the ileocecal valve (Fig. 14-1). Intussusception is one of the most frequent causes of intestinal obstruction in infants and toddlers.

The onset is usually sudden. A previously healthy infant screams out in pain, drawing the legs up to the abdomen. At first the pains are periodic and the infant relaxes between them, but the pain becomes progressively more severe and continuous. Vomiting occurs, first of the contents of the stomach, then of bile-stained matter, and finally of fecal matter. Diarrhea stools may be followed by a bloody mucoid discharge called *currant-jelly stools*, after which no more fecal matter is passed. At first the infant is restless and then prostrate. The temperature may go up to 108°F. with dehydration and shock. A sausage-shaped mass can be felt at the site of the intussusception.

Diagnosis is made on the basis of the physical examination, history, and barium enema. Sometimes the intussusception is reduced by the pressure of the inflowing enema during fluoroscopic examination. Most cases, however, require surgery, during which the surgeon inspects the site and either reduces the intussusception manually or resects the damaged intestine.

After surgery, the infant is maintained on parenteral fluids for several days with gastrointestinal suction to prevent distention and promote healing. Accurate measurement of the drainage is important. Any sudden changes in the vital signs such as pulse rate or temperature may indicate peritonitis and should be reported immediately. As the infant recovers, the suction is stopped and oral feedings are begun cautiously. The infant may be given a pacifier to suck and held to provide the necessary security.

Appendicitis. Appendicitis is an inflamation of the lining of the appendix, the worm-shaped appendage at the base of the cecum. It may be initiated by a fecal obstruction or an infestation of pinworms. Although rare in infancy, the incidence increases during the school years and adolescence.

The chief complaint is abdominal pain, often in the umbilical area, with restlessness, vomiting, low-grade fever, diarrhea, or constipation. The white blood cell count is elevated. If the appendix is removed before it ruptures, recovery is usually prompt and uneventful. But delay, or the dangerous practice of giving laxatives, may result in rupture with the serious complication of peritonitis. Diagnosis is difficult because abdominal pain is also the chief symptom of a wide variety of other conditions, including encephalitis, measles, pneumonia, and urinary tract infection. The physician must take a careful history and make a complete physical examination to establish the diagnosis, because abdominal surgery is never undertaken indiscriminately.

Appendectomy is performed as soon as diagnosis is established. Preoperatively all oral food and fluids are withheld, intravenous fluids and antibiotics may be ordered, and fever-reducing measures are commenced if needed. Uncomplicates surgery is relatively simple and recovery rapid and uneventful.

If the appendix ruptures, generalized peritonitis results. Fever may be high, the abdomen boardlike and painful. Surgery may be delayed until the child's condition improves as a result of parenteral fluids, antibiotics, and cooling measures. Gastric suction may be initiated to relieve abdominal distention and prevent vomiting. At the time of surgery, drains may be placed in the wound and drainage may be considerable. Intravenous feedings may be continued for several days and only ice chips allowed by mouth. Output, including that removed by gastric suction, should be measured accurately. Modern drug and fluid therapy, together with good nursing care, give these patients a good chance of recovery.

Megacolon (Hirschsprung's disease). Megacolon, or large colon, was first described by the Danish physician Hirschsprung in 1880. It is a condition that occurs when there is a congenital lack of intestinal muscle nerve ganglia in the rectal and sigmoid segments of the bowel. As a result, the normal peristaltic action is absent and fecal matter accumulates above the flaccid segment. Symptoms appear early in infancy. The colon becomes increasingly distended and the abdomen progressively enlarged. The child never has normal, intermittent passage of formed stool; instead, the child passes small constipated or liquid stool or may have severe episodes of diarrhea and vomiting.

Diagnosis is made on the basis of the history, palpation of the distended abdomen, rectal examination that reveals an empty rectum, and barium enema that shows a typical picture of a normal rectum and sigmoid but a greatly dilated colon above the obstruction. Biopsy of the rectal muscle wall shows an absence of nerve ganglia.

The only permanent treatment is surgical excision of the aganglionic segment of the bowel, but in children under 1 year of age a temporary colostomy may be performed. Before surgery, enemas are necessary. Absorption of enema fluid from the dilated colon may produce severe water intoxication; therefore, physiologic saline solution (1 teaspoon per 1 pint of water) should be used rather than tap water. A low-residue diet may be ordered to reduce the amount of fecal waste.

Postoperatively the child is fed parenterally and gastric suction maintained until healing takes place. For the infant with a temporary colostomy, care is taken to protect the tender skin around the abdominal opening. For the child who has had a section of the bowel removed and the end anastomosed to the anal canal, the anal sphincter may need to be dilated daily. The presence of bowel sounds and normal stools indicates success and recovery.

In acquired megacolon, or pseudomegacolon, the colon is also distended and full of feces, but the cause is psychic rather than physical. The child resists the normal urges to defecate until the rectum becomes so full that anal control may be inadequate and fecal soiling results. The condition does not develop until after 3 years of age and may be related to severe toilet training. Both the child and the parents need psychiatric help as well as assistance in establishing regularity by means of habit, diet, and bowel-softening drugs.

Parasitic infestations. A parasite lives in or on the body of another living thing. Some common parasites that infest humans are bacteria, one-celled animals called protozoa, plants such as fungi, and insects and worms. Not all parasites cause disease; in fact, the bacteria that normally inhabit the bowel are necessary for health. Among those that do produce disease, bacteria are usually grouped separately. Other parasites are classified according to the body system they most often infest or according to their biological classification.

Intestinal parasites are those that at some stage in their life cycle infest the gastrointestinal tract. The source of infection is often fecal contamination but also may be the uncooked flesh of infected fish or animals, infected plants, or water. Intestinal parasites flourish where there is unhygienic disposal of human excreta, inadequate cooking of food, human crowding, and poverty. They are a worldwide public health problem. This text mentions only the most common of the many varieties that affect children.

Ameba. An infestation of the protozoa *Entamoeba histolytica* is known as *amebiasis*. If severe diarrhea is produced, the condition is called *amebic dysentery*. If the amebas invade the liver, hepatic amebiasis results. Mild amebic colitis may also occur. Some form of amebiasis is found in 1% to 40% of the population in the United States and in some tropical areas it may be greater than 50%. Infection is acquired by the ingestion of encysted amebas in contaminated food or drink. In the small intestine, the cysts break open and the active form, or trophozoites, are expelled. There they multiply by simple division unless limited by the resistive powers of the host. In the colon and rectum they invade the mucosal lining, causing irritation, bleeding, ulceration, and sometimes perforation. They may enter the bloodstream and invade the liver, form abscesses, and spread to the lungs, heart, brain, and other organs. The symptoms produced depend on the extent of the infection. Some children have few or only intermittent symptoms. They may be troubled by abdominal pain, bouts of constipation followed by diarrhea, nausea, and malaise. More severe symptoms are bloody, mucoid stools; fever; vomiting; and dehydration. When the liver is involved, the patient becomes seriously ill with intermittent fever, jaundice, sweats, and weight loss. When the heart and other organs are involved, their functions are seriously impaired and the child becomes critically ill.

When a patient is infected with amebas, some of the trophozoites and cysts are expelled in the feces to carry on their life cycle in other hosts. Carriers of amebic dysentery are an important source of the disease, especially when they are food handlers. Diagnosis is made of both carriers and persons with symptoms by finding the cysts or the trophozoites in their warm stool. Sigmoidoscopy may reveal lesions in the mucous lining of the colon.

The objective of treatment is to eradicate all amebas from all affected tissue. Patients with acute amebic dysentery are treated with specific drugs such as emetine hydrochloride, followed by tetracycline and other potent chemotherapeutic agents. A daily emollient retention enema may be given to promote healing of the ulcerated bowel. Bed rest; high-protein, low-residue diet; supplementary vitamins; parenteral fluids; and whole blood may be ordered. Patients with liver and other organ involvement are given intensive courses of drugs and bed rest. Liver abscesses may be drained. Symptomless carriers are identified by stool examination and given intensive drug therapy. In each case, all family members should be treated. An individual is considered "cured" when at least three stool examinations have been found negative. When possible, stool examination should be repeated 1, 3 and 6 months after treatment.

Tapeworms. Tapeworms are segmented flatworms. Human beings are infected with tapeworms of cattle, pigs, fish, and *Cyclops* (a minute freshwater shellfish). A typical tapeworm consists of a *scolex*, or head, with hooks and suckers for attachment and a series of segments that vary in number from a few to several thousand. New segments, called *proglottids*, bud off the scolex so that a worm is actually a linear colony consisting of immature, mature, and ripe proglottids. Adults live in the intestine of their host. The ripe proglottids break off and pass out of the feces. On disintegration the eggs develop into minute six-hooked *oncospheres*, which, when ingested by an intermediary host, migrate to the muscle tissue and develop into encysted larvae known as *bladderworms*. In the case of the fish, pork, and beef tapeworm, humans become infected when they eat uncooked meat containing the encysted bladderworms. In the case of the *Cyclops*, a nonhuman mammal is the host to the adult tapeworms and the freshwater *Cyclops* is the host to the larval forms. When ingested by a human, the larvae migrate to the lymph nodes, muscles, or subcutaneous tissues, causing an inflamation called *sparganosis*.

A child who is the host to a tapeworm may have no symptoms or may have abdominal pain, dizziness, and diarrhea. The fish variety may cause bowel obstruction and pernicious anemia. Diagnosis is made by finding the eggs in the stool or the proglottids at the anus. Treatment consists of administering various drugs such as quinacrine hydrochloride and hexylresorcinol. Prognosis is usually good.

When sparganosis occurs, the only cure is surgical excision of the encysted worm.

Flukes. Flukes are parasitic worms with complex life cycles involving generations that live in snails, freshwater fish, and pond vegetation. The varieties that affect humans are grouped together according to the body organ they infest, as liver, lung, intestinal, and blood flukes. The sheep-liver fluke is found in sheep-growing countries across the world. In Africa, South America, and the Orient the blood fluke can be found in freshwater streams. It enters a new victim through the skin as the victim swims in infested water. A similar variety found in the United States produces a condition known as "swimmer's itch." Diagnosis is made according to the body system affected and the prevalence of the disease in the region. A number of potent drugs have been found to be effective against all of the flukes. Prevention consists of drinking only safe water and avoiding infested waters for swimming.

Hookworms. Hookworm infestation of children is common in warm, moist climates. The eggs are laid in the intestine of the host and expelled in the feces. They hatch in moist soil into larvae that burrow into the bare skin (usually feet) of a new host. The larvae migrate through the body in the blood and lymph vessels, find their way to the lungs, and crawl up the bronchi and trachea to a point from which they are swallowed. When they reach the intestine, they mature into adults and the cycle is repeated. Because the worms destroy blood cells, the infected child becomes anemic, listless, weak, and without resistance to disease. The abdomen may become distended and there may be blood in the stool (melena). Diagnosis is made by finding the immature eggs in the stool. Treatment includes specific drugs such as tetrachloreothylene and hexylresorcinol and various measures to counter the anemia, including supplementary iron, transfusion if necessary, and a high-protein, highly nutritious diet. Prevention of reinfection is difficult, especially in regions where the incidence is high. Shoes should be worn, infected persons treated, and human excreta processed to prevent contamination of water and food.

Trichinella spiralis. Infection with *Trichinella spiralis* is called trichiniasis or trichinosis. It occurs when a person ingests raw or inadequately cooked pork containing encysted larvae. The cyst wall is digested by the stomach and the freed larvae then penetrate the mucosa of the small intestine. Within 3 or 4 days the larvae mature sexually and mate, the males die, and the females burrow deeply into the intestinal wall, where they discharge young living larvae. The minute larvae enter the lymphatic and blood vessels and are carried to various tissues and organs of the body. Only the larvae that reach striated muscle tissue survive. There they become encysted and cause a myositis that eventually is followed by calcification of the cysts. Elsewhere in the body the larvae cause an inflammation but are destroyed by the body's protective mechanisms. In animals, the encysted larvae constitute the source of infection for the next host.

During the intestinal stage the victim may have nausea, vomiting and diarrhea, but the larvae are not usually found in the stool. Sudden onset of edema of the upper eyelids may signal the sytemic invasion of the larvae. There may be profuse sweating, fever, chills, muscle soreness, particularly of the respiratory muscles, and thirst. If the heart muscle is invaded, symptoms of heart failure may develop. Symptoms gradually subside and by the third month most of the muscle symptoms have disappeared. Prognosis is good in most cases. Treatment consists of bed rest, asperin for pain, and antibiotics for secondary infections of the lungs. Prevention is the best remedy. All fresh pork should be cooked thoroughly before being eaten. The most effective public health measure against this disease is adequate enforcement of laws requiring that all garbage fed to hogs be cooked.

Ascaris lumbricoides. Infestations of the giant round worms (6 to 15 inches long) called *Ascaris lumbricoides* occur commonly among children living in warm climates in poverty and squalor. The infective eggs are swallowed and hatch in the duodenum. The larvae then burrow into the intestinal wall and enter the blood and lymph vessels after which they are carried to the liver, heart, and lungs. In the lungs the larvae penetrate the air sacs, ascend the bronchial tree to the trachea, and are swallowed back down into the intestinal tract. In the small intestine, the now mature worms mate and the female lays eggs that are passed out in the stool to the soil where they mature and are ready to begin the cycle over again. The mature worms live on semidigested food in the child's digestive tract, traveling up and down and occasionally making an alarming appearance at either end. They may cause diarrhea, vomiting, pneumonia, intestinal obstruction, and even perforation. The child may become irritable or exhibit allergic reactions such as a skin rash. Diagnosis is made on finding the eggs in the stool or on seeing the worm emerge from the gastrointestinal tract. Treatment consists of various drugs such as piperazine or hexylresorcinol and general diet therapy to improve the child's nutritional state. Prognosis is good unless there are serious complications such as intestinal obstruction and perforation. Sanitary treatment of sewage, turning the top soil, and treatment of all cases is necessary if infestations of this parasite are to be halted.

Pinworms. *Enterobiasis*, or oxyuriasis, is perhaps the most common parasitic infection of children. It is caused by the small, white, threadlike pinworm known as *Enterobius vermicularis*. The pinworm eggs are ingested, or sometimes inhaled, and hatch in the intestine. They mature in the cecum, where they attach themselves to the mucosa by means of their "lips." Usually during the night the adult female becomes detached, migrates out of the bowel, and lays thousands of eggs in the folds of the anus and perineum. Occasionally, she migrates to the vagina, causing vaginitis in girls. The movement of the worm and the presence of eggs causes local irritation and itching. The child scratches the area, contaminates the fingers, becoming reinfected and infecting others. The interval between ingestion of the eggs and appearance of the female pinworm at the anus is about 6 weeks. There may be very few symptoms, or the anus and vagina may become severely irritated from scratching and secondary infection. The child often becomes irritable and restless. In large infestations, appendicitis may occur. Diagnosis is made on viewing the worms as they emerge from the anus, as they are inadvertently expelled on the surface of stool, or by obtaining the eggs from the anal folds. The Scotch tape test is a practical means of obtaining the eggs. During the night a nurse or parent (if done at home) goes to the bedside of the sleeping child and shines a light on the anal region. Sometimes the female worm can be seen. The nurse or parent then takes a piece of cellophane tape that has been fastened to a tongue blade sticky side out and presses it against the anal area where it picks up eggs. The sticky side of the tape is then placed downward on a slide and sent to the laboratory for examination.

Treatment is aimed at destroying all eggs and worms in all of the family members and infected playmates of the child. Without such treatment, reinfection is almost certain. Gentian violet tablets have been used effectively, but two drugs are now available—piperazine citrate (Antepar), a fruit-flavored syrup that is taken for 14 days, and pyrvinium pamoate (Povan), which may be given in a single dose. Parents should be warned that Povan causes the stool to become bright red in color, and if the child vomits while the medication is in the digestive tract, the vomitus will also be bright red. During the time that the rectal area is irritated, it should be cleansed frequently and a soothing ointment applied as ordered. The child's fingernails should be cut short and mittens or stockings worn during the night. Snug panties or diapers may also reduce the amount of scratching. Bed linens, towels, and clothing of infected persons should be washed in hot water or boiled to prevent infection, and toilet seats should be scrubbed after each use. In the hospital, strict isolation technique is used with special handling of the linens. Prevention lies in teaching good personal and group hygiene.

Diarrhea. Diarrhea is the passage of unformed stool. It is a symptom of many conditions and constitutes a serious threat to very young or debilitated persons because of the dehydration and electrolyte imbalance it produces. The nurse plays an important role in the diagnosis, treatment, and control of diarrhea. In recent years the number of deaths from diarrhea has been reduced with improved sanitation, refrigeration of foods, health education, medical understanding of its pathology, and facilities for treatment.

Diarrhea may be caused by infectious organisms that invade the intestinal tract, such as certain strains of *Escherichia coli*, staphylococci, salmonellas, shigellas, viruses, and amebas. It also may occur as a result of disorders affecting other parts of the body such as respiratory infections, allergic reactions, emotional stress, and generalized fever; or from dietary indiscretions, such as eating too many apricots; or from noninfectious diseases of the digestive tract such as celiac (malabsorption) syndrome; or from a parental fixation on bowel function to "clean out" their child with purgatives.

Diagnosis is directed toward finding the basic cause of the diarrhea, evaluating the child's electrolyte imbalance, and determining whether there are other complications. A history of how the diarrhea started and what factors might have precipitated it are of great importance. If the child's weight was known before the diarrhea began, a weight loss may indicate the degree of dehydration. The dehydrated child's skin is dry and has poor turgor; the face has a tense, anxious expression; the eyes are sunken and lack luster; the child is weak and may be feverish; the stools may be watery and expelled with force. In severe cases, the child may be acidatic and even in shock. Laboratory examination is made of the stool for blood, mucus, or organisms and of the blood to determine the relative cell count, chemical balance, or presence of organisms. In some cases x-ray examination of the chest or abdomen may be ordered to determine complicating diseases.

The body reacts to dehydration with mechanisms that temporarily help but are finally overtaxed. The blood becomes concentrated, arterioles constrict, blood pressure falls, blood flow becomes sluggish, and by the time the oxygen-laden red cells reach the capillaries they have given up their oxygen and have little left for the important metabolism of the cells. The oxygen-starved cells cannot do their job, and the result is incomplete metabolism of carbohydrates, leading to an accumulation of lactic acid and acidosis. Kidney function is hampered by the slow-flowing blood, and if dehydration continues, oliguria is followed by anuria. Normally the kidneys adjust urinary excretion of water and electrolytes to the needs of the body, but in severe dehydration the capacity of the kidneys to concentrate urine is impaired. Only through increasing the blood volume and blood flow will the cells again receive the sustenance they need to perform normally.

Treatment of diarrhea is twofold—correcting the dehydration and chemical imbalance of the body and curing the basic cause of the diarrhea. Because mild cases of diarrhea may become severe, no diarrhea should be ignored. Fortunately, most mild cases can be treated at home by conscientious parents. Children with moderate and severe cases are often hospitalized.

Mild diarrhea is characterized by several loose stools each day without evidence of other illness. There is no vomiting, fever, or weight loss. The stools may appear greenish from bile that has not had time to change color and there may be some mucus. Treatment is conservative. The infant is offered a commercial preparation called Pedialyte that contains electrolytes or dilute formula until the symptoms disappear. Any change in the child's condition should be reported promptly. Most mild diarrheas disappear spontaneously without further treatment.

In moderate diarrhea the child is sicker than in mild cases, has a fever, vomits a few times, may lose appetite, and be fretful, and may pass several loose to watery greenish stools that may be expelled forcibly with flatus and excoriate the buttocks. The child may lose some weight but signs of dehydration are not present. Treatment is modified according to the child's needs.

Severe diarrhea may begin as a mild or moderate case or may be severe from the start. The child is typically feverish, weak, and prostrate, has gassy expulsions of numerous watery stools, vomits, and rapidly develops signs of dehydration, acidosis, and shock. The child should be admitted to the hospital for intensive treatment and observation. All food and fluids may be withheld for varying periods of time to permit the bowel to rest. During the so-called starvation period, water, calories, and electrolytes are given parenterally. Drugs may be given for specific infectious diarrheas. When diarrhea is caused by *Shigella* or *Salmonella* organism, strict isolation technique is maintained. Special skin care to the excoriated buttocks and attention to the emotional needs of the child should be given. Temperature-reducing measures may be necessary. A careful record is kept of all fluids administered by any method, the frequency of voiding, the vital signs, a daily weight, and the frequency and description of the stools. As the child improves and the dehydration and diarrhea are reduced, dilute oral feedings are begun and gradually increased in both amount and concentration. The prognosis of these critically ill children depends on good medical management and conscientious nursing care.

Colon and rectum

Imperforate anus. During embryonic life, the membrane that separates the rectum and anus is normally absorbed, leaving an open, continuous canal. When this fails to occur, imperforate anus results (Fig. 14-7). It is the most common anomaly of newborn infants that is incompatible with life. The colon may end in a blind pouch, or an abnormal tube may form between the rectum and the perineum, called a rectoperineal fistula. A rectovaginal fistula may form in girls or a rectourethral fistula in boys. In these cases meconium may appear on the perineum, in the vagina, or in the urine. When there is no fistula, the infant develops abdominal distention and vomits. The anus may appear as a dimple or may look quite normal but end in a blind pouch. The observant nursery nurse may be the first one to note this abnormality.

The only treatment is surgery. When possible, an anoplasty is performed immediately and the anus and rectum are joined together. If the infant is weak or sick, the anoplasty may be delayed and a temporary colostomy made. In cases of abdominal distention and vomiting, it may be necessary to institute gastric suction before surgery. Postoperative nursing care consists of keeping the site of the anoplasty clean and dry. As the anoplasty heals, regular dilation of the anus may be necessary to prevent stricture. If a colostomy is performed, the skin around the wound must be kept clean and protected from excoriation. This may be accomplished by ap-

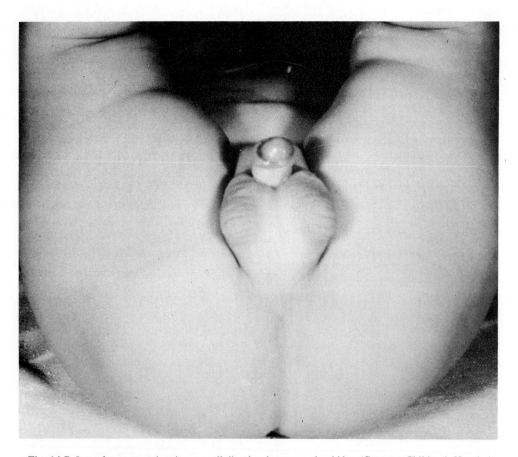

Fig. 14-7. Imperforate anus showing a small dimple where anus should be. (Courtesy Children's Hospital of the East Bay, Oakland, Calif.)

plying a thick pasty ointment such as zinc oxide and by using a folded diaper as an abdominal binder to hold the dressings in place rather than using adhesive straps. The prognosis of these children is good because of modern surgical techniques and good nursing care.

Rectal prolapse and procidentia. *Rectal prolapse* is the abnormal descent of the mucous lining of the rectum out through the anus. *Procidentia* is a descent of all of the tissue layers of the sigmoid and rectum out through the anus. Prolapse and procidentia occur most commonly in infants and toddlers who are malnourished and weak or have diarrhea or constipation. These conditions are precipitated by a sudden increase in internal abdominal pressure such as occurs with straining at defecation when the sphincter is relaxed and the muscles of the pelvic floor are weak. The protruding mass is bright red to dark purple, depending on the length of time it has been prolapsed and the degree to which circulation has been cut off, and it may protrude up to 6 inches. It may recede spontaneously the first few times it occurs but later may require manual replacement. Replacement is accomplished by placing the child's head lower than the body and pressing some toilet paper into the opening of the mass as it is pushed into place. The gloved finger is then quickly removed, leaving the toilet paper in the rectum. The paper becomes soft and is expelled later.

Treatment is aimed at correcting the underlying disorder, such as malnutrition, and in preventing repeated prolapse until the damaged tissue heals and muscle strength is restored. During this period, for prevention of prolapse, it may be necessary to hold the buttocks together manually during defecation and with adhesive tape between defecations. If these more conservative measures do not correct the problem, surgical repair may be required.

Ulcerative colitis. Ulcerative colitis is a chronic, inflammatory condition involving the mucous lining of the colon and rectum. The cause is not known, except that there seem to be emotional (psychogenic) factors in most cases. Part or all of the colon, and the ileum as well, may become involved. Small scattered ulcerations develop, enlarge, and gradually join to form a network that eventually denudes the mucosa, causing fibrosis and a decrease in colon size. The onset may be gradual or sudden and at any age, although it is rare before the age of 8 years. Typically, the stools are small and contain mucus, blood, and pus. Bouts of diarrhea with abdominal cramping may occur. Hemorrhage from the bowel and rectal prolapse are common complications. Appetite is poor; the child becomes listless, emaciated, and anemic and may develop vitamin deficiency symptoms.

There is no specific therapy. In some children, adrenocortical steroids produce impressive but temporary improvement. A soft, bland, low-residue diet with supplementary vitamins and minerals is ordered, but the child needs much encouragement to eat it. Psychotherapy is recommended for both the child and the family. Prognosis is poor. Continued medical supervision is important. When x-ray films of the colon reveal the typical "lead pipe" state of severe mucosal damage, complete surgical removal of the colon (colectomy) and a permanent ileostomy are performed. This drastic surgery is delayed as long as possible.

Hernias

A hernia is the protrusion of an organ or part of an organ through the wall of the cavity that normally contains it. Hernias are caused by a failure of certain normal openings to close during development or from an increase in intraabdominal pressure such as occurs during a cough or when lifting a heavy object. A *reducible* hernia is one in which the protruding organ can be replaced by manipulation. An *irreducible* hernia is one in which the organ is *incarcerated*, or trapped, so that it cannot be returned to its original position out of the hernia sac by manual methods. A *strangulated* hernia is an irreducible hernia so tightly constricted that the blood supply to the organ is cut off. Gangrene will result if circulation is not restored immediately. The most common types of hernias in children are the diaphragmatic hernia discussed earlier in this chapter, umbilical hernia, omphalocele, and inguinal and femoral hernias.

Umbilical hernia. During fetal life, the umbilical vessels pass out through an opening in the abdominal wall. Soon after birth these vessels normally shrivel, the peritoneum and connective tissues close, and the skin heals. If the connective tissue fails to close completely and a circular defect remains beneath the umbilicus, a hernia sac may form that is covered by skin and lined by peritoneum. Most small umbilical defects close spontaneously within the first or second year, but some of the larger ones persist. Surgical repair is needed for these larger ones, and immediate surgery is required for the rare cases when the bowel becomes incarcerated. A curved incision is made in the skin, the hernia sac is excised, and the connective tissue is brought together to cover the defect. The skin is then sutured, but the umbilicus is not removed because it is a normal feature of the abdomen. A pressure dressing is applied. Postoperatively, the child can be as active as desired. A normal diet and fluids are given. Care should be taken to keep the dressing clean and dry until it is removed by the surgeon. Once an umbilical hernia is repaired, it seldom recurs.

Omphalocele. The word *omphalocele* means "umbilical tumor or swelling." It is a herniation of abdominal viscera at the point where the umbilical cord connects to the abdomen because of a failure of the abdominal wall to develop during embryonic life. The infant is born with part or all of the abdominal viscera exposed, covered only by a thin transparent membrane. Sometimes this membrane ruptures before or during delivery. These infants often have other congenital defects.

At delivery, the omphalocele sac should be covered at once with sterile moist gauze to reduce drying and contamination by airborne bac-

teria. Immediate surgery may then be performed, whereby the skin that is present is brought together over the defect (see Fig. 11-2). Even with great care, infections are common and healing is often poor. A nonsurgical method of treatment has been found that has proved less hazardous, especially in cases of large omphaloceles or multiple anomalies. This treatment consists of repeated application of 2% Mercurochrome to the sac. A tough layer of scar tissue (eschar) forms, and over a period of weeks the defect is gradually closed, thus converting the omphalocele into a large ventral hernia which can be repaired at a later date. Because these infants are poor risks, expert nursing care is required.

Inguinal and femoral hernias. Inguinal hernias occur much more frequently in boys than in girls, and although the defect that causes them is present at birth, the actual herniation may occur at any age and may involve one or both sides (Fig. 14-8).

As the testis descends during embryonic life, a sac of peritoneum precedes it into the scrotum, forming a tube. After descent of the testis, the tube normally shrivels up (atrophies); however, if it does not close completely, peritoneal fluid or intestine may descend into it and produce a hernia. A collection of fluid in the sac is called a *hydrocele*. Such hernias vary in size, depending on how far they extend into the sac. In girls the anatomy is different but parallel, in that the inguinal canals are occupied by the round ligaments. An ovary or a loop of intestine may descend into the space.

A herniation of abdominal viscera into the openings created by the femoral vessels as they pass out of the abdomen into the thigh is known as a *femoral hernia*. This type of hernia is more common in girls than in boys and is caused by a sudden increase in intraabdominal pressure. The diagnosis and treatment of femoral hernia is similar to that of inguinal hernia.

When the hernial sac is empty, there are no symptoms. When the abdominal contents are in the sac, incomplete bowel obstruction occurs, casuing the infant to be fretful, lose appetie, and become constipated. If a loop of intestine becomes incarcerated in the sac, all the symptoms of intestinal obstruction appear. The infant becomes irritable, vomits, has a fever, and has a firm, irreducible swelling in the groin. If the hernia cannot be reduced by the physician within 12 hours after it occurs, emergency surgery is necessary. In severe cases in which the blood supply has been cut off from the incarcerated bowel, resection of that portion of bowel may be necessary. Incarceration occurs most frequently in the first 6 weeks of life in infants with inguinal hernia.

Diagnosis is made on the basis of a history of the intermittent appearance of a mass in the groin and on physical examination. Because such defects rarely close spontaneously, the danger of incarceration is great, and surgical repair (herniorrhaphy) is relatively safe for young children, it is planned as soon as a diagnosis is made. The surgical incision is usually made in a natural skin crease to reduce future strains, the collected fluid or herniated part is removed, the sac is tied off, and the connective tissue and skin are closed. The skin line sutures may be sealed with liquid collodion and allowed to dry without application of a dressing. The child usually recovers without incident. Every effort is made to keep the incision site dry. Diapers should not be pinned in place in the usual fashion for at least 24 hours; instead, they may be placed under the child.

If incarceration occurs before the surgical procedure, an ice bag should be applied to the area and the foot of the bed elevated. In cases of infants whose surgery must be delayed because of their poor general condition, various types of trusses may be used to temporarily reduce the hernia. One of the most common types is the yarn truss. To be of value, it must be applied so that it fits snugly and puts pressure on the site to prevent incarceration. The hernia must be kept reduced during truss changes, and the truss must be kept clean and dry. The skin under the truss should be checked frequently for excoriation. If

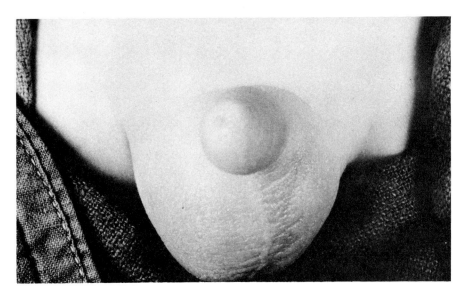

Fig. 14-8. Right inguinal hernia with a collection of fluid in the hernia sac called a hydrocele. (Courtesy Children's Hospital of the East Bay, Oakland, Calif.)

the child is to go home with a truss, the parents should be carefully instructed in its application and use.

Poisonings

A discussion of accidental poisoning, precautions, emergency care, and Poison Control Centers is found in Chapter 3. Fortunately, most children who have ingested poisons are treated successfully as outpatients in emergency rooms and sent home. Of those admitted to the hospital, the most common cases result from the ingestion of petroleum, caustics, salicylates, and lead. Because petroleum ingestion leads to pneumonia, it is discussed in Chapter 12. When caustics are ingested, they cause damage to tissue that may lead to esophageal stenosis, a condition discussed earlier in this chapter. The salicylates and

lead are poisons that cause generalized, systemic effects.

Salicylate poisoning. Of all the thousands of accidental poisonings of children, the salicylates are the most frequent cause. Aspirin, sodium salicylate, and oil of wintergreen are all forms of salicylate. They account for 17% of all deaths from poisons. These drugs are widely used, good tasting, and generally available in large quantities in easy-to-reach places in homes. Most persons do not realize their potential danger. One teaspoon of oil or wintergreen, given instead of cough syrup, contains as much salicylate as 60 grains of aspirin—a potentially fatal dose. Orange-flavored baby aspirin tastes and looks like candy, but to the child who eats too many of them they are lethal. Salicylates are absorbed quickly and excreted slowly. A small

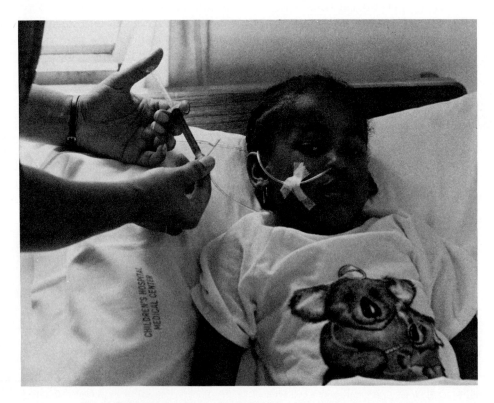

Fig. 14-9. Nasogastric tube is inserted into the stomach for lavage or feeding.

dose repeated too often may cause the drug to accumulate in the system and produce a serious state of poisoning.

The most common sign of salicylate poisoning is an increase in respiratory rate and depth (hyperpnea) and vomiting. Other symptoms of poisoning are restlessness, double vision, dizziness, tremors, high fever, profuse sweating, convulsions, delirium, cerebral hemorrhage, acute pulmonary edema, and coma. Death will follow if immediate steps are not taken to correct the serious acid-base imbalance of the child's body chemistry.

Emergency treatment is aimed at removing as much salicylate from the stomach as possible before it is absorbed. Such treatment means inducing vomiting and gastric lavage, (Fig. 14-9.) The child is admitted to the hospital for close observation and care. Blood specimens are taken periodically to determine the level of salicylate intoxication. Continued treatment is aimed at correcting the acid-base imbalance and removing and neutralizing the salicylates. Such treatments are accomplished by administration of parenteral fluids and calculated amounts of sodium bicarbonate. In more severe cases, *peritoneal dialysis* may be necessary to hasten the removal of salicylates. This is a process of introducing a neutralizing solution into the abdominal cavity where it remains for a period of time and is then removed.

Intense supportive nursing care is necessary. The nurse checks the vital signs every 15 minutes until stable and the pH of the urine is tested and the amount recorded hourly. This information is used by the physician in evaluating and directing the child's care. Fever is reduced with cool sponge baths. Close observation is maintained until the salicylate in the blood falls to safe levels, which may take 3 or 4 days in severe cases. The child remains in the hospital beyond this period for observation and convalescence.

Lead poisoning. Lead poisoning is most often seen in toddlers who live in old homes of the era in which lead pigment paints were widely used indoors. Lead paints are still used outdoors but seldom for indoor finishes and never by U.S. manufacturers of children's furniture and toys. Although lead may be taken into the body through the skin or inhaled into the lungs, in most cases the child ingests small amounts over a long period by chewing or sucking a painted or lead toy, crib rails, window sills, or furniture.

The symptoms develop slowly, except in rare cases of acute poisoning, and are the result of slow absorption of lead into the blood, soft tissue, central nervous system, and bone. Lead is excreted in the urine. The child loses an appetite and becomes irritable. Muscle coordination worsens and development slows. The child may have abdominal pain and intermittent vomiting. If these early symptoms go unnoticed, acute encephalitis may develop, with convulsions, stupor, and death.

Diagnosis is made on the basis of the symptoms, a history of exposure to lead, and confirmed by a 24-hour urine test. It is of great importance that *all* of the urine voided by the child during the test period be collected. This is the nurses' responsibility. X-ray films reveal a typical "lead line" at the end of the long bones where lead has been deposited. There is an excessive concentration of lead in the urine and blood. When encephalitis is present, cerebrospinal fluid pressure and protein levels are elevated.

The object of treatment is to stop further exposure to lead and to rid the child's tissues of lead. The child is hospitalized and an initial catharsis with magnesium sulfate (Epsom salt) may be ordered, followed by a course of the drug edathamil calcium disodium, which aids in the excretion of lead. The drug is usually given intravenously in 3- to 5-day periods, with intervals of 3 to 21 days between courses. To help the body rid itself of lead from the bones, calcium, phosphorus, and vitamin D may also be ordered. Infections and electrolyte imbalance are carefully controlled, because they slow lead excretion. When encephalitis is present with elevated intracranial pressure, hypothermy (lowering body temperature) or surgical decompression may be employed to reduce it.

Nursing care is supportive. Careful observations and recording of data are important. Input and output records are maintained. The child may be hospitalized for several weeks, a long period for a toddler, and the child's emotional needs should be supplied.

Prognosis is poor. About half of the affected children develop encephalitis and one fourth die. Of those who recover, many have permanent brain damage. Prevention is especially important because treatment is not highly successful. The public must be reminded continually of the dangers of lead-containing paints. Standards for the manufacture of safe toys should be promoted on an international level.

DISORDERS OF METABOLISM
Dwarfism and giantism

Dwarfism is stunted growth below normal averages. It occurs as a result of inheritance, as in the pygmies of certain regions, by tumors or disorders of the hypothalamic area of the brain, or from deficiencies in the anterior pituitary, thyroid, or sex glands. In pituitary dwarfism, the child grows at a normal rate for about the first 2 years; then growth slows and, although the child's proportions are normal, the features remain childlike (Fig. 14-10). Secondary sex characteristics fail to develop, and the dwarf remains a child in size and features. Diagnosis is made on the basis of retarded growth, blood plasma tests that indicate low levels of *somatotrophin*, the growth hormone, and reduced levels of 17-steroids in a 24-hour urine collection. Because the growth hormone is not available commercially, treatment is confined to supplying other hormones according to the child's age, sex, and needs. Testosterone and gonadotrophic hormone may be given to boys at about age 17 to induce puberty. Female hormones may be given to girls to induce menstruation although they remain infertile.

Giantism is accelerated growth above normal averages. Although there are certain families in which tallness is an inherited trait, most giantism is caused by the growth of a tumor in the pituitary gland, causing the gland to produce abnormal amounts of somatotrophin. As a result, the child grows rapidly and develops sexually far before normal. If a tumor develops after closure of the epiphyses of the bones, *acromegaly* occurs, a condition in which the facial bones, hands, and feet enlarge, creating a gorilla-like appearance. In the early stages of the tumor, the patient is alert and intelligent and may have increased sexual desire and potency. As the disease progresses, however, the patient becomes dull, easily fatigued, and weak. Their skin becomes coarse and oily, and there is sweating, muscular pain, and headaches. Hypothyroidism and hypogonadism may occur. Diabetes mellitus develops in 25% of the cases with varying degrees of blindness. Diagnosis is made on the basis of the abnormal growth and urinary tests for 17-ketosteroids and plasma somatotrophin, both of which are elevated. Surgical removal of the tumor is difficult and mortality high. Radiation is usually employed; it provides considerable success in arresting the disease and relieving the headaches. Various hormones such as adrenal steroids, thyroid, and estrogen may be ordered to relieve symptoms, but the prognosis is generally poor.

Hypothyroidism

One of the most common endocrine abnormalities in childhood is hypothyroidism. If the child is born with a deficiency, it is called *cretinism*; if the deficiency is acquired, it is called *juvenile hypothyroidism*. Cretinism is caused by an insufficiency of the thyroid gland resulting from embryonic defects, the effects of teratogenic agents, an inadequate intake of iodine, or the production of antithyroid antibodies. The infant appears normal at birth because of having been supplied from the mother's thyroid glands, but symptoms appear in a few weeks or months. Early signs include prolonged physiological jaundice and feeding problems. The infant is pale because of anemia. The infant is chronically constipated, has dry skin and a subnormal temperature and pulse, and develops an umbilical hernia because of poor abdominal muscle tone. The infant sleeps much and cries little, so may be called a "good baby." The infant has a peculiar appearance, with eyes far apart, swollen eyelids, flat nose, and an open mouth with a protruding tongue. The anterior fontanel does not close because of poor bone development, and normal eruption of teeth is delayed; those teeth that do appear decay rapidly. The child's neck is thick and short, the abdomen is enlarged, and the arms and legs are short. Physical, motor, mental, and sexual development is retarded.

Diagnosis is based on the history, physical examination, and laboratory tests. The basal metabolism rate is low; x-ray films of the bones show retardation; cholesterol levels in the blood are usually elevated. A reliable measure of thyroid function is the protein-bound iodine (PBI) level in the serum. Another test of thyroid function is the uptake of radioactive iodine by the thyroid gland as measured by radioactive scanning.

Treatment consists of giving the child desiccated (dried) thyroid in gradually increasing oral

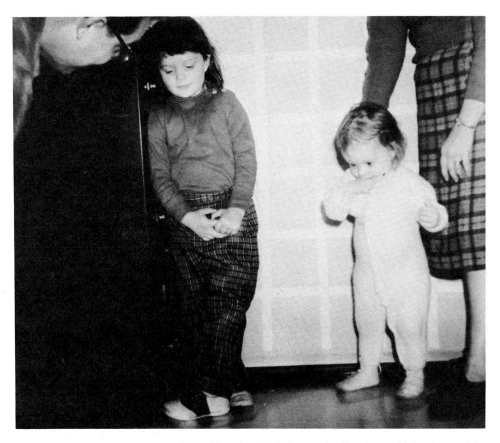

Fig. 14-10. Pituitary dwarfism. The little girl on the right is 4 years old. Her 5-year-old sister's growth is normal. (Courtesy Children's Medical Center, Oakland, Calif.)

doses to a maximum amount that does not produce symptoms of overdosage. This drug must be taken throughout life with increased doses at puberty and during pregnancy. In addition to thyroid, infants should receive added vitamin D in their diet to supply the extra needs caused by stimulated bone growth. Overdosage of thyroid causes rapid pulse, weight loss, vomiting, cramps, diarrhea, elevated temperature, and irritability. Nursing care involves careful observation for the symptoms. Good dental hygiene is of great importance to prevent further dental decay and loss. Children with permanent mental retardation and their parents need special help, so that full potential may be realized. Prognosis of untreated cases is poor—the child becomes a mentally retarded dwarf. The earlier and more effective the treatment, the better the prognosis. Even with treatment, there may be some mental retardation.

Diabetes insipidus

The word *diabetes* in Greek, means "a siphon." *Insipidus* means "lacking savor" or "being dilute." In diabetes insipidus the child passes great quantities of dilute urine and, as a result, is constantly thirsty. The disease is caused by one of the following two defects: (1) a deficiency of vasopressin, the antidiuretic hormone (ADH), as a result of damage or disease to the posterior pituitary gland where it is normally produced, or (2) an inherited defect in the ability of the kidneys to absorb water, called the "nephrogenic type." The diagnosis of *diabetes* is made on the basis of the symptoms of much urine (polyuria) and much thirst (polydipsia); the differential diagnosis of *insipidus* is made on the basis of urine tests showing a low specific gravity with no sugar or acetone. The nephrogenic type is diagnosed when it does not respond to treatment with ADH.

Vasopressin acts on the distal tubules of the kidneys to enhance water absorption (see Fig. 15-1). When this kidney action is inadequate, the child takes in large amounts of water to make up for that lost in the urine. The child who does not do so becomes severely dehydrated. The child becomes undernourished and irritable because of constant thirst and the need to urinate, which interfere with normal rest and appetite.

Treatment for patients with vasopressin deficiency is the lifetime administration of regular doses of the commercially prepared hormone. Prognosis is good when early diagnosis is made and when dehydration does not occur. Prognosis of children with the nephrogenic type is poor. Many die in infancy from severe dehydration. Those who survive are often physically underdeveloped and mentally retarded.

Diabetes mellitus

The word *mellitus*, in diabetes mellitus, means "honey-sweet." This disease is characterized by sugar passing through the body without being used. It is caused by a deficiency in insulin, the hormone produced in the pancreas by the *beta* cells of the islets of Langerhans. Insulin acts to accelerate the transfer of glucose through cell membranes where it can be metabolized. The disease is inherited as a recessive trait, but symptoms may appear at any age during the lifetime. In about 5% of the cases, symptoms appear during childhood. When this happens, the disease is called *juvenile diabetes* and is more serious and difficult to treat than when symptoms first appear in adult life.

In diabetic persons, sugar is absorbed in a normal fashion from the digestive tract into the bloodstream. Without insulin, however, sugar (glucose) cannot pass into the cells, and so it remains in the bloodstream, a condition called *glycosemia*. In the kidneys, some of the glucose spills over into the urine, causing *glycosuria*. To excrete the glucose, the body needs more water. As a result, the child becomes thirsty, drinks large amounts of water, and so produces great quantities of urine. Because the body is not able to use the carbohydrates it digests, the child may have an increased appetite.

When the body does not have enough glucose

to use for heat and energy or to convert to glycogen for storage, it uses up its fats and proteins instead. But because the complete metabolism of fat requires the simultaneous metabolism of carbohydrates, fat is not completely metabolized and ketone bodies (acetone, diacetic acid, and oxybutyric acid) are produced and accumulated abnormally in the blood (ketonemia). The body then attempts to eliminate them from itself. Acetone appears in the urine and in the expired air, giving the breath a fruity order. Diacetic acid and oxybutyric acid must be first neutralized in the body by alkalis (bases); the alkalis are then excreted with the ketones. As a result the body's supply of bases is depleted, the delicate acid-base balance is disrupted, and acidosis develops.

Symptoms. In most cases of juvenile diabetes, the islets produce some insulin for about 2 years before they degenerate. The onset of symptoms is rapid, precipitated by an acute infection or some other stress. The child becomes easily fatigued and excessively thirsty (polydipsia), drinks water freely, which causes increased urinary output (polyuria), may have a greatly increased appetite (polyphagia), but does not gain weight or may lose it. Such typical symptoms may alert those giving medical supervision to the child to possible diabetes. Diagnosis is confirmed by tests showing glucose and acetone in the urine, elevated fasting blood sugar levels, elevated postprandial (after a meal) blood sugar levels, and a glucose tolerance test with prolonged levels of sugar in the blood.

If the diabetes is untreated, the child may go into a state of acidosis. The child feels generally ill, is nauseated, may vomit, and may have abdominal pain. As the acidosis increases, symptoms of dehydration appear, with drowsiness; dry skin; flushed, pink cheeks; cherry red lips; deepening, slow respirations (Kussmaul) with a fruity, acetone odor; lowered blood pressure and temperature; soft sunken eyeballs; and a rigid abdomen. At first the child is irritable; then drowsy, and then lapses into unconsciousness. If emergency treatment is not instituted, deep coma and death follow. Laboratory findings during acidosis show a disturbed blood chemistry, an elevation in blood sugar, hemoglobin, and hematocrit, and an increase in the white blood count. Urine tests show an increase in specific gravity and acidity, and ketonuria.

Treatment. As with other deficiency diseases, the primary treatment is to supply what is lacking; in this disease it is insulin. If there are complications such as acidosis or secondary infections, they must also be treated. Diabetes is especially difficult to treat in children because they react quickly and severely to the slightest chemical imbalance in the body. For this reason their diabetes is described as *brittle*. Insulin dosage is tied to the child's diet, which should meet all nutritional needs. These needs vary from day to day and are increased with physical growth, exercise, local infections, emotional stress, injury, and illness. When a relatively constant balance is found between nutritional needs, diet, and insulin, the child's diabetes is said to be under control, or *regulated*.

After the initial hyperglycemic crisis, there may be a "honeymoon" period when the oral sulfonylurea drugs may temporarily stimulate some remaining *beta* cells to produce enough insulin. The family should understand that eventually the child must return to injectable insulin. They should know and watch for hypoglycemic symptoms.

Urine testing. The urine of a healthy person usually does not contain glucose or acetone. When sugar is present, it indicates that the body cells are not absorbing it and that it is being spilled over into the urine. In a diabetic individual, the amount of sugar in the urine indicates the degree of nonabsorption or the amount of insulin that is deficient. When acetone is present in the urine, it indicates that ketone bodies are being formed as a result of faulty fat metabolism. The amount of sugar in the urine is determined by testing chemicals that change color according to the amount present, from blue-green (none) to bright orange (4+). A color chart is provided with the test as a guide to interpret the results. In the hospital, Clinitest tablets may be employed for this test. In the home, less expensive Benedict's solution or the simple but more costly Clinistix may be used. Acetone is tested by means of Acetest sticks or tablets, which turn bright purple when large amounts of acetone are present in the drop of urine placed on it.

Urine specimens for these simple tests need not be sterile, but they must be freshly voided and clean. They are usually collected and tested 30 minutes before scheduled meals in time to calculate the insulin dosage to be given. Timed fractional specimens may be ordered, during which the child's total urinary output is collected in a single large container and a sample of the whole tested. (See the discussion on the collection of urine in Chapter 9.) The results of tests performed by the nurse should be recorded immediately. When specimens are sent to the laboratory for testing, a notation is also made in the child's chart.

Blood testing. The testing of blood for quantities of glucose has been performed by laboratories for many years. Recently, a quick, semiquantitative test for use by patients and others has been approved by the Federal Drug Administration. It is marketed by such names as Dextrostix and Chemstrip. The test is performed by placing a drop of fresh blood on a test paper and comparing the color change that occurs with a color chart. Values for glucose of 20 to 240 mg per 100 ml are more accurate than those of urine, but this test requires a skin stab, with the attendant pain and danger of infection. If patients and their families are expected to perform these tests, they must be taught aseptic technique.

Diet. The diet of the diabetic child must meet caloric needs for activity and growth and must include all the necessary nutrients, including protein, fat, carbohydrates, vitamins, and minerals. One of two types of diets may be ordered: (1) the strictly measured diet in which the *total available glucose* (TAG) is carefully calculated with a goal of maintaining a sugar-free urine at

all times, and (2) the free or unrestricted diet like that of a normal child, limited only from excesses, with a goal of avoiding ketonuria but allowing some glycosuria. Advocates of the restricted diet believe that excessive sugar in the blood and urine are harmful and are factors in the development of kidney, cardiovascular, and eye diseases. Advocates of the unrestricted diet believe that excessive sugar in the blood is not harmful and that there are fewer reactions and less psychological stress when the child can eat for enjoyment rather than by compliance with the physician's orders. Both types of diet may be used for the same child. The physician may prescribe a carefully measured diet while the child is hospitalized and the diabetes is being brought under control. Then, after it has been stabilized, an unrestricted diet may be instituted. If a measured diet has been ordered, the nurse should make every effort to help the child eat all of the food offered. When such a diet is ordered, the uneaten portions may be sent back to the kitchen to be weighed so that equivalent amounts of nutrients may be added to the next feeding.

Insulin. Insulin was first available to diabetic persons in 1922. Before that time life expectancy for diabetic people was very short. Now there are many insulin preparations, differing chiefly in the speed with which they work. Their action is modified by the addition of various chemicals. Insulin crystals are extracted from beef and pork pancreas. Regular insulin is the unmodified aqueous solution of crystalline insulin. The lente insulins are made from pure beef sources and so are useful for some allergic persons. All insulins should be kept refrigerated and used before the expiration date stamped on the package. In Table 14-2, the characteristics of insulin preparations in current use are described.

Insulin is a potent drug. It must be administered with great caution, observing the five "rights" of medication administration as discussed in Chapter 10 (the right time, drug, dose, patient, and method). In the case of frequently given insulin, a sixth item should be added—the

Table 14-2. Characteristics of insulin preparations in current use

Type of insulin	Time of administration	Onset	Peak effect	Duration	Remarks
Insulin injection, U.S.P. (regular) in strengths of 40, 80, and 100 units/ml; clear and colorless	20 min before meals, subcutaneously, intramuscularly, or intravenously	Rapid, within hour	2 to 3 hours	6 hours	Discard solutions that are not water clear; local tissue reactions can be avoided if no one site is used more often than every 10 days; keep record of injection sites
Insulin zinc suspension, U.S.P. (semilente) in strengths of 40, 80, and 100 units/ml; cloudy suspension	30 to 45 min before breakfast, subcutaneously	Rapid, within hour	5 to 7 hours	12 to 16 hours	A white precipitate on standing is normal; mix thoroughly by gently rotating between palms
Globulin zinc insulin suspension, U.S.P. in the strength of 100 units/ml; clear, yellowish	30 to 60 min before breakfast, subcutaneously	Intermediate, 2 hours	8 to 16 hours	24 hours	A clear yellow solution; similar to NPH in action
Isophane insulin suspension, U.S.P. (neutral protamine Hagedorn, NPH) in strengths of 40, 80, and 100 units/ml; cloudy suspension	30 to 60 min before breakfast, subcutaneously	Intermediate 2 to 1½ hours	8 to 12 hours	24 hours	Useful for patients allergic to other preparations; made up of ultralente 70% and semilente 30%
Insulin zinc suspension, U.S.P. (lente) in strengths of 40, 80, and 100 units/ml; cloudy	60 min before breakfast, subcutaneously	Intermediate, 1 to 1½ hours	8 to 12 hours	24 hours	Useful for patients allergic to other preparations; make up of ultralente 70% and semilente 30%
Protamine zinc insulin suspension, U.S.P. (PZI) in strengths of 40, 80, and 100 units/ml; cloudy suspension	60 min before breakfast, subcutaneously	Long acting, 4 to 8 hours	14 to 20 hours	36 hours	Often given in combination with regular insulin
Insulin zinc suspension, U.S.P. (ultralente) in strengths of 40, 80, and 100 units/ml; cloudy suspension	60 min before breakfast, deep subcutaneously	Long acting, 4 to 8 hours	16 to 18 hours	36 hours	See semilente and lente

right site. The site must be changed because repeated injections into the same site may cause tissue inflammation and damage. To avoid this problem, an injection site chart may be made for planning a sequence of sites on the upper arms and thighs. Even with this care, if a red, swollen, hot, painful area appears, it should be reported at once. No further injections should be made into the site until it is no longer inflamed.

Frequently two types of insulin, one short-acting and one long-acting, are prescribed for simultaneous injection. When this is the case, the following technique is recommended:

1. Inject just enough replacement air into the clear, regular insulin and withdraw the dose.
2. Inject just enough replacement air into the cloudy insulin and remove the dose.
3. Put a bubble into the syringe and rock it back and forth to mix the two types.

Insulin dosage is often adjusted to the urine or blood test made just before the injection. For example, 5 units of regular insulin may be added to the basic order for each "plus" or percent of glucose of the urine tested or for various amounts of glucose of the blood tested. When ordered in this way, the insulin may be referred to according to the "rainbow" (of the color charts), or simply as "rainbow insulin."

As a precaution against human error all nurses would be wise to verify the type and dose of insulin drawn up in the syringe with another nurse before administering it to a patient. In some hospitals the name of the verifying nurse, together with that of the administering nurse, is recorded on the patient's chart.

Insulin reaction. Too much insulin can cause serious reaction and be as dangerous as too little. A balance between the child's nutritional needs, actual food intake, and the amount of insulin administered must be maintained to avoid either diabetic acidosis or the other extreme, insulin shock. Unlike acidosis, insulin shock develops quite rapidly, within a few minutes or hours, depending on the type of insulin being used and

when it reaches its peak of effectiveness (Table 14-2). One of the first signs of too much insulin is a personality change much like a normal person experiences when extremely hungry. The patient becomes excited, irritable, anxious, or sluggish and may have hunger pangs and salivate. If glucose is not supplied, the reaction intensifies; there is weakness, dizziness, double vision (diplopia), dilated pupils, pallor, sweating (diaphoresis), and cold clammy skin. The patient may stagger, be mentally confused, and have tremors. (Adults with these symptoms sometimes have been arrested for drunkenness.) Infants may have apneic spells during which they stop breathing for periods of time. Without treatment, convulsions may occur, followed by deep shock, coma, and death.

All diabetic persons and those who work with them should be familiar with the signs of insulin reaction so that counteraction can be taken early. Children can learn to recognize these symptoms, too. Each diabetic person should carry some rapidly acting source of glucose at all times. A sugar lump or a piece of hard candy is recommended. In the hospital, orange juice is usually kept on hand for this purpose. If there is no improvement in 15 minutes, additional food should be given. If the patient is unconscious or the child cannot take glucose by mouth, it may be given intramuscularly or intravenously. When any diabetic patient has an insulin reaction, the physician should be notified. If there are vague symptoms and a question as to whether the patient is going into insulin shock or acidosis, a blood glucose or urine test should be done at once. In insulin shock, the urine is negative for sugar and acetone. Insulin reactions can be caused by taking too much insulin, skipping a meal, participating in unusual activity that uses up available glucose, or vomiting foods. Table 14-3 shows the effects of too much insulin compared with not enough insulin. In the normal person the body regulates its own needs for both, but in the diabetic individual, these needs must be regulated by outside controls. All nurses should be able to

Table 14-3. Comparison of insufficient insulin and excessive insulin

Insufficient insulin (diabetes mellitus)	Excessive insulin (insulin reaction)
Basic cause	Basic cause
Insufficient insulin production	Too much insulin in the blood
Symptoms appear because of	Symptoms appear because of
Overeating	Eating too little, too late
Stress, physical or emotional	Uncompensated exercise
Infection	Vomiting
Insulin underdose	Insulin overdose
Early symptoms	
Polydipsia	
Polyuria	
Polyphagia	
Fatigue, weight loss	
Symptoms of acidosis	Symptoms of insulin shock
Develop slowly	Develop rapidly
Malaise	Irritability, weakness
Nausea, vomiting, abdominal pain	Hunger pangs
Fruity breath	Sweating
Flushed, warm, dry skin	Pale, cold, clammy skin
Cherry red lips	Drooling moist lips
Deep, slow respirations (Kussmaul)	Shallow respirations
Eyeballs soft and sunken	Diplopia, dilated pupils
Pulse weak and rapid	Pulse full and bounding
Blood pressure and temperature low	Normal blood pressure
Irritability—drowsiness—coma—death	Tremors—convulsions—death
Laboratory findings	Laboratory findings
Glucose in the urine (glycosuria)	No glucose in the urine
Acetone in the urine (ketonuria)	No acetone in the urine
High blood sugar (hyperglycemia)	Low blood sugar (hypoglycemia)
Treatment	Treatment
Administer regular insulin	Administer glucose (if patient is conscious, give sugar, candy, or juice; if unconscious, give by intravenous, intramuscular, or subcutaneous injection)
Correct electrolyte imbalance	
Treat secondary infections	

recognize the symptoms of both extremes so that they can give intelligent care.

General hygiene and nursing care. The general hygiene of the diabetic patient is of great importance because the body is less able to defend and repair itself. A minor infection or a small injury may develop into a major problem. In the hospital the child should be protected from others with infectious diseases and from injury.

If restraints must be used, they should be well padded to protect the child's skin. Technique for administering insulin must be meticulous. Regular bathing, oral hygiene, and close observation for any untoward symptoms are essential. Because the diet plays an important part in treatment, attendants should encourage and assist the child and report any unusual eating habits. Emotional upsets should be avoided.

Health teaching. An important part of the diabetic child's care is health teaching. Both the child and the parents need information in three vital areas: (1) knowledge of what diabetes is and how it affects the body; (2) specific understanding of how to test urine or blood for glucose, prepare insulin, calculate and prepare the special diet, and recognize the symptoms of acidosis and insulin shock; and (3) general understanding of the importance of general and dental hygiene, medical and dental supervision, and moderation in all things, including eating and exercising. In addition, they need to develop an attitude of acceptance of the disease that will allow the child to live a more normal, healthy life. A definite plan for teaching this information should be made so that the nurses, nutritionists and physicians will know just what the others are doing. When possible, written directions should be given as well as verbal ones to reinforce what has been discussed. It is recommended that diabetic patients keep a daily diary in which they record the urine or blood test results, amount of insulin, diet, rest, and activity.

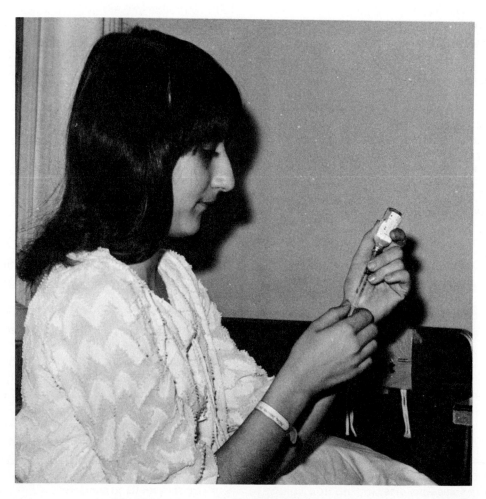

Fig. 14-11. Adolescent girl learns to give her own insulin.

Information about diabetes and how it affects the body is available from many sources. The American Diabetic Association, Inc., and various drug companies and public health agencies have published a number of excellent pamphlets and books specifically for children and their parents. Local chapters of the ADA provide a variety of services. Nurses should remember that a great deal of health teaching is done by example as they care for the child in the hospital.

The child should be taught how to test the urine or blood and interpret the results. Even a child of 6 years of age can do these tests. A child of 8 to 10 years can be taught to draw up the insulin dosage and administer it under supervision. The parents should also learn to do these things. Increasing responsibility can be given as the child grows older. By adolescence the child should be able to regulate diet and insulin with a minimum of supervision (Fig. 14-11). If a nutritionist is not available to teach parents how to adapt the child's diet to the family menu, the nurse may be asked to do so. Practical-vocational nurses are seldom expected to give the initial instruction in these techniques; however, they may be asked to give continuing supervision as the child tests blood and urine or administers insulin.

The child, the parents, and all those who work with diabetic children should know and be able to recognize the early symptoms of acidosis or insulin shock. The child should wear some identification (a card or Medic-Alert tag) of being a diabetic and should carry sugar in case of insulin reaction. The child should be allowed freedom and outdoor exercise, but when there is additional exercise, additional glucose may be needed and possibly more insulin to adjust the exercise-glucose-insulin balance.

Because resistance to disease is reduced in diabetics, immunization against communicable diseases and protection from infections are of great importance. Parents should be alerted to possible sources of problems such as ill-fitting shoes, neglected abrasions, and dental caries. As the child grows, insulin and nutritional needs change. Continuing medical and dental supervision is vital. The prognosis of a diabetic child depends on how well the disease is controlled and how adequately complications are prevented and treated. As diabetic children reach the teenage years, they sometimes rebel against the restrictions placed on them by their disease. These adolescents need special help to accept their disability and to lead a full and productive life.

Tay-Sachs disease (amaurotic family idiocy)

Tay-Sachs disease is one of a group of diseases characterized by an accumulation of fats in the cells of various organs. In this one, the brain is primarily affected. Tay-Sachs disease is caused by an inherited recessive gene most commonly found among eastern European Jews. The child appears normal at birth, but by about 6 months of age becomes listless, with progressive brain damage. By about 1 year of age the child is flaccid, fat, and blind. The disease continues with muscular degeneration, seizures, malnutrition, and death within 3 years. There is no treatment. Both the infant and parents need much supportive care. Genetic counseling about future children should be made available to the parents.

Phenylketonuria (PKU)

Phenylketonuria is an inborn error of metabolism that occurs in about 1 in 9,000 births. It is caused by a deficiency of an enzyme in the liver that changes phenylalanine into tyrosine. Phenylalanine is an essential amino acid present in all natural protein foods. As the newborn takes in food, the phenylalanine is not metabolized and so accumultes in the blood; the excess is excreted in the urine and through the skin. High levels of this potent amino acid prevent normal brain development. The defect is transmitted by the inheritance of a recessive gene that is carried by about 1 in 40 of the population. If two such persons marry, the chances are 1 in 4 that one child will be normal, 2 in 4 that the child will be a carrier as were the parents, and 1 in 4 that the child will have the disease. In some families the proportion of affected children is unfortunately higher.

The child with PKU appears normal at birth. The child often has blond hair and fair skin, a trait thought to be related to a lack of tyrosine, a necessary component of pigment. After about 6 weeks, the urine begins to have a strong musty odor caused by the phenylketones. At about 4 to 6 months the mother may notice a lack of normal development. The baby becomes increasingly irritable and resists cuddling. The baby vomits frequently and convulses. A patchy rash may appear on the skin. Mental and motor retardation continue. The child displays erratic, bizarre behavior, and may not accept toilet training or learn to feed alone until 10 years old, if ever. By school age the child may have become such a severe management problem that institutional custody is required. The IQ of these children ranges from 10 to 50.

Diagnosis is made by finding phenylketone bodies in the urine or by a serum test for phenylalanine in the blood. Because the urine test is not valid until about the sixth week of life, the serum test is preferred. At birth the serum level of phenylalanine may be normal (1 to 4 mg/100 ml), but as soon as the PKU baby begins to take milk the serum level rises rapidly to 15 to 100 mg/100 ml. Serum tests are currently done 12 to 48 hours after birth on all infants born in California as a public health measure. Similar screening tests are being used in other states. To confirm the diagnosis the physician may perform a repeat test 4 to 6 weeks later. When urine tests are used, they are done at least three times during the infant's first year.

The only known treatment is a low phenylalanine diet. Because children need a certain amount of phenylalanine for normal growth some must be allowed in the diet. The amount is carefully calculated by the physician at regular checkups. A synthetic food providing sufficient protein for growth and repair yet containing little phenylalanine may be substituted. Ketonil and Lofenalac are two commercial products used for infants. As the child grows older, foods low in phenylalanine are used to meet the child's protein requirements. A nutritionist may be asked to help the family plan and prepare the special diet required for these children.

The prognosis of PKU children is directly related to how soon they are placed on the low phenylalanine diet. The objective in early diagnosis is to begin treatment sooner and thus prevent mental retardation. Once brain development has been retarded, the process cannot be reversed, only arrested. Even children with brain damage, however, respond to therapy and show improvement in behavior patterns. As yet it is not known whether PKU patients must continue on their diets indefinitely; current recommendations are that they continue at least until the sixth year of life.

Malnutrition (marasmus, kwashiorkor, failure to thrive)

Malnutrition is caused by an inadequate dietary intake or the inability of the infant to use the food received (Fig. 14-12). The result is that reserve food elements in the body are used instead. Some of the more common specific causes for inadequate intake are severe poverty, famine, or child neglect; physical defects that interfere with intake, such as cleft palate; infections that produce anorexia or severe vomiting; and emotional problems. Some of the causes for an inability to use the food received are celiac syndrome diseases, parasitic infestations, and diarrhea. *Marasmus* is emaciation and wasting usually following an acute disease such as diarrhea. *Kwashiorkor* is a type of malnutrition that results from a high-carbohydrate, low-protein diet. *Failure to thrive* is a term used to describe malnutrition that occurs during periods of rapid growth, from unknown causes, or from a disturbed mother-child relationship. *Undernutrition* is a term used to describe a state resulting from a chronically inadequate, but not starvation, diet.

Diagnosis is made by physical examination, social and family history, and specific laboratory tests such as stool cultures for parasites. Typical symptoms begin with the child's failure to gain weight, followed by weight loss. The body uses up its fat and protein in an effort to maintain metabolism. The skin becomes loose and wrinkled. At first the sucking pads of the cheeks remain, giving a false roundness to the face, but when these are gone, the features take on the appearance of an old man with sunken eyes and prominent bones. The abdomen may become bloated, but the head and skeleton continue to grow, with the result that the body proportions become distorted. The infant is weak, the muscles are flabby, and the cry is shrill. As the blood

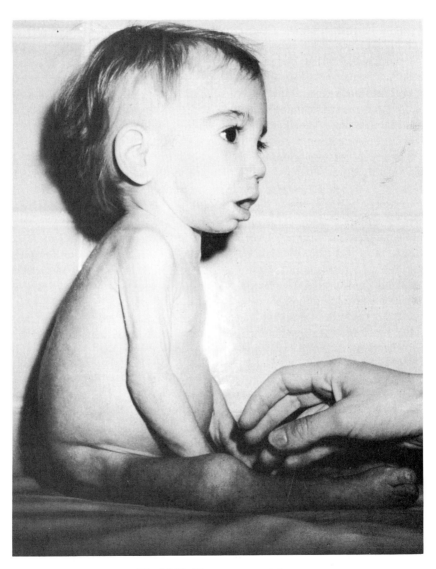

Fig. 14-12. Marasmus, emaciation.

volume diminishes, the child becomes anemic, pale, and often edematous because of fluid imbalance. The basal metabolism is reduced, temperature subnormal, and pulse slow. Starvation diarrhea, in which the stool contain mucus and bile, may occur. The infant is subject to infections because resistance is low. There may be evidence of specific deficiency diseases such as rickets or scurvy. Death comes as the child succumbs to disease, dehydration, or both.

Treatment is directed toward the special cause, general state of malnutrition, and dehydration and infection when they are present. Intravenous fluids and whole blood may be given in some cases. The first oral feedings may be dilute breast milk or lactic acid milk given frequently in small amounts. Gradually other foods are added in increasing amounts according to the child's response. Specific treatment for the various causal diseases is also begun. Care is highly individualized. The prognosis depends on the severity of the condition and its underlying cause.

There are few conditions in which nursing care is more demanding or rewarding. Except when the malnutrition results from physical defects or diseases, the parent is usually not available to meet the child's nurturing needs. Nurses must supply these needs in addition to their other responsibilities. With tenderness and patience they hold, cuddle, feed, and care for the weakened child. Serious bedsores may be present when the child is admitted to the hospital; additional ones may develop if special skin care is not given. Gradually the child begins to respond to treatment. Because such children are often hospitalized for long periods of time, strong bonds develop between them and those nurses who provide care. As the time for dismissal approaches, these children will need help to shift emotional ties to the ones who will be nurturing them. These persons may be asked to come to the hospital frequently to assume an increasing part in the child's care. Nurses must then give up the role of parents and continue on as teachers, supporters, and friends. This shift may be more

difficult for the nurses than for the child. It is best to recognize the difficulty and to deal with it candidly.

SUMMARY OUTLINE

  I. The digestive system
    A. Function
    B. Structure
  II. The endocrine system
 III. Disorders of the digestive system
    A. Mouth
      1. Abnormalities of the teech
      2. Dental caries and stains
      3. Trauma
      4. Stomatitis
      5. Cleft lip and palate
    B. Esophagus, stomach, and small intestine
      1. Esophageal atresia and tracheoesophageal fistula
      2. Esophageal stenosis
      3. Foreign body ingestion
      4. Congenital pyloric stenosis
      5. Hiatal (diaphragmatic) hernia
      6. Meckel's diverticulum
      7. Malabsorption (celiac) syndrome
        a. Celiac disease (gluten-induced enteropathy)
        b. Cystic fibrosis (mucoviscidosis)
          (1) Digestive and nutritional involvement
          (2) Respiratory involvement
          (3) Sweat, salivary, and lacrimal gland involvement
          (4) Prognosis
          (5) Nursing care
    C. Large intestine
      1. Intussusception
      2. Appendicitis
      3. Megacolon (Hirschsprung's disease)
      4. Parasitic infestations
        a. Ameba
        b. Tapeworms
        c. Flukes
        d. Hookworms
        e. *Trichinella spiralis*
        f. *Ascaris lumbricoides*
        g. Pinworms
      5. Diarrhea
    D. Colon and rectum
      1. Imperforate anus
      2. Rectal prolapse and procidentia
      3. Ulcerative colitis
    E. Hernias
      1. Umbilical hernia
      2. Omphalocele
      3. Inguinal and femoral hernias

F. Poisonings
   1. Salicylate poisoning
   2. Lead poisoning
IV. **Disorders of metabolism**
   A. Dwarfism and giantism
   B. Hypothyroidism
   C. Diabetes insipidus
   D. Diabetes mellitus
      1. Symptoms
      2. Treatment
      3. Urine testing
      4. Blood testing
      5. Diet
      6. Insulin
      7. Insulin reaction
      8. General hygiene and nursing care
      9. Health teaching
   E. Tay-Sachs disease (amaurotic family idiocy)
   F. Phenylketonuria (PKU)
   G. Malnutrition (marasmus, kwashiorkor, failure to thrive)

STUDY QUESTIONS

1. Trace the path of an olive from the mouth to the anus and describe how its nutrients are used in the body.
2. Describe the postoperative nursing care of a child having had cleft palate and lip repair. Discuss the problems of therapy and nursing care.
3. What is congenital pyloric stenosis? What is the chief symptom? Describe the conservative and surgical treatment.
4. Discuss the effect mucoviscidosis has on the digestive, respiratory, and Integumentary systems; describe the treatment for each involvement.
5. What is the life cycle of *Trichinella spiralis*? of pinworms? How can the cycle of each be broken?
6. Define hydrocele, inguinal hernia, incarcerated hernia, femoral hernia.
7. What are the symptoms of insufficient insulin and too much insulin in the blood? How does childhood diabetes differ from adult diabetes?
8. What is PKU? How is it detected? What can be done to reduce its brain-damaging effects?

15
Conditions of the urinary and reproductive systems

The urogenital system consists of the urinary organs and the reproductive organs. They are grouped together in this text because they are closely related; in fact, in the male some of the parts serve both systems.

THE URINARY SYSTEM

The urinary system includes two kidneys, two ureters, the bladder, and the urethra (Fig. 15-1). Together these organs excrete metabolic waste products and other substances from the body.

Kidneys. The kidneys are located just in front of the "floating ribs" but outside the peritoneal cavity. They are bean shaped and reach nearly full size by about the tenth year of life. A cushion of fat and connective tissue helps protect and anchor them in place. Tough, fibrous tissue encasing each kidney makes the surface smooth and rounded except for the indentation on the inner part, called the *hilum*, through which pass the ureter, renal vessels, nerves, and lymphatics. Located atop each kidney is a small mass of endocrine tissue that forms a *suprarenal* (or *adrenal*) *gland*.

Structurally the kidney is composed of two regions, the functional part (parenchyma) and the collecting part (pelvis). The parenchyma is made up of two parts, the outer *cortex* and the inner *medulla*. The cortex is composed of *nephrons*, the structures that produce urine. The medulla consists of pyramids—bundles of collect-

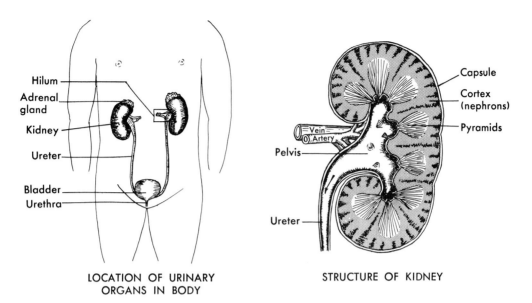

LOCATION OF URINARY
ORGANS IN BODY

STRUCTURE OF KIDNEY

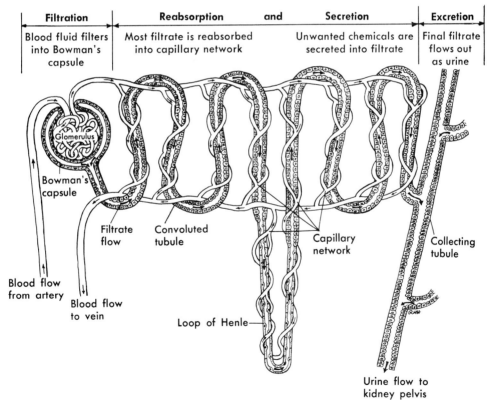

DIAGRAM OF NEPHRON, THE FUNCTION UNIT OF THE KIDNEY

Fig. 15-1. The genitourinary system.

ing tubules that drain the urine into the pelvis, which funnels it into the ureter.

The functional unit of the kidney is the nephron. There are about 1 million nephrons in each kidney. Each one is composed of a *renal corpuscle* (malpighian body) and its tubules. The renal corpuscle consists of the *glomerulus*, a coiled arterial capillary, and *Bowman's capsule*, a double-walled funnel leading to the *convoluted tubules*. Blood is brought to the nephron through microscopic branches of the *renal artery* and returns to general circulation by the *renal vein*.

Within the nephron the amazing process of filtration, reabsorption, secretion, and elimination of water and unwanted substances from the blood takes place. This complex mechanism is diagrammed in Fig. 15-1 and occurs in the following way:

Filtration Blood flows into the glomerulus under considerable pressure. Some water and solutes are forced out by so-called filtration pressure into Bowman's capsule.

Reabsorption As this essentially cell-free, protein-free filtrate moves along through the convoluted tubules, 97% to 99% of this water and solutes are reabsorbed back into the capillary network surrounding the tubules.

Secretion To the filtrate is added certain substances such as electrolytes, nutrients, and water that are secreted by specialized cells located in the lining of the convoluted tubules.

Excretion The remaining filtrate—urine—then passes out into collecting tubules and on to the kidney pelvis.

The kidneys of children are immature and do not function as efficiently as those of adults. The excretion rate of adults is 100 to 125 ml per minute. That of children is 10 to 15 ml per minute per square meter of body surface.

The ability of the kidney to clear blood and body fluids of unwanted substances is called *renal clearance*. A simple test often used to determine this ability is the PSP test, in which a red dye called phenosulfonphthalein is injected into a vein and clocked to see how much time it takes for the dye to appear in the urine. Healthy kidneys clear most of the dye in 1 hour and all of it in 2 hours. If it takes much longer for the dye to clear, one or both kidneys are probably damaged. More definitive tests are then employed to determine where the damage has occurred.

Ureters. The ureters are funnel-shaped tubules that begin with the renal pelvis and convey the urine from the kidneys to the bladder. Each is composed of three layers—an inner mucous, a middle muscular, and an outer fibrous coat. Beginning at the kidney, the muscular coat produces peristaltic waves that push along the urine into the bladder, where it is held until voided.

Urinary bladder. The urinary bladder is a tough muscular storage sac whose size, shape, and position vary with the amount of urine it contains. It lies just below the peritoneum and behind the pubic bone. The wall is composed of an outer serous coat, a muscular layer, a submucous layer, and an inner mucosa. There are three openings—two through which the ureters deliver urine and one through which the urethra expels urine. They are located in the triangular-shaped floor called the *trigone*. An internal sphincter guards the urethral opening.

Urethra. The urethra is a thin-walled tube extending from the bladder to the *urinary meatus*, the external opening. In the female, the urethra is a short tube opening between the clitoris and the vaginal opening. The male urethra is five to six times longer than that of the female and is divided into three parts—the prostatic, which runs through the prostate gland; the membranous, which pierces the body wall; and the cavernous, which extends the length of the penis to the meatus.

Urination (micturition). The urge to urinate, or micturate, comes when the bladder is distended with urine (about 250 ml in adults, lesser in children) and the nerve endings in the bladder wall, called "stretch receptors," send stimuli to the spinal cord. They initiate reflex contraction of the bladder and simultaneous relaxation of the internal sphincter, followed by relaxation of the external sphincter and emptying of the bladder. Although 92% of newborn infants void within their first 24 hours, it is important to report those who do not. By means of a complex nervous process, an individual can learn to overcome the relaxation of the external sphincter, contract it, and therefore control urination. Infants and young children do not have sufficient nerve development to exercise such control, nor do persons with damage or disease to the nervous pathways.

MALE REPRODUCTIVE SYSTEM

The male reproductive system consists of the testes and scrotum, ducts, glands, and penis. Together these structures produce sperm, seminal fluid, and testosterone and carry out the act of copulation that makes possible fertilization of a prepared ovum.

Testes. The *testes* are the primary male sex organs (gonads). They are small oval bodies supported in the *scrotum*, the saclike pouch suspended from the pubic and perineal regions. In the fetus, they lie within the lower abdominal cavity until about 2 months before birth, at which time they descend through the inguinal canal into the scrotum, carrying with them the seminal duct, blood vessels, lymphatics, and nerves bound together with connective tissue to form the *spermatic cord*. If they do not descend, sterility results because sperm cannot thrive unless their environment is below body temperature.

Within the testes are a number of wedge-shaped lobes, each containing the convoluted *seminiferous* ("seed-bearing") *tubules*. Along these tubules are found the Sertoli cells, which produce *spermatozoa*, the male gamete, and also other cells that secrete the major part of the *seminal fluid* (semen) in which sperm are transported. Leydig cells, found in the interstitial tissue, secrete various male hormones called *androgens*, the chief of which is *testosterone*. The testes remain dormant until puberty, at

which time gonadotrophic hormones from the anterior pituitary gland stimulate the Leydig cells to produce androgens. These hormones cause the secondary male characteristics such as deepened voice and beard growth to develop; they also stimulate the testes to produce sperm, a process called *spermatogenesis*.

Excretory ducts. A series of ducts carry the semen from each testis to the urethra and then to the outside. The tiny seminiferous tubules, in which sperm are formed, empty into the *vas efferens*, which empties into the *duct of the epididymis* where the sperm develop tadpole-like tails and are stored. From the epididymis they pass into the *vas deferens*, a tube about 12 inches long that enters the body as part of the spermatic cord through the inguinal canal and arches around behind the bladder to the prostate gland where it joins the duct from the seminal vesicle to form the *ejaculatory duct*. This duct passes through the prostate gland and empties into the *urethra*.

Male accessory glands. The male accessory glands are the seminal vesicles, prostate gland, and bulbourethral (Cowper's) glands. Their secretions are added to that from the testes to form *semen*, a whitish fluid, a drop of which is said to contain as many as 300 million sperm. The two *seminal vesicles* are coiled pouches that lie along the lower part of the bladder. Each joins a vas deferens and in so doing forms an ejaculatory duct that goes to the urethra. The *prostate gland* is a pyramid-shaped organ that lies just below the bladder. Through its tissues course the urethra and the two ejaculatory ducts. It adds its secretions directly to the urethra through several small ducts. The two *bulbourethral glands* resemble peas in both size and shape and lie just below the prostate gland. Each adds its secretions through a duct connected to the urethra.

Penis. The *penis* is composed of three columns of erectile tissue enclosed in separate fibrous coverings and held together by a covering of skin. The urethra is embedded in the lowest one and just opposite, running along the top, are the blood vessels and nerves. The penis is divided into three parts—the root or base, the shaft, and the glans penis at the distal end. The *glans penis* is a slightly bulging structure over which skin is folded doubly to form a more or less loose-fitting, retractable casing called the *foreskin*, or *prepuce*. If the foreskin fits too tightly about the glans, a circumcision may be necessary to relieve the constriction. Erectile tissue consists of many irregular cavernous spaces that fill with blood, under certain nervous stimuli, causing the organ to become large, rigid, and erect. At the peak of sexual excitement, the seminal vesicles and ducts convulsively contract, forcibly ejecting 3 to 7 ml of semen in an action called *ejaculation*. The blood then gradually leaves the cavernous spaces and the penis returns to its flaccid state. Beginning in puberty, spontaneous ejaculations, called night emissions or wet dreams, occur at intervals unless the buildup of semen is relieved by copulation or masturbation.

Copulation. Biologically speaking, the chief purpose of the male reproductive organs is to manufacture and deliver sperm, the male gamete, to the mouth of the female uterus. This is accomplished by the act of copulation, or coitus, when the erect penis, inserted into the vagina, ejaculates semen. Impotency is the inability to copulate. Infertility is the probable inability to procreate because of a low sperm count. Sterility is the complete lack of viable sperm. Potency is not synonymous with fertility and may begin in early adolescence. Fertility is believed to gradually increase during adolescence, reaching its maximum about 22 years of age.

FEMALE REPRODUCTIVE SYSTEM

The female reproductive system consists of the ovaries, uterine tubes, uterus, vagina, glands, vulva, and breasts. Together these structures produce ova, the hormones progesterone, and the estrogens. They provide a repository for the male semen, a nesting place for the fertilized egg to grow into an infant, and milk to nourish the newborn baby.

Ovaries and ovarian cycles. The *ovaries* are the primary female sex organs. They are about the size and shape of almonds and are situated on each side of the uterus, behind and below the uterine tubes, but not connected to them. The ovaries are anchored in place by ligaments through which come their nerve and blood supply. During fetal life they develop from the broad ligaments whose epithelial cells are modified to become germinal cells of the ovaries. By repeated division of these cells, thousands of primitive ova are present at birth within microscopic structures called graafian or *primordial follicles*. During childhood these follicles and their enclosed ova remain dormant, but beginning at puberty, great changes take place as the monthly *ovarian cycles* occur.

Under the influence of the follicle stimulating hormone (FSH) of the pituitary gland several follicles begin to develop each month. The follicular cells secrete *estrogens*, a group of hormones that promote growth of the uterine lining and secondary female characteristics. Usually only one follicle at a time matures and migrates to the surface of the ovary. At *ovulation* the ripe ovum bursts from the follicle into the pelvic cavity and enters a uterine tube. The cells of the follicle then grow inward to form the *corpus luteum*, which grows for 7 days, during which it secretes estrogens and progesterone in increasing amounts. *Progesterone* acts to further prepare the uterine lining for implantation of the ovum. If the ovum is not fertilized, it disintegrates; the size and amounts of secretions of the corpus luteum decrease, causing the uterine lining to slough away in *menstruation*. Another follicle then begins to develop and the cycle is repeated approximately every 28 days for the remainder of the woman's reproductive life. If the ovum is fertilized, it moves into the uterus, embeds itself in the lining, and grows. As a result of the pregnancy, the corpus luteum continues to produce hormones, and ovarian cyclic changes are suspended until the pregnancy is terminated, at which time they begin again.

Uterine (fallopian) tubes. The uterine tubes are long, slender oviducts that extend out from the top of the uterus. Their funnel-shaped fingered ends, called fimbriae, open toward the ovary so that when the ovum ruptures it can easily find its way into the cilium-lined oviduct. The combined action of these hairlike cilia and the undulating smooth muscles of the tube wall moves the ovum along to the uterine cavity. If free-swimming sperm are traveling up a uterine tube and an ovum is moving down toward the uterus, *fertilization* may occur whenever they meet. Usually the fertilized egg continues down into the uterine cavity before embedding itself. Occasionally, however, the egg embeds itself in the lining of the tube. This is called a *tubal pregnancy*. More rarely a fertilized egg, failing to find its way into the tube, may attach itself to the peritoneal cavity. When this happens, it is called an *abdominal pregnancy*. All such extra-uterine pregnancies are abnormal and may be called *ectopic*.

Uterus. The uterus is located in the pelvis between the urinary bladder and the rectum. In cross section it looks like a tiny hollow pear lying on its side with the upper *body* tipped forward and the narrow lower *cervix* projecting down into the vagina. The *fundus* is the bulging prominence above the level at which the uterine tubes enter. Several ligaments hold the uterus in place but allow its body considerable movement, a characteristic that may lead to various malpositions. The walls of this ever-changing organ are made of smooth muscle called *myometrium*. They are covered on the inside by secretive tissue called *endometrium* and only partially covered on the outside by *parietal peritoneum*, leaving the cervix and part of the body outside the peritoneal cavity. The muscle fibers extend in all directions, with the thickest portion at the fundus. The endometrium undergoes cyclic changes that are closely related to those of the ovaries. These are called *endometrial* or *menstrual cycles*.

Vagina. The vagina is the canal leading from the cervix to the outside, into which the erect penis deposits semen at copulation and through which the infant passes at birth. It also serves as the excretory canal for the placenta and for postpartum and monthly endometrial sloughing. The vagina is composed of smooth muscle lined with mucous membrane arranged in folds called *rugae*. The *hymen*, one of these rugae, may partially close the mouth of the vagina of virgins. Occasionally, it completely closes the outlet and must be perforated to allow discharge of the menstrual flow. Folklore taboo about the "maidenhead" persists in some localities, making it a symbol of virginity. This taboo is becoming less important, however, with the widespread use of tampons during menstruation, which stretch the hymen, the participation of girls in active sports, which tear it, and the relatively common practice of cutting it under anesthesia if it presents a potential problem.

External genitalia and glands. The female external genitalia are collectively called the *vulva*. They are the mons pubis, labia majora, labia minora, and clitoris. Closely associated with and located nearby are the urinary meatus, vaginal opening, rectum, and Bartholin's and Skene's glands. The *mons pubis* is a skin-covered mound of fat padding the pubic bone. At puberty, coarse hair begins to grow over the mons and down over the labia majora. The *labia majora*, or larger lips, are the large folds of skin and fatty tissues that extend backward and down from the mons to about 1 inch from the rectum. The *labia minora*, or smaller lips, lie within the labia majora. These two small folds of modified skin extend back from the clitoris. The area between them is called the *vestibule*. The urethra and vagina open into the vestibule. The *clitoris* is a small elongated body of erectile tissue just above the anterior angle of the labia minora. It corresponds to the penis in the male and responds to sexual stimulation by erecting. It is probably the most erotic area in the female body. The ducts of the two *Skene's glands* empty their lubrication secretions through openings on each side of the urinary meatus. On each side of the vaginal orifice are the ducts of the *Bartholin's glands*. The secretions from these and from Skene's glands are normally alkaline. They maintain the constant moisture necessary for healthy mucous membranes. The glands sometimes harbor stubborn infestations of pinworms, yeast, and gonorrhea. Although nurses often refer to the whole area of the external genitalia as the perineum, strictly speaking the *perineum* is the region between the vaginal opening and the anus.

Breasts. The breasts, or *mammary glands*, are the milk-secreting organs of the body. Although they are present in both sexes and remain dormant until puberty, they normally develop only in females and function only after pregnancy. Occasionally, both girls and boys are born with extra nipples located on the abdomen, back, or thighs. Breast tissue grows in response to hormone stimulation. This response can be seen in some newborn infants whose breasts are temporarily swollen from the effect of hormones that crossed the placenta from the mother's blood. Boys experience some breast swelling during early adolescence in response to an androgen increase in their systems. Girls experience profound breast growth, first during puberty when estrogens promote fat deposition and mild duct development and, later, during pregnancy when progesterone stimulates the development of milk-secreting cells. After delivery of the baby, the levels of estrogens and progesterone in the woman's blood are sharply reduced, as is the inhibiting effect on the pituitary gland to produce *luteotrophin*, the hormone that stimulates milk production (*lactation*).

The breasts are composed of glandular tissue organized into lobes that are separated by septa of connective tissue. Each lobe consists of several lobules in which are embedded the mild-secreting cells arranged in grapelike clusters (*alveoli*) around minute ducts. The ducts from the various lobules unite to form a single excretory duct for each lobe of the sixteen or more lobes of each breast. These main ducts converge to-ward the nipple, enlarging slightly before reaching it, into *ampullae*, and then ending in a tiny opening on the nipple surface. The whole glandular system is embedded in fatty tissue. Breast size depends on the amount of this fat. The ability to produce milk depends on the glandular tissue. There is no relation between breast size and the ability to produce milk. Around the nipple is a circular area of pigmented skin known as the *areola*. It contains numerous oil glands that appear as small nodules under the skin. The oils help protect the skin from milk gland secretions.

Menstruation. Menstruation, menses, or the menstrual flow is the periodic discharge of blood, water, and dead cells from the vagina as a result of the sloughing away of the endometrium of the uterus. The beginning of the menstrual cycles (menarche) occurs when a girl is about 10 to 14 years of age. Although the cycles may occur irregularly at first, they normally become established on a regular 28- to 32-day cycle and continue throughout reproductive life until about 45 years of age when they cease (menopause). The only normal interruption of these cyclic changes occurs during pregnancy. (See the discussion of ovarian cycles above.)

DISORDERS OF THE URINARY AND REPRODUCTIVE SYSTEMS
Abnormalities

Of all congenital deformities, those of the urogenital system are the most common, comprising 30% to 40% of all inborn defects. Treatment is surgical. In most cases, the sooner the surgery, the better the prognosis because most defects are obstructive and lead to kidney failure. External ones can be detected at birth. Internal ones are not as apparent but may be suspected if the infant fails to void within the first 24 hours after birth. Abdominal enlargement or swelling in the area of a kidney also warrants immediate attention.

Renal agenesis. Failure of the kidney to develop is called *renal agenesis*. When there is bilateral agenesis so that both kidneys fail to develop, the infant cannot survive. When agenesis is unilateral, the infant can live, but the single kidney is often mislocated in the pelvis and associated with defects of the ureter and so is more likely to become overloaded and diseased.

Double kidney. Normally, each individual has two kidneys. Sometimes, one or both of them are doubled; that is, the kidney is formed with two halves, a constriction between them, and two separate ureters leaving each half. These ureters may remain double throughout their length and open into the bladder through different orifices; or, they may join in a Y somewhere along the way to the bladder. The anomaly does not create problems unless there are obstructions along the way or one of the ureters opens somewhere other than the bladder (ectopically). Obstructions of the ureter may cause hydronephrosis or ureterocele with abdominal enlargement and infections. Ectopic placement of the ureteral opening into the vagina or urethra may lead to constant dribbling of urine, even when the child has learned bladder control. Diagnosis is made by intravenous pyelograms that give x-ray films of the collecting system of the urine. Surgery is performed when there is obstruction or functional need.

Horseshoe kidney. A horseshoe kidney results when the two kidneys fuse into one, forming a horseshoe-shaped mass. The kidney lies centrally and lower than separate kidneys. There may be no symptoms, but complications such as infections are common.

Congenital cystic (polycystic) kidneys. The cause of congenital cystic kidneys is unknown but is believed to be inherited. Both kidneys are filled with innumerable cysts that compress the tissue, causing great enlargement and varying degrees of malfunction. The condition often occurs with other anomalies such as hydrocephalus and heart defects. Such kidneys are more prone to obstructions, infections, and stone formation, and there is usually progressive renal insufficiency, hypertension, and signs of congestive heart failure. Some children live for years before these symptoms appear. Others die of uremia within the first year of life. Treatment is supportive and palliative. There is no known cure.

Exstrophy of the bladder. Exstrophy of the bladder is an extensive defect in the midline closure of the lower abdomen, leaving the pubic bone separated and the bladder completely exposed. In boys the defect may extend from the umbilicus to the tip of the penis. In girls the clitoris may be cleft, the labia separated, and the vagina absent. Associated defects may be indirect inguinal hernias and undescended testicles. The condition is in itself compatible with life, but complications are serious and treatment involves complicated plastic surgery. The infant is constantly soaked with urine that drains directly from the ureters, causing excoriation of the skin and considerable discomfort. Infections and ulceration of the exposed mucosa may occur, as well as pyelonephritis from an extension of infection into the kidneys.

The initial surgery is delayed until the infant is several months old and may involve many years of successive operations. When it is possible, the abdominal and bladder walls are closed and an anatomic reconstruction is made. The penis or the vagina is reconstructed. In severe defects when such surgery is impossible, the ureters may be transplanted to the colon or an artificial bladder may be constructed from a segment of ileum or rectum. A permanent colostomy may then be used for fecal elimination. Prognosis depends on the injury to the kidneys from back pressure and whether the child has suffered damage from urinary tract infections.

The nursing care of these children is extremely important. Good hygiene is necessary to prevent infections and damage to the surrounding skin. The parents need support and instructions in caring for their infant during the months before the first operation and after the many subsequent ones. The community nurse is a valuable ally of the hospital nurse in providing the continuity of nursing supervision and care so necessary if these children are to survive and to finally reach adulthood with a degree of normal adjustment.

Hypospadias. Hypospadias is a common deformity in which the urethra of the male opens somewhere along the lower surface of the penis (Fig. 15-2). Because the sphincter is not affected, the child can learn urine control. In the more extensive defects a cordlike anomaly (chordee) may bow the penis downward so that the tip of the glans lies near the abnormal open-

ing. At birth, when the defect is first diagnosed, a plastic surgeon may be called upon to plan the repair. If the meatus is near the glans, a high circumcision may be all that is required. For more extensive defects circumcision is not performed because the foreskin may be needed in the urethroplasty that may involve several successive operations. Repair is usually planned before school age to avoid the psychological damage that ridicule might cause the boy. The

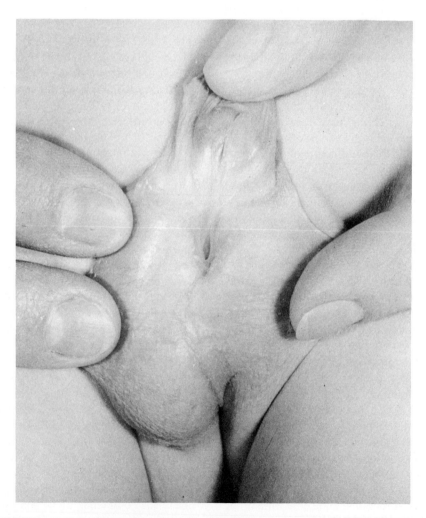

Fig. 15-2. Hypospadias with an undescended left testicle. Defective closure involved foreskin and urethra near head of penis. (Courtesy Children's Hospital of the East Bay, Oakland, Calif.)

chordee is released early to help straighten the penis and allow for normal urination and growth.

After surgery the penis is wrapped in petroleum gauze and then covered with a dry gauze bandage. Ice may be ordered to help reduce the swelling, pain, and bleeding. A catheter drains the bladder during the healing period. The penis should be observed frequently for signs of swelling and bleeding. The child is kept on his back and may require hand and arm restraints. A bed cradle helps prevent pressure on the operative area. Some form of diversion is recommended during the immediate postoperative days to help occupy the boy's attention.

Epispadias. In epispadias the urethra opens on the upper surface of the penis. Various degrees of epispadias may occur. The urethral meatus may lie just behind the glans, or the urethra may lie open along the full length of the penis. It is a relatively uncommon anomaly, except in conjunction with exstrophy of the bladder. Treatment is surgical. The psychological problems are similar to those of hypospadias.

Cryptorchidism (undescended testicles). Cryptorchidism, or "hidden testes," is the absence of one or both testes from the scrotum. It occurs in about 2% of the male population and results from a failure of the testicles to descend from within the abdomen before birth. The missing testicle may be found at any point along the way, and it is more subject to trauma, tumor formation, and developmental failure than is the descended one. There may be torsion, or twisting, of the vas deferens causing it to be occluded (closed). Inguinal hernia occurs in more than half the cases. If both testes remain in the body until after puberty, sperm cannot develop normally and sterility results; male characteristics will develop, however, because the testes continue to release androgens into the blood. The developing boy may suffer serious psychological damage from ridicule and a distorted self-image.

Spontaneous descent sometimes occurs during the first year of life. If it does not occur, some physicians recommend waiting until the boy is 5 to 7 years of age and then giving a 6-week trial of gonadotropin injections in the hope that this hormone will encourage spontaneous descent. Other physicians recommend surgical descent (orchiopexy) at any age from 2 to 7 years. Inguinal hernia must be repaired surgically when present.

After orchiopexy, when the child returns from the operating room, there will be a suture in the lower part of the scrotum fastened to a rubber band attached to the thigh. The nurse should not disturb this tension device. An indwelling catheter may also be in place. Antibiotics may be ordered to prevent infection. When healing has advanced sufficiently, the tension band and catheter are removed and the child is allowed increasing activity. The prognosis for these children is good if the testes can be placed in the scrotum and no permanent damage has been done to them before surgery.

Intersexual anomalies. When a child is born whose sex is not immediately obvious, an extensive examination is first made by the physician. If there is still a question, chromosome studies may be made from buccal smears or skin biopsy. This determination of sex should be done before the parents announce the child's sex to their friends and before the birth certificate is filed. Although this anomaly has little effect on physical health, it is of great importance to the psychological health of both the child and the parents. The social role of a boy is much different from that of a girl. It is harmful for a child to be reared as one sex and later find that the other is the correct sex. Once the sex, or potential sex after treatment, is determined, the child should be identified as such. Treatment is highly individualized and may be surgical, medical, or both. The parents need to understand the issues involved and the treatment that is planned so that they can better help the child adjust to this profound somatopsychic problem.

Three types of intersexual anomalies are well recognized—true hermaphroditism, female pseudohermaphroditism, and male pseudohermaphroditism. The term *hermaphrodite* comes from the name of a Greek god who was the son of Hermes and Aphrodite and became both male and female after uniting with a nymph.

True hermaphroditism. The true hermaphrodite has both male and female gonads. The chromosomal sex may be either male or female. Fortunately the condition is rare, but in all intersexual cases the possibility of this condition must be considered. Treatment consists of removing the gonads of one sex. Because acceptable female

genitalia can be formed by relatively simple surgical procedures, the male gonads are usually removed and the child is made a female. This surgery should be done as soon as possible to increase the child's opportunity for a successful adjustment to life.

Female pseudohermaphroditism. In the condition of female pseudohermaphroditism the child is a true female possessing two ovaries, but with ambiguous external genitalia (Fig. 15-3). The condition results from the effects of andro-

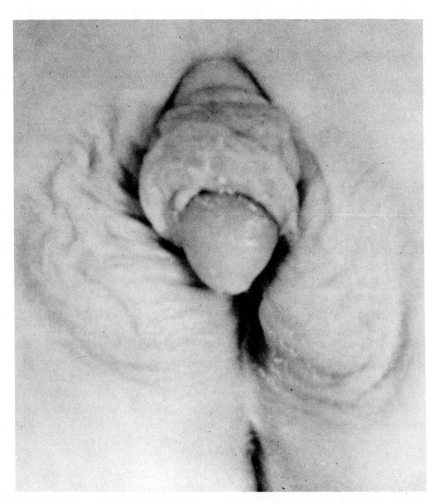

Fig. 15-3. Female pseudohermaphrodite. This child is a true female with an enlarged clitoris. (Courtesy Children's Hospital of the East Bay, Oakland, Calif.)

gens from sources other than the gonads. The clitoris becomes enlarged, the labia may fuse and appear as a scrotum with an associated hypospadias. The most common cause is an overgrowth (hyperplasia) of the adrenal cortex in response to a deficiency in hydrocortisone. Recently a number of cases have been seen in infants whose mothers were treated with progesterone agents during pregnancy. Treatment is both medical and surgical. If the child has a deficiency in hydrocortisone, it is administered; if the anomaly was caused by the mother's drug ingestion, no additional drugs are needed. Plastic surgery is performed between the ages of 1½ and 4 years to restore the child's female genitalia.

Male pseudohermaphroditism. Children having male pseudohermaphroditism are chromosomal males, regardless of the appearance of the external genitalia. One type is causes by a failure of the testes to grow because of damage during fetal life. Another type is characterized by normal female external genitalia but with testes, not ovaries, internally. In cases in which the male external genitalia are absent, or nearly so, making surgical reconstruction impossible, the testes are removed and the child is reared as a girl. At puberty estrogens are given to cause female characteristics to develop. In cases in which the external genitalia are male but there is also a vaginal opening, it is closed and the child is reared as a boy. Androgens may be administered at puberty for those children with deficiencies.

Disorders and diagnostic procedures

Enuresis. Technically, the word *enuresis* means "urination in" (as in a bed); however, the word has come to mean incontinence or involuntary urination after the age when one normally gains control. It may be caused by mental retardation, neurological disease or injury, local irritation, small bladder capacity, systemic disease such as diabetes, emotional disturbances, or a combination of any of these conditions. Nocturnal enuresis is usually caused by fears, anxieties, or circumstances that can be overcome during

the day but not at night. As with any disorder, the underlying cause must be found before treatment can be instituted. Urinary tract infections and other diseases can be identified by physical examination, urinalysis, and other laboratory tests. Mental retardation may be diagnosed by intelligence tests and other objective evidence. When these causes have been ruled out, the enuresis probably results from psychological disturbances. Parents' help must be enlisted in finding the root of the difficulty. They must understand that the child is not bad or mean and that punishment and public ridicule only increase anxiety. The solution may be as simple as providing a nightlight to overcome fear of the dark or withholding fluids after supper, or it may be as complex as overcoming deep hostility brought on by strict toilet training or sibling rivalries. Conditioned-reflex devices that ring bells when the child wets the bed are only useful for a limited number of cases. Whatever the specific cause, treatment should include acceptance of the child as is, recognition of accomplishments in other areas, and unwavering love and security. Enuresis is more common than most parents admit, especially among boys. If it continues beyond the age of 12 years, however, it is probably caused by serious emotional maladjustment and psychiatric help should be sought.

Cystoscopy. Cystocopy is the direct visualization of the bladder and lower urinary tract through a small scope inserted through the urethra. It is carried out in a specially equipped room in the surgical suite by a physician. An operative permit must be signed by the parents; the child is prepared as for other surgeries. Postoperatively the child may experience bladder spasms or hematuria, depending on the reasons for cystoscopy. A notation should be made of the first postoperative voiding and accurate intake and output record maintained.

Pyelonephritis and infection of the urinary tract. Urinary tract infections affecting the urethra (urethritis), bladder (cystitis), ureters (ureteritis), and kidneys (pyelonephritis) are common in children. Because these infections are rarely limited to any one part, they are usually referred to as pyelonephritis. The urinary tract is normally sterile. Bacteria may invade from below, through the urethra, or from the bloodstream. About 80% of the infections are caused by gram-negative bacteria of the colon bacillus group. Other organisms are in the *Proteus, Pseudomonas*, and *Staphylococcus* families. One of the predisposing factors of infection is *stasis*, which means that the urine stays still, or nearly so, allowing bacteria to multiply. Stasis occurs because of congenital obstructions in the urethra or ureters and because of spinal nerve defects that reduce normal muscle contractability. Other factors that predispose the child to urinary tract infections are chronic systemic potassium deficiency, steroid therapy, diabetes, and malformed kidneys.

Acute pyelonephritis occurs most often in girls between the ages of 2 months and 2 years. The onset may be gradual or abrupt. Symptoms are chills, fever, pallor, anorexia, vomiting, prostration, back tenderness, irritability, and sometimes convulsions. The child may have frequent voiding, urgency, and pain on voiding; however, these urinary symptoms are not always present, making diagnosis more difficult. Pus and blood are found in the urine. The white blood count is elevated (leukocytosis). Chronic pyelonephritis may follow an acute infection after many months or years. The symptoms are often nonspecific—abdominal pain, enuresis, dribbling, and recurring episodes of fever and backache. Although urinalysis reveals bacteria, albumin, and casts, voiding may not give discomfort. There is progressive renal failure with hypertension and other cardiovascular symptoms. Diagnosis of both acute and chronic pyelonephritis is made from a history of symptoms, physical examination, urinalysis, and blood tests. X-ray films of the urinary tract using radiopaque dye are useful in identifying abnormal strictures that may cause urinary stasis and continued infection.

Treatment consists of rest, large amounts of fluids, blood transfusions for those with anemia, and specific drugs. Chemotherapy and antibiotic therapy is given to shorten the course of illness and to avoid progressive renal damage. Methenamine mandelate and nitrofurantoin are urinary antiseptics that are effective against common urinary pathogens.

Acute glomerulonephritis (Bright's disease). Acute glomerulonephritis is the most common type of nephritis found in children and young adults. It affects 3- to 17-year-old boys most often and results from an allergic-like reaction begun by infectious organisms, usually hemolytic streptococci. This complex immune reaction may follow scarlet fever, "strep throat," or streptococcal infections of the skin such as impetigo. The disease starts as an acute generalized condition affecting capillaries throughout the body, with the chief lesion in the kidneys. Glomerular damage is diffuse and characterized by inflammatory changes that interfere with the essential function of the kidney, which is to purify the blood and excrete urine. Diagnosis is made on the basis of history, symptoms, urinalysis, positive streptococcal throat culture, and a high antistreptolysin O blood titer.

Symptoms of acute glomerulonephritis appear a few days to several weeks after the original bacterial infection. The child becomes lethargic, loses an appetite, and may develop a mild fever. The facial tissue around the eyes (periorbital edema), becomes puffy, and edema may appear in the legs or become generalized. Blood and albumin appear in the urine, which may become scant (oliguria) or cease completely (anuria). Twitching, headaches, and loss of consciousness may occur as a result of cerebral edema. Hypertension of a moderate degree (140 to 200 systolic and 90 to 140 is diastolic) present in more than half the cases. The duration of symptoms varies from a few days in mild cases to 6 weeks in more severe cases. Microscopic blood in the urine (hematuria) and protein in the urine (albuminuria) may continue for 1 or 2 years or be followed by healing and recovery. When abnormal laboratory findings of the urine continue beyond 2 years, the condition has become subacute (chronic) and may progress to acute renal failure.

Subacute (chronic) glomerulonephritis follows the acute condition in about 5% of children and in 25% to 60% of young adults and older persons. It is characterized by a progressive loss of kidney function as the glomeruli and tubules gradually degenerate. Symptoms may develop slowly or be made worse during upper respiratory infections. The disease usually follows several stages that may occur over a few months or several decades, beginning with the latent, then nephrotic, then hypertensive, and finally uremic stages. Most deaths are caused by uremia, but death from hypertensive heart failure or cerebral hemorrhage is common.

There is no specific treatment that will reverse or eliminate the hypersensitivity reaction causing the glomerular damage. Fortunately, the original reaction usually subsides by itself and the lesions heal. Therefore, treatment of the acute disease consists mainly of general supportive care combined with prevention of complications. If the disease becomes chronic, the complications, such as hypertensive heart failure, are treated specifically.

Most cases of uncomplicated nephritis in children require only a short period of hospitalization for diagnostic workup, evaluation of kidney function, and observation for potential complications. Bed rest is recommended during the early phase of about 2 to 3 weeks unless complicated by oliguria, hypertension, cardiac failure, or brain involvement. Regular diet without added salt is usually permissible. Fluids are not restricted unless there is increased edema or oliguria. Antibiotics are not usually given unless a residual infection is identified by culture of the throat or of skin lesions.

Nursing observations are extremely important so that complications can be discovered early. These observations include the vital signs, daily weight, accurate measurement of fluid intake and output, and symptoms of central nervous system irritation such as nausea, vomiting, drowsiness, double vision, muscle twitching, and convulsions. Regular urinalysis and blood counts are done to determine progress of healing. Only emergency surgery is performed until the child is well. If complications such as hypertension, cardiac failure, or brain tissue involvement (encephalopathy) develop, they are treated specifically. Recovery from acute glomerulonephritis is related to the age of onset. When it occurs in childhood or adolescence, the cure rate is 80% to 100%. In older persons, it is 40% to 75%.

Nephrotic syndrome (nephrosis). A syndrome is a group of symptoms that appear together. The nephrotic syndrome is characterized by massive generalized edema (anasarca), proteinuria, reduced blood protein, and increased blood cholesterol. It occurs because glomerular damage allows the escape of large amounts of protein (mainly albumin) into the urine. As a result, fluid shifts into the space between cells, causing edema. Nephrotic syndrome may appear secondary to diseases such as lupus erythematosus, anaphylactoid purpura, and syphilis, exposure to poison oak, bee venom, mercury, and drug ingestion (Fig. 15-4). When it occurs without any known cause, it is called primary nephrotic syndrome.

The nephrotic syndrome seems to occur more often in boys than in girls and most frequently between the ages of 2 and 7 years. The outstanding symptom is edema that may first be noted as a puffiness around the eyes. As the edema increases, the arms, legs, and abdomen reach massive proportions and the child may double in weight. Fluid collects in the peritoneal cavity (ascites) and thoracic cavity (hydrothorax), causing the child to lose an appetite and to become increasingly dyspneic. Urinary output decreases as edema increases. Stretch marks (striae) may appear in the pale, taut skin. Malnutrition is common, although it is masked by the edema. The child is prone to skin infections, pneumonia, and peritonitis. The edema may last from several weeks to months. There may be remissions, such as occur if the child contracts measles, but the edema then returns. Prognosis of untreated cases is generally poor, with death caused by pneumonia or other infections or by cardiac or renal failure.

The objective of treatment is to reduce edema, control infection, prevent complications, provide good nutrition, and promote good mental health. The nurse works together with the physician and parents to achieve these goals.

In recent years the management of nephrosis has been greatly simplified and the prognosis improved as a result of steroid therapy. Prednisone is the drug often prescribed, initially, in large doses, several times a day. After about 10 days, fluids begin to be eliminated from the child's swollen body (diuresis). As the edema

and ascites are reduced, so are many of the associated problems. When the urine has been free of protein for 2 weeks, the dosage is halved and then administered on an intermittent schedule. Intermittent therapy is continued during the course of the disease, sometimes for several years, with the steroid dosage based on the degree of proteinuria.

The nephrotic child must be protected from exposure to infectious diseases because resistance is poor. Eyes should be washed with irrigant to prevent infection. The child should have adequate rest, but prolonged bed rest is to be avoided for both physical and mental health. Antibiotics may be administered for infections. During the acute period the child's skin must be given special attention. It should be kept dry and clean, especially in the folds of skin. Usually the

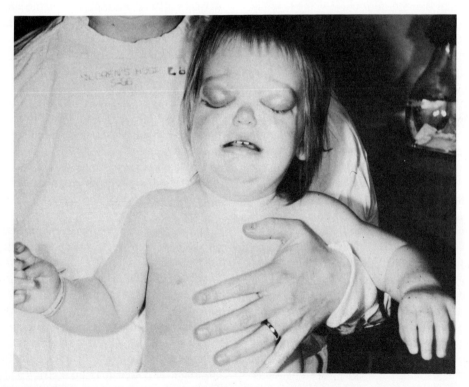

Fig. 15-4. Nephrotic syndrome as a result of a drug reaction. (Courtesy Children's Hospital of the East Bay, Oakland, Calif.)

child breathes more easily in a semi-Fowler position, but should not be left in any one position too long without movement.

The edematous child is too uncomfortable to be hungry, yet needs a well-balanced nutritious diet with adequate protein to make up for the constant loss. It is currently believed that it is better to give the child a liberal diet that will be eaten than a strict, salt-free diet that will not. Salty foods such as potato chips are avoided, but fluids are not restricted. Nurses need to keep accurate records of the intake of all fluids and the output of urine, because these fluids, together with the daily weight, provide valuable information about the fluid retention status of the child.

During times of massive edema the child's self-image may be seriously impaired. Modern treatment with steroids has helped reduce the period of such gross distortion, but the child still needs much reassurance. Parents, too, need encouragement. Steroid therapy is effective in about 80% of these children, but they require constant care and medical supervision for many years.

Acute renal failure. Sometimes called a "kidney shutdown," acute renal failure is a severe reduction of the kidney's excretory function characterized by scant urinary output (oliguria) or no output (anuria). In children, renal failure is caused by a great variety of disorders including acute nephritis, poisoning with heavy metals such as mercury, transfusion and drug reactions, severe shock, hypoxia, dehydration, heart failure, overwhelming infections, congenital kidney malformations, collagen disease, purpura, severe burns, and kidney trauma. It is life threatening. Treatment is directed toward eliminating the underlying cause and correcting the chemical imbalance within the body caused by the loss of kidney function. Blood chemistry studies and urinalysis are done at once. Urinary output is carefully measured and fluid intake calculated according to the output. Daily weight measurement of the blood pressure and assessment of

edema are essential. A low potassium diet is ordered. Foods high in potassium that should be avoided are bananas, lentils, and fish. Peritoneal dialysis may be instituted to control edema, remove potassium, and correct other chemical imbalances. Hemodialysis, whereby the blood is purified in a special water bath outside the body and then returned to the bloodstream, is also effective. Packed cells may be administered in cases of severe anemia. The prognosis depends on the cause and how soon treatment was begun. These children require intensive nursing care of the most expert quality.

Uremia. Uremia is a toxic condition associated with renal insufficiency and the retention of nitrogen urinary wastes in the blood, called *azotemia*. It is caused by nephritis, pyelonephritis, polycystic kidney disease, urinary tract obstructions, collagen disease, severe dehydration, acute renal failure, and severe systemic infections. The condition may develop rapidly or slowly over weeks or months. Blood urea nitrogen (BUN) and creatinine are elevated. Often there is progressive anemia, anorexia, dyspnea, and general wasting. The patient has headaches, nausea, vomiting, diarrhea, nosebleeds, pruritus, and dry skin. The mouth is foul smelling, sore, and bleeds easily. Retinal hemorrhages cause visual loss. Kussmaul (deep and slow) respirations develop, followed by muscle tetany, restlessness, stupor, and sometimes convulsions, coma, and death.

Treatment is directed toward the underlying disease. Dietary restrictions of protein may be made with an increase in carbohydrate and fat. Anemia is treated with blood transfusions. Nursing care is supportive, aimed at relieving the child's discomfort—the dry skin, bleeding mouth, and general misery. In cases of acute uremia in which the causal illness, such as acute glomerulonephritis, is successfully treated, the prognosis is favorable. In other cases, however, the course is generally downhill and the prognosis poor.

Wilms' tumor (nephroblastoma). Wilms' tumor is a highly malignant adenosarcoma of the kidney. It develops from abnormal tissue in the embryo that begins to grow before or after the infant is born. Most cases are diagnosed before 3 years of age. Wilms' tumor is one of the most common intraabdominal neoplasms of childhood, occurring unilaterally in 90% to 95% of the cases. It usually grows silently, with few symptoms, until the abdominal mass is discovered by accident during routine care or physical examination. Pain and hematuria seldom appear until the tumor is in an advanced stage after the prognosis has become grave. Diagnosis is confirmed by intravenous pyelograms that show the distortion and displacement of the affected kidney's pelvis. After diagnosis is made, care must be taken not to palpate the child's abdomen, because handling might dislodge cells and increase the likelihood of their spread (metastasis). With time the tumor extends through the kidney to the renal vein and then spreads to other areas of the body by way of the bloodstream, especially to the lungs. Without treatment, the condition is fatal.

Treatment usually consists of both surgical excision and radiation. If the tumor is localized and encapsulated, surgery may be performed immediately. If the tumor is large and involves many other abdominal structures, radiation may be used before surgery to reduce its size. Actinomycin D may be given intravenously to sensitize the child to x-ray therapy so that a smaller dose will be effective. After surgical excision radiation may be continued intermittently over a period of 2 years. With treatment, children with localized tumor have a 90% chance of cure. In those with metastasis survival rates are about 50%.

Nursing care before and after surgery involves special attention to nutrition, care not to palpate the abdomen, and normal postoperative care. Actinomycin D and x-ray therapy often produce toxic symptoms, such as malaise, loss of appetite, nausea, and vomiting. When more severe toxic signs such as hair loss, peeling skin, and ulcerations in the mouth appear, the therapy is temporarily discontinued. Any of these toxic signs should be reported to the physician as soon as they appear. As with all potentially fatal conditions, the parents need information, practical means for working out their grief, and understanding support.

Neuroblastoma. Often confused with nephroblastomas, neuroblastomas are malignant tumors that arise from neural ectoderm, the embryonic precursor of nerve tissue. They may be found wherever sympathetic nerve cells migrate, but most often arise near the adrenal glands. They often have grown quite large and have metastasized by the time they are discovered, often by mothers before children are 5 years of age. The first symptoms may be from destruction of tissue or tumor growth at the metastasized site, such as weakness of the legs caused by spinal cord involvement or protusion of an eye caused by a retro-ocular tumor. When the adrenal gland is involved, high levels of catecholamines are excreted in the urine. Diagnosis is made by laboratory tests and x-ray examination. During the treatment stage when children are ill from potent chemotherapy and radiation, general supportive care of both parents and children is essential.

Venereal diseases. The chief venereal diseases were syphilis and gonorrhea until recently when a third one, herpes simplex, appeared. These diseases are named "venereal" from Venus, the goddess of sensual love, because they are most often transmitted by sexual contact with infected persons, but not always. Venereal diseases have been a scourge of humans for centuries. With the discovery of penicillin it was believed that they eventually would be eradicated. And so it seemed, as the number of reported cases of syphilis gradually declined to an all-time low in 1957 of 6,251 cases in the United States. Then there was an abrupt reversal of the trend, with a worldwide resurgence and steady increase in every socioeconomic and ethnic group, particularly the teenage population. This resurgence has been attributed to false confidence in the "wonder drugs," ignorance, and reluctance to seek treatment. Until immunization vaccines are developed against these diseases, their control will continue to depend on early detection, adequate treatment, and educational programs.

Syphilis. Syphilis is an infection by a tiny spiral organism called *Treponema pallidum*. The spirochete enters the body through a break in the skin or mucous membrane or across the placenta from the mother into the blood of her developing fetus. Once in the body the spirochete may attack any kind of tissue. When children are born with the disease, it is called congenital syphilis. When they are infected with it later, it is called acquired syphilis.

Congenital syphilis. The mother must have syphilis to give it to her fetus. Fortunately, *T. pallidum* does not infect the baby before the fifth month, which affords time to test and treat the syphilitic mother before her baby can be harmed. If the mother contracts the disease later in pregnancy, however, and goes undiagnosed and untreated, the fetus can be infected. For this reason, some physicians advise a serologic test for syphilis late in pregnancy as well as early.

Because the spirochetes enter the fetal bloodstream directly, they have access immediately to all the body tissues, particularly the central nervous system, liver, lungs, bones, skin, spleen, kidneys, and pancreas. They may produce symptoms immediately, and the fetus may die in utero or be born with obvious disease. More often their effects appear at a later time. For this reason congenital syphilis is classified as "early" or "late" according to whether symptoms appear during the first 2 years of life or later. In early congenital syphilis, even in infants that appear normal at birth, 75% show signs of the disease within 1 month. Typical symptoms are a failure to thrive, anemia, persistent rhinitis called "snuffles," a typical skin rash, ulcers of the mucous membrane, especially of the mouth, lips, anus, and genitals, joint inflammation, enlarged liver and spleen, and inflammation of the retina with later damage to the optic nerve. In late congeni-

tal syphilis typical symptoms are destruction of the bones of the nose, called "saddle nose"; inflammation of the periosteum of the tibial bones of the legs whereby the bones develop a sharp forward curve, called "saber shins"; deformity of the permanent incisor teeth with a characteristic V-shaped notch, called "Hutchinson's teeth"; formation of radial scars from the early lesions around the mouth and nose, called "rhagades"; inflammation of the cornea of the eye at about 6 to 12 years, causing photophobia and impaired vision; and neurosyphilis, causing hemiplegia, spastic paralysis, mental retardation, and behavioral disorders.

Diagnosis is confirmed by serologic tests. At birth blood is obtained from the cord of all infants whose mothers had positive serology. A repeat test at 6 months of age is more definitive than that made from the cord blood. All infants with abnormal serology should have repeated tests at various intervals throughout childhood and early adulthood. Tests of cerebrospinal fluid, such as the colloidal gold reaction, are of value in the diagnosis of neurosyphilis.

Treatment of congenital syphilis is both specific and supportive. Penicillin is the drug of choice. It is given in large doses immediately upon diagnosis. Follow-up blood and spinal fluid tests are done at intervals after treatment. Supportive care includes blood transfusions for anemia, regulated feedings for malnutrition, prevention and treatment of secondary infections, immobilization of inflamed joints, and fever control.

Nursing care during the initial period when spirochetes are found in the skin lesions and nasal discharge begins with strict aseptic technique. Nurses may be required to wear gloves to protect themselves from infection. No pins should be used in the infant's clothing because of the possibility of pricking with a contaminated pin. After about 2 days of treatment the infant is no longer infectious. Because of the snuffles, the nasal passages should be suctioned before feedings, the upper lip kept clean, and a soothing ointment applied. If an older child shows signs of photophobia because of eye inflammation, the room should be darkened or the child should be allowed to wear sunglasses. These children need cuddling and love just as any other child. Judgmental attitudes and feelings of loathing may be reflected in the nursing care. These emotions should be faced honestly. Ward conferences for the nursing staff may be helpful in airing them.

Prevention is the key to control. All pregnant women should be tested for syphilis early in pregnancy and then again near term. Repeated follow-up testing should be done for both mothers and infants. A serious attempt should be made to help solve the socioeconomic and emotional problems that so often accompany syphilis.

Acquired syphilis. Syphilis may be acquired in infancy from the kiss of a person with an oral lesion, from transfusions of infected blood, or, rarely, from infected objects. (Spirochetes die if they become dry or come in contact with antiseptics.) As the child grows older, sexual contact becomes the chief means of contracting the disease. As in the case of congenital syphilis, the acquired disease is described as "early" or "late," depending on when the symptoms appear. A latent period may separate the early symptoms from the late ones by many years. Early syphilis is divided into two stages, primary and secondary. Late syphilis is called tertiary, or third stage.

The primary stage of early syphilis begins about 3 weeks after infection. At the site of the entrance of the spirochetes, a painless sore called a *chancre* develops. Occasionally there are more than one such lesion. The chancre is swarming with live spirochetes and is highly infectious; however, the blood serology test is still negative. In about 1 to 2 months, with or without treatment, the chancre heals. The patient has not been cured. The spirochetes have merely gone "underground" where they multiply and invade the bones, eyes, kidneys, liver, nervous system, skin, and mucous membrane.

Typically, the secondary stage begins soon after the primary stage, with a general feeling of malaise and the appearance of a rosecolored rash. Flattened, moist lesions, called *mucous patches* or *condylomata lata*, may also appear on the skin and mucous membranes. These lesions contain spirochetes and are infectious. The patient often has a sore throat and aching muscles and joints. The hair may fall out, causing spotty baldness called *alopecia*. These symptoms fade away and never return, or they may reappear at irregular intervals for 2 to 4 years. During this second stage the blood serology test turns positive.

The latent period begins when active symptoms have disappeared and the patient is no longer infectious. It may extend for 2 to 20 years, with positive blood serology as the only evidence of disease. In a tragic 20% of the cases, tertiary, or third stage, syphilis develops. This state is characterized by destructive changes in the nervous, cardiovascular, and integumentary systems. In neurosyphilis, mental acuity, motor coordination, and vision are seriously affected. In cardiovascular syphilis the aorta and other large vessels are damaged. In tertiary syphilis tumorlike masses called *gumma* may develop in almost any tissue, such as the lymph nodes, liver, bones, testes, pharynx, and stomach. The spinal fluid and blood serology tests are positive.

The most effective treatment for syphilis at any stage is penicillin. Highly resistant strains, however, have developed that require larger doses for longer periods of time or different drugs such as tetracycline. There is also grave danger that the patient with early syphilis will not receive adequate treatment so that symptoms are masked and the spirochetes are not fully destroyed. With adequate treatment, prognosis for early syphilis is good. If the patient goes on to tertiary syphilis (and some do even with standard treatment), the vital organs are seriously damaged so that the prognosis is poor and treatment becomes largely symptomatic.

Prevention, as with congenital syphilis, is the key to control. Widespread educational programs especially for youths should be instituted to help lift the veil of ignorance and superstition that surrounds this disease. Once diagnosed, prompt and adequate treatment should be given with repeated follow-up testing.

Gonorrhea. Gonorrheal infections are caused by the diplococcus *Neisseria gonorrhoeae*, a highly infectious organism that can live for hours outside the body if kept moist and below 106°F. It thrives in the moist warmth of the mucous membrane of the genitourinary tract and other similar tissue such as the rectum, cervix, and conjunctiva of the eye. Although gonococci are passed along most often by sexual intercourse, they also may be spread by contaminated fingers and objects, such as rectal thermometers. The eyes of an infant may be infected while passing through the birth canal of an infected mother. Gonorrheal infections may be acute or chronic. The acute infection is typically one of marked inflammation and edema with a profuse, greenish yellow exudate. A chronic infection may follow an acute one and be almost symptomless. These infections leave thick scar tissue that produces many serious complications.

A gonorrheal infection of the male typically beings as an acute, purulent urethritis with dysuria. The urinary meatus becomes red and swollen. The penis may be bowed down (chordee) if the inflammation involves the deeper tissue. If the infection becomes chronic, the foreskin may be bound by scar tissue so that retraction is restricted (phimosis). The infection may spread up the urethra to the prostate gland, bladder, and seminal vesicles and then down to the testes, causing scar formation and a variety of complications.

A gonorrheal infection of the female involves the urethra, cervix, and vulvovaginal glands. The primary infection may be severe, but frequently it is moderate or so mild that it goes undiagnosed. The gonococci remain in the folds of the vagina as a constant source of the disease, making the woman an asymptomatic carrier. The infection may spread to the endometrium of the

uterus and the fallopian tubes and proceed into the pelvis, causing pelvic inflammatory disease. Resultant scar tissue may produce abdominal adhesions and stricture of the fallopian tubes that may result in sterility.

Gonorrheal vaginitis in female infants and children is usually an acute inflammation with thick purulent discharge. The vulva and vagina become swollen and red. There may be dysuria, fever, and excoriation of the skin of the thighs. Without treatment the infection may spread inward and upward, eventually becoming chronic and producing scar tissue.

Gonorrheal conjunctivitis is discussed in Chapter 18 under the subject of disorders of the eye.

The diagnosis of gonorrhea is based on the symptoms, history, and laboratory examination of exudate by a direct smear or a culture made from a smear. Gram stain may be used to identify the gram-negative diplococci. A flourescent antibody (FA) test is useful for specimens of vaginal exudate in which the gonococcal organism may be difficult to locate.

Most strains of gonococci are vulnerable to penicillin. For this reason it is the drug of choice. A highly resistant strain, however, called "beta," recently evolved that destroys penicillin. Infections of this strain must be treated with large doses of new antibiotics to which the cocci are not yet resistant. To be sure the disease is cured, two follow-up smears or cultures should be done 1 and 3 weeks after treatment. In cases of chronic or severe inflammations such as pelvic inflammatory disease (PID), more extensive antibiotic therapy may be necessary. Usually patients are considered no longer infectious 24 hours after therapy and, except in complicated cases, are not usually hospitalized. The nurse should recognize the possibility, however, that patients who are hospitalized for other conditions might have a gonorrheal infection and should treat all purulent discharge, especially from the genitourinary tract, as potentially infectious.

Prevention depends on public education and prompt treatment of all diagnosed cases before they can infect others.

Herpes simplex. Herpes simplex infections are caused by the *herpes simplex virus hominis* (HVH), usually type II. It is a virus that causes ulceration of the mucous membrane in the mouth and genitourinary tract of both men and women. The ulcers appear in crops, cyclically, and there is no known cure, although intensive research is underway to find one. The incidence of cervical cancer is much higher in women infected with herpes than in noninfected women. If ulcers are present in the birth canal during delivery, the baby may be infected and may develop generalized viremia, with multiple organ involvement and death. To avoid such serious consequences cesarean sections are advised for women with herpetic vulvovaginitis during the third trimester of pregnancy. Regular Papanicolaou smears to detect early cervical cancer are also recommended.

Abnormal sexual development. Although most children follow the average normal sequence of sexual development, there are a surprising number who do not and yet end up as normal adults. Their nonaverage pattern of development results from variations in the relative time at which the endocrine glands arrive at productivity and not to basic defects, tumors, or disease. In such individuals the delay or acceleration of sexual development may cause social and emotional problems and require medical evaluation and counseling, but it is not considered an abnormal condition.

Normal sexual development depends on a complex chain reaction beginning with the hypothalamus, which stimulates the pituitary gland, which secretes gonadotrophins, which stimulate the gonads to produce their respective hormones, and which finally cause the primary and secondary sex characteristics to develop. The adrenal hormones also play an important part in the maturation of both boys and girls. An abnormality at any point in the system results in abnormal sexual development.

Sexual infantilism is a failure of sexual development. It may be caused by tumors or congenital defects of the hypothalamus, by pituitary defects, chromosomal defects that affect the gonads, or removal of the ovaries or testes (orchidectomy) before puberty. Diagnosis of sexual infantilism is made on the basis of history, a careful physical examination, and hormone and chromosome studies. When the defect is caused by a tumor, radiation or surgery may be indicated. If it results from deficiency because of orchidectomy, the missing hormones are supplied.

Sexual precocity is described as "true" or "false (pseudo-)." In true precocity the sexual development is normal but accelerated (Fig. 15-5). In pseudoprecocity the sexual development does not proceed in the usual orderly fashion and is often not complete; for example, the breasts may not develop or the gonads may not mature. A girl's puberty is considered precocious if it begins before 8 years of age or if menstruation begins before 9 years of age. A boy's puberty is considered precocious if it begins before 9 years of age.

True sexual precocity is caused by abnormal stimulation of the hypothalamus or pituitary gland. Tumors, encephalitis, and congenital brain defects may stimulate the hypothalamus abnormally. 90% of female precocity and 45% of male precocity, however, is caused by pituitary stimulation of unknown origin. The onset may be as early as 3 months of age. At first these children are taller than their peers, but ultimately they are shorter because the growth of the long bones stops at sexual maturity.

False precocity (pseudoprecocity) is caused by abnormal stimulation of the gonads or adrenal glands. Hyperplasia of the adrenal glands or benign or malignant tumors of both the gonads and adrenals may produce abnormal sexual development.

Diagnosis is based on history, physical examination, hormonal levels, x-ray examination of the bones, vaginal smear to determine estrogen effects, and biopsy in cases of suspected tumors.

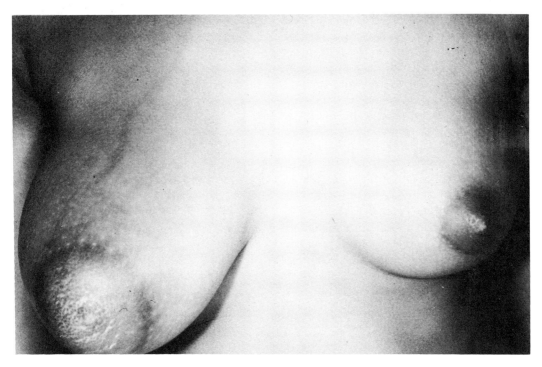

Fig. 15-5. Precocious puberty in an 8-year-old girl with fibroadenoma (a benign connective tissue tumor) in the right breast. (Courtesy Children's Hospital of the East Bay, Oakland, Calif.)

Treatment is based on the cause. Tumors should be removed surgically or with x-ray therapy if possible. Adrenal lesions are treated with cortisone, which inhibits the production of corticotropin with a resultant decrease in the production of adrenal androgens. In true precocity involving the pituitary the child is observed closely over a period of years. Counseling may be needed to help the child cope with some of the emotional problems that such an abnormal development create. The nurse seldom sees these patients in the hospital except for other problems or for surgery or radiation therapy, but when they are in the hospital, they are cared for as individuals, not as freaks or specimens. Such children may appreciate a degree of privacy not usually afforded children of their age.

Menstrual irregularities. Although menstruation usually begins between 11 and 15 years of age, it may not occur on a regular schedule at first. This results in part from the fact that these initial cycles are anovulatory; that is, ovulation does not take place. As a result, the normal formation of a corpus luteum does not occur and the rise and fall of hormones is not as great. Other factors that affect the menstrual cycle are emotions and physical activity, both of which may be quite intense in the adolescent girl. If such irregularity does not correct itself within a year after menarche, the physician may prescribe oral estrogen and progesterone to regulate the hormone levels. Usually these drugs are taken for 3 weeks and then stopped for 1 week during which menstruation takes place; then the cycle is repeated again.

Menstrual cramps (dysmenorrhea) may cause the adolescent girl much difficulty. They may be caused by varying degrees of malpositioned uterus or infantile uterus. They are *not* caused by bathing or washing one's hair. Mild cramps can be treated by moderate exercise, heat, muscle relaxants, and analgesic drugs. When dysmenorrhea is so severe as to interfere with normal life, a careful medical workup is indicated. When the cause is malposition of the uterus, a pessary may be inserted, or in some cases a uterine suspension operation may be necessary. When the cause is a narrow cervical canal, dilation may relieve the painful symptoms. Occasionally an imperforate hymen may obstruct the menstrual flow and cause cramping. This can be corrected quite simply by a small incision. Often the mental attitude of a girl about her developing body affects the degree of menstrual discomfort she experiences. When a girl understands what is going on within her, she is usually less subject to folk myths, which create fear and mystery, and more likely to have a healthy response to the changes she is experiencing.

SUMMARY OUTLINE

I. The urinary system
 A. Kidneys
 B. Ureters
 C. Urinary bladder
 D. Urethra
 E. Urination (micturition)
II. Male reproductive system
 A. Testes
 B. Excretory ducts
 C. Male accessory glands
 D. Penis
 E. Copulation
III. Female reproductive system
 A. Ovaries and ovarian cycles
 B. Uterine (fallopian) tubes
 C. Uterus
 D. Vagina
 E. External genitalia and glands
 F. Breasts
 G. Menstruation

IV. Disorders of the urinary and reproductive systems
 A. Abnormalities
  1. Renal agenesis
  2. Double kidney
  3. Horseshoe kidney
  4. Congenital cystic (polycystic) kidneys
  5. Exstrophy of the bladder
  6. Hypospadias
  7. Epispadias
  8. Cryptorchidism (undescended testicles)
  9. Intersexual anomalies
   a. True hermaphroditism
   b. Female pseudohermaphroditism
   c. Male pseudohermaphroditism
 B. Disorders and diagnostic procedures
  1. Enuresis
  2. Cystoscopy
  3. Pyelonephritis and infection of the urinary tract
  4. Acute glomerulonephritis (Bright's disease)
  5. Nephrotic syndrome (nephrosis)
  6. Acute renal failure
  7. Uremia
  8. Wilms' tumor (nephroblastoma)
  9. Neuroblastoma
  10. Venereal diseases
   a. Syphilis
    (1) Congenital syphilis
    (2) Acquired syphilis
   b. Gonorrhea
   c. Herpes simplex
  11. Abnormal sexual development
  12. Menstrual irregularities

STUDY QUESTIONS

1. What is the functional unit of the kidney? Define filtration, reabsorption, and secretion as these terms relate to kidney function.
2. What are the male and female gonads? What hormones do they secrete?
3. Discuss the defect and nursing care of exstrophy of the bladder.
4. Define cryptorchidism. Why and when is it corrected surgically?
5. Compare the cause and symptoms of acute glomerulonephritis and nephrosis. Discuss the nursing care for each condition.
6. Describe the course of acquired and congenital syphilis. What measures do you believe could be taken to reduce the numbers of cases?
7. Discuss menstrual irregularities, their causes, and nursing approaches.

16
Orthopedic devices, principles, and nursing care

Orthopedics literally means "that pertaining to straight child." It is that branch of medicine originally concerned with childhood deformities but now includes the prevention and treatment of all types of disorders of locomotion in persons of all ages. These disorders affect the normal posture and movement of the body and involve the nervous, muscular, and skeletal systems. These systems and their disorders are discussed in Chapters 17 and 18. The treatment of orthopedic conditions, however, requires the use of a variety of special devices that in themselves represent a challenge to those who are giving nursing care. These devices are traction, braces, casts, crutches, and prostheses. So that needless repetition is avoided, what these devices are, why and when they are used, the principles upon which they work, and the nursing care associated with their use are discussed in this chapter before a discussion of various disorders of locomotion.

TRACTION
Definition and uses

Traction is a process of exerting pull. It is used for the following reasons: (1) to bring a broken bone back into alignment and immobilize the parts, (2) to correctly align nonfractured but dislocated bones such as at the hip or knee joints, (3) to relieve muscle spasm and pain, and (4) to prevent or treat contracture deformities caused by muscle shortening.

Principles and their practical application

For traction to take place there must be a point of attachment to the body. From this point pull must be exerted in one direction. This is called *traction*. At the same time there must be a counterpull in the other direction, called *countertraction* (Fig. 16-1). Traction is usually provided by means of weights connected to the attaching device by ropes suspended from a frame through pulleys. Countertraction is provided by (1) weights attached to ropes pulling in the opposite direction from the traction, (2) restraints to hold the body at a fixed point, and (3) the friction of the patient's body on the bed. Countertraction may be increased by tilting the bed so that gravity pulls the body away from the traction.

Methods of attachment

There are three ways to attach pulling devices to the body—by adhesive strips to the skin, by halters and straps to the body frame, and by pins, wires, and tongs to the bony skeleton. Each of these methods has its special uses, advantages, and disadvantages.

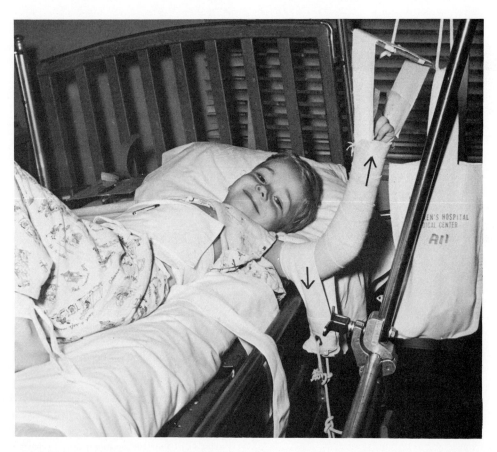

Fig. 16-1. Traction and countertraction (arrows). Weight (in sack at right) is attached to the skin of the forearm by a rope running through a pulley to produce traction. Note spacer over the boy's hand. Countertraction is exerted by a weight attached to the strap on the upper arm. Body restraint about the boy's abdomen keeps him from falling out of bed. (Courtesy Children's Medical Center, Oakland, Calif.)

Skin traction. Skin traction is most often used on an extremity. The skin should be unbroken and usually is painted with a protective coat of tincture of benzoin. Long, wide strips of adhesive tape are then attached to the prepared skin and secured with roller bandage bindings. The ends of the adhesive strips are attached to a spacer bar that is connected to the desired weights by rope.

Skin traction is relatively simple to apply and involves no surgical operations; however, only a limited amount of pull can be exerted on it. The adhesive tape may irritate the skin or interrupt circulation. The nurse should inspect the skin at the edge of the adhesive for signs of redness and check the bindings to be sure they are smooth and dry. The traction must never be discontinued nor the adhesive strips removed without specific prescription by the physician.

Harness traction. Cervical or head halters made of canvas and pelvic girdles made of strong web straps are used as harnesses to exert pull to the body frame. They provide a means for a strong pull without surgical operation but are only useful in special instances such as to provide traction to the vertebral column. The skin under these devices must be observed frequently for excoriation or circulatory disturbance. These devices should be kept clean and dry and changed during periods when traction may be released. It may be helpful to rub cornstarch onto the skin to protect it from the rough material of the harness. If continuous traction must be maintained, any change of device should be prescribed by the physician.

Skeletal traction. Skeletal traction is made possible by inserting some mechanical device such as wire, pins, or tongs into or through the bone (Fig. 16-3). Skeletal traction provides greater pull than is possible with skin traction, and there are no bulky wrappings or irritating adhesive strips. There is greater danger of infection, however, because the devices must be both inserted and removed through the skin. The skin

area where the holding device is inserted must be inspected frequently for signs of inflammation (heat, pain, redness, and swelling). Skeletal traction is always continuous. It must not be released until the injured part is stabilized in some other way as prescribed by the physician.

Other parts of the traction apparatus

To the beginning student nurse a traction setup may appear extremely complex and perplexing, but every part has a purpose and, when understood, it is not particularly mysterious. The maintenance of traction depends on the direction and amount of pull exerted through the use of ropes, pulleys attached to a fixed frame, and weights. Shock blocks may be placed under one end of the bed to increase the amount of countertraction. Additional apparatus such as a trapeze, sling, or positioning device may be added to facilitate patient care and prevent deformities. All these parts should function properly and safely.

Frame and pulleys. A rigid frame is essential to traction. To it are attached the pulleys through which the weight-carrying ropes pass. The frame may be part of the traction device itself, a simple bar at the foot of the bed, or a large overbed frame to which are attached numerous other rigid arms. Sometimes these protruding arms constitute a danger to hospital personnel and visitors. They should therefore be covered by foam protectors or it may be necessary to move the bed about in the room.

Pulleys are grooved wheels mounted in frames in which they turn freely. They are attached to the rigid frame by clamps and never moved by the attending nurse. Their function is to increase the amount of pull and change the direction of pull. The rope passing through the pulley should ride in the intended groove and move freely.

Ropes and weights. The rope should be in good condition and checked frequently for signs of wear. Knots should not be placed near pulleys and should be taped to ensure that they hold.

Weights may be lead or heavy metal made into various shapes or simply measured amounts of sand or water in bags. They may be tied to a rope directly or placed on a weight carrier, a device that allows specially notched metal weights to be added or removed without tying or untying the rope. Weights should hang freely and be checked frequently to be sure they are not resting on the floor or on a piece of furniture. In the case of fractures, too much weight may cause nonunion of the break; too little may cause overriding and nonalignment. No one but the physician should add to or subtract from the amount of weight on any part of the traction apparatus. Traction should be applied continuously unless ordered otherwise.

Trapeze, slings, and positioning devices. In addition to the actual apparatus that creates the traction and countertraction, some of the devices found about the patient are provided to increase comfort and to aid the nurse in giving care. The overhead trapeze is one of these devices. It is a bar hung from the frame just above the patient's shoulders. The trapeze is used for older children and adolescents whose upper extremities are free and who are allowed to lift themselves off the sheets for linen changes, bedpanning, and change of position.

Another device that is used to facilitate care and relieve pressure on the affected part is a slinglike attachment of various types that suspends the part above the bed. This device creates what is called *balanced traction* or *balanced suspension*.

A number of deformity-preventing attachments may also be added to the apparatus, such as positioning devices to prevent internal or external turning of the extremity or to prevent foot drop. These attachments consist of various pads, sandbags, restraints, or rope-pulley-weight traction devices. Whatever the attachment, nurses should understand its purpose and correct position so that they may keep it functioning as intended.

Types of traction equipment

There are a great many traction devices, many of which bear the name of their inventors. Only those used most commonly for orthopedic correction in children will be described here.

Bryant's traction (vertical suspension). Bryant's traction is often seen on the pediatric unit for the treatment of fractures of the femur. It is always applied bilaterally and is attached to the lower legs by skin traction. The hips are flexed at the joints and the legs drawn up by ropes through pulleys attached to the overbed frame. The weight of the child's body provides the countertraction (Fig. 16-2). The buttocks should just clear the bed, with the shoulders and upper back resting on the bed. The child is usually younger than 3 years of age and is placed in diapers with a protective pad over the bed linens. This type of traction allows the child considerable freedom of movement and facilitates nursing care.

An adaption of this traction may be employed to progressively flex the hip joint outward (abduct) when it is dislocated. Initially, the legs are suspended vertically from a large A-shaped overbed frame. Then the pulleys for the two legs gradually are moved apart down the frame until both legs are abducted at right angles to the body. (See discussion on the dislocated hip in Chapter 17.)

Buck's extension (leg traction). Buck's extension is a rather simple type of traction used for the treatment of the lower extremity or back. It is applied to both leg or back traction. By means of skin traction the lower leg or legs are pulled directly away from the body by weights that hang at the foot of the bed. Countertraction is provided by the friction of the body against the sheets. The heel should not press on the mattress and may be lifted off the sheet by a small pad or pillow. The nurse should see that the child does not slip down in bed so that the foot rests against the end of the bed.

Russell's traction. Russell's traction is similar to Buck's extension in that skin traction is at-

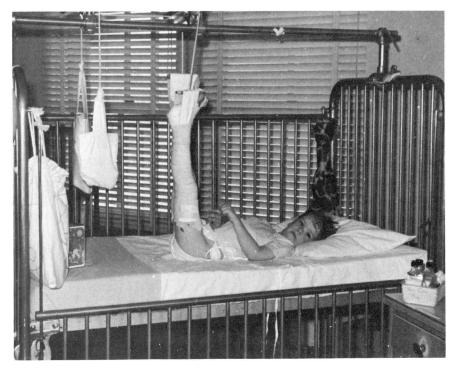

Fig. 16-2. Bryant's traction. Toys are stored in a bag at the foot of crib. (Side rail should be raised except when care is given.)

tached to the lower leg, which is pulled away from the body toward the foot of the bed, except that a sling is added under the knee by means of a pulley attached to an overbed frame. This sling provides lift or suspension. Russell's traction is used to treat various knee injuries and fractures of the femur and hip. Nursing care includes keeping the heel off the mattress to prevent pressure and maintaining the knee sling wrinkle-free to prevent pressure on the nerves and soft tissue.

Thomas leg splint and Pearson attachment. A Thomas leg splint is a rigid frame that fits around an extremity and to which the leg can be attached by either skin or skeletal traction (Fig. 16-3). It may have a complete ring that fits around the leg at the groin, or it may be made with a halfring. A canvas sling supports the leg within the splint. The friction of the thigh against

the upper part of the splint and the pressure of the ring at the groin provide the countertraction. The leg is pulled to the foot of the bed by weights. To the splint may be added a Pearson attachment, which lifts the splint by means of ropes and pulleys to the overbed frame and suspends, or balances, the whole apparatus. Nursing care includes checking the skin under the ring for excoriation and circulatory disturbance. The area should be washed, dried, and massaged regularly. The heel, as well as the skin at the knee, should be protected from pressure from the sling or metal parts.

Putti board. The Putti board is a frame on which an infant with a congenitally dislocated hip may be placed for progressive abduction traction. The angle of the padded wedge between the legs is gradually increased to produce greater

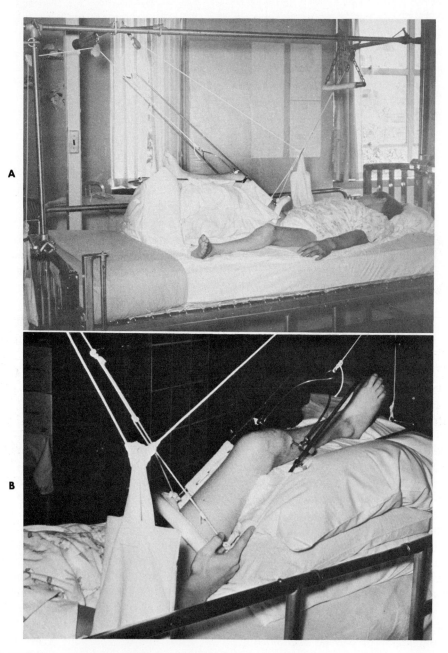

Fig. 16-3. Thomas leg splint with Pearson attachment. **A,** Overbed frame supports traction apparatus and trapeze bar. Pillows help support thigh and leg. **B,** Close-up shows position of pin that provides skeletal attachment and ring of Thomas splint.

and greater outward flexion at the hip joint, causing the head of the femur to move into its correct position in the socket of the hip bone. When the correct position is reached, the child's hips and legs are put in a plaster cast for continued treatment. An adaptation of Bryant's traction (described previously) is also used for progressive abduction but requires that the child remain on the back during the period of traction. The Putti board, on the other hand, permits the child to be carefully turned onto the abdomen if prescribed by the physician. The nurse should check the skin frequently for signs of circulatory disturbance such as cool, swollen, or blotchy-looking toes or delayed return of skin color after pressure to the toenail beds. The pedal pulse should be checked for strength and regularity. Frequent back care and diaper changes are necessary.

Cervical traction. The cervical or neck vertebrae are sometimes fractured or dislocated. A common treatment for these conditions is cervical traction, either by means of a harness that goes under the chin and back of the head or by skeletal traction using Crutchfield or Venke tongs, which go into, but not through, the cranial bone. These attaching devices are then connected to weights at the head of the bed. Countertraction is provided by the weight of the patient's body against the mattress and may be increased by elevating the upper part of the bed. The amount of movement allowed is specified by the physician. Usually flexion, or bending the head forward, is not permitted. Although skeletal traction to the skull may be frightening to the nurse, it is not normally painful to the patient and, in fact, usually provides great relief from severe pain. Skeletal traction is always continuous. When halter traction is used, it may be permissible to release it at intervals. Care must be taken to keep the halter clean and dry from food and saliva. Some patients experience pain in their jaws. Gum chewing may help relieve this aching.

Pelvic traction. Pelvic traction pulls the lumbar vertebrae apart and relieves pain caused by muscle spasm, nerve root disorders, or minor fractures of the lower spine. A pelvic girdle of strong fabric is applied directly to the skin much like a garter belt. The girdle is then attached to weights at the foot of the bed by a strap. Countertraction is provided by a thoracic belt attached to the upper part of the bed or by the weight of the patient's body. It may be increased by raising the knee lift (gatching the bed) at the knees or by placing shock blocks under the foot of the bed. Pelvic traction may be continuous or intermittent, depending on the patient's needs. For traction to be effective, however, the feet must not rest against the end of the bed and the girdle strap must be free of interfering pillows and bedding that might block the pull or make it uneven. The skin under girdle should be observed for excoriation. Cornstarch rubbed into the skin may reduce friction between the skin and the rough girdle material.

Plaster traction. Occasionally a plaster cast is used to maintain the distance and traction between a skeletal pin and an opposing point, such as the groin. The plaster cast is applied over the skeletal pin, which is embedded in or through a bone. The cast is then extended up to the opposing point and down to below the pin. When the plaster dries, the weights, ropes, pulleys, and frame can be removed and the patient is freed except for the cast, which remains on the part, usually the lower extremity. The nursing care of these patients will be discussed in the section on plaster casts.

General nursing care

Although each type of traction equipment requires special knowledge and precautions, there are certain general understandings and concerns that apply to the nursing care of all children in traction.

Duration of traction. Traction is ordered either continuously or intermittently, depending on the purpose and type. Skeletal traction is *always* applied continuously. Skin traction is *usually* applied continuously, and harness traction is often applied *intermittently* with the duration of the interval specified by the physician. Unless there are orders to the contrary, the traction should never be discontinued nor should the amount of pull be adjusted by adding or removing weights.

Traction is continued until healing is complete and further treatment is unnecessary or until other means of fixation are instituted (such as plaster casting of the affected part or surgical placement of pins or plates internally).

Activity and body position. The amount and direction of movement permitted in traction should be clearly understood by the nurse and, when possible, by the child. Certain conditions allow almost no movement whereas others allow for considerable activity. Mobility may be safely increased by various types of balanced traction devices and by the trapeze, both of which are prescribed by the physician whenever possible. In general, the child should be encouraged to move about and exercise as much as possible without disturbing the affected part. Such activity benefits every body system and improves emotional health. For example, by lifting the body by the trapeze the child increases respiratory effort, exercises back, arm, and abdominal muscles, improves circulation, and improves the overall perspective. Even when movement must be severely restricted, the slightest change of position can relieve muscle spasm and fatigue.

Foot drop is a problem for all patients who are bedridden for long periods of time and especially for those whose legs are in traction. It occurs because the strong muscles at the back of the leg contract when the foot is not used for walking and cause the foot to extend, or "drop" forward. Because of pain or neglect, the foot becomes fixed in a nonfunctioning position. When the legs are not in traction, a padded footboard can be positioned so that the feet can be pressed against it at right angles, thus counteracting the natural dropping of the foot. For patients whose legs are in traction, a footboard may not be used. Instead, other devices such as a harness type of traction apparatus may be used to flex the foot and prevent this deformity.

Other deformities may occur as a result of long-standing malpositions of the extremities, particularly those caused by incorrect turning of the part, called internal or external rotation. Special apparatus can be employed to prevent these deformities for patients both out of and in traction. The nurse must be aware of the problems of foot drop and internal and external rotation. Patients should be checked regularly for correct positioning and whole-body alignment.

Circulation and skin care. The skin of any bedfast person must be observed frequently and protected from pressure that blocks circulation, friction that causes excoriation, and moisture that breaks down normal skin.

Pressure areas commonly occur over bony prominences such as the ankles, heels, or hip bones. To prevent skin breakdown, these areas should be massaged, padded, and protected from wrinkles and bed crumbs. A number of excellent paddings have been developed, such as foam supports and real and synthetic lamb's wool pads.

Friction occurs when there is constant rubbing of the skin such as occurs at the groin by a Thomas splint or of the good heel from digging into the mattress. The skin at these places should be protected by rubbing cornstarch onto it or by covering it with padding. Moisture from urine or saliva breaks down normal skin. Diapers should be changed frequently and drool wiped from around the mouth. A soothing ointment may be applied to protect the skin from constant moisture.

Bedmaking. Bedmaking on the orthopedic unit requires considerable nursing ingenuity because of the irregular shapes and sizes of traction equipment. To guide the nurse in this task, the following goals of bedmaking are suggested:

1. Maintenance of positioning of the affected parts as intended by the physician.
2. Promotion of patient comfort and privacy.

3. Economic use of linens and supplies.
4. Conservation of the nurse's energy.
5. Prevention of injury to nurse by use of good body mechanics.

To help accomplish these goals, many hospitals have specially designed linens for their orthopedic units. Others use standard linens in special ways. In preparing a bed for a traction patient, bed boards are always placed under the mattress to give strength and rigidity. One very satisfactory method of making up the bottom portion of the bed is to place three half-sheets crosswise over the mattress pad. Then, if any part becomes soiled, it can be changed without disturbing the rest of the bedding, thus conserving linen and nursing energy. Modesty can be maintained by dressing the patient in pajamas, diapers, loin cloths, or specially designed jumpers or gowns. Top covers may be draped over the chest or unaffected leg but should not interfere with the traction device or weights. Generally, bath blankets are easier to hold in place than slippery ironed sheets and separate blankets, which become displaced very easily. Extremities often become cold at night. One way to warm them is to increase the room temperature. Another is to wrap them in a blanket, taking care not to disturb the traction.

Diet, fluids, and feeding. The diet of an immobilized patient should be high in fluids and supplied with natural laxative foods and adequate fluid, because constipation is a common problem.

An infant who must be immobilized, such as for progressive abduction traction, cannot be held and cuddled during feedings. To help make up for this lack, the person who does the feeding should make every effort to provide some bodily contact during this time. Contact may be provided by holding the bottle in the infant's mouth with one hand and placing the other one around the shoulders so that the child can feel the warmth and comfort of physical contact that is necessary for normal emotional development.

Intellectual and emotional support. Traction is a valuable therapeutic tool for orthopedic conditions, but it requires some degree of confinement. For an active person of any age such restriction is boring and lonely. Boredom and loneliness are potent stressors. When these stressors are coupled with pain and grief for lost experiences, patients may not be able to adapt and may develop various stress responses such as ulcers, depression, and antisocial behavior. Nurses should be alert for these problems and seek ways to intervene, using diversion, education, and interpersonal measures.

Weights and other apparatus. Nurses are held responsible for the maintenance of traction. A rope slipping off a pulley or the weights resting on the floor or a chair will interrupt traction and could cause great harm.

Assessment checklist. Regardless of the type of traction, the following is a checklist for nurses to use for assessing patients in traction:

1. The whole body is in normal alignment and the parts of the body in traction are aligned as prescribed.
2. The apparatus is attached correctly and the weights are hanging free.
3. The bed linens are clean, smooth, and dry.
4. The patient looks comfortable and relaxed.
5. Intake of fluids and foods and output of urine and stool are adequate.
6. The patient demonstrates mental and emotional health.

CASTS
Description and purposes

A cast is a mold. Casts are made of various kinds of materials that undergo rapid, but controllable, physical and chemical change from being soft and pliable to becoming hard and rigid. In medical and dental practice, casts are used for two rather different reasons: (1) to copy the shape and size of a body part, such as a tooth, and (2) to limit the movement (immobilize) of some part of the body.

When teeth must be extracted, a cast first may

be made of them. The dentist does so by pressing molten plastic around them. When the plastic cast sets, the resultant mold is removed and poured full of another material that hardens to form the new teeth. The new teeth are the same size and shape as the original ones and so fit perfectly in the space left when the original ones are extracted.

The second use for casts in medical practice is to immobilize a part of the body. Various quick-setting plastics may be used for this purpose. One of the oldest materials is crinoline bandage impregnated with plaster of Paris. Plaster of Paris is a substance made from gypsum, which is a water-heavy form of calcium sulfate. One of the first large deposits of gypsum was found near Paris, France, hence the name "plaster of Paris." When gypsum is heated, 75% of the water in it evaporates, leaving the white powder, calcium sulfate. If water is again added to this powder, it hardens quickly, a property that makes it well suited for making casts of all kinds, and especially for those used to immobilize a body part. When the physician wishes to apply a cast, the part is first positioned, then protected with padding, and then the moistened plaster bandages are wrapped around it. In a relatively short time the plaster sets and, when dry, forms a rigid shell that immobilizes the encased part, Such a cast may be left in place for many weeks or months until its usefulness is over, at which time it is cut off and discarded.

Application

The nurse may be assigned to assist in the application of a cast and should be familiar with the cast room, equipment and supplies, preparation of the patient, process of casting, and responsibilities of the casting assistannt.

Cast room and cast cart. Although the purpose of casting a part for immobilization is quite different from casting molds to copy famous statuary, both tasks have certain similarities. Neither task is tidy. Both require special supplies and equipment. Because of these features, cast application in the hospital, like mold making in the artist's studio, is best done in a room set aside for the purpose. In many hospitals a *cast room* is located in or near the surgical unit. In hospitals with large orthopedic units, a cast room may be located there. Whether or not there is a cast room, most hospitals have a portable *cast cart*, which holds all the necessary supplies for the application of simple casts.

Equipment and supplies. Because cast application involves splashing about water and plaster, only necessary equipment should be kept in the cast room. Such equipment consists of a table on which the patient can be positioned (a specially adjustable one is used for complex or large body casts), a work surface, stools, an x-ray film view box, lighting fixtures, newspaper-lined wastecans, and a sink with a plaster-catching trap. When a general anesthesia is to be administered, this equipment is brought into the room. A portable x-ray machine may also be brought in for temporary use. In addition to these items, a well-labeled cupboard that contains the following supplies should be provided:

1. Materials used to protect the skin from the plaster, such as sheet wadding and stockinette
2. Plaster of Paris bandages in various width rolls and various sized strips, called splints
3. Materials to reinforce or protect the cast or body, such as felt, yucca board, wire netting, and rubber heels for walking casts
4. Special tools for cast shaping and cutting such as cast knives, shears, spreaders, and cutters
5. Bucket for tepid water to moisten plaster
6. Protective gowns and caps for the personnel, sheets and pillows for the patient

Preparation of the patient. The child who is to have a cast applied may be an inpatient or an outpatient. The child may have just undergone a surgical operation, may have come to the cast room directly from the emergency unit, may have been in traction in the hospital for days or weeks, or may be a child with a long-term condition that is being treated with casts on an outpatient basis. Whatever the child's status, preparation for casting consists of skin care, withholding of food and fluids, and preoperative medication.

When possible, the skin should be clean and free of abrasions because the cast is usually left in place for many weeks.

Food and fluids are usually withheld for 6 to 8 hours before casting is scheduled to reduce the likelihood of stress-produced vomiting, especially if a general anesthesia is to be administered.

Preoperative medications are given before casting to help reduce the fear, tension, and pain so commonly experienced by the patient.

Casting procedure. Regardless of the size or location of a cast, the following sequence is usually followed: administration of anesthesia, manipulation of the part, protection of the skin, application of the cast, finishing of the surface, and checking for alignment.

Anesthesia or analgesia. Some type of anesthetic is usually administered because the manipulation and positioning of a part before immobilization may be quite painful. Local anesthesia may be used when the procedure is relatively simple. For this type the physician uses sterile needles and a syringe and injects a local anesthetic directly into the site. For more extensive manipulation, general anesthesia is administered by an anesthetist. If the child has had general anesthesia for orthopedic surgery, the cast is applied while the child is still under anesthesia, usually in the operating room. Naturally, all precautions against sparks and explosions must be taken when gaseous anesthetics are employed.

Manipulation. The manipulation and positioning of a part is done by the physician using a variety of means, such as mechanical traction devices, slings, pillows, the physician's own hands, and the hands of assistants. Traction may have been applied many days before in preparation for casting. An x-ray film may be taken after manipulation to check the alignment of bones.

Protection. When the part is in correct alignment, the skin is wrapped or covered with soft protective material such as stockinette or sheet wadding. It is important to pad bony prominences especially well because plaster becomes rough and hard and can cause serious damage if it contacts or rubs a skin area.

Application. When the part has been sufficiently protected, the plaster bandages are moistened with tepid water and immediately wrapped around the part. Plaster splints, yucca board, and other materials may be incorporated in the cast to add strength. Special attachments may also be added, such as a rubber heel to a leg-and-foot cast to make it possible for the patient to walk without crushing the plaster (Fig. 16-4).

Finishing. When all the attachments have been incorporated and sufficient plaster has been added to provide immobilization without excessive weight, the person applying the cast wets the hands and smooths the entire surface of the cast to give it a hard, even finish.

Checking. After the cast is applied, an x-ray film is taken to check the alignment of the bones. Only rarely is it necessary for the cast to be removed immediately and replaced.

Responsibilities of the nurse. The nurse assisting the physician in the cast room is responsible for preparing the room, making all the equipment and supplies available, assisting in the positioning and application of the cast, and cleaning the room afterward. When all is in readiness for the plaster to be applied, the nurse removes the wax-paper wrapper from a roll of plaster bandage and immerses it end down into water of about 105°F. When bubbles no longer rise from the bandage, it is lifted from the water and gently squeezed. The loose end is then unrolled slightly and the bandages are handed to the physician. Only one roll of plaster should be dipped in water at a time and then just before it is to be applied because moistened plaster begins to change immediately and sets in a few minutes. Once set, it cannot be dried and reused. Because casting supplies are expensive, waste should be avoided.

During the process of casting, the nurse may

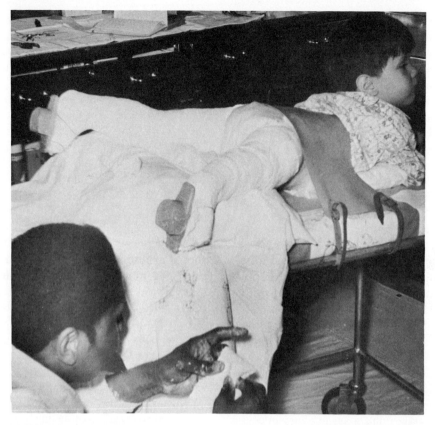

Fig. 16-4. Technician adds rubber attachment to each casted foot so that the plaster will not be crushed when it bears weight.

be asked to hold an extremity or to support a newly casted part. In doing this the nurse should remember to use the palms of the hands rather than the fingers to prevent indentations into the soft plaster.

When the cast is complete and the patient has left, the cast room nurse is responsible for ensuring that all of the equipment is cleaned and returned to its proper place. Prompt action is necessary because plaster is rather easy to wash away when it is fresh, but when it dries it becomes hard and difficult to remove. Newspaper lining the wastecans and covering the floor under the area where plaster is likely to be splashed help reduce the cleanup task.

A record of all supplies used in forming the cast must be kept. Some nurses keep a running account during application, others count the empty plaster wrappers at the conclusion. Regardless of how a record is made, a charge slip must be sent to the business office for each cast so that supplies will be replenished. The cast room is left clean, stocked, and ready for reuse.

Nursing care

The care of the newly casted patient and the cast is most critical during the first 24 hours. The patient may be recovering from anesthesia, trauma from the procedure, and, in some cases, open surgery. The tissue of the newly positioned part is reacting, and the cast is undergoing rapid change. During this initial period special observation and care of the child and the cast are essential. After this period, continuing nursing care is necessary for many weeks or months.

New casts. New, or "green," plaster is damp and still undergoing chemical change. As a result it gives off considerable heat. It smells musty and is grayish white, soft, and easily indented. It is particularly susceptible to soiling and damage until it becomes hard and dry. For this reason the new cast should be protected and dried as promptly as possible. Because cast care is so closely associated with the care of the child, they are discussed together in the following section.

Newly casted patients

Preparation of the unit. The unit must be prepared before the patient is transferred to it. Bed boards are placed under the mattress to prevent sagging. An overhead trapeze is added if it will facilitate care. The mattress and pillows should be covered with plastic to protect them from cast moisture. If special frames or devices are to be used, they should be in place.

Transfer and positioning. When the unit is ready, the child is transferred to the prepared bed. The cast should be lifted by the palms of the hands and not with the fingers. Finger pressure may cause indentations in the soft plaster and may damage the underlying tissue and disturb circulation. If the child is in a large body cast, many hands make the transfer smoother and more efficient. Once the child is in bed, the casted part is positioned on pillows or slings and the body is aligned in a natural position in relation to the part. Generally, a casted part should be elevated to reduce circulatory congestion and pressure on heels and elbows relieved by lifting them off the mattress. The initial positioning of the patient is often done by the physician. If not, it should be checked by an experienced supervising nurse.

Protection of the cast from soiling. Protection of the cast and the child from soiling with urine and feces is of immediate concern. Nurses have devised a number of ingenious methods to ensure this protection. For an older, continent child a flat fracture pan is used. It slips under the buttocks with relative ease and does not crush the cast. For the younger child or infant, a cast board is very satisfactory (Fig. 16-5). It is a wooden frame on which the child's casted body is suspended off the mattress sufficiently for a bed pan to be positioned under the buttocks. Plastic is placed over the perineum and into the pan to deflect the urine downward. Plastic is also tucked under the cast around the buttocks in the back to protect the cast from fecal soiling. Pillows may be used instead of the cast board to lift the cast off the mattress. For infants, a urine specimen—catching apparatus may be placed over the penis or female urethra and left in place.

Drying the cast. To expedite drying, one should expose green casts to the air of a well-ventilated room. Cast-drying machines, which blow warm air over the cast, are sometimes used. If the cast comes up to or surrounds the perineum, a loin cloth, diapter, or plastic sheet should cover the genitalia. Casts usually dry in 24 hours.

Postanesthesia care. The nurse must remember that the newly casted patient had preoperative relaxation and sedation medications. The child may also have had a general anesthesia. If so, normal postanesthesia care must be given, such as taking the vital signs and making observations about them, protecting the patient from aspiration of mucus and vomitus, and preventing the patient from falling out of bed or from harming the new cast.

Observations for circulatory disturbances. Because of the body's natural defenses and process of healing, the site of manipulation or operation normally swells. If not enough space is allowed under the new cast for this process, circulation is impaired and serious tissue damage can result. The following signs and symptoms indicate circulatory disturbance:

1. Swelling of the tissue so that the cast is tight against the skin, producing unusual coldness of the toes or fingers of a casted extremity
2. Paleness, cyanosis, or a mottled appearance
3. Absence of the blanching sign (the immediate turning white, or blanching, of the nail bed on

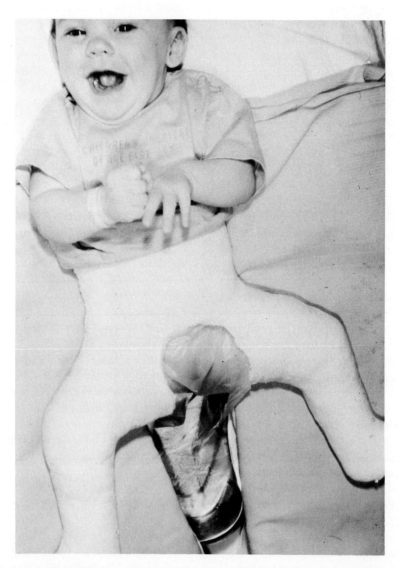

Fig. 16-5. A padded cast board suspends this little girl over a bedpan. Urine and feces are directed into the pan below by the plastic tucked under the cast edges. This child was born with a dislocated hip joint. Casting is one stage of her treatment.

pressure, followed by a return to the normal color on release of pressure)

4. Weak or absent pulse in a casted extremity
5. Inability of the patient to move the toes or fingers of a casted extremity
6. Neurological symptoms in the casted part (numbness, tingling, pain, or a burning sensation)
7. Bleeding excessively into the cast after a surgical procedure (amount is difficult to evaluate; periodically, nurse should measure the area of bleeding, noting its size and the time in the record; the amount and significance of the bleeding can then be judged by the physician on the basis of the information provided by the nurses)

The absence of these signs of circulatory disturbance should be recorded in the child's chart at regular intervals, for example, "toes warm and pink, no swelling noted." The presence of any of these signs should be reported at once to the supervising nurse or physician. Immediate action must be taken to relieve the constriction or else it could result in gangrene. The usual emergency procedure involves cutting the cast in half, forming an upper and lower shell. The inner wrappings must also be cut because they may also be cutting off the blood supply. The extremity is then maintained in the shell with the halves held opposite one another by elastic bandages. Such a cast is said to be *bivalved*. Occasionally, the physician intentionally plans to bivalve a cast to allow some movement but still to provide support to the part. Such casts act as splints and greatly facilitate skin care.

Skin care. The care of the skin around the newly casted part includes not only observation but also cleansing. Plaster is harsh and irritating. If some has been splashed on the exposed skin during cast application, it should be washed away with a damp cloth.

Movement. Until the cast is dry, only necessary position changes should be attempted, and then with adequate help. Nurses, however, should encourage the patient to move the toes or

fingers and to use the overbed trapeze if it is present. The nurse can adjust the pillows under an elevated part or smooth the sheet under the shoulders. Even small movements help relieve muscle strain and fatigue.

Dry casts. When the cast is dry, it is chalk white and hard but still has considerable weight. It must be protected from blows that would crush it and from moisture that would soften and soil it. The child must be protected from the cast's raw edges and the effects of its weight and shell-like nature. The patient needs continuing care for many days and weeks to come. Both the patient and the cast are so closely associated that they are discussed together in the following section.

Patients in dry casts

Edging the cast. The edges of the dry cast should be covered, either by the stockinette, which was folded back on the plaster while the physician was forming the cast, or, after the cast is dry, by petaling. *Petaling* is the name given to adhesive pieces of tape that are cut into wedges, circles, or chevrons and placed side by side around the edges of the dry plaster cast. They keep small bits of plaster from falling under the cast and protect the child's skin from excoriation. They also improve the overall appearance of the cast, because they neatly border the cast edges with petals.

Maintaining the cast. A soiled cast is unsightly and may become offensive if urine or feces has been allowed to soil it. To prevent soiling, one should protect the cast from excreta by the various means described in the care of the newly casted patient. If the cast is grimy from dirty fingers, white shoe polish may be used to whiten it again. Some physicians recommend that casts be sprayed or painted with clear plastic or shellac to give them a soil-resistant surface.

Although a dry cast is quite hard, it can be crushed by blows and by pressure. When the physician intends for a child to walk with a leg cast, a walking heel may be incorporated in the plaster or special walking boots are ordered. A crushed cast is of little value. The child should be instructed in cast care if old enough to understand.

Protecting the skin. Plaster is harsh and irritating. Cast crumbs should be removed from the sheets and every effort made to prevent them from falling into the cast. There they cause irritation and make the child want to scratch. Scratching can produce serious consequences. When back scratchers and the like are pushed under the cast, they can disrupt a suture line or break the skin and initiate an infection. Objects may be "lost" under the cast, produce inflammation, or even become embedded in the tissue. To prevent these dangers *nothing should be pushed under the cast!*

Turning, moving, and supporting. As soon as the cast is dry, the child can move about more freely. The nurse should ask the child to assist by using the overhead trapeze when possible. Those in body casts should be turned at least every 3 hours. Such turning helps prevent pressure areas, encourages digestion, and improves respiration. Casts are heavy, however, and great care must be taken to see that the child does not fall from the bed. The following precautions should be used when turning and moving a patient and supporting the cast:

1. Unless contraindicated, turn the child toward the nonoperated side.
2. Do not attempt too much alone; be prepared before beginning the turn.
3. When turning a patient in a body cast, begin by pulling or lifting to the side of the bed so that the turning side is placed toward the center of the bed. Have patient lift an arm above the head, or if this is impossible, place a cloth between the cast and the arm.
4. Do not use the crossbar (abduction bar) that separates the legs of a body cast as if it were a lift bar. It is there to give the cast stability but is not a handle.
5. Position the child so that the cast edges do not press against the skin and disturb blood circulation.

6. Use pillows to support the patient and the cast, preferably positioning them before the beginning of a turn. When the patient is prone, a small flat pillow should be placed just below the chest to help chest expansion, and a small pillow should also be placed under the head. When the patient is supine, a small pillow should be placed under the head and the space that occurs as a result of the curving of the cast should be supported by a small pad or pillow. Heels should be lifted off the mattress. Pillows may be used to position the child on a side or over a bedpan in the place of a cast board.

Casted parts should be elevated (Fig. 16-6). If a child with a leg cast is permitted to be up in a wheelchair or easy chair the leg should be placed on the leg rest or on a footstool. When a child with an arm cast is permitted to be up, the arm should be supported in a sling. There are a variety of slings, but the classic one is formed by a triangular bandage. The hand should be held higher than the elbow, with the wrist supported and the fingers exposed. The knot should *not* rest over the cervical spine. This is uncomfortable and may cause a pressure area.

Food and fluids. For prevention of constipation and urinary stasis, the casted child should have a liberal fluid intake and laxative foods. The diet should be rich in protein and minerals to further healing of the bones and soft tissue. Usually it is better to offer the child small portions frequently than to offer large meals spaced several hours apart, because the appetite may be dull. Children in body casts can feed themselves and swallow with greater ease if they are positioned on the abdomen for meals.

Daily hygiene. The casted child has all the same needs for daily hygiene as the noncasted one, such as bathing, oral hygiene, care of the hair, elimination, and that personal contact with a nurse that makes the child feel important. The only difference is the presence of the cast. It must be protected from damage and moisture, and the child must be protected from injury that

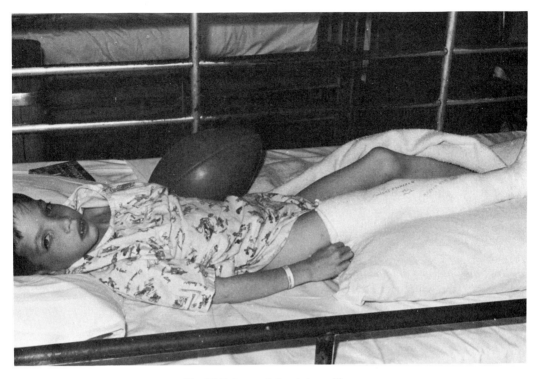

Fig. 16-6. Leg cast elevated on pillow.

may occur as a result of the cast. The skin should be inspected carefully for signs of pressure or irritation. The body alignment should be checked to see that it is not being positioned abnormally as a result of the cast. Children who must remain in body casts for many weeks or months need to have their hair shampooed regularly. Shampoos can be given by placing the child on a gurney with the head near the edge over a basin or by positioning the child near the edge of the bed over a rubber or plastic protector. Self-help for daily hygiene should be encouraged, but the nurse should remember that hospitalized children are like other children—they tend to go light on such things as washing the neck and brushing the teeth—and must be checked from time to time. A record should be kept of bowel movements to avoid constipation and its result-

ant problems. Adequate fluid intake is usually sufficient to prevent constipation in younger children, but mild laxatives may be necessary in older ones.

Education and diversion. A child with a small arm cast or a walking leg cast usually can resume normal schooling soon after the part is immobilized. When the child must remain in the hospital or at home for a long period of time, some provision should be made to provide for education and diversion. An occupational therapist may be asked to help the child fill long hours with interesting things to think about and do. A visiting teacher may be requested from the public schools. Hospital nurse or family members can contribute to the child's diversional needs by talking or playing games, reading aloud, and encouraging visits with other children in the hospital. The television and radio are useful sources of education and diversion, but they cannot substitute for the personal interest of one person in another.

Home care. A great many children are dismissed from the hospital soon after their casts are applied or soon after they are dry. These children have the same needs for care at home as those in the hospital. The hospital personnel and the physician are responsible for seeing that parents are instructed in the care of the child and the cast and how to obtain assistance if they have questions. A visiting nurse may be asked to supervise the home care of the casted child.

Cast removal, revision, and changes

The decision to remove, revise, or change a cast is made by the physician on the basis of the progress of healing or correction of the part, the rate of growth of the child, and the condition of the cast. X-ray and physical examinations aid in this decision. When a cast was applied for a fracture and the x-ray film reveals that the bone has healed, the cast is removed and not replaced. When the cast was applied for correction of bony alignment at joints, such as for clubfoot, a wedge of cast may be removed, the joint positions altered, and new plaster added to fix the foot in the new position. When the cast cannot be revised

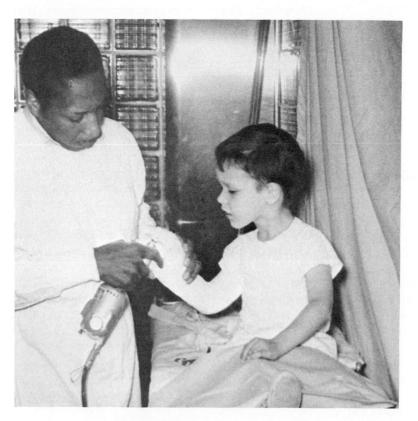

Fig. 16-7. The electric vibrating-blade cast cutter is noisy and somewhat frightening, but it really does not hurt. (Courtesy Shriners Hospital for Crippled Children, San Francisco, Calif.)

because of its condition or because the child has outgrown it, the entire cast is removed and a new one applied almost immediately.

Cast removal. The child whose cast is to be removed or revised may be a patient in the hospital or may be brought as an out-patient specifically for the purpose of cast removal. If the child is to have a cast revision or change with manipulation of a joint, a preoperative medication is given. If the case it to be removed, the child may not be sedated.

The nurse prepares the cast room for the procedure by setting out the special instruments needed on the work table. If new plaster is to be applied immediately, those supplies are also made ready. The physician decides where to cut the cast. The child is positioned accordingly. The cast may be cut by a *cast knife*, which is shaped like a short kitchen paring knife, by a hand *cast cutter*, which looks like huge snub-nosed bandage scissors, or by an *electric vibrating-blade cast cutter*. The electric-powered vibrating blade is noisy and frightening but will not cut the underlying skin. The child (and parent, if present) may need to be convinced of its safety (Fig. 16-7). When the cast is cut, *cast spreaders* of various sizes are used to open the space. Then the padding below is cut with large *bandage scissors*. The sections of the cast are then gently lifted from the part.

Support and skin care. The part that has been casted has been supported and protected for many weeks by the cast. Its muscles are weak and wasted and the skin is tender. In some cases a joint has been held in a fixed position. When the cast is removed, some other support must be provided to reduce the likelihood of repeated injury. In a surprisingly short time with a gradual resumption of activity, the muscles regain their strength and the affected part can be moved without discomfort.

When skin is covered for several weeks, sebaceous material and old skin accumulate on its surface in crusty patches. If these crusts are rubbed or pulled off without first being softened, the lower layers of skin can be damaged and exposed to infection. Because of this concern, some physicians recommend repeated water soaks or baths followed by applications of oil until the crusts are removed. If the part is to be recast immediately, some physicians believe the least handling possible is the best choice, whereas others recommend a thorough cleansing of the skin. All wish to avoid trauma to the skin that would lead to problems during the subsequent casting period.

BRACES

Description and purpose. Braces are removable, external supports used to maintain a position or to provide support. They are made of a variety of materials such as leather, metal, plastic, felt, and lacings. Skilled brace makers create them according to the physician's specifications to meet the individual needs of the patient. Each one provides support by exerting pressure on at least three points.

Braces are made for many areas of the body. Neck braces are for the cervical spine and back braces such as the Milwaukee brach are used to treat curvature of the spine (scoliosis) (Fig. 16-8). Shoulder and arm braces, short below-the-knee braces, and full-leg braces are also used. A leg brace is often attached to a shoe and frequently includes movable joints that can be locked into certain fixed positions (Fig. 16-9). Because of their important function, complexity, and expense, braces should be used exactly as intended and maintained conscientiously. The skin under them must be observed closely for evidence of injury.

Care of the brace. Both the nurse and the parents should know how to maintain the brace in the best possible condition, as in the following manner:

1. Protect the metal parts from moisture, clean lint from all movable parts, and oil joints and locks

weekly. Remove the surplus oil immediately so that leather or clothing is not stained.

2. Clean the leather parts periodically with saddle soap and the felt pads with cleaning fluid.
3. Inspect the brace for worn or missing parts, and elastic straps for loss of resilience. Report any such part to the brace maker for replacement.
4. Do not tie broken laces into knots. Replace them. If the tips come off, mend them with collodion.

Care of the child who wears a brace. The nurse, parents, and child (when old enough) should understand the purpose of the brace, the correct way it should be applied, and when and how long it should be worn.

Application of a body brace and some leg braces is facilitated if the patient is lying in good position on the bed. Back braces are buckled or laced from the bottom up. They are adjusted as necessary with the patient in a standing position.

The skin under a brace should be inspected frequently for pressure areas or evidence of bruising. "No-hole" socks should be worn inside shoes and a cotton shirt under a body brace.

Before a child is discharged from the hospital with a new brace, the parents should have an

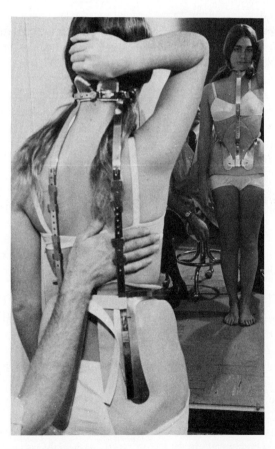

Fig. 16-8. The Milwaukee brace is adjusted for each child to exert pressure at specific points with the goal of straightening the spine. (From American Academy of Orthopaedic Surgeons: Atlas of orthotics: biomechanical principles and application, St. Louis, 1975, The C.V. Mosby Co.)

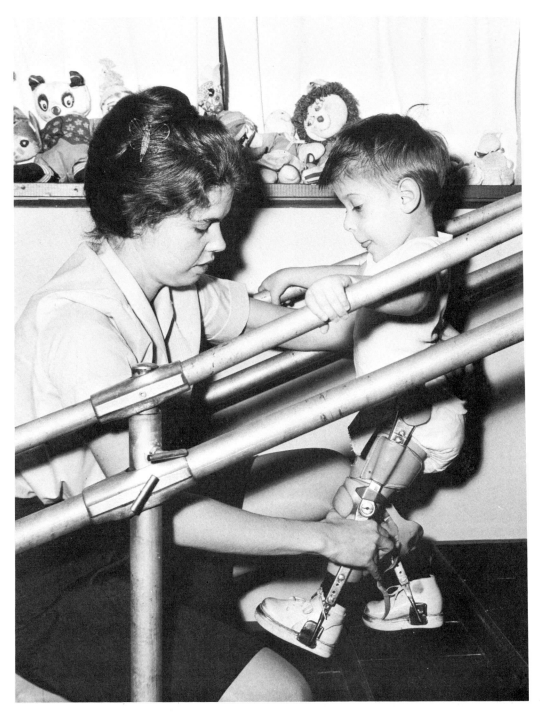

Fig. 16-9. Full leg braces permit this boy, paralyzed from birth by a myelomeningocele, to walk. A physical therapist is teaching him to go down stairs between parallel bars. (Courtesy Children's Medical Center, Oakland, Calif.)

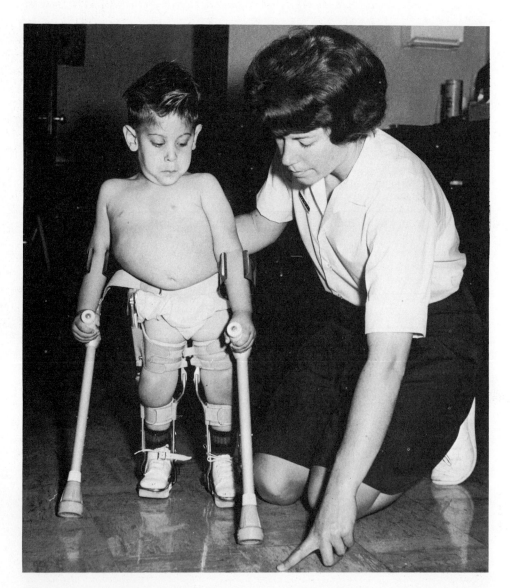

Fig. 16-10. Crutch-walking is hard work for this boy, paralyzed from birth by a myelomeningocele. Large rubber tips on these Canadian crutches keep them from slipping. (Courtesy Children's Medical Center, Oakland, Calif.)

opportunity to apply it under supervision. The child's progress is then followed by the physician at regular intervals. As the child grows, the brace must be adjusted to changing needs and increasing size. Although braces are often difficult to apply and are heavy and ungainly, their use enables many children who would otherwise be helplessly confined to bed to move about and take care themselves.

CRUTCHES

Crutches are devices used to support the patient while walking. They are made of wood or lightweight metal and are of two basic types—the full-length ones with underarm and hand bars and the Canadian crutch with an upper armband and a handpiece (Fig. 16-10). Both types are made in adjustable versions. The full-length type is usually employed by patients who need them only temporarily, whereas the Canadian type is usually preferred for long-term use because it is smaller and less cumbersome.

A child may be required to use crutches whenever one or both legs cannot bear weight. If possible, the child should be prepared beforehand by exercising the muscles of the arms, shoulders, chest, and back. Such exercise can be accomplished by pulling up on an overhead bar, by moving the nonaffected leg through the full range of motion, and by doing pushups with the palms of the hands flat on the bed. The patient should learn to balance by the side of the bed, to sit down, and to stand up from a sitting position. When possible, the child should also work with parallel bars (Fig. 16-9) to further strengthen the arm muscles and to learn balance. The physical therapist is usually asked to teach crutch-walking according to the gait best suited to the patient. The nurse may be asked, however, to measure the patient for crutches and to supervise continuing practice.

Measuring for crutches. A standard procedure for measuring for the full-length type of crutch is as follows: (1) Measure the distance from the patient's axilla to the sole of the foot while the child is lying flat in bed or standing upright, and (2) add 6 inches to allow for the slant of the crutches away from the body during walking.

Safety factors. The two greatest dangers with crutch-walking are that the patient may fall or may injure the axillary nerves. To avoid falls the crutches should be the correct length, and each one should have a new rubber tip to keep it from sliding on the floor. The child should be carefully supervised until skill in crutch-walking is developed. During this period the nurse should walk behind the patient and be ready to grasp the waist if there is any difficulty. Most children learn quickly and, if anything, become overconfident, swinging along at almost reckless speed.

To avoid injury to the axillary nerves from pressure, nurses should teach the child to use the hand bar and the arm muscles rather than to rest the body weight on the armrest. To discourage incorrect use, some doctors recommend against padding the armrests.

PROSTHESES

A prosthesis is an artificial substitute made to replace a body part (see Fig. 17-6). In children the most common types are artificial arms, legs, and eyes. As with braces, prostheses are individually designed to fit the size and meet the special needs of the patient. A variety of materials are used, such as molded plastic, glass, leather, metal, and felt. After a part is made, it is carefully adjusted to the patient. For leg or arm prostheses an occupational therapist then painstakingly works with the child until able to make use of the appliance. The therapist also teaches parents and hospital nurses how to apply and care for prostheses.

An artificial eye should be cleansed and the eye socket irrigated daily with normal saline solution. If any redness or irritation is noted, it should be reported to the physician. Before the child is discharged from the hospital the parents should be instructed in this care. Eventually the child is able to assume personal eye care.

SUMMARY OUTLINE

I. **Traction**
  A. Definition and uses
  B. Principles and their practical application
  C. Methods of attachment
     1. Skin traction
     2. Harness traction
     3. Skeletal traction
  D. Other parts of the traction apparatus
     1. Frame and pulleys
     2. Ropes and weights
     3. Trapeze, slings, and positioning devices
  E. Types of traction equipment
     1. Bryant's traction (vertical suspension)
     2. Buck's extension (leg traction)
     3. Russell's traction
     4. Thomas leg splint and Pearson attachment
     5. Putti board
     6. Cervical traction
     7. Pelvic traction
     8. Plaster traction
  F. General nursing care
     1. Duration of traction
     2. Activity and body position
     3. Circulation and skin care
     4. Bedmaking
     5. Diet, fluids, and feeding
     6. Intellectual and emotional support
     7. Weights and other apparatus
     8. Assessment checklist

II. **Casts**
  A. Description and purposes
  B. Application
     1. Cast room and cast cart
     2. Equipment and supplies
     3. Preparation of the patient
     4. Casting procedure
        a. Anesthesia or analgesia
        b. Manipulation
        c. Protection
        d. Application
        e. Finishing
        f. Checking
  C. Responsibilities of the nurse

  D. Nursing care
     1. New casts
     2. Newly casted patients
        a. Preparation of the unit
        b. Transfer and positioning
        c. Protection of the cast from soiling
        d. Drying the cast
        e. Postanesthesia care
        f. Observations for circulatory disturbances
        g. Skin care
        h. Movement
     3. Dry casts
     4. Patients in dry casts
        a. Edging the cast
        b. Maintaining the cast
        c. Protecting the skin
        d. Turning, moving, and supporting
        e. Food and fluids
        f. Daily hygiene
        g. Education and diversion
        h. Home care
  E. Cast removal, revision, and changes
     1. Cast removal
     2. Support and skin care

III. **Braces**
  A. Description and purpose
  B. Care of the brace
  C. Care of the child who wears a brace

IV. **Crutches**
  A. Measuring for crutches
  B. Safety factors

V. **Prostheses**

STUDY QUESTIONS

1. Define traction, countertraction, and balanced traction. What are the uses of traction? How is it applied to the body? How is countertraction provided?
2. Describe Bryant's traction, Buck's extension, Russell's traction, Thomas leg splint, and Pearson attachment.
3. What are the purposes of casts? Describe the responsibility of the nurse during their application.
4. Discuss the nursing care of the newly casted patient. What are the signs and symptoms of circulatory disturbance?
5. What is the procedure for measuring for crutch length?

17
Musculoskeletal conditions

The muscular and skeletal systems are inseparably related because together they provide the body with shape and movement. In this chapter we will first discuss the functions and structure of the skeletal and muscular systems and then the disorders that affect them most commonly during childhood.

SKELETAL SYSTEM

The skeletal system of the body is a living, ever-changing structure made up of bones and joints that together form the skeleton, without which the body would be a formless mass.

Function

The function of the skeleton is to support, protect, and permit positioning and movement of the body. Its bones also produce most of the blood cells of the body and store and release calcium according to the body's needs. The tissues, bones, and joints of the skeletal system carry out this necessary and complex function.

Structure

Tissues. The skeletal system is composed chiefly of fibrous connective tissue, cartilage, bone, and reticuloendothelial tissue. All of these tissues are classified as connective tissue, although their appearance and function are quite different.

Fibrous connective tissue. Fibrous connective tissue is characterized by a high proportion of fibrous strands that may be especially strong,

443

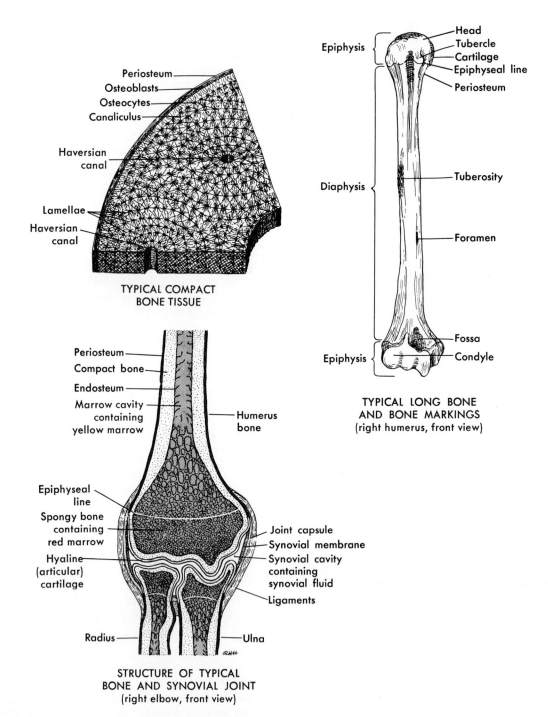

TYPICAL COMPACT
BONE TISSUE

TYPICAL LONG BONE
AND BONE MARKINGS
(right humerus, front view)

STRUCTURE OF TYPICAL
BONE AND SYNOVIAL JOINT
(right elbow, front view)

Fig. 17-1. Structure of typical bone, synovial joint, and bone tissue.

elastic, or both, depending on their location. Fibrous connective tissue composes the ligaments, tendons, muscle sheaths, coverings of bones, and deep fasciae between organs and is found within the walls of large arteries such as the aorta.

Cartilage tissue. Cartilage is an opaque, bluish white tissue that consists of a firm, rubbery material called a *matrix*, which is secreted by *chondrocytes*, the embedded cells. It is covered by a dense membrane called the *perichondrium*, which serves to nourish and repair the tissue by the *chondroblast cells* found within it. *Hyaline cartilage* is the specialized glasslike cartilage found at the end of bones (articular cartilage) and in the larynx and trachea; it forms the nasal septum. *Fibrous cartilage* is hyaline cartilage with interlacing bundles of fibers running through the matrix. It forms the symphysis pubis and the shock-absorbing pads found between spinal vertebrae.

Bone tissue (Fig. 17-1). Except for the bones of the face and skull, most bone is hyaline cartilage that has "turned to stone" by the deposit of calcium in the matrix. Unlike the isolated chondrocytes of cartilage, embedded bone cells called *osteocytes* lie within tiny spaces called *lacunae* and are supplied with blood by an interconnecting system of *haversian canals*. Each canal is surrounded by concentric *lamellae*, which are rings of bony matrix. In *compact bone tissue*, the rings of matrix are put down layer upon layer. In *cancellous bone tissue*, the rings form delicate lacy patterns with a spongy appearance. Bone tissue is composed of about two thirds inorganic matter (calcium) and one third organic matter (bone cells and blood vessels).

Reticuloendothelial tissue. The marrow found within all bone is classified as reticuloendothelial tissue. Marrow may be of the red or yellow type. *Red marrow* is a specialized *hemopoietic tissue* that generates millions of blood cells each day, hence its color; these include erythrocytes, leukocytes, and platelets. Of all blood cells, only lymphocytes are not manufactured in the red marrow. Red marrow is found in many bones of infants and children. With age, the number of sites and the total amount of red marrow gradually decrease until by adulthood it is found only within the ribs, sternum, vertebrae, and cranial bones and at the near ends of the femurs and humeri. *Yellow marrow* is not hemopoietic, contains fat, and is used for storage. By old age, yellow marrow has replaced all red marrow except at the ends of the long bones.

Bones

Types. The 206 bones of the body are classified according to their shape into the following four groups: (1) long bones, such as the femur and humerus; (2) short bones, such as the carpals and tarsals, (3) flat bones; such as the scapulae; and (4) irregular bones, such as the vertebrae and mandible.

Markings (Fig. 17-1). In orthopedic manuals students may find strange-sounding words that describe the markings found on the surfaces of bone. For clarification of some of these terms, a brief description follows:

DEPRESSIONS AND OPENINGS

foramen hole
fossa depression
meatus tube-shaped opening
sinus cavity or space

PROJECTIONS OR PROCESSES THAT FIT INTO JOINTS

condyle rounded knob at the end of a bone
head rounded projection beyond a necklike portion

PROJECTIONS OR PROCESSES TO WHICH MUSCLES ATTACH

crest ridge
spine sharp projection
trochanter very large projection
tubercle small, rounded eminence
tuberosity large, broad process

Parts of a typical bone (Fig. 17-1). The various types of bone have certain distinguishing features. The typical long bone consists of a *diaphysis*, or main shaft, composed of compact bony tissue; the *epiphyses*, or bulbous ends, composed of cancellous bony tissue to which muscles are attached; the *articular cartilage*, a thin layer of hyaline cartilage, which cushions shock; the *periosteum*, a dense fibrous membrane that covers bone except at joint surfaces at which the articular cartilage forms the covering; the *marrow cavity*, a space that runs the length of the diaphysis and contains the bone marrow; and the *endosteum*, the lining within the marrow cavity.

The short, flat, and irregular bones consist of an inner core of cancellous tissue in which marrow is found, an outer layer of compact bone, and a covering of periosteum.

Formation (ossification). Growth from an embryonic skeleton to a full-sized adult skeleton takes about 25 years. It is a complex process. Actually, the "bones" of the embryo are not real bones but are skeletal structures composed of hyaline cartilage or fibrous membranes. As growth continues, the membranes take the form of certain of the flat and irregular bones, and the cartilage forms the other bones of the skeleton. The soft spots (fontanels) of the infant's head are fibrous membranes that have not yet turned to bone (ossified).

Ossification of the cartilage of long bones starts at the two bulbous ends (epiphyses) and in the midst of the shaft (diaphysis) and progresses in all directions. The cartilage that remains between the diaphysis and the epiphyses is called *epiphyseal cartilage*. As long as this cartilage remains and is visible in x-ray films, the physician knows that the child is still growing because growth occurs by a continual thickening of the epiphyseal cartilage, followed by ossification. When the cartilage finally disappears, the external line of junction between the epiphysis and the diaphysis is referred to as the *epiphyseal line*.

The process of ossification is accomplished by the osteoblast cells, located chiefly under the periosteum. These cells first secrete a protein substance that forms a tough mesh. Then they secrete an enzyme, *alkaline phosphatase*, that acts chemically on phosphate and calcium to bring about their deposition in the mesh to form a marblelike substance, *carbonate apatite*, the chief material of bone.

Repair of a broken bone takes place because the osteoblasts in the vicinity of the fracture are stimulated to multiply and become very active. As a result large quantities of the protein matrix and alkaline phosphatase are made available for ossification.

The formation of bone is not irreversible. Bone is constantly being dissolved and the calcium resorbed into the body fluid. This process occurs when the calcium levels in the body fluid fall below the normal level as a result of the action of giant bone cells, called *osteoclasts*. These cells are stimulated to secrete an enzyme that digests the protein mesh and releases the calcium salts so they can be absorbed.

Two important substances regulate the formation and dissolution of bone—vitamin D and parathyroid hormone. Vitamin D accelerates the absorption of calcium and phosphate from the digestive tract into the blood, thus making these ions available to the bone tissue. Parathyroid hormone regulates the concentration of ionic calcium in the body fluids. It does so by increasing both the size and number of osteoclasts. If the concentration of calcium in the body fluids falls below the normal 10 mg/100 ml, the parathyroid glands are triggered to secrete their hormone. A severe deficiency of either calcium or vitamin D will stimulate the glands and bring about the release of calcium and phosphate ions from the bony matrix, thereby weakening their structure.

Joints (articulations). A joint is the point at which bones come together. Because the Greek name for "joint" is *arthron*, the prefix "arthro" refers to joints. They are usually classified according to the degree and variety of movement they permit.

Synarthroses are those joints with a close contact between two adjacent bones and no movement or joint cavity. The sutures of the skull are of this type and characterized by a thin layer of fibrous tissue uniting the margins of the near bones.

Amphiarthroses are partially movable joints. Fibrocartilage of the two bones forms the contact, and ligaments bind the joint together. There may be a joint cavity. The joints between the vertebrae, the two pubic bones, and the sacrum and ilium are of this type.

Diarthroses are joints that move freely. At a typical diarthrosis, the place where bones come together (articulating surface) of each bone is covered with hyaline cartilage and the entire joint is bound together with ligaments. There is usually a joint cavity lined by a synovial membrane and filled with synovial fluid. Diarthroses are thus often referred to as *synovial joints* (Fig.

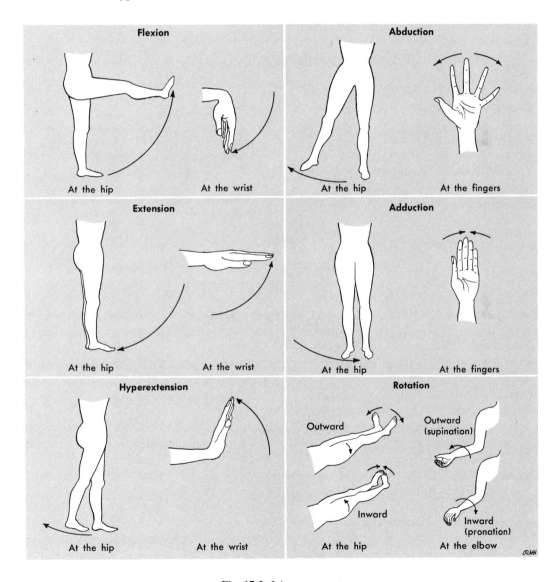

Fig. 17-2. Joint movement.

17-1). This type of joint is described according to the degree of movement as follows: (1) ball and socket—permits full movement, as hip joint; (2) hinge—permits movements in one plane, as elbow joint; (3) pivot—permits movement in the long axis of a bone, as joint between the radius and ulna; (4) gliding—one bone moves or glides across another, as joints between the carpals; and (5) biaxial or rotating—permits movement in two planes at right angles to each other, as wrist and saddle joint at base of the thumb.

Movement at these joints has been given various descriptive names. Some of the more common ones are pictured in Fig. 17-2 and are defined as follows:

flexion bending or decreasing the angle of a joint
extension straightening or increasing the angle of a joint
hyperextension bending a joint backward or increasing its angle beyond the normal degree
abduction drawing a part away from the central plane of the body
adduction drawing or "adding" a part toward the central plane of the body
rotation turning a part on an axis

Two positions that the body or parts of the body may assume are the prone position (face down or palm down) and the supine position (face up or palm up). *Pronation* is the motion placing any part of the body in a prone position; *supination* is the motion placing any part of the body in a supine position (see Fig. 17-2).

Bursae. *Bursae* are small sacs lined with synovial membrane containing synovial fluid. They develop in connective tissue wherever pressure is exerted over a moving part such as between bones and tendons, muscles, ligaments, or skin. Bursae act as cushions, relieving pressure. If they become inflamed, a painful bursitis results.

Skeleton. The two main divisions of the skeleton are the axial and the appendicular. An axis is the center around which other parts turn. The *axial skeleton* consists of the bones that form the central portion of the body, such as the skull,

Table 17-1. Bones of the body

Cranium (skull)	Upper extremity
Frontal	Clavicle (2)
Parietal (2)	Scapula (2)
Occipital	Humerus (2)
Temporal (2)	Radius (2)
Sphenoid	Ulna (2)
Ethmoid	Carpus (16)
Face	Metacarpus (10)
Nasal (2)	Phalanges of hand
Lacrimal (2)	(28)
Maxilla (2)	**Vertebrae**
Inferior nasal concha	Cervical (7)
(2)	Thoracic (12)
Zygoma (2)	Lumbar (5)
Palatine (2)	Sacrum (5 fused)
Vomer	Coccyx (4 fused)
Mandible	**Lower extremity**
Ear and neck	Hip (2)
Ossicles of ear (3	Femur (2)
pairs, 6)	Patella (2)
Hyoid	Tibia (2)
Thorax	Fibula (2)
Ribs (24)	Tarsus (14)
Sternum	Metatarsus (10)
	Phalanges of foot
	(28)

backbone, ribs, and sternum. Appendages are attachments to a central portion. The *appendicular skeleton* consists of the bones of the upper and lower extremities. A listing of the bones of the skeleton is provided in Table 17-1.

MUSCULAR SYSTEM

The muscular system is made up of all the muscle tissue in the body, including that which helps form the walls of various internal structures, such as that of the heart and intestines. The greatest portion of this tissue is in the form of skeletal muscle. Because of this preponderance of muscle tissue and because the muscles act as separate organs, the skeletal muscles are of major concern in any study of the muscular system.

Function

The outstanding characteristic of muscle tissue is its ability to contract. By contracting, the muscle tissue (1) provides external movement of body parts for locomotion and provides internal movement of portions of body organs for their proper function, (2) maintains body posture by partially contracting the skeletal muscles, and (3) produces a large share of body heat as a result of chemical changes.

Structure

Muscle tissue

Types. There are three types of muscle tissue—*skeletal* or *striated*, *visceral* or *smooth*, and *cardiac* or *branching*. Because the special function of muscle tissue is contraction, its structure is suited to its function. The cells are long and slender with numerous contractile fibers running lengthwise through them. Because of their elongated shape, muscle cells are often spoken of as fibers.

Skeletal muscle cells are bound into numerous small bundles by a membrane of connective tissue called the *sarcolemma*. The dark and light bands along the cells give them a striped or striated appearance and are called *sarcomeres*. Sarcomeres are caused by the presence of different chemical substances in the filaments arranged in an orderly striped pattern.

Visceral muscle tissue is made of tapering spindle-shaped cells that do not have stripes and are not bound together in bundles like the skeletal cells. These "smooth" muscle cells are found in the walls of the intestine, blood vessels, and other internal structures.

Cardiac muscle cells, like skeletal muscle cells, have cross striations, but, unlike them, cardiac cells are not separate and distinct fibers but branch into each other. This branching characteristic makes them especially suited to form the walls of the heart.

Nerve supply (innervation). The nerve supply of the three types of muscle tissue is of considerable importance. Visceral and cardiac muscle tissues are innervated by autonomic nerve fibers and are therefore called *involuntary* muscles. They possess an inherent ability to contract rhythmically. Skeletal muscles receive their nerve stimuli from the cerebrospinal nerves and are under the control of the will, and so are called *voluntary* muscles. They contract only as a result of stimulation. If the nerves to the skeletal muscles become diseased or are injured so that impulses cannot reach the muscle, the muscle cannot contract and thus it is paralyzed.

Characteristics. Muscle tissue has certain characteristics that make it especially suited for its specialized task. An understanding of these properties will help the student better understand the effects of activity and disease on the muscles.

Muscle tissue is in itself irritable. The cells respond to stimulation independently of their nerve supply. For example, if an electric shock is given to a paralyzed muscle, it will contract.

Muscle tissue is contractile. On stimulation it contracts, causing it to shorten and become thicker.

All healthy muscle tissue is in a state of continual partial contraction, called *tonus*. Muscle tone is caused by a small fraction of the total number of fibers of any one muscle contracting at all times. Complete relaxation of a muscle occurs only when a person is sleeping or the nerve supply has been interrupted.

Muscles respond to excessive and continuous contraction by becoming fatigued. Complete fatigue is the state in which a muscle has lost its irritability and contractility and is unable to contract. It is believed that muscle fatigue is caused by an accumulation of waste products such as lactic acid and a temporary exhaustion of the energy-supplying adenosine triphosphate (ATP) molecule.

Exercise of muscle tissue causes the cells to multiply and the muscle to enlarge (hypertrophy). Disuse of a muscle causes atrophy. This atrophy is aptly described as "wasting" and can be seen in the child who has been too ill to move about actively.

Skeletal muscles. Skeletal muscles vary in size, shape, arrangement of fibers, and mode of attachment. They range from extremely tiny strands to large masses such as those of the buttocks. Some muscles are composed of a great many fibers and others of only a few. Fibers may be parallel to the long axis of the muscle, or oblique, or curved. The direction of the fibers is significant because it determines the direction of pull on the bones when the muscle contracts.

Parts of a muscle. Each muscle consists of a central portion called the *body* and two ends called the *origin* and *insertion*. These ends are attached by fibrous connective tissue to bones, cartilage, or skin. A fibrous tissue *sheath* covers each muscle. In some cases the sheath extends into a strong cordlike *tendon* that terminates in the periosteum of a bone, thereby attaching the muscle firmly to it. In other cases, the sheath continues on as a broad, flat, fibrous sheet, called an *aponeurosis*, to become attached to a bone or cartilage. Extensions of the sheath also form partitions between muscles. Tendons are so strong that they are seldom torn, even when a bone is fractured, although they may be pulled away from bone if the force is sufficient.

Action. Muscles move the various parts of the body much as strings move the various parts of a puppet. Shortening of a string attached to a puppet part causes the part to move. When a muscle contracts, it shortens and causes the bone to which it is attached to move. The type of movement produced depends on the place the muscle is attached to the bone and the type of joint involved. By so moving, bones function as levers and joints as pivots (fulcrums) for these levers. The muscle creates the power so that motion results. As the muscle contracts, one bone must remain stationary to act as an anchor for the muscle to pull against as it draws the other bone toward it. By definition, the *origin* of a muscle is the end attached to the bone that remains stationary when the muscle contracts. The *insertion* of a muscle is the end attached to the bone that moves when the muscle shortens. The insertion is pulled toward the origin. In many cases the origin and insertion are interchangeable; that is, the end that acts as origin in one movement acts as the insertion in another.

Muscles act in groups, not singly. Any given movement is produced by the coordinated action of several muscles so that whereas some muscles of a group contract, others relax. Names have been given to the special function of each muscle as it relates to others in group action, as follows:

prime mover the muscle or muscles whose contraction actually produces the movement

synergist muscles that contract at the same time as the prime mover but act on neighboring joints to steady them and thus help the prime mover produce a more effective movement

agonist muscles that act together to produce a movement

antagonist muscles that relax while the prime mover is contracting (exception: when some part needs to be held rigid, such as the knee joint when standing, the antagonist contracts at the same time as the prime mover)

Names and groupings. There are 327 paired and 12 unpaired skeletal muscles of the body. They are named for various descriptive features, such as their action, location, shape, points of attachment, number of divisions, and direction of the fibers. Although nurses are not expected to memorize the names of all of the muscles, they should learn to identify the most prominent ones such as the deltoid of the upper arm, the gluteal muscles of the buttocks, the rectus femoris of the thigh, and the gastrocnemius of the lower leg.

DISORDERS OF THE MUSCULOSKELETAL SYSTEM

The most common musculoskeletal disorders of children are discussed in the following section, whereas those neuromuscular disorders that result from damaged nerves are included in Chapter 18, together with other neurological conditions. In studying all these disorders the student is urged to refer to Chapter 16 in which the various orthopedic devices and the specific nursing care related to them are discussed.

Congenital deformities

Clubfoot (talipes). A clubfoot is one that is twisted out of its normal position. The word *talipes* comes from *talus*, meaning "angle," and *pes*, meaning "foot," and refers to all deformities of the ankle and foot joints (Fig. 17-3). Talipes may result from an abnormal intrauterine position, from a deformity-producing (teratogenic) agent in the mother, or from a defective inherited trait. Clubbing may involve one or both feet, may be mild or severe, and may be associated with other defects or occur alone. Clubfoot deformities are given descriptive names according to the distorted position of the foot. The two chief types are equinus and calcaneus. *Equinus* means horselike with the toes down and the foot in plantar flexion. *Calcaneus* means heel prominent with the toes elevated and the foot in plantar extension. Each of these types may be bent in (varus) or bent out (valgus) (Fig. 17-4). Talipes

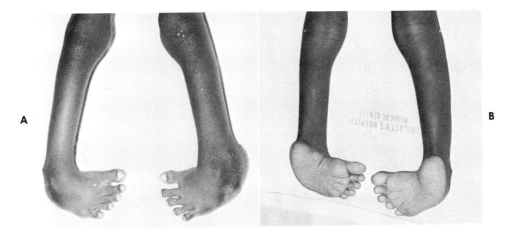

Fig. 17-3. Talipes equinovarus (horselike and bent in) is the most common type of clubbed feet. **A,** View of feet from top. **B,** View of feet from bottom.

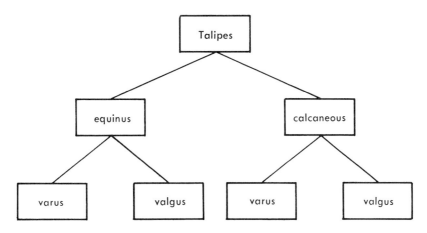

Fig. 17-4. Types of clubfoot deformities.

equinovarus (horselike and bent in) is the most common congenital defect and accounts for 95% of all clubfoot deformities. Talipes calcaneus (heel prominent and bent out) is the next most common. Other types occur only rarely.

Without treatment, the afflicted child may eventually learn to ambulate on these twisted, painful clubs much as the little girls of ancient China learned to hobble about on their wrapped and purposely deformed feet. Today, however, such deformities are neither desirable nor necessary. The sooner diagnosis is made, the sooner treatment can be instituted, and the better will be the chances for a more perfect correction. To this end, the feet of all newborn infants should be examined carefully. Usually, if corrective positioning is started soon after birth, surgery is not necessary. If treatment is delayed beyond the age of 2 years, surgery may be necessary.

In cases of early diagnosis, various splinting devices such as the Dennis Browne brace are used with considerable success. The feet are secured to foot plates or in shoes that are attached to a metal cross bar. This device has many advantages. Hip and knee movement is not restricted. As the infant moves, the leg muscles are exercised and the bones do not become porous from disuse. Gradually, the tendons and muscles of the ankle joint are stretched, and correction takes place. When the child is ready to walk, the shoe soles are built up to continue the correction. The child may need to sleep in the brace for some time to maintain the corrected position, and orthopedic shoes may be required for several years. Complete correction is achieved when the feet are in normal alignment without external support.

When diagnosis is delayed beyond the age of 2 years, correction becomes more difficult with the passage of time. Repeated manipulation and plaster casting every 3 weeks may be necessary. The feet are eventually positioned in a hyperextended and adducted position to allow for some flexibility when the casts are eventually removed. In certain cases surgery may be required

to elongate the Achilles tendon or otherwise free the ankle joint. In severe cases of prolonged neglect, muscle transplants may be required. After many months and years of casting, bracing, and special shoes the clubfeet may eventually assume normal alignment.

Dislocated hip. Congenital dislocations of the hip are believed to be caused by incomplete embryonic development of the joint. Newborn infants seldom have a complete dislocation; instead the head of the femur is displaced so that it does not lie entirely within a shallow socket (acetabulum). When the child begins to walk, weight-bearing may produce a true dislocation. The abnormality is seven times more common in girls than in boys and occurs in some regions such as northern Italy much more frequently than in others. It is rare in the Orient where infants are carried with their legs astride their mother's back so that if the condition occurs it is corrected in the course of normal child-rearing.

A positive diagnosis may not be possible in the newborn infant but should be looked for at the monthly physical examinations during the first year. The first sign of difficulty is usually limitation of abduction (bending out) of the hip joint involved. When the infant is lying supine, the flexed thighs and knees normally can be pushed outward to almost the level of the examining table. This flexion cannot be done if the child has a "congenital hip." Diagnosis is confirmed by x-ray examination. If diagnosis is missed and the child begins to walk and bear weight, the affected leg will be shorter and gluteal folds of skin will appear on the affected side.

Treatment should be started as soon as diagnosis is made. Delay prolongs treatment and may result in a partial dislocation becoming a complete one. The object of treatment is to place the head of the femur within the acetabulum, which position by constant pressure enlarges and deepens the socket with ultimate correction of the dislocation. Treatment is achieved by placing both of the infant's legs in abduction. Sometimes a bulky double diaper or pillow (Frejka) splint is used. Sometimes it is necessary to admit the child to the hospital for gradual reduction of the defect through use of skin traction and a Putti board or modified Bryant's traction on a A-frame as described in Chapter 16. Traction is followed by the application of plaster casting or abduction braces for continued treatment at home (Fig. 16-5).

Osteogenesis imperfecta. Osteogenesis imperfecta is an inherited disease caused by a mutant, or changed, gene. It is characterized by soft, fragile bones with abnormally low calcium deposition. The symptoms may be present at birth (congenital) or may appear later. Fortunately, the congenital form is rare. The infant's bones may fracture while still in utero or during the birth process. The skull is soft and the whites of the eyes are typically blue colored. Depending on when symptoms appear, the lack of bony growth causes dwarfism, poor tooth development, progressive deafness, various skin lesions, and muscle weakness. A variety of deformities may result from the multiple fractures.

Diagnosis is made by examination and confirmed by x-ray films of the fractured and poorly calcified bones. Treatment is supportive because there is no known cure. The infant or child must be handled with great care to prevent further damage to the bones. Fractures are treated by means of casts and orthopedic procedures. A nutritious diet with adequate vitamins and minerals is given. Emotional support is very important. Prognosis is especially poor for infants born with symptoms but improves with the age of onset of symptoms. A greater number of these children are surviving longer periods as a result of continuous medical supervision and improved treatment techniques.

Torticollis (wryneck). Although wryneck may occur after the newborn period as a result of injury, inflammation, or emotional disturbance, the congenital variety is caused by a retardation in the lengthening of the sternocleidomastoid muscle of the neck. Soon after birth a firm fibrous lump can be felt in the affected mus-

cle. The lump may disappear, but restriction of the neck movement continues and tends to worsen. If the condition is not corrected, the face becomes distorted, the child's vision adjusts to the deformity, and eventually the neck and shoulder bones are displaced, causing a curvature of the upper spine (thoracic scoliosis) and an abnormal elevation of the shoulders.

Early diagnosis and treatment prevent complications. An alert parent may be the first to notice the lump and restricted neck movement and bring the child to the physician for examination. At first, conservative treatment may be attempted. This consists of passive stretching of the neck. The parents are taught to do this three times a day for several weeks with frequent review by the physician. If there is no improvement, surgical lengthening of the affected muscle is performed, followed by casting the neck in an overcorrected position until healing occurs. After the cast is removed, passive stretching and exercises are continued for some time. Medical supervision should continue beyond puberty to check for recurrence.

Nursing care in the hospital usually involves a brief preoperative period and postoperative care until the cast is dry. If the nurses are expected to give the passive stretching exercises of the neck, they should receive individual instruction by the physical therapist or physician.

Developmental anomalies of the extremities. Congenital anomalies of the extremities vary in severity from a slight defect of a finger to the complete absence of all four extremities. These defects are caused by changes in the normal embryonic development as a result of unknown factors, inherited traits, and teratogenic substances taken by the mother such as the drug thalidomide (see Chapter 2). The following are some of these deformities:

Syndactyly (joined-together digits) is manifested by fingers or toes that are partly or completely fused. Only the skin may be involved, or the bones themselves may be joined.

Polydactyly (many digits) is the presence of

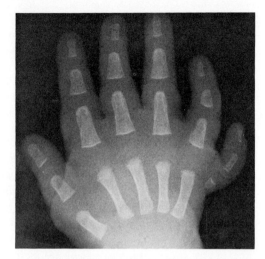

Fig. 17-5. Polydactyly. This child was born with six fingers on each hand and six toes on each foot. The presence of three bones in the extra digit is not usual.

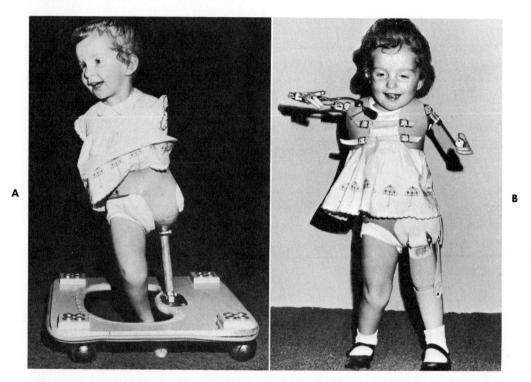

Fig. 17-6. A, Ectromelia of three limbs showing a walking platform created to permit this child to ambulate during her toddler years. **B,** Same little girl as pictured in **A** after she learned to walk with a full leg prosthesis, using her prosthetic arms for balance. (Courtesy The National Foundation–March of Dimes.)

more than the normal number of fingers or toes. The condition may be inherited (Fig. 17-5).

Adactyly (absent digits) is the absence of one or more fingers or toes.

Amelia (no limbs) is the complete absence of all extremities.

Ectromelia (abortive limbs) is the absence of a limb or limbs (Fig. 17-6).

Micromelia (small limbs) is severe shortening of a limb as a result of the absence of the shaft of an extremity.

Hemimelia (half limbs) is the absence or a defect in the distal portion of a limb.

Phocomelia (seal limbs) is the absence of all but the most distal portion of an extremity.

All of these deformities are usually obvious at birth. When they are present, the physician examines the infant with great care because other defects may be present. Simple defects may be treated immediately. Extra digits may be amputated or merely tied off with a tight suture to eventually drop off. Major complex defects require the careful planning and cooperation of the whole medical team, composed of the pediatrician, orthopedist, prosthetist, social worker, psychologist, occupational therapist, physiotherapist, nurses, educators, and other professional persons. The objective of all treatment is to help the child grow to adulthood with a minimum of dependency and a maximum of emotional and physical health. The parents and the child must be included in the plan of therapy. As soon as possible the child is fitted with a prosthesis to promote more normal development, reduce atrophy of the parts that are present, and help both the child and parents accept the prosthesis.

The impact of a congenital limb deficiency on the parents and the afflicted child is profound. The parents must be told the truth about their child as soon as possible after birth. This difficult task usually falls upon the physician. The future for such children today is not nearly as bleak as in the past. Tremendous strides have been made in the fields of prosthesis and occupational and physical therapy. Public funds are available to help families who need them. But even with these facts, the parents may need help to accept their feelings of guilt, fear, helplessness, and rejection of the child. Talking about these feelings seems to relieve some of the intensity. Nurses, too, may need to talk out their feelings of helplessness, horror, or rejection with other members of the nursing team.

Searching for causes, with the goal of preventing such tragedies, has been the major thrust of much research in recent years. One of the largest private organizations devoted to this cause is the National Foundation–March of Dimes. Originally formed to fight poliomyelitis, it now spends millions of dollars in research, care, direct assistance to patients, education, and public information to fight birth defects.

Traumatic injuries

Traumatic injuries are those caused by a forceful impact. They include soft tissue injuries, fractures, and joint injuries. Most traumatic injuries are unplanned and require emergency treatment before the child arrives at the hospital. The student is referred to Chapter 3 where accidents are discussed briefly and a list of first-aid priorities is provided.

Soft tissue injuries. When soft tissue is torn (lacerated), cut (incised), or bruised (contused) there is always bleeding. If a large vessel is cut, there is danger of hemorrhage. If the skin is broken, there is danger of infection. When bleeding occurs within tissue, it causes a contusion and sometimes, if the blood pools in one place, a blood "tumor" (hematoma) may form. Emergency care consists of control of the bleeding by direct pressure (only rarely by tourniquet, as a last resort) and covering the exposed flesh with a clean cloth. In the hospital the child is evaluated and treated for shock, the wounds are cleansed, bleeders are tied off, and tissue is sutured as needed. If a hematoma forms, the surgeon may aspirate the accumulated blood to relieve pressure and promote healing. Ice may be applied to help constrict the blood vessels. Depending on the seriousness of the injuries, the child may be admitted to the hospital or sent home.

Fractures and joint injuries. Bones tend to break at sites of natural or disease-produced weakness. Breaks that occur as a result of bone tumors or disease such as osteogenesis imperfecta are called *pathological fractures*. Breaks that occur as a result of excessive pressure are called *traumatic fractures*. Fractures are classified according to (1) whether the skin is broken (open) or not (simple); (2) the relative position of the broken bones to one another, as when one segment is overlapping (overriding) the other, is twisted (rotated), or is at an angle (angulated); and (3) the contour of the fracture line—straight across (transverse), angled across (oblique), angled across and around (spiral), fragmented (comminuted), or only partially severed and bent (greenstick), often seen in children because their bones are quite pliable (Fig. 17-7).

Whenever a child has a severe fall or is involved in a traumatic accident of any kind, the child should be examined for evidence of fracture as follows:

1. Pain or tenderness at a possible fracture site
2. Loss of function or abnormal mobility
3. Deformity in alignment or swelling
4. A grating sensation (crepitus) at the suspected break point
5. Discoloration of tissue about the site

Indications of joint injury are as follows:

1. Pain and tenderness
2. Splinting of the nearby muscles
3. Swelling
4. Discoloration of the tissue about the joint

Serious damage can be caused if an injured joint or broken bone is carelessly moved; a simple fracture can be compounded. For transportation to the hospital the affected part must be immobilized below and above the injured area. Protruding bone ends should be covered with a sterile or clean cloth.

When the child is brought to the emergency room with a possible fracture, the general condition is evaluated. Vital signs, level of consciousness, and pupils of the eyes provide valuable information. Elevated blood pressure and fixed or unequal pupils may indicate concussion. Depressed blood pressure and dilated pupils may mean shock. The physician evaluates these findings and prescribes medications and treatment as necessary. Drugs to control pain may be needed. When the child is ready, x-ray films are taken of all suspected fracture points. Positive diagnosis is made by x-ray examination, but until proved otherwise, all possible fractures should be treated as positive.

When diagnosis is established, the orthopedist decides how best to align the bones. If overriding or angulation of the fracture has occurred, the displaced bone must be pulled into alignment by some form of traction. This is called "setting a bone" or "reducing a fracture." If the bones can be positioned without surgical exposure, the procedure is called *closed reduction*. If the site must be exposed to direct view or if some type of internal immobilization must be used such as a pin, plate, nail, or screw, the procedure is called an *open reduction*. Sometimes alignment is not disturbed by the fracture, and x-ray examination reveals a break, but the bony segments are still in proper relationship. If this is the case, no traction is needed. A plaster cast or splint is applied to maintain the correct position and assure healing.

Sometimes a fracture is of such a nature that the strong muscles nearby tend to displace the bony segments. In this case traction may be applied until sufficient new bone is formed at the fracture site to help hold the segments in place. When the segments stay in place, traction is discontinued and a cast applied to immobilize the part.

Joint injuries are especially serious because so many interrelated structures are involved. They are often followed by continuing pain and limitation of movement. *Ankylosis*, or abnormal immobility of a joint, may occur as a result of

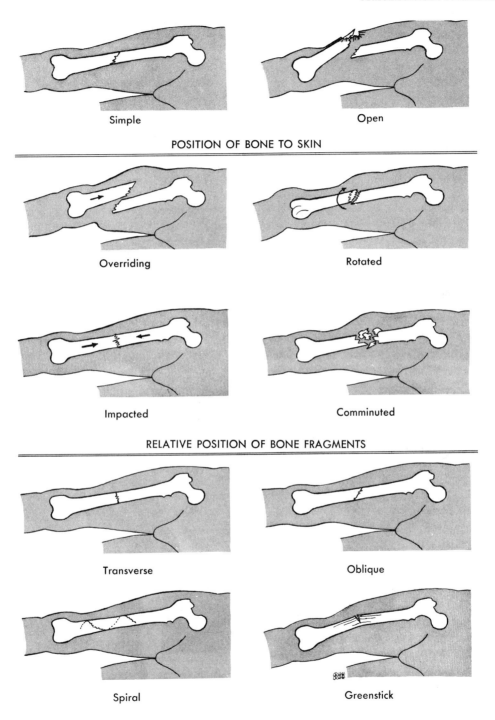

Simple

Open

POSITION OF BONE TO SKIN

Overriding

Rotated

Impacted

Comminuted

RELATIVE POSITION OF BONE FRAGMENTS

Transverse

Oblique

Spiral

Greenstick

CONTOUR OF FRACTURE LINE

Fig. 17-7. Types of fractures.

disease or purposeful surgery in which the articular cartilage is destroyed. As a result the bones grow together in a fixed position. When such fixation is done surgically, the joint is first placed in a useful position and a cast applied for immobilization.

The nurse should remember that any injury or surgical procedure involving a joint is extremely painful. This pain causes muscle spasm, which produces even more pain. For this reason medications to control pain should be administered. The affected joint is usually elevated and ice applied to reduce congestion of blood. Normal cast care is given.

Refer to Chapter 16 for a discussion of the nursing care of children in casts and other orthopedic devices.

Battered child syndrome. A battered child is one who has been beaten, burned, stabbed, neglected, sexually molested, or otherwise abused. Over 50% of the victims are under 2 years of age and 90% are under 10 years of age. Three fourths of the time the parents are responsible, many of whom were abused by their parents. Immaturity, personal unhappiness, frustration, lack of parent-child bonding, and chronic poverty seem to be the root causes for such desperate action.

In the typical case the child is brought to the hospital or physician with many injuries in various stages of healing—bruises, fractures, burns, lacerations, stab wounds, concussion, or ruptured internal organs. More than one fourth of those brought for care die. Unknown numbers are never diagnosed or rescued, and some grow up to inflict similar cruelties on their own children.

Diagnosis is made from a number of clues, such as x-ray films showing old and new fractures, injuries that could not have been accidental, and parental evasiveness to questioning, together with anger at the child for being injured.

Hemorrhage, serious burns, shock, infections, and fractures are immediate concerns of the medical team for the abused child. Treatment of physical and emotional malnutrition follows.

Because many of these children have been neglected, they may be listless and without appetites. A battered child represents a tremendous nursing challenge. The child may have never known a trusting relationship with an adult, and may be apathetic, furtive, or openly frightened. The school-aged child may defend the parents, fearing that known security will be taken away. As nurses care for the estranged child, they use continuity of care and increasing bodily contact to communicate tenderness and caring. Gradually and ideally, the child becomes more active and responsive and begins to grow physically and emotionally.

All 50 states now have laws that encourage or require the reporting of suspected cases of child abuse and provide legal immunity to the reporting person. Legal charges are filed against the accused persons, and as soon as physically able, the child may be placed in a foster home until the parents are able to provide care. Continued support for convicted parents who are freed and help for others with abusive tendencies are available at organizations such as Parents Anonymous through group and individual counseling. Prevention of this tragic syndrome involves removing the root causes, providing mental health services to all, and increasing public awareness of the need to report suspected cases.

Infections and inflammations

Osteomyelitis. Osteomyelitis is an inflammation of the bone caused by such organisms as *Staphylococcus aureus*, *Streptococcus pyogenes*, and sometimes *Mycobacterium tuberculosis*. These bacteria may reach the bone directly, as in a compound fracture, or, more commonly in children, by the bloodstream from some other acute infection such as a boil (furuncle), otitis media, or active lung tuberculosis. Often a history of local bone injury reduces resistance to the blood-borne bacteria.

Typically, the bone marrow becomes involved first, usually near the end of the shaft if it is in a long bone. Then the infection spreads in any or all directions. It may involve the entire shaft or may be arrested at any point. The periosteum becomes separated from the inner dead bone and begins to lay down new bone over it. The area of separated dead bone is called a *sequestrum*. A tube of new bone around the old is called an *involucrum*. Through this layer, openings may form through which pus can escape to the surface. If the infection is near a joint, the infection may spread there so that the purulent exudate soon destroys the articular cartilage. If the condition becomes chronic, draining sinuses open through the skin and some of the sequestra may be cast out during periods of increased infectious activity.

In acute osteomyelitis symptoms develop rapidly. There is a sharp rise in temperature, pain in the affected bone with local tenderness, and pain on movement. The nearby joint may also be affected with septic arthritis. The white blood count increases (leukocytosis) and blood cultures reveal the causative organism. X-ray examination may not give early evidence of osteomyelitis.

Treatment involves the prompt administration of antibiotic agents, particularly penicillin, and immobilization of the affected bone in plaster or traction. These measures are continued until all symptoms have subsided for at least a week. If an abscess forms or a joint becomes involved, the exudate must be aspirated or drained and antibiotics injected locally. In chronic osteomyelitis, treatment involves open incision and drainage, antibiotic therapy, and immobilization.

Nursing care of the child with osteomyelitis consists of taking the child's temperature at regular intervals, administering antibiotics as ordered, giving cast or traction care and special skin care, moving the affected part with great gentleness to avoid further trauma, encouraging the child to drink fluids and eat a nourishing diet, and, in cases of open drainage, observing wound and skin isolation technique until the exudate is no longer infectious. Fortunately, because of the prompt use of antibiotics to treat the common infections of childhood, acute osteomyelitis is less common and chronic cases are rare.

Juvenile rheumatoid arthritis (Still's disease). Rheumatoid arthritis is a chronic systemic disease with major involvement of the musculoskeletal system. It is characterized by nonbacterial inflammations, or lesions, in which there is an infiltration of lymphocytes and an overgrowth of connective tissue. These lesions occur in joints, tendons, cartilage, the periosteum of bones, muscles, and the outer covering of the heart and lungs and may form into subcutaneous nodules over pressure areas. There is no known cause. Girls are more often afflicted than boys.

Symptoms of the disease may appear gradually or abruptly, with high fever and many painfully swollen joints (*polyarthritis*). The joint pain causes muscle splinting with resultant spasm. Movement is restricted. The child tends to hold the joints in flexion, which may cause them to become fixed in what are called *flexion contractures*. If the muscles are also inflamed, they become weak and wasted. Characteristic subcutaneous nodules may appear. As the disease progresses, the fingers become spindle shaped as the muscles atrophy on either side of swollen joints. The child loses an appetite and prefers to be left alone. Growth is stunted. A birdlike face may result from impaired jawbone growth. The disease is characterized by *remissions*, when the symptoms subside, and *exacerbations*, when they become worse. Fortunately about 80% of children with rheumatoid arthritis have complete remissions; about 20% continue to adult life with intermittent episodes of the disease.

There is no "cure" and the course of the disease for each child is unpredictable. Therapy, therefore, is aimed at promoting normal growth and development, maintaining motion, and preventing deformities of affected joints. Certain drugs are used to relieve symptoms, particularly steroids and aspirin. Passive and active exercises are used to prevent contracture deformities.

Nursing care during the acute phases may involve feeding, bathing, and dressing. As soon as possible activity is resumed. Joints should be put through the full range of motion at least every day. The child should lie flat on the back rather than curl up on a side. The legs may be placed in half-shell casts at night to prevent contractures and foot drop. Hospitalization is kept at a minimum to promote a more active and more normal life.

Parents should be taught how best to care for their arthritic child at home. Measures that will relieve pain include placing bed boards under the mattress and giving a hot tub bath in the morning followed by passive or active exercises of all the joints. The child should be encouraged to lead as normal a life as possible, attending school and participating in play and nonstrenuous activities to full capacity. The services of the community health nurse and various other community resources may be needed by the family because the disease may last for many years. The Arthritis Foundation is a national organization devoted to meeting the needs of arthritic persons.

Coxa plana (Legg-Calvé-Perthes disease). Coxa plana, or Perthes disease, is a peculiar condition of unknown etiology in which the blood supply to the hip joint is temporarily disturbed, causing the tissue to die (necrose). It affects children from 5 to 10 years of age, usually boys, which suggests that trauma may be a cause. The course of the disease is usually divided into the following three stages, each lasting about 9 to 12 months: (1) necrosis, or death of the tissues; (2) revascularization as the blood vessels grow again; and (3) reossification, as new bone reforms the acetabulum and head of the femur. If the joint is forced to carry weight before the third stage is well along, the head of the femur tends to become flattened and mushroom shaped, hence the name *coxa plana*, meaning "flat hip." Later this abnormal shape causes degenerative changes in the hip.

The first symptoms are those caused by synovial inflammation (synovitis)—a limp and pain in the hip joint. Diagnosis is confirmed by x-ray

films showing typical bony changes. Treatment consists of preventing weight-bearing until the bone is regenerated. Such prevention is accomplished first by bed rest and traction and later by casts, splints, or braces. Eventually the child is allowed up on crutches, but no weight is to be placed on the affected hip. Muscle exercises are begun early to prevent atrophy and decalcification of the affected bones from disuse.

Nursing care in the hospital while the child is in traction or in a cast is like that of other children in traction or casts. Passive and active exercises of the muscles should be carried on as directed by the physician and physiotherapist. When the child is to be dismissed to go home, the parents will need specific instructions and help to provide the physical care and emotional support needed during a long period of immobility. A community health nurse is a valuable member of the health team for such a child. When allowed up on crutches, the child should have instructions on how to use them without placing *any* weight on the affected hip. The importance of no weight-bearing cannot be overemphasized.

Prognosis depends on how perfectly the hip bones are reformed during the reossification stage. Two factors affect this stage: how young the child is at onset and how little the amount of weight borne by the femur. With imperfect reformation of the bones, degenerative changes take place that cause permanent disability.

Slipped femoral epiphysis. Slipped femoral epiphysis occurs most often in overweight boys between the ages of 12 and 15, and the condition often affects both hips. Although trauma usually causes the actual displacement, these children all have some deficiency in calcium metabolism and probably also in thyroid and pituitary gland function.

There are three successive stages to the disease, as follows:

1. In the preslipped stage, the child limps and has a slight limitation of hip movement. The x-ray films show little or no displace-

ment of the head of the femur from its normal position but may show some change in the bone on the femoral side of the epiphysis.

2. Through trauma, the epiphysis slides further upward and greater displacement occurs.

3. In the advanced, untreated stage, there is more extensive slipping of the epiphysis with even greater displacement. X-ray films show more bone damage. There is a marked limp and the child has increased limitation of movement, but pain is not severe.

Treatment varies with the stage and the philosophy of the physician and includes internal fixation with pins and nails and manipulation under anesthesia and casting. Preoperatively the child is placed on bed rest with no weight-bearing. Postoperatively, the child usually returned to the ward with a wet cast. Close observation for possible circulatory disturbance is important. When the condition has stabilized after surgery, the child is usually discharged to go home with crutches and with instructions not to bear any weight on the affected hip.

Postural defects

Postural defects are abnormal positions of the spine, shoulders, and pelvis that are not caused by disease or trauma. Common during adolescence, they are caused by rapid bone growth compared with the relatively slower muscle development of the period and by a physical response to emotional stress. They may also result from structural defects such as an untreated clubfoot or a short leg.

The following are some of the more common postural defects:

kyphosis hunchback or an outward curving spine
lordosis curved spine with the pelvis tilted forward
scoliosis an S-shaped, sideways-curving spine
swayback curved spine with lordosis and kyphosis, the "posture of fatigue"

Diagnosis of postural defects in adolescents is aimed at finding the cause. Disease and trauma must first be ruled out. This is done by examination and x-ray films. The physician then determines the group of muscles that are weak and cause the poor posture. Treatment is directed toward strengthening these muscles and helping the youth to establish new posture habits. If emotional factors are the basis for poor posture, professional counseling may be needed to help resolve the conflicts. Parental nagging serves no useful purpose. It merely antagonizes and hinders therapy.

Adolescent kyphosis. Hunchback of adolescence is a chronic disease producing bone damage to the affected vertebrae. It is caused by pathological changes of the intravertebral disks of unknown origin. Diagnosis is made by x-ray examination. Mild cases are treated by means of harness traction attached to the head for about 20 minutes daily. In more severe cases patients may be required to wear a special brace during the day with regular exercises. Serious cases may require a stay of several months in a plaster bed (a bivalved body cast) with gradual correction by felt pads and hourly hyperextension exercises. Some physicians recommend that all patients sleep in a plaster bed. Success of treatment depends on the extent of the defect when treatment was commenced

Scoliosis. Scoliosis is an S-shaped sideways curvature of the spine that develops most often during a period of rapid growth. When it results simply from poor posture and not from spinal disease or trauma, it is called *functional scoliosis* and is classified as one of the postural defects. When the curvature results from defects or disease of the muscles, bones, or nerves of the spine, it is called *structural scoliosis*, and there is usually an associated rotation or twisting of the vertebral column. This type most often occurs during the growth spurt of puberty.

Scoliosis may go unnoticed for several years because of the absence of pain and may finally be observed by the presence of a higher shoulder or a protruding hip. Diagnosis is confirmed by physical examination and x-ray films. The absence of specific defects indicates that the scoliosis is functional. The presence of defects indicates structural scoliosis.

Treatment is aimed at arresting further curvature and correcting that which has already occurred. Functional scoliosis is treated by retraining and exercises. The treatment of structural scoliosis begins with bed rest. Various braces and plaster splints may then be used until vertebral growth is complete. Ultimately, surgical fusion of the vertebrae must be performed to correct structural defects. In some cases, when there is pain or bone destruction in a young child, a short fusion may be done at the time and extended later when vertebral growth ceases.

One of the more common devices used both before and after spinal fusion is the *Milwaukee brace* (see Fig. 16-8). This brace exerts pressure on the chin, pelvis, and outcurving (convex) side of the spine to achieve correction. The number of hours each day and the total period of time the brace is worn are ordered by the physician depending on the stage of the child's treatment.

Another common device is the *turnbuckle cast*. It begins as a heavy body cast that extends from the chin and back of the head down to the hip on one side and the knee on the other. When the cast is thoroughly dry, a large pie-shaped wedge extending to the midline both back and front is cut out of the cast on the convex side of the scoliosis curve. A crosscut is also made on the concave side of the curve, allowing movement of the top part of the cast. Hinges and a turnbuckle are then attached to the cast to control the amount of lateral angulation of the top to the lower part of the cast. Over a period of time the physician gradually tightens the turnbuckle, forcing the deformed spine into a corrected position. When the desired position is attained, the open areas of the cast are plastered shut and a window is cut in the cast over the vertebrae to be fused. The child is then taken to surgery and a spinal fusion perfomed through the window.

This fusion often involves the use of bone grafts from the child's own iliac or tibial bones or from a bone bank.

Another commonly used device is the *Risser localizer cast* applied by using the Risser table or frame. The frame helps straighten the spine by both pulling the child in vertical traction and by pushing against the protruding side. The child is supported on the frame after being protected with layers of stockinette and padding, and plaster casts are applied to the pelvis and head in two separate sections. Traction is then applied to the head by a halter and to the pelvis by a special girdle. At the same time pressure is exerted on the convex side of the curvature by padded plaster-backed localizers. When maximum correction at that time is achieved, the cast is completed by joining the head and pelvic portions with a plaster cast of the trunk, including the localizers. Successive castings are followed by spinal fusion.

Nursing care of the child in a large body cast must be comprehensive. Exercises of the non-casted parts may be ordered to prevent muscle wasting. Skin care is vital, as is the diet and adequate fluid intake, because constipation is often a problem. When the patient is ready for a spinal fusion, preoperative and postoperative care is similar to that for all surgical patients. In addition, great care must be taken turning and moving the child. When there has been a bone graft, the site should be handled carefully for at least 8 weeks until healing has taken place.

Although many spinal fusion patients return from surgery with a cast, some do not. When there is no cast to stabilize the operative site nurses must exercise great care to avoid twisting or bending the spine. The bed is kept flat unless there are specific orders to allow a slight incline while the patient is supine. The patient being turned from abdomen to back should be rolled like a log. A turning sheet greatly facilitates turning. If the patient is to lie on a side, a pillow should be placed between the thighs to maintain constant hip-spine alignment.

The long involved treatment of scoliosis places a great burden on both parents and patient, especially because the patient often is an adolescent. Such teenagers are benefited by being hospitalized in teen units and by maximum participation in normal living experiences when outside the hospital. Every effort should be made to help them mature intellectually and emotionally in spite of the physical restrictions of the prolonged treatment. Information about community services should be provided for the family.

The muscular dystrophies

The muscular dystrophies are a group of inherited disorders characterized by progressive muscular weakness and wasting. They are caused by an inherited disturbance in the metabolism of the muscles and not by nervous system disease as are the muscular atrophies. In the dystrophies the skeletal and cardiac muscle fibers degenerate and are replaced by connective tissue and fat. The type of dystrophy depends on the muscle groups affected and its inherited characteristics. The most common ones are the pseudohypertrophic (Duchenne), facioscapulohumeral, and limb-girdle types.

The *pseudohypertrophic (Duchenne) type* is the most severe. It occurs in boys by means of a sex-linked recessive gene (Chapter 2). Muscle weakness appears during the first year, with slowed motor development. Although eventually learning to walk, the child falls frequently, has a waddling gait, and has a typical self-climbing method of getting up to a standing position, called Gower's sign. The child may toe-walk and develop large calf muscles as a result of fat deposition rather than muscle fiber growth, hence the name *pseudohypertrophic*, meaning "false enlargement." The disease progresses throughout childhood. By early adolescence the victim is confined to a wheelchair and eventually to bed. Near the end the child is unable even to turn over because of weakness. Scoliosis and flexion contractures are common in advanced cases. Death

comes from congestive heart failure or respiratory complications.

The *facioscapulohumeral type* affects both sexes. It is caused by both dominant and recessive autosomal (non–sex chromosomal) genes. The symptoms of facial and shoulder muscle weakness appear in adolescence and progress so slowly that the patient may be barely aware of them. Eventually the pelvis and leg muscles are involved, but life expectancy is normal and not affected by the disease.

The *limb-girdle type* may appear in either sex, at any age, although it is more common in young adults. It affects the pelvic girdle and shoulder muscles and may progress rapidly, with severe disability a few years after onset, thus lowering life expectancy.

Diagnosis of muscular dystrophy is made on the basis of family and personal history, physical examination, serum enzyme studies, electromyography, and muscle biopsy. There is no cure. Treatment consists of giving general supportive care. As soon as the diagnosis is made, a systematic plan of physical therapy is instituted to prevent contractures and maintain ambulation as long as possible. Daily exercises are vital. Lightweight leg braces may be used to maintain heel-cord length and correct foot-leg alignment. A torso brace may be employed to prevent scoliosis when there is shoulder muscle weakness. Antibiotics are valuable in combating respiratory infections, and digitalis may be necessary if congestive heart failure develops.

Nurses usually see the child in the hospital only when diagnosis is made, when there are acute health problems, and when orthopedic devices are being evaluated. Care is adjusted to patient needs at the time and includes normal hygienic measures, diet, elimination, and maintenance of a daily exercise schedule. Physical therapists plan, demonstrate, and supervise exercises and the use of orthopedic devices as they become necessary. When the child is not hospitalized, the parents must assume responsibility for care. Both the parents and the child need emotional support as well as practical assistance during the long worsening course of the disease. Every member of the health team should be aware of these needs and seek to meet them. Parents may be encouraged and helped by meeting with other parents of muscular dystrophy children to share their common burden and learn from one another. The Muscular Dystrophy Association sponsors such groups on the local level, and on the national level promotes research into the treatment and eradication of this tragic disease.

Bone tumors (sarcomas)

Malignant tumors are colonies of altered cells that produce destructive changes in nearby tissues and spread (metastasize) via the bloodstream to distant tissues where they initiate other sites of malignant change.

Sarcomas are malignant tumors of connective tissues such as bone and cartilage. Although they are rare, the most common types are osteogenic and Ewing's endothelioma.

Osteogenic sarcoma occurs more often in preadolescents and adolescents. It arises in the metaphyses of long bones (Fig. 17-1) and is characterized by slowly increasing bone pain, local tenderness, and swelling. The child gradually refuses to use the affected extremity, leading to muscle atrophy and contracture of the nearby joint.

Ewing's endothelioma is a rapidly growing, highly destructive sarcoma that occurs in young children as well as older ones. It arises in the diaphyses of long bones (Fig. 17-1) and is characterized by pain and local swelling.

Both types of sarcomas spread to the lungs and other bones. Diagnosis is made by biopsy of bone tissue, and x-ray studies are made to determine the extent of bone involvement and possible metastasis.

Treatment consists of radical surgical amputation when it is believed metastasis has not yet occurred. Although ineffective for osteogenic sarcoma, radiation of the affected bone and ad-

ministration of certain alkaloid drugs have produced some palliative effects for Ewing's endothelioma. Prognosis is poor for both types, and death within 5 years is common.

The child admitted for diagnostic evaluation must undergo various tests, including biopsies and x-ray studies. These procedures are frightening, exhausting, and often painful. The child needs support and comfort. If a positive diagnosis of malignancy is made, the surgeon, parents, and sometimes the patient must decide the course of action—whether to forego surgery and accept sure death or to undergo surgery and its mutilation for uncertain life.

If the decision is for surgery, normal orthopedic preparations are made. Postoperatively the amputated stump should be elevated and protected from trauma. Close observation for hemorrhage and of vital signs is made during the first 24 hours. In the days and weeks following amputation, the child may experience "phantom" pains in the absent foot and leg. Nurses should remember that such radical surgery creates tremendous emotional conflicts within both the child and the parents. Their acceptance of the malignancy and the drastic surgery may be slow. Nurses may be able to help by showing sincere concern.

When radiation and chemotherapy are administered, nausea or vomiting are common side effects. Maintenance of adequate fluid intake and nutrition are especially important.

When treatment does not halt the malignancy these children may be hospitalized during the last days of life. For a discussion of children with terminal illnesses see Chapter 7.

Rickets (osteomalacia)

Rickets or bone softening (osteomalacia) is a malformation of bones as a result of inadequate deposits of calcium in developing cartilage and bone (Fig. 17-8). It is primarily caused by vitamin D deficiency. Vitamin D is synthesized in the skin by the action of the sun or ultraviolet rays or is obtained preformed from animal fats such as milk and fish oils and some plants. It may also be obtained from "vitamin-enriched" breads, cereals, and milk. Vitamin D affects the absorption of calcium and phosphorus from the intestine and the reabsorption of phosphorus by the kidneys. A deficiency usually results from an inadequate intake of vitamin D–rich food, or in some cases to poor utilization of the vitamin by the tissues, called *refractory rickets*.

Infants with early rickets are restless and may develop a slight fever at night. They perspire freely, are pale, and seem to have soreness and tenderness of the body. They do not sit, crawl, or walk early, and there is a delay in closure of the fontanel. Weightbearing bends the bones and causes characteristic bowed legs, knock-knees,

and pigeon breast. Diagnosis is difficult in early cases because of the many other conditions with similar symptoms. Typical x-ray findings of more advanced rickets show defective calcification of growing bones and overgrowth of the epiphyseal cartilage. Blood studies of calcium, phosphorus, and serum phosphatase are done to confirm the diagnosis. Treatment consists of supplying the deficient vitamin D. Dosage depends on the condition and response of the child to treatment. Refractory cases require massive doses for correction of defects. When large doses of vitamin D are administered, however, special tests must be made to guard against renal overload. Prognosis is usually good, with deformities disappearing in 90% of the cases if treatment is begun before the final growth spurt of adolescence.

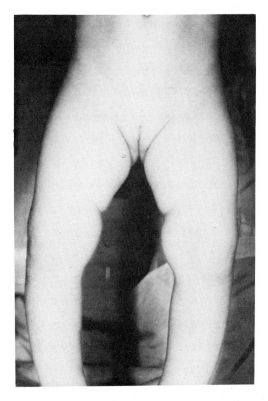

Fig. 17-8. Rickets (osteomalacia). Bowed legs are caused by weight bearing when the bones are soft as a result of inadequate deposits of calcium.

SUMMARY OUTLINE

  I. Skeletal system
    A. Function
    B. Structure
      1. Tissue
        a. Fibrous connective tissue
        b. Cartilage tissue
        c. Bone tissue
        d. Reticuloendothelial tissue
      2. Bones
        a. Types
        b. Markings
        c. Parts of a typical bone
        d. Formation (ossification)
      3. Joints (articulations)
      4. Bursae
      5. Skeleton
  II. Muscular system
    A. Function
    B. Structure
      1. Muscle tissue
        a. Types
        b. Nerve supply (innervation)
        c. Characteristics
      2. Skeletal muscles
        a. Parts of a muscle
        b. Action
        c. Names and groupings
 III. Disorders of the musculoskeletal system
    A. Congenital deformities
      1. Clubfoot (talipes)

    2. Dislocated hip
    3. Osteogenesis imperfecta
    4. Torticollis (wryneck)
    5. Developmental anomalies of the extremities
B. Traumatic injuries
    1. Soft tissue injuries
    2. Fractures and joint injuries
    3. Battered child syndrome
C. Infections and inflammations
    1. Osteomyelitis
    2. Juvenile rheumatoid arthirits (Still's disease)
    3. Coxa plana (Legg-Calvé-Perthes disease)
    4. Slipped femoral epiphysis
D. Postural defects
    1. Adolescent kyphosis
    2. Scoliosis
E. The muscular dystrophies
F. Bone tumors (sarcomas)
G. Rickets (osteomalacia)

STUDY QUESTIONS

1. Describe how the "bones" of the embryo become bones of an adult. Discuss the process of bone growth, repair, and dissolution.
2. Describe the three types of joints. Give an example of each.
3. Describe the three types of muscle tissue. Discuss the characteristics of each.
4. What are the causes of clubfeet? What is the most common position of clubfeet? How is this condition treated?
5. What simple test is used to identify a possible congentially dislocated hip? Describe three methods of treating a dislocated hip and the nursing care for each.
6. List the evidences of fractures. What is the emergency treatment of a fracture? Define internal fixation.
7. Discuss the battered child syndrome, the causes, legal aspects, nursing care, and prevention.
8. Discuss the emotional impact of leg amputation on a 10-year-old child and the parents.

18
Neurosensory conditions

NERVOUS SYSTEM

The nervous system is made up of the central nervous system (brain and spinal cord) and the peripheral nervous system (nerves and sense organs).

Function

The nervous system regulates and coordinates body activities in response to various internal and external changes in the environment. It also makes possible all conscious experience such as emotions, sensations, and learning.

Structure

Nervous tissue. Nervous tissue is composed of *neurons* (nerve cells and their processes, called fibers) and *neuroglia* (special nervous connective tissue). Each neuron consists of a *cell body*, one or more branching *dendrites*, and one elongated *axon*. Dendrites carry nerve impulses toward the cell body; axons conduct them away from cell bodies. Except for the "naked" nerve fibers found in specialized end organs and in the central nervous system, each nerve fiber is encased in a *myelin sheath* surrounded by a thin outer covering, the *neurolemma*.

The myelin sheath is a fatty coat that serves to speed up the rate of impulse transmission. It is not present on all nerve fibers at birth, and until myelination occurs, nerves are not fully functional. For example, the motor nerves that provide voluntary control of the anal sphincter do not myelinize until well into the second year of life. Until they do, toilet training is of little value. The *white matter* of the nervous system consists chiefly of myelinated nerve fibers. The *gray matter* consists of nonmyelinated nerve fibers and cell bodies.

The *neurolemma* is the outer covering that surrounds the myelin sheath. It serves the important function of regeneration. When a nerve is cut, the distal portion dies. Within a few days the neurolemma cells begin to grow, the nerve fiber follows, and finally, new myelin is laid down. Such growth and restoration of function takes about 2 weeks for each inch of length. Because nerve regeneration is dependent on the neurolemma, naked nerve fibers and cell bodies of the central nervous system cannot be restored if they are severed or die.

There are three types of neurons—sensory or afferent, motor or efferent, and internuncial or connecting (Fig. 18-1). *Sensory neurons* transmit impulses from receptors in the body to the spinal cord and brain; *motor neurons* transmit impulses from the brain and cord out to the muscles and glands; *internuncial* neurons conduct impulses from sensory neurons to motor neu-

rons. Bundles of nerve fibers of the sensory and motor neurons within the central nervous system are called *tracts*. There are both sensory and motor tracts, each with specific areas of origin and termination. Some of the nerve fibers cross over from one side to the other (decussate) at some point in the brain or spinal cord. In decussation, damage to right-side neurons will be evident on the left side, and vice versa. Bundles of nerve fibers, small blood vessels, and lymphatics held together by connective tissue are called *nerves*. Most nerves are *mixed*, that is, they carry both sensory and motor fibers.

Nerve cells have a high rate of metabolism and therefore require a great deal of oxygen. Any lack of oxygen makes nerve calls incapable of conducting impulses. A continued lack of oxygen produces cell damage and death. In fact, the higher the location of the nerve cell in the nervous system, the greater its susceptibility. At normal body temperature, cerebral cells are permanently damaged if deprived of oxygen for a very short time, probably 5 minutes. For this reason, hypoxia of the infant or child is of great concern.

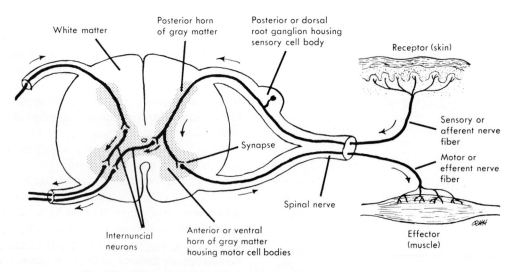

Fig. 18-1. Nervous pathways to and from the spinal cord showing a reflex arc.

Nervous pathways. Nerve impulses are conducted over nervous pathways (Fig. 18-1). They begin in the endings of dendrites, called *receptors*, and travel to the cell body and then to the branching end of the axon. In the simplest pathway, called a two-neuron *reflex arc*, the ends of the sensory neuron contact the dendrites of a motor neuron. This place of contact is called a *synapse*. From the synapse the nerve impulses travel along the dendrites of the motor neuron to the cell body and from the axon to the *effector*. A knee jerk is this type of reflex arc. In a three-neuron reflex arc the sensory neuron synapses with internuncial neurons that synapse with motor neurons. There are many more complex reflex arcs. The place where incoming sensory impulses become outgoing ones in a reflex arc is called the *reflex center*.

Impulses not only travel over reflex pathways, but they also travel to specific sensory areas of the brain. There, with computerlike complexity, a decision is reached and motor impulses are sent out along motor pathways down the spinal cord to the appropriate level and out to the gland or muscle for action.

Central nervous system. The central nervous system consists of the brain and spinal cord (Fig. 18-2). These organs are contained within the cranium and the vertebral column and are continuous with each other through a large opening at the base of the skull called the *foramen magnum*.

Coverings. Because the brain and spinal cord are so delicate and vital to life, they are provided with two protective coverings—an outer one of bone and an inner one of membrane, the *meninges*. The meninges are made up of three distinct layers of tissues—the dura mater, arachnoid membrane, and pia mater. The *dura mater* is the outermost covering. It is tough and fibrous and serves as both an inner periosteum of the cranial bones and the outer layer of the meninges. *The arachnoid membrane* is a delicate cobweblike layer that attaches to the pia mater below it. The *pia mater* is a transparent layer adherent to the

outer surface of the brain and spinal cord. It contains blood vessels that nourish the various parts of the central nervous system. Between the dura mater and the arachnoid membrane is a potential space called the *subdural space*. Between the arachnoid and the pia mater is the *subarachnoid space*.

Fluid spaces and cerebrospinal fluid. In addition to the coverings of bone and membrane, the brain and spinal cord are further protected by a cushion of fluid, both within and without, called *cerebrospinal fluid*. The fluid is contained in the subarachnoid space around the brain and cord and in cavities, called *ventricles*, and *aqueducts* inside the brain and in the spinal canal.

There are four ventricles within the brain—two lateral ones (the *first* and *second*), located within each cerebral hemisphere, the *third*, situated in the middle as a lengthwise slit, and the *fourth*, lying below the third. The lymphlike cerebrospinal fluid continually seeps from the blood plasma through capillary tufts known as *choroid plexuses*, located in the ventricle walls. The fluid passes from ventricle to ventricle through aqueducts into the spinal cord and also through openings in the roof of the fourth ventricle out into the subarachnoid space where it is reabsorbed by the blood. In an adult there is only about 135 ml of fluid at any one time. Because about 550 ml is secreted each day, the fluid must be reabsorbed at about the same rate as it is secreted. If there is a blockage of the normal circuit so that reabsorption is prevented, the fluid accumulates and pressure increases (see the discussion on hydrocephaly, p. 482).

Brain. The brain is the seat of the personality, the center of intelligence, and the controller of bodily functions, yet it weighs only 3 pounds when fully grown. Although the most rapid growth occurs during the first 9 years of life, it reaches full size and weight by the eighteenth year. The brain, or *encephalon*, is composed of nervous tissue divided into the *cerebrum*, *cerebellum*, and *brainstem*. Each part is complex in

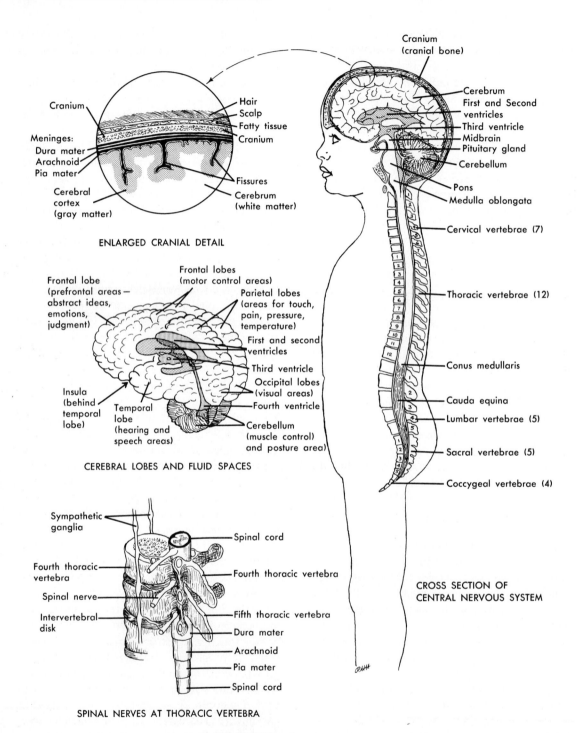

ENLARGED CRANIAL DETAIL

Cranium

Hair
Scalp
Fatty tissue
Cranium

Meninges:
Dura mater
Arachnoid
Pia mater

Cerebral cortex (gray matter)

Fissures

Cerebrum (white matter)

CEREBRAL LOBES AND FLUID SPACES

Frontal lobe (prefrontal areas— abstract ideas, emotions, judgment)

Frontal lobes (motor control areas)

Parietal lobes (areas for touch, pain, pressure, temperature)

First and second ventricles

Third ventricle

Occipital lobes (visual areas)

Fourth ventricle

Insula (behind temporal lobe)

Temporal lobe (hearing and speech areas)

Cerebellum (muscle control) and posture area)

SPINAL NERVES AT THORACIC VERTEBRA

Sympathetic ganglia

Fourth thoracic vertebra

Spinal nerve

Intervertebral disk

Spinal cord

Fourth thoracic vertebra

Fifth thoracic vertebra

Dura mater

Arachnoid

Pia mater

Spinal cord

Cranium (cranial bone)

Cerebrum
First and Second ventricles
Third ventricle
Midbrain
Pituitary gland
Cerebellum

Pons
Medulla oblongata

Cervical vertebrae (7)

Thoracic vertebrae (12)

Conus medullaris

Cauda equina

Lumbar vertebrae (5)

Sacral vertebrae (5)

Coccygeal vertebrae (4)

CROSS SECTION OF CENTRAL NERVOUS SYSTEM

Fig. 18-2. Central nervous system.

both structure and function and is interrelated with the other parts within the relatively small space of the cranium.

Cerebrum. The cerebrum consists of the right and left *cerebral hemispheres* connected by bands of nervous tissue of which the *corpus callosum* is the most prominent. Projecting from the undersurface of each hemisphere is an olfactory stalk to which is attached the *olfactory nerve* (cranial I) of each side. (The 12 paired cranial nerves are discussed under the topic of the peripheral nervous system.)

Each hemisphere is divided into five lobes. The *frontal, parietal, temporal,* and *occipital* are located adjacent to similarly named cranial bones. The *insula* is hidden below the frontal and temporal lobes.

The cerebrum is formed by an outer layer of gray matter called the *cortex* and an inner portion of white matter in which are embedded areas of gray matter made up of cerebral nuclei called *basal ganglia.*

The cortex is largely composed of cell bodies of neurons. Its area is greatly increased by rounded eminences or *convolutions* between which are large grooves called *fissures* and smaller ones called *sulci.* Experiments have shown that the specific areas of the cortex are related to particular body functions. For example, the parietal lobe is primarily concerned with the appreciation of touch, pain, temperature, pressure, and the sense of position. The temporal lobe contains the primary center for hearing and language formation. The occipital lobe is the visual area. The motor part of the frontal lobe contains pyramidal cells that give rise to pyramidal tracts through which are transmitted impulses responsible for voluntary muscle movement. The prefrontal area of the frontal lobe is concerned with abstract ideas, emotions, and judgment (Fig. 18-2).

The white matter of the cerebrum, which lies below the cortex, is composed of nerve fibers that interconnect within the cortex and then connect the cortex with other parts of the nervous system. The basal ganglia help control voluntary movements by influencing impulses leaving the motor areas of the cortex.

Cerebellum. The cerebellum, or "little brain," is a large mass of nervous tissue that lies beneath the back part of the cerebrum. It has two hemispheres that are joined together by a wormlike bridge called the *vermis.* The outer surface of the cerebellum is composed of gray matter arranged in shallow grooves. Within the inner white matter are islands of gray matter. Three paired nerve tracts, called the *cerebellar peduncles*, connect the cerebellum with the rest of the brain. The chief function of the cerebellum is to regulate the strength of contraction of voluntary muscles and thus provide the body with smoothness of motion and steadiness in body posture.

Brainstem. The brainstem is the upward extension of the spinal cord, with the cerebrum resting above and the cerebellum behind. It is composed of the diencephalon, mesencephalon, pons, and medulla oblongata.

The *diencephalon* is that part of the brainstem located between the cerebral hemispheres. Its walls surround the third ventricle. It is composed of the epithalamus, thalamus, subthalamus, and hypothalamus. The epithalamus consists of the pineal body (which controls timing of puberty) and a group of nuclei that are part of the olfactory apparatus of the brain. The *thalamus* consists of numerous nerve cell groups and is a reception center for all types of sensory stimuli. The *subthalamus* consists primarily of two paired nuclei that function to coordinate and regulate body movement. The hypothalamus forms the floor of the third ventricle and is composed of the *pituitary gland* (hypophysis), the *infundibulum* (the stalk that attaches the pituitary to the brain), and the nuclei of the hypothalamus, which have to do with sleep, emotions, and regulation of body temperature and blood pressure.

The *mesencephalon,* or midbrain, is a constricted portion of the brainstem that acts as a passageway. Through it pass the aqueduct that connects the third and fourth ventricles and a variety of important nerve fibers. Two *superior* and two *inferior colliculi* are centers for optic and auditory reflexes. In the lower portion are the nuclei of the *oculomotor* and *trochlear* (cranial III and IV) *nerves*.

The *pons* also acts as a passageway for nerve fibers. It contains the nuclei for the *trigeminal*, *abducens*, and *facial* (cranial V, VI, and VII) nerves.

The *medulla oblongata* lies at the lower end of the brainstem. It is continuous with the spinal cord below and the pons above and contains the *respiratory center* and the *auditory, glossopharyngeal, vagus, spinal accessory*, and *hypoglossal* (cranial VIII, IX, X, XI, and XII) *nerves*.

Spinal cord. The spinal cord lies within the vertebral column and extends from the foramen magnum to the lower border of the first of five lumbar vertebrae where it tapers to a point called the *conus medullaris* (Fig. 18-2). The cord, like the brain, is protected by three layers of meninges; an *epidural space* containing fat, connective tissue, and veins cushions it from the bony vertebrae. The innermost covering, the pia mater, adheres closely to the cord down to its point. There the pia mater becomes the *filum terminale* and continues down within the fluid-filled subarachnoid space to the level of the sacrum and the dural sac, disappearing into the tailbone (coccyx). The extension of the meninges below the cord makes possible the removal of cerebrospinal fluid. By insertion of a needle into the subarachnoid space at the level of the fourth or fifth lumbar vertebrae, cerebrospinal fluid can be withdrawn without danger of injury to the spinal cord.

In fetal life the spinal cord fills the entire length of the vertebral column and the spinal nerves emerge from the cord in pairs and exit through the vertebrae at right angles to the cord. As the vertebral column elongates with growth, the lumbar, sacral, and coccygeal nerves must pass down the spinal canal below the cord for varying distances before exiting. As a result the lower portion of the spinal canal becomes filled with an array of nerves and the filum terminale, giving the appearance of a horse's tail, hence the name *cauda equina*.

The spinal cord is an oval-shaped cylinder. Its outer layer is composed of myelinated fibers. Six lengthwise grooves divide this white matter into long columns made up of large bundles of nerve fibers, or tracts. Proceeding out from the cord are the 31 pairs of spinal nerves.

The inner core of the cord is composed of gray matter shaped like a three-dimensional letter H, the projections of which are called the dorsal and ventral horns.

Dorsal, or *posterior*, horns are composed of sensory neurons that receive impulses from sensory nerve fibers entering via the posterior root of a spinal nerve. *Ventral*, or *anterior*, horns are composed of motor neurons through which impulses course from the higher centers of the brain or from reflex centers in the spinal cord. The fibers of these motor neurons pass out of the cord via the *anterior root* of a spinal nerve and on to muscles or glands.

As one can see from its structure, the spinal cord acts as a great conduction pathway between the brain and the peripheral nerves. It also contains many reflex centers that are responsible for the vital unconscious responses that protect and maintain the body. If the spinal cord becomes diseased or is injured, impulse transmission will be affected. When the sensory impulses of some area cannot reach the central nervous system, the situation is like a dead telephone—the isolated part of the body can no longer report what is happening to it. When motor impulses are interrupted, a part can no longer respond with action. Loss of function to the body depends on the degree and site of damage to the spinal cord.

Peripheral nervous system. The peripheral nervous system is composed of the cranial and spinal nerves with their many branches and specialized portions, including the autonomic nervous systems and the special sense organs.

Cranial nerves. Twelve pairs of cranial nerves arise from various parts of the brain. They are given descriptive names and are numbered in the order in which they emerge, from front to back, as follows:

I   Olfactory nerve for reception of sense of smell
II   Optic nerve for reception of sight
III   Oculomotor nerve for movement of several eye muscles
IV   Trochlear nerve for movement of one eye muscle
V   Trigeminal nerve for reception of sensations from the face and movement of chewing muscles
VI   Abducens nerve for outward movement (abduction) of one eye muscle
VII   Facial nerve for movement of the facial muscles, reception of sense of taste, and secretion of saliva
VIII   Auditory nerve for reception of the senses of hearing and equilibrium
IX   Glossopharyngeal nerve for reception of taste and for movement of pharyngeal muscles
X   Vagus nerve for control of activity in many abdominal and thoracic organs
XI   Spinal accessory nerve for movement of some neck muscles
XII   Hypoglossal nerve for movement of tongue muscle

Spinal nerves. There are 31 pairs of spinal nerves, named according to the region of their spinal cord attachment, as follows:

8 pairs of cervical nerves
12 pairs of thoracic nerves
5 pairs of lumbar nerves
5 pairs of sacral nerves
1 pair of occygeal nerves

Each spinal nerve leaves the cord in two branches or roots, a dorsal root and a ventral root (Fig. 18-1). Neurons of the dorsal or posterior root carry sensory impulses from the peripheral areas of the body to the spinal cord. The cell bodies of these neurons are found outside the spinal cord in an enlargement on each dorsal root called the *dorsal root ganglion*. A ganglion is a collection of nerve cells outside the central nervous system. The dendrites of these neurons go out into the body tissue where their end receptors pick up stimuli.

Neurons of the ventral root of each spinal nerve serve a motor function, carrying impulses from the cord to the peripheral tissues of the body. Unlike the dorsal neurons, the cell bodies of the ventral root neurons are located within the spinal cord in the ventral horn.

Just before the dorsal and ventral roots of each spinal nerve pass out from the between the vertebrae into the body, they join to form a single mixed nerve. All spinal nerves are mixed (both motor and sensory nerves). The spinal nerve then splits into two branches called *anterior* and *posterior primary rami*. The posterior rami runs down the back, supplying the posterior of the body with sensory and motor nerves. Most of the anterior rami fuse into a complex network called a plexus. Here the nerve fibers are rearranged into new groupings different from those in the primary rami. There are four plexuses—cervical, brachial, lumbar, and sacral. The *cervical plexus* lies deep in the neck. The *brachial plexus* is located in the shoulder region and is sometimes stretched or torn at birth, causing paralysis or numbness of the baby's arm. The *lumbar plexus* lies within the chest muscles and the *sacral plexus* lies deep in the buttocks.

Autonomic nervous system. The autonomic nervous system is composed of those nerve fibers that transmit motor impulses to the glands and smooth muscles, causing them to act automatically and involuntarily. Its fibers are intermingled with others in the spinal nerves, and it is influenced by the higher centers of the brain and by endocrine secretions.

The autonomic system is made up of a *sympathetic* and a *parasympathetic division*. The ganglia of the sympathetic nerves lie on each side of the spinal column like beads on a chain of connecting fibers (Fig. 18-1). Short fibers connect the sympathetic ganglia, or thoracolumbar ganglia, to the thoracic and lumbar regions of the cord. The parasympathetic ganglia, or craniosacral ganglia are located on or near the various structures they innervate. Their connecting fibers are long, running from the brain to sacral regions of the cord.

In general, the sympathetic system prevails in times of stress, the parasympathetic in times of quiet. Although both cause smooth muscle to contract in one structure and to relax in another, the systems are generally antagonistic to each other. A balance between the two systems is maintained by coordinating centers believed to be located in the hypothalamus.

The autonomic nervous system functions on the same reflex-arc principle as the voluntary nervous system, with receptors and effectors. Sometimes the effectors are other smooth muscles or glands and sometimes they are skeletal muscles, demonstrating that the nervous system is all interrelated.

Sense organs. Sense organs or receptors are actually the beginnings of dendrites of sensory neurons. They are of several different types, each adapted to receiving one kind of stimulus. The *general sense organs* are found all over the body and receive such sensations as pain, temperature, touch, pressure, and position. The *special sense organs* are located in specialized tissues in particular places in the body and consist of the olfactory epithelium of the nasal cavity, the taste buds of the tongue, the retina of the eye, and the organ of Corti of the ear. The eye and the ear are of special concern to the pediatric nurse.

Eye. The eye is the organ of vision. Often described as a ball, the eye is round with a clear circular window in the front to permit the entrance of light (Fig. 18-3). The optic nerve comes off the back portion and carries impulses from the light-sensitive retina to the brain. The

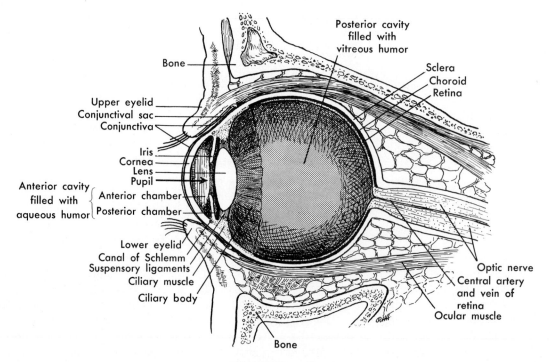

Fig. 18-3. The eye.

eye is contained in a bony socket of the skull called the *orbital cavity* and is cushioned from blows by an underlying bed of loose fatty tissue. It is protected in the front by a fleshy *eyelid* and lubricating *tears*. Skeletal muscles are attached to the eyeball to provide it with movement.

Vision, or the act of seeing, results from the reception of nerve impulses at the visual areas of the cerebral cortex. (See the preceeding discussion on the cerebrum.) These impulses begin in the special receptors of the retina—the light-sensitive *rods* and *cones*. For the rods and cones to send meaningful impulses to the brain, an image must be focused on the retina. *Focusing* is therefore the central function of the eye, involving refraction, pupil constriction, and eye conver-

gence. *Refraction* is the bending of light rays and involves the cornea and the anterior and posterior surfaces of the lens. *Constriction of the pupil* occurs when the smooth muscle of the iris contracts to control the amount of light entering the eye. *Convergence* is the working together of the two eyes so that an image falls on corresponding areas of the retina. If convergence does not occur because the eye muscles do not work together, the child will see double, or experience *diplopia*. Some of the more common optical defects are discussed later in this chapter.

Ear. The ear is the receptor of sound and the gauge of balance. It is a complex organ consisting of many tissues and usually divided into three parts—an external, middle, and inner ear (Fig. 18-4).

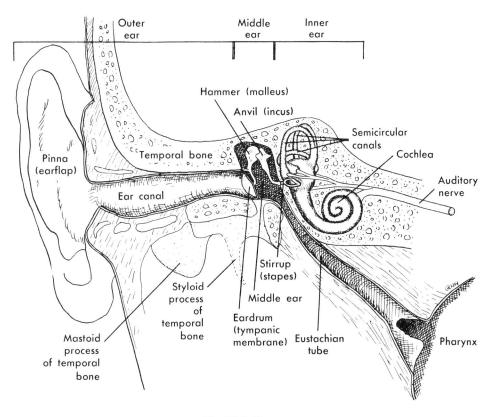

Fig. 18-4. The ear.

The *external ear* consists of the pinna (earflap, or auricle) and the ear canal. The ear canal is a curving tube in the temporal bone that leads to the eardrum, a thin membrane separating the external ear from the middle ear.

The *middle ear* is a small cavity within the temporal bone connected to the pharynx by the eustachian tube. Three tiny bones, the hammer, anvil, and stirrup, are suspended between the eardrum and the oval window, which leads to the inner ear. The bony walls of the middle ear and the small bones are covered by mucous membrane. This mucous coat continues into the mastoid air cells and down into the eustachian tube and the throat, which accounts for the rapid spread of infections up from the throat into the middle ear and mastoid cells.

The *inner ear* consists of several membrane-lined channels deep in the temporal bone. They make up the cochlea, the organ of hearing, and the semicircular canals, collectively the organ of equilibrium.

The *cochlea* is a coiled tubular structure resembling a snail shell, from Latin *cochlea*. It is filled with lymph, which effectively transmits sound waves arriving from the three middle ear bones to the organ of Corti. The sound vibrations are picked up by the organ of Corti, transformed into nerve impulses, carried to the auditory cortex of the brain, and interpreted as sound.

The *semicircular canals* are three horseshoe-shaped tubes arranged so that they lie at right angles to one another. They are lined with connective tissue that divides them into two lymph-filled channels. When the head or body is moved, the fluid in the canals moves the hairlike processes of special cells, which in turn stimulate receptor cells that send impulses to the brain by way of the auditory nerve. By this mechanism a person becomes aware of body movement and is able to maintain balance (equilibrium). Disturbance of this mechanism causes dizziness or inability to maintain a body position.

DISORDERS OF THE NEUROSENSORY SYSTEM
Neurological symptoms

Disorders of the neurosensory system produce typical symptoms, including altered sensations, changes in the level of consciousness, seizures, and signs of increased intracranial pressure. Although these symptoms vary with the disease process and age of the child, they all require knowledgeable nursing care.

Altered sensations

Touch. Normally touch relays two kinds of information: (1) an awareness of the nature of the contact (degree of pressure, size of area) and (2) the location of the contact, called proprioception, The capacity to feel touch may be affected by toxins, drugs, tumors, infections, trauma, and degenerative diseases. Four types of altered touch may result:
1. *Paresthesia*—burning, tingling, prickling, crawling
2. *Hypesthesia*—dulled or decreased sensations
3. *Hyperesthesia*—exaggerated sensations
4. *Anesthesia*—absent sensations

Nursing interventions are aimed toward prevention of muscle atrophy, joint contractures, and tissue damage resulting from lost sensations. They include such measures as range of motion exercises, positioning, and skin care.

Pain. Pain is a protective sensation that signals bodily harm from distention, pressure, friction, cell destruction, muscle fatigue, and inflammation. Stimulated by such harm, specialized nerve endings pick up and transmit impulses via the posterior horn cells and the thalamus to the somatesthetic area of the parietal lobe of the brain. Pain is experienced as severe, dull, throbbing, burning, or aching. When pain is felt in a different area than the actual stimulus, it is called *referred pain*. Pain can be experienced when no physical cause exists and may be exaggerated by fear.

Nursing assessment of pain includes its location, intensity, character, and duration. Nurses obtain such information verbally and also learn to recognize body language. For example, children may pull on their earlobes when they have an earache. Pain can be stopped by removing the cause or by blocking its reception in the brain. Nursing measures include the application of heat or cold, administration of drugs, repositioning, interpersonal interaction, and assisting with medical treatment.

Changes in level of consciousness

The level of consciousness is the most important indicator of cerebral function. It can be affected by general anesthesia, tumors, trauma, toxins, and metabolic disorders. Alternations in level of consciousness vary from the normal alertness of a healthy child to total lack of responsiveness to the environment, as follows:

1. Normal behavior for age, alert, responsive; oriented to person, place, and time
2. Restless, irritable, can be comforted by parent; oriented to person and place, but may not be oriented to time
3. Irrational or drowsy; oriented to person, but may not be oriented to place and time
4. Very drowsy, responds to commands; not oriented to person, place, or time
5. Unconscious, but responds purposefully to painful stimuli
6. Unconscious, nonpurposeful response to painful stimuli
7. Unconscious, flexion response to painful stimuli
8. Unconscious, extension response to painful stimuli
9. Unconscious, decorticate posturing (arms and fingers adducted in rigid flexion with hands in internal rotation)
10. Unconscious, decerebrate posturing (all extremities in rigid extension and adduction, back arched, toes pointed inward)
11. Cessation of heart and lung action, death

Nursing assessment of the level of consciousness should be made at regular intervals and according to objective signs such as turning the head in response to a loud noise. Nursing interventions are aimed at preventing the complications of immobility and at providing sensory stimulation to maximize such brain activity as is present.

Seizures

Seizures are abnormal, involuntary neuromuscular activity that may affect the body in part or whole, and may cause a loss of consciousness and fecal and urinary incontinence. Motor activity is described as tonic (rigid) or clonic (alternately flaccid and rigid). Seizures are triggered by irritation to certain areas of the brain caused by infections, congenital defects, tumors, metabolic disorders, and elevation of body temperature. They are common in children because of the immaturity of their nervous systems. Convulsive disorders are discussed later in this chapter together with nursing assessment and interventions.

Increased intracranial pressure

Because the cranium (skull) is a relatively closed box, an increase in the amount of cerebrospinal fluid (CSF), blood, or tissue increases the intracranial pressure. Such conditions as blocked CSF passageways, tumor growth, and trauma cause increased pressure and produce a variety of symptoms. These have been classified according to when they develop, as follows:

Early symptoms Irritability, restlessness, anorexia, and headache

Intermediate symptoms Projectile vomiting, bulging fontanel in child under 18 months of age, severe headache, slow or unequal response of pupil to light, blurred vision, papilledema, diplopia, decreased pulse, increased blood pressure, seizures

Late symptoms Decreased level of consciousness, decreased reflexes, decreased respirations, elevated body temperature, herniation of optic disk, fixed eyes, decerebrate rigidity, death

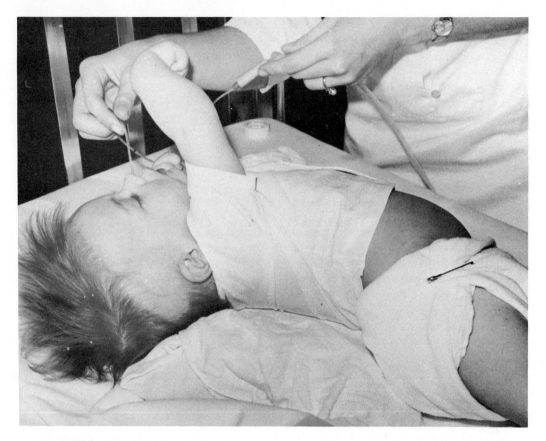

Fig. 18-5. Opisthotonos infant with brain damage caused by anoxia. Nurse is suctioning mucus from nose.

Nursing assessment of neurological responses (a neuro check) includes checking the following:

1. *Level of consciousness:* determine the degree of alertness, orientation to time, place, and person, and ability to respond to stimuli.
2. *Pupillary response:* determine if pupils are equal and react to light (PERL) and if eyes move together purposefully.
3. *Vital signs:* determine if temperature, pulse, respirations, and blood pressure are within normal range for age of the child.
4. *Motor activity:* determine the strength, equality, appropriateness, and control of movement. Opisthotonos is a dorsal arched position of the body caused by tetanic spasm (Fig. 18-5).

Nursing interventions are aimed at making accurate observations, preventing injury to the child, and carrying out medical prescriptions.

Injuries

Children suffer a variety of injuries to the head and other parts of the body at birth and later in life. The most common ones are forceps marks, caput succedaneum, cephalohematoma, intracranial hemorrhage, subdural hematoma, cerebral concussion, skull fracture, brachial plexus palsy, and facial nerve paralysis.

Forceps marks. Forceps marks are bruises made by the pressure of forceps on the infant's head. Although they may trouble the parents, they usually disappear in a few days and leave no scarring or after effects.

Caput succedaneum. Caput seccedaneum is an accumulation of tissue fluid within the scalp making it puffy and edematous. It is caused by pressure to the area during delivery. The swelling usually disappears in about 3 days.

Cephalohematoma. Cephalohematoma is an accumulation of blood between one of the skull bones and its membranous covering, the periosteum. Because it is limited by the attachment of the periosteum to the bone affected, the margins are well defined. It is a soft, movable mass that may not be evident the first day after birth because of the presence of a large caput succedaneum. It may then increase in size for about 2 to 3 days. A cephalohematoma is not aspirated because the needle might cause a dangerous infection and the blood will be absorbed eventually. Though it is not serious, the presence of cephalohematoma may be quite distressing to the parents, who need information and reassurance.

Intracranial hemorrhage. Intracranial hemorrhage is the most common and by far the most serious birth injury. It is seen most often in premature infants with bleeding tendencies and in full-term infants born of difficult deliveries. Rupture or tearing of the vessels cause bleeding between the layers of the meninges or in the brain mainly over the cerebral cortex. It produces symptoms of increasing intracranial pressure. These symptoms may appear at birth or several hours thereafter. The infant becomes irritable or lethargic and may twitch, convulse, or vomit, become feverish and cyanotic, and have a bulging fontanel, difficulty in sucking or breathing, or a shrill cry. The diagnosis is made by the physician on the basis of the birth history, symptoms, and a lumbar puncture, which shows increased pressure and bloody spinal fluid.

The infant is usually placed in an incubator with the head slightly elevated, and is kept somewhat dehydrated to help relieve intracranial pressure. Oxygen is administered for cyanosis. Vitamin K is given to enhance clotting, antibiotics to prevent infection, and sedation to control convulsions. The infant is fed by gavage when there is poor sucking ability.

Sometimes the bleeding stops spontaneously and the child recovers with no ill effects. In other cases the pressure becomes so intense that it must be relieved by aspiration or surgery. A common complication of intracranial hemorrhage is hydrocephalus. Mental retardation, epilepsy, cerebral palsy, and behavioral disorders may appear later.

Subdural hematoma. A subdural hematoma is a collection of blood and fluid in the potential space below the dura mater. The acute form occurs immediately after head trauma. The chronic form occurs in children with bleeding tendencies such as produced by meningitis or lack of vitamin C.

At the time of the injury, the veins passing through the dural space are torn. Fluid collects and a sac is formed that enlarges as fresh blood is added to the accumulated old blood and fluid. The brain beneath is compressed and may atrophy. In an old hematoma, even though the fluid may be gone, the membrane remains and prevents normal brain growth.

In the acute form, symptoms of increased intracranial pressure develop rapidly. In the chronic form, they develop more slowly and include anorexia, irritability, vomiting, convulsions, recurrent fever, bulging fontanels, and enlarged head. When these symptoms appear, diagnosis is confirmed and treatment instituted by the withdrawal of old blood and fluid through a needle inserted in the angle of the anterior fontanel. The procedure is repeated at intervals for several weeks to allow for brain expansion and healing. If blood continues to fill the hematoma capsule, a drain may be inserted through holes made in the skull bone (trephination, or trepanation) or a craniotomy may be necessary to remove the capsule.

Nursing care consists of preparing the child's scalp for the subdural taps. The hair is usually shaved and the skin cleansed thoroughly. The nurse should hold the child securely during the aspiration to avoid injury from sudden movement. After the procedure the dressings should be observed for drainage. Frank bleeding should be reported at once. Other important observations include the level of consciousness and the posture assumed by the child. Postoperative craniotomy nursing care is discussed in the section on brain tumors. Prognosis depends on the degree of brain damage before treatment. For this reason early diagnosis is of great importance.

Cerebral concussion. A concussion is a sudden blow to the head. It may cause damage to the blood vessels and nervous tissue within the brain with loss of consciousness, headache, pallor, vomiting, and irritability.

Nursing care for the first 12 to 24 hours should include bed rest, with observations every 2 hours for level of consciousness, degree of restlessness, eye movement, equality of the pupils and whether they react to light, and vital signs. A full bladder may contribute to restlessness, so it, too, should be checked for distension. If the child appears to have no untoward signs or symptoms, the physician usually prescribes a gradual return to normal activity with continued close observation. If the child is dismissed to the family, the parents should be instructed to report immediately any change in the child's level of consciousness, convulsions, or head pain to the physician.

Skull fracture. Although serious brain injury can occur without a skull fracture, no skull is fractured without some internal brain injury. The most common sites for fracture are the parietal bones on the sides of the head. A fracture can occur at any age, even at birth. Positive diagnosis is made by x-ray examination, but it may be delayed if the patient's condition is grave and surgery is not planned. At least 90% are lineal or comminuted and nondepressed, and so operation is not needed. A depression fracture must be elevated by surgical techniques. Treatment is individualized and fitted to the degree of intracranial damage. Nursing care includes close observation for signs of increased intracranial pressure and implementation of the medical treatment. It is the same as for concussion or craniotomy, if one is performed.

Brachial plexus palsy (Erb-Duchenne paralysis). Brachial plexus palsy is a paralysis of the upper arm caused by damage to the fifth and sixth cervical spinal nerves. The injury occurs when the infant's shoulder is pulled away from the head during delivery. The injury causes the arm on the affected side to lie near the body and turn inward. The hand and fingers of the arm are not affected. If the paralysis is caused by edema and hemorrhage around the nerve fibers, function will gradually return. If it is caused by tearing the nerves, permanent paralysis may result although surgical neuroplasty may be attempted to restore function.

The initial treatment consists of positioning the arm so that it is abducted and externally rotated. This positioning may be done by restraints fastened to the bed to pull the arm out from the body or by splints. Manipulation and massage may also be ordered to prevent contracture deformities.

Because of the widespread knowledge of the causes of this condition, physicians and midwives responsible for delivering babies make every effort to ease the shoulders out of the birth canal during delivery.

Facial nerve paralysis (Bell's palsy). The left and right facial nerves (cranial VII) enervate the facial muscles of expression. In Bell's palsy one or both of these nerves is damaged so that muscles on the affected side do not contract. The eye remains partially open, the cheek droops, and sucking is impaired (Fig. 18-6). Injury may occur at birth from forceps pressure to the nerves or unknown factors associated with the immune

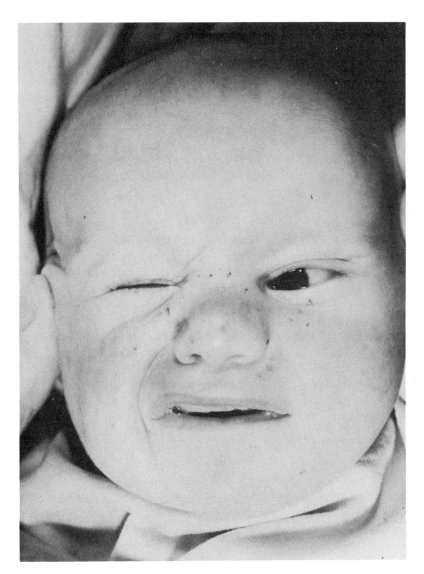

Fig. 18-6. Facial nerve paralysis (Bell's palsy).

mechanism following bacterial or viral infections. Function may return gradually. If not, surgical neuroplasty may be attempted.

Nursing care includes taking special care with feedings because the infant may not be able to suck a nipple, covering the exposed eye to prevent the conjuctiva from drying, holding and cuddling the infant whose twisted face may repel the parents, and relating positively with the parents who must cope with feelings of revulsion, anger, and guilt.

Malformations

Craniosynostosis. In the normal newborn infant the bones of the skull are separated by fibrous membranes called sutures that gradually fill in with bone by the age of 6 months. The soft spot (anterior fontanel) usually closes by the ninth to sixteenth month. In craniosynostosis one or more of the sutures close before or soon after birth. When a suture closes, the bone on both sides stops growing; where open sutures remain, growth continues. Such uneven growth causes the skull to grow into various deformed shapes. *Scaphocephaly* (long and narrow skull) is the deformity caused by premature closure of the sagittal suture, located along the midline of the skull. *Oxycephaly* (pointed skull) is the deformity caused by premature closure of the coronal sutures, located on the two sides of the skull (Fig. 18-7).

Craniosynostosis is serious, not because of the odd-shaped head that results, but because the increased intracranial pressure it produces interferes with normal brain growth and causes mental retardation, loss of vision, headaches, convulsions and protruding eyeballs. Thus, the sooner diagnosis is made and treatment begun, the better will be the child's prognosis. Diagnosis is made by manual palpation of the skull and is confirmed by x-ray films.

Treatment consists of surgically opening the suture lines (craniotomy) in the hope of reducing the mental and visual damage. Craniotomy may need to be repeated if bone growth is too rapid.

Postoperative nursing care is similar to that after a craniotomy for brain tumor as discussed later in this chapter.

Microcephaly. Unlike craniosynostosis, in which the brain is prevented from growing, *microcephaly* is a condition in which the brain fails to grow and, as a result, neither does the skull. It is caused by heredity, infection with rubella, or irradiation of the mother during pregnancy. The infant is born with a small head (microcephalus) and severe mental retardation. There is no cure, and care is directed toward providing for basic needs and making full use of present capacities.

Hydrocephaly. Hydrocephaly is a condition involving an accumulation of cerebrospinal fluid within the cranium. *Hydrocephalus* means "water head." It can occur in an infant both before and after birth. The head enlarges from the pressure within because the cranial sutures are not yet closed and the bones are soft.

Cerebrospinal fluid normally oozes out from the blood vessel tufts in the ventricles within the brain and flows through aqueducts. In the fourth ventricle it passes out into the subarachnoid space that surrounds the spinal cord and brain. There the fluid is absorbed back into the bloodstream.

When cerebrospinal fluid collects in the ventricles because of a blockage somewhere before it reaches the subarachnoid space, the hydrocephaly is called *noncommunicating*. Such obstructions may be caused by congenital defects or hemorrhage. The fluid distends the ventricles so that they get larger and larger. The head size increases; the cranial bones thin; the fontanels bulge; the sutures separate; and the brain tissue gradually thins as it is compressed against the skull (Fig. 18-8). When hydrocephaly occurs before birth, the infant may die in the uterus or its head size may necessitate cesarean section. After birth, increase in head size becomes noticeable and the scalp becomes shiny because the skin is stretched. The infant is increasingly helpless and unable to lift the head. The neck muscles weaken

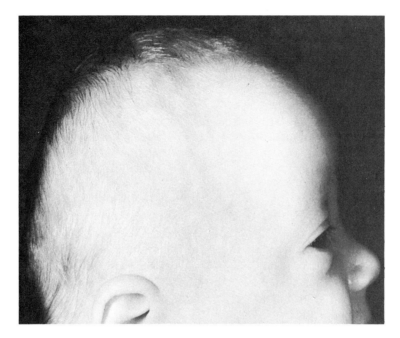

Fig. 18-7. Craniosynostosis of the coronal sutures on the two sides of the skull, called *oxycephaly.* (Courtesy Children's Medical Center, Oakland, Calif.)

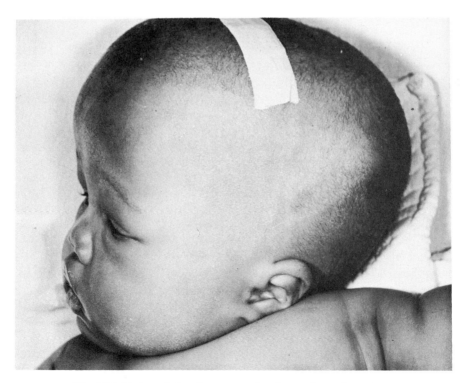

Fig. 18-8. Hydrocephalus. Tape covers site of recent fontanel puncture.

from disuse. The eyes seem to be pushed downward and protrude slightly (sunset eyes). The cry is shrill. Muscle tone throughout the body is poor, and as the condition worsens, the body becomes emaciated. The child convulses and has little resistance to infection. Without medical or surgical intervention, the head becomes enormous and the child dies from malnutrition and infection.

In *communicating hydrocephaly* the cerebrospinal fluid can find its way to the subarachnoid space but cannot be absorbed because of congenital malformations, hemorrhage, or scars from meningitis. The result is an accumulation of fluid outside the brain. The convolutions become flattened. The nervous tissue of the brain cannot grow. Usually the pressure of the fluid does not enlarge the head as much as it does in the noncommunicating type because in communicating hydrocephaly the brain atrophies, making more space for the fluid. The fontanels are tense and wide. The child becomes irritable and loses an appetite. Death comes from malnutrition and infections.

Diagnosis of both types of hydrocephaly is made on the basis of the family and child's history, a fontanel puncture, ventriculograms, the transillumination procedure, and pneumoencephalograms (see the diagnostic tests in Chapter 9). The usual treatment is to bypass surgically the obstruction or nonabsorbing tissue. Several "shunt" procedures have been devised to make this bypass. They all involve placing a small plastic tube in a ventricle and draining off the excess fluid to other areas of the body such as the vena cava, right atrium of the heart, peritoneal cavity, and ureter of a kidney that has been removed. The child may outgrow the device and the tubing may become blocked. Each procedure has certain drawbacks such as clot formation when the tube is placed in a blood vessel, ascending infection, or excessive loss of body salts. Perhaps most discouraging is that if the increased intracranial pressure is not relieved quickly after it commences the child suffers permanent brain damage, regardless of subsequent surgery. Even with a brain-damaged child, surgery may be performed to halt or slow head enlargement so that nursing care will be less difficult.

Preoperative and convalescent nursing care is directed toward maintaining the child's nutrition, protecting the skin from breakdown, and preventing pneumonia and other infections. These children are often fed by gavage since their sucking reflex may be weak. Because of the weight of the head, it may not be possible to hold them. The skin must be cleansed carefully and kept dry. The ears and scalp may develop pressure sores and so should be moved often and placed on a soft flexible pad.

Postoperative shunt care requires considerable skill and experience. Nurses play an important role in giving care during the acute phase and when the child's condition stabilizes. Close observations are made of the vital signs, state of consciousness, the degree of fontanel bulging, measurement of the head circumference, and amount of restlessness. The head is usually elevated. Intravenous fluids are given, usually through a venous cutdown (Fig. 18-9). Special instructions regarding the type of shunt and the devices used are provided to the nursing staff. Special skin care and positioning are important. Sometimes a one-way valve is placed somewhere along the draining tube and orders are left for it to be pressed at certain intervals.

As the child recovers from the surgery, preparations are made for care, either at home or at an institution. If the parents are to provide care, they should be encouraged to come to the hospital beforehand to observe and take part in the child's care. After dismissal, follow-up supervision by a community health nurse may be of great help. The parents may have difficulty accepting the reality of their child's condition. They may feel guilty, especially if it becomes necessary to place the child in an institution. The nurse should be considerate of their feelings, encourage them to talk, and allow them to do

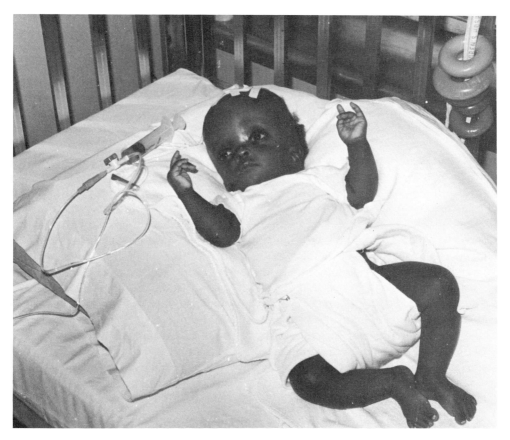

Fig. 18-9. Hydrocephalic infant with head elevated on pillow. Intravenous fluids are being administered in scalp vein. Position is changed frequently. Note toys at right.

physical things for their child, thus providing them with an outlet for their emotions.

Spina bifida. The spinal canal is enclosed in a flexible tube made up of individual vertebrae. Spina bifida, or "divided spine," is the congenital failure of the arches of one or more vertebrae to unite at the center of the back so that the bony wall normally surrounding the spinal canal at that place is missing. This defect occurs most often in the lumbosacral region just below the spinal cord, although it occasionally occurs at higher levels.

When the defect is small, marked only by a dimple, port-wine birthmark, or tuft of hair, and when the spinal cord and meninges are normal, the condition is called *spina bifida occulta*, or "hidden." Unless neurological symptoms develop there is usually no need for treatment.

When the defect is larger, the meninges may protrude through it, forming a sac filled with cerebrospinal fluid. This condition is called *spina bifida cystica*. Such a sac or tumor is called a *meningocele*. Because the defect contains no nerve tissue the child is usually not paralyzed and is able to develop bladder and bowel control. A meningocele is a cosmetic problem, however, and is a potential opening for infection if it becomes injured. For these reasons surgical correction is made as soon as possible.

When a portion of the spinal cord herniates

into the meningocele, the condition is called a *myelomeningocele* or a *meningomyelocele* (Fig. 18-10). The sac is covered by a thin skin or membrane subject to ulceration and leakage of spinal fluid. The child often suffers partial or complete paralysis below the defect, incontinence, and sensory disturbances. Urinary tract infections are a common complication. Hydrocephalus may develop before or after cosmetic surgery from a downward displacement of the brain into the spinal canal, causing obstruction of the normal fluid flow.

Before corrective surgery, nursing care is directed toward giving the child adequate nourishment, protecting the sac from pressure, injury, or infection. The infant should be held for feedings whenever possible in a sitting position with no pressure on the sac, or with the head over a nurse's shoulder while being fed by another nurse holding the bottle. Careful observations are made of vital signs, degree of incontinence, activity of the legs, signs of increased intracranial pressure, and for leakage of CSF.

When not being held, the child should be positioned on the abdomen or propped on a side. Diapers are not pinned in place but may be placed beneath the child. A plastic sheet may be taped to the back below the meninocele to prevent feces from contaminating the exposed sac. Sometimes the infant is placed on a Bradford frame over a bedpan. Urine and feces fall through the slit in the frame into the bedpan below. A gauze dressing may be placed over the meningocele. For prevention of foot deformity, when the child is on the abdomen, the ankles should be supported by a pad so that the toes do not rest on the bed. A mild ointment may be applied to the knees, elbows, and face to prevent chafing. Manual expression of urine may be prescribed to prevent distention and infection. This is accomplished by pressing firmly, but gently, on the abdomen with the side of the hand at the umbilicus and slowly rolling the hand toward the pubic bone. Remember to give intramuscular injections into nonparalyzed muscles to enhance absorption.

After corrective surgery, the infant is kept flat until the sutures are removed. There may be no

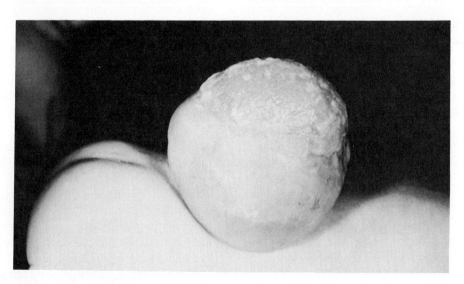

Fig. 18-10. Large myelomeningocele on newborn infant. (Courtesy Children's Medical Center, Oakland, Calif.)

dressing or only a light dry dressing over the incision. The area should be kept clean until healing occurs. Feedings may be given by gavage until the infant can be lifted. Because hydrocephalus frequently follows repair of myelomeningocele, the circumference of the infant's head should be measured regularly to determine any increase in size.

Although surgery rarely improved function, it greatly facilitates nursing care. Even if hydrocephalus does not develop, the patient continues to need special care throughout life because bowel and bladder sphincters and the legs are usually paralyzed. The procedure described earlier for manual expression of urine is taught to the parents and the child. By the age of 7 to 10 years the child can learn to express urine at intervals appropriate to bladder capacity. A series of orthopedic procedures may be necessary even before the child is ready to walk with braces. Recurrent bladder infections are common. Emotional dependency is a natural result of physical dependency. The goal of treatment is to help the child achieve maximum mental and physical health.

Encephalocele. An encephalocele is a protrusion of the brain through a congenital defect in the skull. It occurs because the bones of the fetal skull fail to unite normally. It is commonly found in the midline in the occipital region but may also occur anywhere in the skull, including the orbit of the eye or in the nose. Other abnormalities of the nervous system and abdominal organs may be associated with this defect. Symptoms depend on the degree of involvement, size, and location of the encephalocele. It is covered by only a thin layer of skin or meninges. If large and in danger of rupturing, early repair is attempted. Otherwise, repair may be delayed for about a year. Prognosis depends on the extent of involvement and location. Meningitis is a grave danger if the sac ruptures. Nursing care is the same for these infants as for normal ones with special caution to avoid pressure on the sac.

Infections

Meningitis. Meningitis is an inflammation of the meninges, the membranous coverings of the brain. It is caused by a variety of bacteria and viruses that invade the tissues directly or indirectly from the bloodstream. The most common organisms, by age group, are as follows:

Newborn infants	*Escherichia coli* and herpesvirus
6 months to 3 years	*Haemophilus influenzae*, type B
3 to 8 years	*Meningococcus, Pneumococcus, Streptococcus, Neisseria gonorrhoeae*
8 to 12 years	Rubella virus, mumps virus

Bacterial infections of the meninges usually produce considerable pus and spread rapidly over the brain and the spinal cord, causing cloudiness in the CSF. If the patient survives, widespread damage and scarring of the arachnoid tissue may interfere with normal absorption of the CSF, with resulting hydrocephalus.

Typical symptoms include irritability, high fever, vomiting, headache, delirium, neck and back rigidity, involuntary arching of the back (opisthotonos), twitching, convulsions, and death (Table 18-1). In severe cases of meningococcal meningitis a purpuric rash may appear, hence the name *spotted fever* sometimes given the disease.

Medical diagnosis is made on the basis of the history, physical and neurological examinations, and laboratory tests of CSF and blood. CSF is especially important because from it the causal organism can be identified and treatment made more specific. CSF is obtained by lumbar puncture. Because meningitis is such a serious complication, and the symptoms may not be obvious immediately, lumbar puncture may be performed on infants with infections such as otitis media. Medical treatment includes antibiotics and intravenous fluids.

Nursing care is of great importance. Strict isolation is instituted until the child is no longer

Table 18-1. Signs and symptoms of meningitis

Cause	Infants	Older children
Increased intracranial pressure	Bulging fontanel Projectile vomiting Shrill cry Seizures Coma	Headache Vomiting Delirium Seizures Coma Cranial nerve involvement
Infection	Fever	Fever
Meningeal irritation	Opisthotonos (Fig. 18-5) Hyperesthesia (increased sensitivity to light, noise, etc.)	Muscle rigidity Hyperesthesia

infectious. If the organism is highly contagious, as is *Meningococcus*, prophylactic drugs may be given to exposed staff or family members. Vital signs and neurological signs are checked at regular intervals. Urinary output is measured accurately. Side rails are padded to prevent injury from convulsions, and the child is placed in a quiet, nonstimulating environment. Oral hygiene, skin care, range of motion exercises, and proper positioning must be conscientiously performed by the nurse.

During the convalescent period, parents should be encouraged to continue nursing measures aimed at returning the child to full recovery. Home health supervision may be helpful.

A great many complications besides hydrocephalus may follow meningitis. Otitis media and infections of the eyes and lungs may occur. Headaches may persist. Mental retardation and paralysis of muscle groups may result from nerve damage. Each of these complications must be treated according to the needs of the individual child.

Encephalitis. An inflammation of the brain (encephalon) is called *encephalitis*. If both the brain substance and meninges are involved, the condition is called *encephalomyelitis*. Encephalitis may be a specific disease entity caused by the viruses of mites, mosquitoes, or mice, or of mumps, rabies, or poliomyelitis. It may occur as a sequel to upper respiratory infections, chickenpox, measles, or German measles. It may follow immunizations against smallpox or diphtheria-pertussis-tetanus (DPT), or it may result from the ingestion of lead, which is readily absorbed by nerve tissue causing serious damage. (See the discussion of lead poisoning in Chapter 14.)

Symptoms of encephalitis vary widely, depending on the extent of the inflammation and its location in the brain. In children the onset may be marked only by lethargy or irritability. In infants, it may be mostly gastrointestinal with severe cramps and pain. Mild symptoms are headache, stiff neck, fever, and delirium. More severe manifestations are convulsions, coma, twitching, paralysis, and abnormal eye movement. Sometimes the coma continues for weeks or months, hence the name *sleeping sickness* often given the disease. Return of speech, thought processes, and motor control may be very slow. Permanent brain damage with cerebral palsy and mental retardation may result.

Diagnosis of encephalitis is made on the basis of history of the illness, neurological examination, and laboratory tests of blood, spinal fluid, and urine. There is no specific treatment for encephalitis caused by virus. Corticosteroids may be given for postinfectious or postvaccination types. Broad-spectrum antibiotics may be given to prevent secondary infections. Symptomatic care is provided. Nutritional needs are met by intravenous infusions and gavage, elimination needs by cathartics, enemas, and catheterization. Inhalation therapy may be ordered to prevent or treat hypostatic pneumonia, and physiotherapy to prevent contracture deformities. Sedatives of various types may be used to control convulsions.

Nursing care of the delirious, convulsing, or comatose child is of great importance. The room should be kept quiet and the light subdued to reduce the stimuli for convulsions. There should be close observation of symptoms and changes in the state of consciousness, special skin care, oral hygiene, conscientious recording of intake and output, and range of motion exercises of extremities. When lumbar punctures are performed, a nurse positions the child and assists the physician. As soon as possible the parents should be included in the child's care, so that they will be better prepared to understand, accept, and assume responsibility for meeting the child's needs during the long period of convalescence.

Landry-Guillain-Barré syndrome. This strange disease produces temporary paralysis that begins in the legs and moves upward, sometimes involving all but the eyelids. In mild cases the paralysis disappears in a few days with complete return of muscle function. In severe cases recovery may take a year or more. If cardiac or respiratory failure occurs, emergency tracheostomy and mechanical cardiopulmonary assistance is necessary to prevent death. There may be urinary retention, incontinence, and constipation during the paralytic period. The disease usually follows a viral respiratory infection and is associated with an autoimmunological response. It occurs most often in children between the ages of 4 and 10 years and in adults of all ages. Because function usually returns spontaneously, nursing care is directed toward maintaining the life processes during the paralytic period. This includes skin care, tracheostomy care, bowel and bladder care, attention to nutritional needs, observation for changes in vital signs or degree of paralysis, emotional support, and encouragement. Parents need to become a part of the care-giving team with information, education, and support.

Tumors

Most brain tumors in children are caused by the abnormal growth of cells from within the brain; few are caused by metastasis to the brain from neoplasms elsewhere in the body. They produce symptoms that result from increased intracranial pressure and damage to specific areas of the brain. The most common types are medulloblastoma, astrocytoma, craniopharyngioma, and brainstem glioma.

Medulloblastoma is the most common brain tumor found in children and often occurs in children between 3 and 6 years of age. It originates in the cerebellum, grows rapidly, destroys the tissue, occludes the aqueduct, and invades the brainstem. It may spread via the spinal fluid to other areas of the nervous system. Death usually results in less than 1 year.

Astrocytoma is the second most common tumor. It occurs at any age but especially in older children. It originates in the cerebellum and appears in two forms—solid and cystic. The solid form is highly malignant, causing death within 1 year. The cystic type can occasionally be removed surgically with complete cure.

Craniopharyngioma occurs more often in 5- to 15-year-old children. Because of its location near the pituitary gland, various hormonal disturbances such as myxedema, delayed puberty, and diabetes insipidus often develop. Visual, memory, and personality changes also occur. Surgical removal of the entire tumor is usually not possible, but with radiation its growth may be controlled for many years.

Brainstem glioma occurs most often in the early school years. A glioma is the abnormal growth of neuroglia cells that make up the special connective tissue of the nervous system. Motor nerves are especially affected. The tumor grows slowly but is inoperable and eventually fatal.

Early diagnosis of brain tumor is difficult because specific symptoms may not become obvious until major damage has been done. Diagnosis is based on symptoms of increased intracranial pressure and localized disturbances. Electroencephalogram (EEG), ventriculogram, arteriogram, and x-ray studies of the skull are employed to help locate the tumor (see the diagnostic tests in Chapter 9). Lumbar puncture is not done when there is the possibility of increased intracranial pressure because of the danger of pushing the medulla down into the spinal canal.

Treatment consists of surgically removing the tumor or as much of it as possible and giving radiation therapy. Even when a complete cure is not possible, the symptoms may be reduced and the child's life prolonged.

Nursing care is directed toward providing for the nutritional and other physical needs of the child and toward maintaining the morale of both the child and the parents. Observations by the nurse are important in helping the physician localize the tumor and appraise the increasing intracranial pressure. Any muscle weakness, visual disturbance, or subjective compliant of the older child, such as headache, should be noted and reported, as well as vomiting, convulsions, changes in the vital signs, irritability, or drowsiness. Emergency oxygen, suction, drugs, and ventricular tap tray are kept on hand.

Preoperative preparation for a craniotomy includes cutting the hair and shaving the scalp. A special permit for this, signed by the parents, is required by many hospitals. The cut hair should be saved and given to the parents with a notation made on the chart. All the other normal preoperative care is given.

Immediate post craniotomy care requires great skill and experience. It is provided in an intensive care unit whenever possible. At first the child is positioned on the unaffected area with the head to the side to prevent aspiration of mucus and vomitus. As soon as the danger of aspiration is passed, the position should be changed frequently, but with great care. The child should be turned slowly and steadily, with the head well supported and the body in a straight line. Vital signs are taken until stable. Fever-reducing measures may be necessary. Hypothermia may be used to reduce intracranial edema, bleeding, or disturbances of the heat-regulating center. The rate of intravenous fluid absorption is carefully controlled. Too rapid administration may produce a dangerous increase in intracranial pressure. Restraints are used only if absolutely necessary because if the child struggles against them, intracranial pressure may be increased. As a result of the surgery the area around the eyes may become "black" and the face swollen. This discoloration gradually disappears. The perineum should be kept clean and dry. Skin areas where there is pressure should be massaged and padded to prevent tissue breakdown. Foot drop and other contracture deformities must be guarded against by proper positioning and movement.

While recovering from surgery, the child should be encouraged to assume as many normal activities as possible. Regression to behavior of a younger child is common. Residual paralysis, blindness, and speech impairment require special therapy. The parents need emotional support and practical assistance as they assume the care of the child after surgery. (See the discussion on children with terminal illnesses in Chapter 7.)

Degenerative disorders

These disorders are characterized by a progressive course that ends in death. Those most frequently seen are diffuse sclerosis, multiple sclerosis, and neuroymelitis optica. In all these diseases the insulating myelin sheath of the nerves degenerates with sclerosis (scarring) so that the capacity of the nerve to carry impulses is impaired.

Diffuse sclerosis (Schilder's disease) usually

occurs before 10 years of age, and involves personality changes, blindness, progressive ataxia (muscle noncoordination), deafness, and seizures. Biopsy of brain tissue is diagnostic and reveals generalized demyelinization. Progressive deterioration continues until death.

Multiple sclerosis usually appears in later childhood or early adulthood. Included are attacks of optic neuritis with visual disturbances, ataxia, and sensory changes in various parts of the body. Remissions and exacerbations occur, but the course of the disease generally progresses from blindness and progressive loss of function to death.

Neuromyelitis optica appears in children between 5 and years of age, with fever, radiating pain in the affected eye, visual disturbances, and increased gamma globulin in the spinal fluid. One third of affected children later develop multiple sclerosis.

Nursing care for victims of all of the degenerative disorders is individually planned to assist the patient and family to cope with and adjust to the increasing limits of the disease. The goal is maximum independence, and fulfillment for each member of the family. A variety of community resources are available to aid in this task, including the National Multiple Sclerosis Foundation.

Convulsive disorders

The term *epilepsy* was once used to describe all conditions accompanied by *convulsions (spells, fits,* or *seizures).* Many people continue to use it as a general term, but as more is learned about these disorders more precise terms are being developed to describe them. A single episode is called a *convulsion, spell, fit,* or *seizure.*

Causation. Convulsions result from abnormal electric discharges produced by irritated or injured nerve cells in the cerebrum. The discharges can be demonstrated by electronencephalogram (EEG). Nerve irritation may be caused by known organic causes such as infection, fever, tumors, edema, hemorrhage, trauma, brain tissue dis-

ease, congenital malformation, and systemic poisoning. When the cause is not known, the condition is termed *cryptogenic* (hidden) or *idiopathic* (self-originated). Conditions that precipitate seizures by lowering the convulsive threshold include electrolyte imbalance, stress, fever, infection, and fatigue.

Classification. Convulsions have been classified by the International League Against Epilepsy into two major groups, *centrencephalic* and *focal-cortical.*

Centrencephalic convulsions. Centrencephalic convulsions emanate from the central portion of the brain and produce generalized grand mal, petit mal, myoclonic, and kinetic convulsions.

Generalized grand mal convulsions may occur in children at any age, but those that occur after 4 years of age are not as likely to indicate serious mental or motor defects. The typical seizure begins with a warning *aura* experienced by the victim, such as a visual image, nausea, headache, or odd feeling. There is a cry as the air rushes out of the lungs and the person loses consciousness and *falls*; the eyes roll up, the head is extended, the body stiffens, the jaws clamp shut, sometimes biting down on the tongue, and breathlessness causes increasing cyanosis. Following this *tonic phase,* the muscles begin to twitch in what is called the *clonic phase.* There may be salivation and incontinence of urine and stool. The tonic and clonic phases last about 5 minutes and are followed by several hours of confusion or deep sleep. When one grand mal seizure follows another in rapid succession the condition is called *status epilepticus.*

Petit mal seizures consist of a transient loss of consciousness, sometimes with a rolling of the eyes, lip movements, and head and limb movement. The attack lasts from 1 to 20 seconds with or without loss of muscle tone. The child just stops activity and may not realize that a seizure has occurred and may have as many as 100 or more such attacks a day. Petit mal seizures occur most often between the ages of 5 and 12 years.

They have serious consequences and require diagnosis and treatment.

Infantile myoclonic seizures are seen in infants between 3 and 12 months of age. A typical episode consists of a rapid flexion and extension of the head, trunk, or limbs; the eyes may roll up or in with no apparent loss of consciousness. Several of these seizures may occur each day. The convulsions usually occur in infants with severe brain injury caused by meningitis, microcephaly, and cerebral anoxia.

Kinetic seizures usually occur between the ages of 3 and 12 years. The child momentarily loses trunk and limb muscle tone, often followed by a sudden muscle spasm, resulting in a fall. The child does not lose consciousness. These episodes may occur hundreds of times a day. Such repeated interruptions interfere with the child's capacity to think and function. A number of drugs have been found effective in controlling these seizures.

Focal-cortical convulsions. Focal-cortical convulsions emanate from the outer portion of the brain. They include focal-sensory, focal-motor, and psychomotor seizures.

Focal-sensory seizures are rarely identified in children younger than 8 years of age. They describe a variety of sensory aberrations such as flashing colored lights, prickling pain, or numbness of the face or limbs. Odd movements or posturing may occur. The causative lesions are located in the parietal sensory cortex.

Focal-motor seizures originate in various cortical areas of the cerebrum causing motor, sensory, psychic, or visceral episodes. Jacksonian or "march" seizures consist of alternate tonic-clonic seizures of one side of the face or body, which then spread to the other. After the seizure, transient weakness may occur.

Psychomotor (limpic or temporal lobe) seizures are commonly seen in children 3 to 15 years of age. They are characterized by bizarre behavior and by motor and sensory manifestations and are associated with memory loss lasting from minutes to hours. Although these seizures vary from one child to another, in most the child remains conscious during the episode, then sleeps for long periods afterward.

Mixed convulsions are common in children 2 to 10 years of age. They are a combination of focal-motor and psychomotor seizures with generalized or myoclonic manifestations. It is as if the electric discharge that fired in one area of the brain spreads and fires the whole. Mental retardation and learning and behavior disorders are frequently associated with this disorder.

Diagnosis and care. Diagnosis of a convulsive disorder is based on a medical and family history, electroencephalogram, and x-ray studies of the skull. Pneumoencephalography and cerebrospinal fluid examination may also be done. It is important that the physician have an accurate description of convulsive attacks. If the child is admitted to the hospital for study, the attending nurse should be especially observant of the child's normal behavior, any signs preceding a seizure, where and how it began, whether there was incontinence, and how long the convulsion lasted. All this information is important in localizing the brain lesion.

Treatment consists of anticonvulsive drugs, physical care to maintain general hygiene and nutrition, psychological support, neurosurgery in selected cases, and protection during convulsions and periods of unconsciousness.

The choice of the drug, or drugs, is made by the physician from a large selection of anticonvulsants according to the individual needs of the child and the type of seizure experienced. Some of the most common ones are:

The *barbiturates* (phenobarbital, mephobarbital, metharbital, primidone) are effective anticonvulsants, especially for centrencephalic seizures. The chief disadvantages are that they cause sleepiness and addiction. They may produce skin rashes and loss of motor coordination.

The *succinimides* (methsuximide, phensuximide, ethosuximide) are used for petit mal, psychomotor, and myoclonic seizures. Side effects of these drugs include skin rash, nausea, lethargy, and loss of motor coordination.

Diphenylhydantoin (Dilantin) is an effective anti-convulsive for all types of seizures except peti mal. It should be given with food to reduce stomach irritation. Overgrowth of gum tissue may develop with prolonged use.

Diazepam (Valium) is a tranquilizer used for myoclonic and generalized seizures and status epilepticus. Side effects include ataxia and lethargy.

Trimethadione (Tridione) is one of the drugs used to control petit mal seizures. Phenobarbital and Dilantin may be given with it. Because Tridione depresses blood cell production, monthly blood studies are ordered to watch for anemia. Skin rash and photophobia may also develop.

When drug therapy is first begun, the dosage must be individually adjusted to the child. It is important to follow the prescription exactly and to observe and report the child's reaction carefully. Excessive drowsiness, skin eruptions, nausea, other untoward reactions, or the event of a convulsion should be reported. To avoid stomach irritation and to establish a regular time, drugs should be given at mealtimes. Both the child and the parents should understand the need for regular and consistent medication.

When a convulsion occurs in the epileptic child or a child with an acute illness, what should be done? The convulsion cannot be "stopped." The chief responsibility of those nearby is to prevent the convulsing child from injury as a result of a fall, uncontrolled jerking, or biting the tongue. In the hospital the side rails should be kept up and padded. In some hospitals, a padded tongue blade is kept at the bedside to be placed between the teeth during convulsion. After a seizure the child should be allowed to rest quietly.

Although a high-fat diet is prescribed for epileptics by some physicians, others order a regular, balanced diet appropriate to the age of the child. All authorities recommend against excesses in food or drink and moderation in all things with good personal hygiene. Excessive fatigue, anxiety-producing situations, and over-stimulation should be avoided. The child should not be overprotected, however, but should be encouraged to participate in social and school activities and to lead as normal a life as possible. The parents and the child need factual information about epilepsy to face its realities and cope successfully with them. They need to know exactly what to do (and not do) during a convulsion. They should understand the expected action of the prescribed drugs and be in continuous communication with their physician to report any untoward symptoms. Regular medical checkups are important because of the child's changing needs.

One of the more difficult things the epileptic child and the parents face is the social stigma attached to epilepsy. Some of the facts both they and the general public should be given are as follows:

1. Epilepsy is caused by brain damage, not "bad genes" or "sins."
2. Death rarely occurs during seizures.
3. Seizures do not cause deterioration of normal mental activity.
4. With continuous medical supervision and modern drug therapy, seizures can be controlled and sometimes eliminated.
5. Archaic legal restrictions on the epileptic are gradually being repealed. In some states driver's licenses are granted seizure-free epileptics.
6. Epilepsy is like any other physical disability. Although its limitations must be recognized, it need not prevent the person from leading a full life, including education, adventure, travel, marriage, and professional accomplishment.

Neuromotor disorders (cerebral palsy)

Neuromotor disorders, commonly called *cerebral palsy*, result from damaged brain tissue causing loss of voluntary muscle coordination or sensation. The damage may be caused by developmental defects, birth trauma, metabolic abnormalities, infections, tumors, hemorrhage, toxicity, or hypoxia of the newborn. Such damage may occur at any time in life, but most often it occurs before or shortly after birth. It is permanent and does not become progressively greater, but all of the symptoms may not appear until the child is fully developed. Symptoms vary from mild to severe. The chief characteristics are lack of muscle coordination, muscle spasms of various types, and lack of balance (ataxia). There may also be convulsions, blindness, deafness, and speech difficulties. About two thirds of patients suffer some degree of mentally retardation. Those with normal mental capacity may have such severe physical problems that they appear to be retarded. Emotional development is often hampered because of the restrictions of the physical disability.

In more severe cases diagnosis may be made soon after birth. The infant nurses poorly, may have convulsions, and is slow to develop motor coordination. Blindness and deafness may also be evident. Mild cases may go unnoticed until the child is a toddler or of school age.

Cerebral palsy is classified according to the region of the brain affected and the muscular symptoms it produces as follows: spastic, dyskinetic, ataxic, rigid, and mixed types.

In the *spastic type* certain muscle groups are in a state of great tension or spasm. The *dyskinetic type* is characterized by tremors and involuntary, snakelike (athetoid) motions that interfere with normal movement (Fig. 18-11). The *ataxic type* is a disturbance in the sense of balance so that the child staggers in attempts to walk. The *rigid type* is characterized by stiff extension of the legs, flexion of the arms, and hyperextension of the neck, and the *atonic type* by lack of muscle tone. Most cases have symptoms of more than one type and so are called *mixed*. When only the legs are involved, the condition is described as *paraplegia*. When one half of the body is involved, it is called *hemiplegia*, and when all four extremities are involved it is called *quadriplegia*. Occasionally one limb may be under normal control and three involved, or three limbs may be under normal control and only one involved.

Because of the great varieties of disability,

each child having cerebral palsy must be evaluated individually. A whole team of professionals is involved in helping the child develop capacities to the fullest extent; such a team is composed of the pediatrician, social worker, surgeon, orthopedist, psychologist, speech therapist, physiotherapist, occupational therapist, teacher, nurses, and the parents. Because no treatment can restore a damaged brain, the aim in therapy is

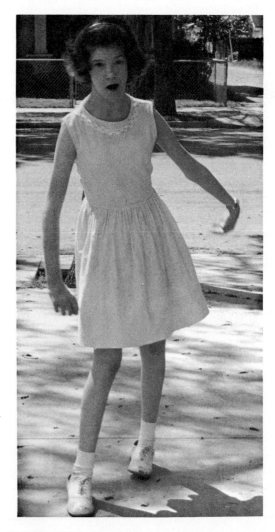

Fig. 18-11. Girl with cerebral palsy with the excessive motion of dyskinetic type.

habilitation, or establishing new habits whereby the muscles are used for new functions. A great variety of techniques and mechanical devices are employed, and untold hours of laborious effort are expended. Progress is slow. The eventual degree of self-sufficiency attained by the child depends on the disability and response to habilitation.

When a child with cerebral palsy is admitted to the hospital, it is important that the staff know about the child's capabilities. Information about feeding, dressing, toileting, the use of special orthopedic appliances, ability to communicate, and history of convulsions is needed. The parents are usually the best source of this information. When possible, it is best if the child continues to do as much personal care in the hospital as at home. If the child has difficulty swallowing, suction should be available immediately. The child should be cared for with gentleness and deliberateness; sudden movements and overstimulation increase tension. The child finds it difficult to relax and becomes fatigued easily. Even the simplest controlled movement may require tremendous amounts of energy and concentration. Nurses cannot be in a hurry. They must take time and exercise great patience. It is extremely frustrating to the child not to be able to make the muscles do what is desired. Recognition and praise for even small accomplishments should be given. The nursing staff should seek the guidance of the occupational therapist and other specialists in working with the child.

Because cerebral palsy affects so many persons and constitutes a lifelong disability, it is a matter of public as well as private concern. The United Cerebral Palsy Association, Inc. is a voluntary agency devoted to this condition. Special educational programs are available in most communities. Workshops and recreational facilities are also provided. No longer are these persons locked away in institutions; instead, they are integrated into the community. Special classes within public schools make it possible to begin

this integration early in life, thus increasing independence and a feeling of self-respect.

Mental (psychiatric) disorders

Mental disorders are those manifested by behavior that fails to meet the expectations of society. They have perplexed medical science for centuries because of the wide range of symptoms and complex nature of their causes. As a step toward understanding and treating these diverse conditions, the medical community has devised various classification systems. The World Health Organization publishes *The International Classification of Diseases*, currently in its ninth edition. The American Medical Association published a modified version, entitled *The International Classification of Diseases: Clinical Modification, ed. 9*, in 1979. In 1980 the American Psychiatric Association published *The Diagnostic and Statistical Manual III*, a system whereby each patient has a five-part diagnosis. In DSM-III the first major category of disease is entitled, "Disorders that usually first manifest themselves in infancy, childhood, or adolescence." Those conditions are further classified as follows:

Mental retardation
Attention deficit disorders
Conduct disorders
Anxiety disorders of childhood or adolescence
Other disorders of infancy, childhood, or adolescence
Eating disorders
Stereotyped movement disorders
Other physical disorders
Pervasive developmental disorders

Mental retardation. Mental retardation is an interference with intelligence that limits the child's ability to adapt to surroundings. It is not a disease in itself but is the result of many different factors that affect mental capacity. Some of the causes include intracranial hemorrhage, endocrine disorders as in hypothyroidism, hypoxia of the newborn, metabolic disorders as in phenylketonuria, infections such as encephalitis, poisoning as with lead, neoplasms, chromosomal defects as in Down's syndrome, and heredity. About 3.5% of the children born in the United States have intelligence below "normal." To better understand mental retardation, the student is urged to review the discussion of normal mental development provided in Chapter 2.

Diagnosis of mental retardation is made only after thorough study of a child's mental and motor development and the medical and family history. In recent years greater attention has been given to early detection and treatment of conditions leading to retardation, such as phenylketonuria, discussed in Chapter 14, or craniosynostosis, discussed earlier in this chapter. Severe retardation may be recognized early when the infant fails to respond or suck during the first weeks of life. A slowness to follow the normal pattern of smiling, grasping, sitting, or walking may also be noticed. Mild retardation may not become apparent until the school years when a child is unable to understand abstract ideas. The parents may be reluctant to accept a diagnosis of mental retardation and may go to several physi-

cians or agencies in a vain attempt to find another explanation for their child's lack of progress.

When the diagnosis of mental retardation is made, the physician seeks to help the parents make realistic plans for their child's care based on the degree of disability, home situation, and available community resources. In Table 18-2 the various classifications of intelligence are given. The student will notice that for each degree of intelligence various levels of achievement expected are listed.

The decision of whether to place the child in an institution or to provide care in the home is difficult. The entire family's physical and emotional capacity to cope with such responsibility must be considered. The retarded child needs constant supervision, special training, and the same love and security as the normal child, but for a longer period. The availability of special classes in public schools and recreational and vocational programs in the community is another consideration. The profoundly retarded child may be best cared for in an institution, whereas the moderately or mildly retarded child may

Table 18-2. Classification of intelligence

Classification	Intelligence quotient*	Level of achievement
Profoundly retarded	0 to 24	Completely dependent; may walk; needs nursing care; behavior of 0 to 2 year old
Severely retarded	25 to 39	Trainable in repetitive tasks; needs supervision; behavior of 3 to 7 year old
Moderately retarded	40 to 54	Educable; travels alone in familiar places; needs some supervision; behavior of 8 to 12 year old
Mildly retarded	55 to 70	Educable; simple vocational and social skills adequate for self-maintenance; needs help in stressful situations
Normal	71 to 110	Majority of population is in this group
Above average	111 to 130	Technical and professional occupations
Gifted	131 to 150	Superior ability to understand abstract concepts and solve complex problems
Genius	151 and up	Rare ability; the Michelangelos and Albert Einsteins of the world

*Wechsler Adult Intelligence Scale.

thrive at home. The child's presence may even enrich the lives of the family and community by providing a noncompetitive object of love and concern.

When a retarded child is hospitalized for acute illness, nurses care for physical needs just as they would for a normal child. Nurses must also be careful to protect the child from injury, and must communicate, select toys, and give recognition and praise appropriate to mental, rather than chronological age.

Except for the profoundly retarded child, life expectancy is about the same as for one with normal intelligence. This makes it especially important these these children be educated and trained to the fullest extent of their capacities and that every effort be made to prevent mental retardation. Many private and public research projects are currently in progress to discover the causes and eventually hope to discover a way to prevent mental retardation. One of the conditions that has undergone considerable investigation recently is Down's syndrome.

Down's syndrone (mongolism) is a form of mental retardation with certain typical physical characteristics that give the child a somewhat Oriental appearance, hence the name "mongolism" (Fig. 18-12). It is caused by chromosomal abnormalities, the most common being trisomy of chromosome 21. As a result the child has a total of 47 chromosomes instead of the normal 46. Down's dyndrome occurs once in every 625 births with 80% of the affected children born to mothers over 35 years of age.

Because of their typical appearance, these children are usually diagnosed soon after birth. The face is round, ears set low, nose flat, eyes somewhat slanted, mouth open and drooling, tongue protruding, fingers short, a wide space between the first and second toes, birth weight low, and behavior lethargic. Mental capacity varies from profound to mild retardation. After the newborn period other signs become apparent. The teeth are slow to erupt and growth is stunted. Congenital umbilical hernias and heart defects are common. Resistance to infections is poor. Mongoloid children are usually affectionate and happy-go-lucky. As with other forms of mental

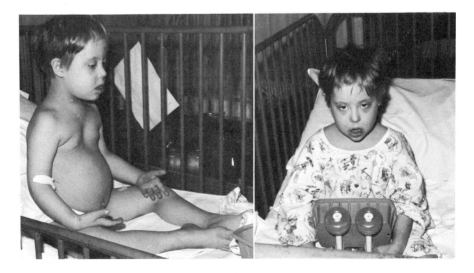

Fig. 18-12. Down's syndrome showing typical open mouth, protruding tongue, lethargic behavior, and slant eyes. This child also has a serious heart defect.

retardation the child needs the same care as a normal one and, in addition, special training and education appropriate to ability to learn.

Minimal brain dysfunction. Some children have apparently normal physical, motor, and mental development with normal electroencephalograms, but they are excessively active and are said to suffer from *hyperkinetic syndrome*. Others behave quite normally but cannot learn to read or write as other children and are described as having *learning disabilities*. Both groups are classified as having minimal brain dysfunction.

Attention deficit disorders. Some children have normal electroencephalograms and normal physical, motor, and mental development, but they are easily distracted, cannot seem to listen, have difficulty concentrating, and act impulsively. Some are also hyperactive, constantly moving as if "driven by a motor." When these symptoms occur before 7 years of age and last for 6 months or more, the child may be diagnosed as having an attention deficit disorder. Various drugs are used both to confirm the diagnosis and to treat the condition. Ritalin (methylphenidate hydrochloride), a cerebral stimulant, sometimes produces dramatic results in the hyperactive (hyperkinetic) child. A few minutes after administration the child becomes calm, is able to exercise control and concentrate, and exhibits normal response to others. This drug is given three times a day, with a dosage adjusted to the age and needs of the child. Tranquilizing drugs may also be prescribed. Drug therapy is continued indefinitely into adulthood until it is no longer needed.

Such children are rarely hospitalized for hyperkinosis, but they may be hospitalized for other conditions. It is important that drug therapy be continued exactly as ordered and that any excessive drowsiness or excitability be reported to the physician by the nursing staff.

Conduct disorders. This group of childhood disorders include those behaviors that violate the rights of others. Sometimes these children are able to form friendships with peers and sometimes they are not. Sometimes their behavior is aggressive and sometimes it is not. Because the behavior of these children violates the societal standards and is against the law, they receive attention from the authorities and social agencies. Various psychotherapeutic approaches are attempted to change their behavior, including individual counseling, behavior modification, and milieu (environmental) therapy. Their medical and dental health needs may be neglected except when they are in the custody of the courts.

Anxiety disorders of childhood or adolescence. The anxiety disorders include separation anxiety, avoidant disorder of childhood or adolescence, and overanxious disorders. These disorders are characterized by excessive fear, avoidance, and need for reassurance to a much greater degree than the average person. They are treated with individual and family therapy.

Other disorders of infancy, childhood, or adolescence. This is a miscellaneous group that includes attachment disorder of infancy which affects children 3 years of age or younger; schizoid disorders of childhood or adolescence; elective mutism (refusal to speak); oppositional disorder characterized by provocative opposition to authority; and identity disorder in which there is severe distress over such issues as moral values, sexuality, and career choice. This diverse group of disorders is treated with individual, group, and family therapy.

Eating disorders. The eating disorders include anorexia nervosa in which the child or adolescent loses at least 25% of original body weight; bulimia in which there is a pattern of episodic binge eating; rumination disorder of infancy (regurgitation of food without physical cause); and atypical eating disorders. All of these disorders are treated with diet therapy, psychotherapy, and behavior modification. Occasionally these children are admitted to the hospital for treatment of these or other conditions. When they are admitted, nursing interventions need to be planned together with the medical and dietary treatment plan.

Stereotyped movement disorders. This group of disorders are characterized by recurrent, repetitive, involuntary, purposeless motor movement. They affect children from 2 to 15 years of age and are distinguished from atypical stereotyped movement disorders that are voluntary and that give the child pleasure.

Other physical disorders. This group of mental disorders includes stuttering, functional enuresis (voiding urine at inappropriate times and places), and atypical stereotyped movement (such as head-banging or rocking that can be stopped at will), functional encopresis (passing formed stool at inappropriate times and places), sleep walking, and sleep terrors. All of these disorders are treated with individual and family therapy and with behavior modification.

Pervasive developmental disorders. This group includes infantile autism (with onset before 42 months of age), childhood autism, and atypical pervasive developmental disorder.

Infantile autism is characterized by self-absorption (autism), by a pervasive lack of responsiveness to other human beings, by gross deficits in language development, and if speech is present, by peculiar speech patterns such as echoing and metaphoric language. There are bizarre responses to the surroundings such as resistance to change and peculiar interest in objects. In the childhood disorder there may be self-mutilation such as biting themselves; acute, excessive anxiety manifested by such symptoms as unexplained panics; and peculiar posturing and hand movements. These children usually learn to walk at an early age and are highly mobile and active. About the age of 5 to 7 years most become more manageable, more affectionate, less given to needless fears, and more aware of real dangers. Two thirds of autistic children remain so handicapped into adulthood that they require special living and working conditions.

The care and education of these children are enormous tasks. Communicating even the simplest concept is a major problem requiring patience, understanding, and skill. Behavior modification techniques have been used with some success to lead these children from isolation to the world of people and ideas.

Other major psychiatric disorders. In addition to those disorders identified by DSM-III as first manifesting themselves in infancy, childhood, or adolescence, there are many other categories of psychiatric disorders which describe conditions that afflict children and adolescents. While such patients are seen in the pediatric and medical-surgical units for various physical conditions, their mental illnesses are usually not identified or treated there. Instead, psychiatric disorders are treated in psychiatric units or through outpatient clinics. These other major categories of psychiatric disorders are as follows:

Organic mental disorders (substance-induced)
Substance use disorders (alcohol abuse and dependence, etc.)
Schizophrenic disorders
Paranoid disorders
Affective disorders (manic, depressive, bipolar, chronic minor, etc.)
Psychotic disorders not elsewhere classified (schizoaffective, etc.)
Anxiety disorders (phobias, anxiety neurosis, post-traumatic stress)
Factitious disorders (falsifying disease conditions)
Somatoform disorders (conversion hysteria, hypochondriasis, etc.)
Dissociative disorders (amnesia, multiple personality, etc.)
Psychosexual disorders (gender confusion, paraphilias, dysfunctions)
Disorders of impulse control not elsewhere classified (pyromania, etc.)
Adjustment disorders
Nondisorders that are a focus of treatment (parent-child problems, uncomplicated bereavement, antisocial behavior, etc.)

Disorders of the eye

In studying the disorders of the eye the student is urged to refer to Fig. 18-3. The following professionals specialize in this field:

ophthalmologist a physician who specializes in the study and treatment of disorders of the eye
oculist another term for ophthalmologist
optometrist one who is licensed to test for visual acuity and to prescribe corrective lenses
optician one who grinds lenses and makes and sells optical apparatus

Infections

Conjunctivitis. Conjunctivitis is an inflammation of the conjunctiva of the eye. It may be caused by bacteria, viruses, or allergy, but the ordinary type is caused by bacteria such as staphylococci and streptococci. The infection begins suddenly, with burning, redness, and mucopurulent discharge, hence the common name "pink-eye." It is highly contagious, spreading easily from one eye to the other and from child to child. If untreated, the infection is self-limiting and lasts up to 2 weeks. Diagnosis is confirmed by smears taken from the discharge. Bacterial infections usually respond quickly to penicillin and other antibiotics locally or systemically.

Gonorrheal ophthalmia neonatorum. Gonorrheal ophthalmia neonatorum is a gonococcal infection of the conjunctiva of a newborn infant acquired while passing through the birth canal of an infected mother. It is first noticed 2 to 5 days after delivery. The baby's eyelids become swollen and a profuse purulent discharge develops. Diagnosis is made by smears of the discharge. Treatment with penicillin effectively overcomes the infection if given promptly and in large doses. Strict isolation technique must be practiced because the condition is highly contagious. The uninvolved eye may be protected by a shield.

Without treatment there is danger of ulcers of the cornea with perforation and destruction of the eyeball. Because of these serious complications, prophylactic instillation of silver nitrate 1% into the eyes of all newborn infants is required by law in all of the 50 states. As a result gonorrheal conjunctivitis is relatively rare.

Blepharitis. Blepharitis is a common infection of the lid margins and conjunctiva with characteristic crusting and redness. Severe cases may involve ulceration and loss of eyelashes. In children it is usually caused by an allergic reaction to staphylococci and their toxins. Treatment consists of a thorough cleansing and removal of the crusts followed by the local use of antibiotic ointment instilled into the eye and rubbed onto the base of the lashes.

Hordeolum (stye). A hordeolum is an acute infection of the glands of the lid margin that results in a small abscess. Being superficial, it usually comes to a head rapidly, ruptures by itself, and heals completely. Hot moist compresses hasten the outcome and relieve some of the discomfort.

Injuries. In spite of the natural protection afforded the eye by its bony orbit, cushion of underlying fat, and lids and lashes, children suffer many eye injuries. Particles of dirt may scratch or become embedded in the cornea; sharp sticks, arrows, and exploding firecrackers may damage the eye; and chemicals or heat may burn it. Immediate care is of great importance. If a particle of dirt does not work itself out of the eye right away, the lid should be everted and the particle removed with a moist cotton swab. If the foreign matter cannot be removed readily, the eye should be covered with a clean cloth and the child taken to a physician. In like manner, any large embedded object should be left in place, the eye covered with a clean cloth, and the child taken to an emergency room. If strong chemicals get into the eyes, they should be irrigated immediately with a large stream of water from the faucet.

When the child is seen in the emergency room, the ophthalmologist may first instill a local anesthetic in the eye before examining it. The nurse is responsible to see that there is a good light and that the child is restrained during this examination. The nurse may need to obtain help or to use a mummy restraint. Complicated repair of a lacerated cornea or removal of a foreign body from the eye is usually performed in surgery. After such procedures infection is a major concern. Nursing care requires much patience and constant attention. The nurse should enlist the help of the parents when possible, instructing them in any precautions regarding the child's care. Special treatments and dressing changes are usually done by the ophthalmologist with the nurse assisting.

Congenital defects

Ptosis of the eyelids. Ptosis, or drooping, of the eyelids is usually congenital in children. It may affect either one or both eyes. It is caused by weak levator muscles. As a result of the defect, the child tilts the head back to see beneath the upper lids (Fig. 18-13). If the pupil is covered, vision may fail to develop. When such a condition occurs, the child should be referred to an ophthalmologist for evaluation. Treatment is surgical by shortening the levator muscles or by connecting the upper lid to the frontalis muscle of the forehead by means of connective tissue. Nursing care is similar to that for cataract operations.

Cataracts. The lens of the eye is situated just behind the pupil. Its function is to maintain accurate focus of the light rays that pass through it to the retina. When a lens becomes cloudy, the condition is called a *cataract.* Congenital cataracts in children may be caused by infectious agents such as the virus of rubella during the mother's pregnancy, metabolic disorders in the child, or heredity. The only treatment for cataract is removal of the affected lens. One of the procedures is pharmoemulsification, by which high-frequency ultrasonic vibrations dislodge the lens. These are combined with controlled irrigation to maintain normal ocular pressure and aspiration of lens fragments through a needle. Removal is carried out between the ages of 1 and 2 years to prevent permanent impairment of vision. Lenses may be implanted surgically or the

child may be fitted with glasses that act to focus light rays on the retina in place of the removed lens. Contact lenses made of "soft" plastic are sometimes prescribed.

The child is admitted to the hospital and given routine preoperative care. After returning from surgery, both eyes are bandaged. The amount of movement permitted depends on the physician's orders and the type of procedure performed. Some physicians require jacket and elbow restraints, with sandbags placed at the sides of the head and maintenance of a supine position. Others permit more movement, believing that it re-

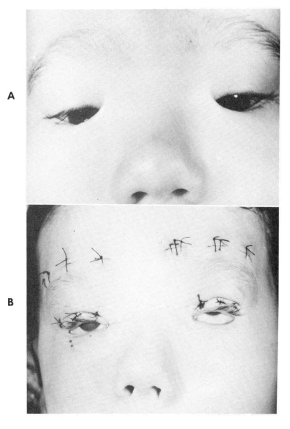

Fig. 18-13. Congenital ptosis of the eyelids. **A,** Before surgery and, **B,** immediately after, showing sutures. (Courtesy Children's Medical Center, Oakland, Calif.)

duces agitation. Every effort should be made to reduce crying and prevent vomiting because they increase intraocular pressure, bleeding, and suture strain. Great care must be taken to prevent the aspiration of food and mucus. Parents can be a help to the nurse and a comfort to the child during this time but should be instructed about special precautions regarding the child's care.

Strabismus (squint). Strabismus is an inability of the eyes to work together. It is one of the most common ocular abnormalities in children, occurring at birth or soon after in 1% of all children. Strabismus is variously called squint, cross-eyes, and wall-eyes, because the eyes may turn in, out, up, or down (Fig. 18-14).

At birth, coordination of the two eyes is not completely developed. There may be deviation and wandering of the eyes. By the age of 3 months, however, the eyes should work together and follow a moving object. If, by the age of 6 months, the eyes still deviate instead of converging on an object, the child should be seen by an ophthalmologist.

When the two eyes develop normally, they work as a unit. Images are focused on the retina of each eye and passed on to the brain as two sets of nervous impulses. There they are fused as one. In strabismus this ability to fuse the two images is faulty or absent. The child is unable to use the two eyes together because two images are present in the brain and double vision (diplopia or ambiopia) results. To overcome this distortion, the brain suppresses the images of one eye. It soon finds that if one eye is not centered, its image is less intense and more easily suppressed. This suppression may be only of one eye, called *monocular strabismus*, or of each eye alternately, called *alternate strabismus*. In monocular strabismus the child uses the same eye all the time and the other one is crossed.

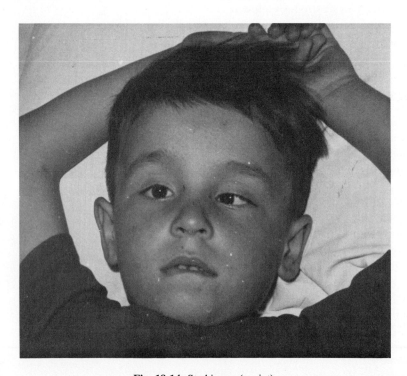

Fig. 18-14. Strabismus (squint).

Because vision normally develops during these early months, when one eye is not used, vision fails to develop in it and permanent visual impairment results. In addition to this fusion difficulty, many children also have astigmatism, a refractory error described later.

Treatment should begin early. The ophthalmologist can determine whether the infant, at 1 year of age, is using both eyes. If the infant is not using both, the most-used eye is covered to assure that vision develops in the deviating one. By the age of 18 months the child can be tested for astigmatism and glasses prescribed as necessary. Eye muscle exercises (orthoptic treatment) are sometimes ordered for the deviating eye, but ultimately most cases of strabismus require operation on the extraocular muscles to realign the eyes. This surgery is postponed until about 5 years of age to permit more accurate measurement of the degree of deviation. It should be performed before the child enters school to avoid the emotionally damaging taunts of other children.

The child should be prepared for hospitalization and surgery, as discussed in Chapter 7, and should experience having the eyes covered and the arms restrained beforehand so that upon returning from surgery there will be less anxiety. Postoperative care is similar to that of the cataract patient described previously. The nurse should speak before touching the child to avoid startling when the eyes are bandaged. Recovery is usually uneventful and prognosis is good if visual acuity was not impaired before treatment.

Errors of refraction. The most common abnormality of the eyes is an error of refraction (bending of light rays). In children this abnormality is a special problem because of the demands of school. The child may become irritable, have poor relationships withclassmates, and do poorly in schoolwork. The basis for the difficulty may be discovered by periodic vision screening carried out as part of school health program.

Normal refraction (emmetropia) exists when parallel light rays are focused clearly on the retina. Abnormal refraction (ametropia) may be of three types in children—hyperopia, myopia, and astigmatism. The type of error is determined by the shape of the eyeball. This shape is an inherited trait just as a large nose or small ears. As the eyes grow with the child, refraction may undergo marked change, hence the importance of periodic testing.

Hyperopia, or farsightedness, is the most frequent abnormality. In this condition the image is focused behind the retina. To bring the focus forward to the retina, the curvature of the lens of the eye must be changed. To do so, the ciliary muscles contract. If these muscles must contract constantly, they become fatigued and symptoms of eye strain such as tension and headache develop. Correction of this error is accomplished by prescription of convex lenses for eyeglasses.

Myopia, or nearsightedness, occurs because the eyeball is too long and the focus falls in front of the retina, producing a blurred image for distance. In severe cases the child may hold the print very close to the eyes to obtain a clean image. Prescription of concave lenses for eyeglasses corrects this abnormality.

In *astigmatism* the curvature of the cornea is not the same in all areas. As a result the rays of light are not focused evenly on the retina and the image is distorted like that seen in a mirror in a carnival funhouse. The error is corrected by a specially ground lens that compensates for the abnormal curvature of the cornea.

The child with a visual impairment should be examined by an ophthalmologist or optometrist to determine the cause. Testing (Fig. 18-15) for glasses, called "refraction," is usually carried out with the focusing power (accommodation) of the eyes at rest. To do so, drugs that produce temporary paralysis of the ciliary muscles (cycloplegic), such as atropine, are dropped into the eyes. The opthalmologist or optometrist then tests and prescribes the exact lens for each eye. These lenses are placed in an eyeglass frame appropriate to the child's needs. As the child

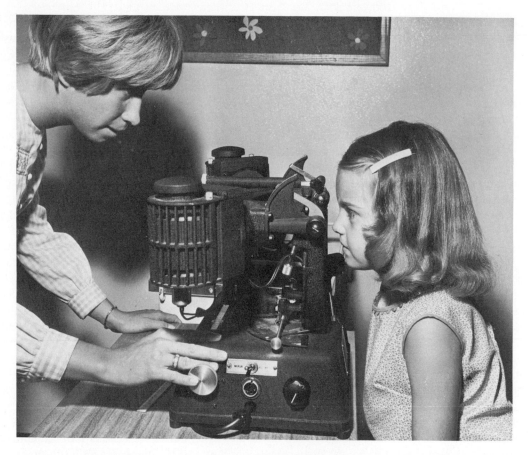

Fig. 18-15. Vision testing. (Courtesy Children's Medical Center, Oakland, Calif.)

grows, both the lenses and the frame need to be changed periodically. The child may cease to need them entirely. Contact lenses are seldom prescribed for children during their growing years. They may be a tremendous boon, however, to the emotional well-being of an older adolescent or young adult who continues to need refractory correction beyond childhood.

Blindness. In the United States there are about 34 legally blind school-aged children for every 100,000 persons. A child may be born blind or may acquire blindness from hereditary factors, intrauterine or postnatal infections, retrolental fibroplasia (as a result of high oxygen concentra-

tions in the care of premature infants), and trauma. The child who is blind or who has extremely poor vision requires special education and training. Instruction is given through the other senses. A number of useful devices have been created to help these children learn about the world outside, including braille, an alphabet of raised dots, tape and disk recordings, music, touch perception, and a new system of "tactile vision substitution," using a small television camera and a device for converting the television image to electrical impulses and transmitting them to electrodes on the child's back or abdomen.

The sightless child has all the normal adjustments to life to make as the sighted child. The parents may need help to understand this situation, avoid overprotectiveness, and yet make realistic demands. A great deal of literature and several organizations are devoted to meeting the needs of blind children and their parents.

Disorders of the ear

In studying the disorders of the ear the student is urged to refer to Fig. 18-4. The following professionals specialize in this field:

otologist a physician who specializes in the study and treatment of disorders of the ear

otolaryngologist a physician who specializes in the study and treatment of disorders of the ear, nose, and throat

audiometrist a technician who tests hearing by using an audiometer

Otitis externa. An inflammation of the external ear may be caused by bacteria or fungi. It often follows fresh-water swimming. The swollen ear canal becomes extremely painful and the child may be brought to the hospital emergency room. There the physician examines the ear, takes a recent medical history, may take cultures to determine the cause, and then inserts a gauze packing in the ear, leaving the end exposed to act as a wick. The parents and nurse are instructed to keep the packing moist for 48 hours with a solution of aluminum acetate. This treatment reduces swelling. The packing is then removed and ear drops of antibiotics or fungicide are administered for several days until the inflammation recedes.

Foreign body in the ear. Many things become lodged in children's ears. Insects crawl in; little fingers poke in paper, peas, stones, and sharp objects. If an object remains, it irritates the tissue and may become embedded. Often parents do not know anything is amiss until the child pulls at the ear, complains of pain, or drainage appears. Amateurs should not try to remove anything from the ear because of the danger of pushing it deeper or damaging the eardrum. The child should be taken to the physician, who has the skill and equipment to remove the object safely. Sharp objects must be removed with forceps; other objects may be removed by irrigation. Alcohol is used for water-absorbing items and normal saline solution for others.

In assisting the physician the nurse sets out an otoscope with fresh batteries, irrigating syringe, bowl, solutions of saline and alcohol 70% (warmed by placing their containers in a pan of hot water), and forceps. The child is then positioned with the affected ear up. Every effort should be made to gain the child's cooperation, but because the procedure is both frightening and painful, it may be necessary to restrain the child with various holds or a mummy restraint (see Chapter 8). Antibiotic eardrops may be prescribed to overcome infection.

Otitis media. Otitis media is an inflammation of the middle ear by various bacteria and viruses. It is the most common complication of upper respiratory infections in infants and children because their eustachian tubes are relatively short and straight with a wide opening, permitting ready access of pathogens to the middle ear.

The child usually has an upper respiratory infection or is just recovering from one, and may or may not have a fever and hearing loss. The older child may complain of an earache, and an infant may indicate pain by rolling the head, pulling the ear, or becoming irritable and vomiting. Sometimes the first indication of otitis media is purulent drainage from the ear, indicating a ruptured eardrum.

Diagnosis is based on the history, symptoms, and a bulging eardrum (tympanic membrane) on examination with an otoscope. Treatment is begun at once and consists of large doses of antibiotics, nasal decongestant drops, and sometimes eardrops. After 3 days of drug therapy, the eardrum is examined again. Anti-infective therapy should be continued for the full length of time prescribed by the physician to ensure that the infection is actually eradicated.

When the eardrum ruptures, a ragged tear results. On healing, the scar may impair hearing. To avoid this danger, if it appears that the eardrum will rupture spontaneously in spite of antibiotic therapy, the physician may lance a tiny opening at the edge of the drum to release the pressure safely. This procedure is called a *myringotomy*. Purulent matter then drains from the ear. After a few days the myringotomy incision heals with minimal scarring. In cases of repeated otitis media, the physician may implant a tiny tube in the eardrum, called a tympanic membrane (TM) button, to act as a drain. Eventually the button falls out into the outer ear canal. When a child has chronic otitis media or repeated rupture of the eardrums, a conductive deafness may result.

Untreated infections of the middle ear may spread to the inner ear and temporal bone, causing acute and chronic infections. Fortunately such infections are becoming rare as a result of widespread antibiotic therapy for otitis media.

Deafness. Deafness is a total or partial impairment of hearing as a result of birth defects, congenital syphilis, meningitis, encephalitis, or chronic otitis media. Because hearing plays such an important part in a child's mental, emotional, and social development, early diagnosis is essential. If an infant fails to startle at loud noises, or a 1-year-old child ceases to vocalize, or an 18-

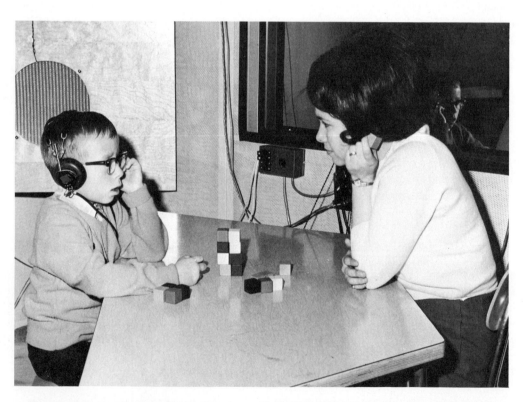

Fig. 18-16. Every means is used to communicate with the deaf child. This specially prepared teacher is using colored blocks to teach abstract ideas. Earphones amplify sound to make use of even minimal hearing ability. (Courtesy Children's Medical Center, Oakland, Calif.)

month-old child neither speaks nor responds to words, hearing should be investigated. Many children with impaired hearing are identified by audiometric testing in school health programs. When children cannot be tested because they are mentally retarded or autistic, *averaged electroencephalic audiometry* is used. The test is based on encephalogram findings altered by perceived sound.

The deaf child is cut off from communications with others except by overt physical acts. Although of average or above-average intelligence, without special help the child is isolated from the world by a wall of silence. Unable to mimic sounds that cannot be heard, the child is mute and needs special education to break the barrier. To this end a great variety of techniques are used to teach communication with finger and sign language; lip, facial-expression, and word reading; and speech therapy (Fig. 18-16). Children with even a minimal degree of hearing are fitted with hearing aids. In many cities there are special schools or classes for the deaf, staffed by trained teachers. These teachers must exercise great patience and deaf students enormous effort. Parents must learn to communicate with their child as together they all work toward the goal of a full and productive life.

SUMMARY OUTLINE

I. **Nervous system**
  A. Function
  B. Structure
    1. Nervous tissue
    2. Nervous pathways
    3. Central nervous system
      a. Coverings
      b. Fluid spaces and cerebrospinal fluid
      c. Brain
        (1) Cerebrum
        (2) Cerebellum
        (3) Brainstem
    4. Spinal cord
    5. Peripheral nervous system
      a. Cranial nerves
      b. Spinal nerves
      c. Autonomic nervous system
      d. Sense organs
        (1) Eye
        (2) Ear
II. **Disorders of the neurosensory system**
  A. Neurological symptoms
    1. Altered sensations
      a. touch
      b. pain
    2. Changes in level of consciousness
    3. Seizures
    4. Increased intracranial pressure
  B. Injuries
    1. Forceps marks
    2. Caput succedaneum
    3. Cephalohematoma
    4. Intracranial hemorrhage
    5. Subdural hematoma
    6. Cerebral concussion
    7. Skull fracture
    8. Brachial plexus palsy (Erb-Duchenne paralysis)
    9. Facial nerve paralysis (Bell's palsy)
  C. Malformations
    1. Craniosynostosis
    2. Microcephaly
    3. Hydrocephaly
    4. Spina bifida
    5. Encephalocele
  D. Infections
    1. Meningitis
    2. Encephalitis
    3. Landry-Guillain-Barré syndrome
  E. Tumors
  F. Degenerative diseases
  G. Convulsive disorders
    1. Causation
    2. Classification
      a. Centrencephalic convulsions
      b. Focal-cortical convulsions
    3. Diagnosis and care
  H. Neuromotor disorders (cerebral palsy)
  I. Mental (psychiatric) disorders
    1. Mental retardation
    2. Attention deficit disorders
      a. Depression
    3. Conduct disorders
    4. Anxiety disorders of childhood or adolsecence
    5. Other disorders of infancy, childhood, or adolescence
    6. Eating disorders
    7. Stereotyped movement disorders
    8. Other physical disorders
    9. Pervasive developmental disorders
    10. Other major psychiatric disorders

J. Disorders of the eye
  1. Infections
    a. Conjunctivitis
    b. Gonorrheal ophthalmia neonatorum
    c. Blepharitis
    d. Hordeolum (stye)
  2. Injuries
  3. Congenital defects
    a. Ptosis of the eyelids
    b. Cataracts
    c. Strabismus (squint)
    d. Errors of refraction
  4. Blindness
K. Disorders of the ear
  1. Otitis externa
  2. Foreign body in the ear
  3. Otitis media
  4. Deafness

STUDY QUESTIONS

1. What is the function of the central nervous system? Identify the coverings, fluid spaces, and divisions of the brain. Consider the 12 cranial nerves. How would a tumor or blood clot near each one affect the person?
2. Describe the symptoms of increased intracranial pressure.
3. What is the most common and most serious birth injury? Describe the symptoms and nursing care.
4. What causes the head to enlarge in hydrocephalus? Describe nursing care after a "shunt" operation.
5. How are convulsions produced? What factors lower the convulsive threshold? What are the important observations the nurse should make in reporting a seizure?
6. What is cerebral palsy and what are the treatment goals?
7. What are the central disabilities in autism? Compare autism with congenital deafness and mental retardation.
8. Name three classification systems of mental disorders and the organizations that publish them.
9. What is otitis media? What surgical procedure is performed to avoid ruptured ear drums? What is a "TM button" and why is it implanted?

19
Integumentary, generalized, and communicable conditions

VOCABULARY

Melanin
Bleb
Sclerosing
Débridement
Granulation tissue
Autografts
Hyposensitization
Endemic

The skin not only suffers injury and inflammation, it also manifests many generalized conditions that affect the body as a whole. For this reason, in this chapter we have grouped together conditions affecting the skin and a number of generalized disorders, including those commonly classified as communicable.

INTEGUMENTARY SYSTEM
Function

The skin, or integument, is a soft flexible membrane that covers the entire surface of the body. It serves many important functions: *protection* against injury, infection, and loss of life-sustaining water; *excretion* of wastes via the sweat and sebaceous glands; *regulation* of body temperature by evaporation through the sweat glands and conduction through the circulation of blood; *reception* of sensations via a variety of nervous receptors; and *absorption* of ultraviolent rays, which act on 7-hydrocholesterol in the skin to provide vitamin D_3.

In addition, the skin bathes, oils, and gives itself a new coat when the old one wears off.

Structure

The skin is composed of two distinct layers—the epidermis, or false skin, and the dermis, or true skin (Fig. 19-1). The dermis is attached to subcutaneous tissue and the subcutaneous tissue is attached to muscle and bones. Skin thickness varies in different parts of the body and under different circumstances. It is naturally thicker on the soles of the feet and palms of the hands and becomes thicker when there is continual pressure or rubbing.

Epidermis. The epidermis is composed of layers, or strata, of cells; but only in the lowest one, located just above the dermis and appropriately called stratum germinativum, do these cells multiply. Because blood vessels do not extend beyond the dermis, as new cells are formed, they are pushed upward and away from their source of nourishment. As a result they die and become

dry and horny, a quality that makes the surface of the skin water resistant and also protects the underlying layers of cells. Normally, the outermost cells flake off (desquamate) at the same rate as new cells are formed in the stratum germinativum. If there is unusual skin damage as from a sunburn, high fever, or metabolic disturbance, desquamation may be greatly accelerated. If there is irritation or pressure to a circumscribed area, a horny layer of dead cells builds up, producing a *callus*.

Color is only epidermis deep and depends on varying amounts of pigment, called *melanin*,

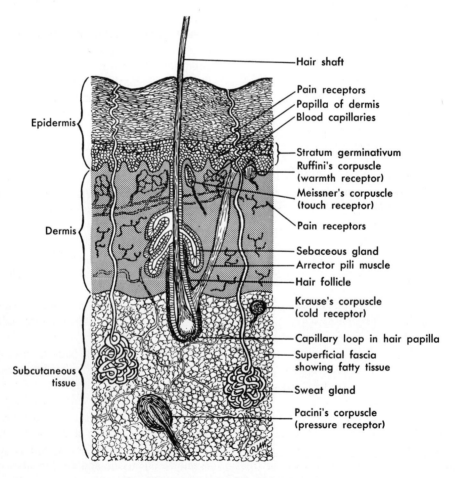

Fig. 19-1. The skin and subcutaneous tissue.

formed in the stratum germinativum and dispersed throughout the epidermis. Blushing is caused by a sudden dilation of blood vessels just beneath the epidermis. Nervous receptors of pain extend into the lower layers of epidermis but not up into the horny layers.

Dermis. The dermis lies just below the epidermis and is composed of connective tissue laced with elastic fibers, blood vessels, lymphatics, nerves, roots of hairs, and secreting portions of sebaceous and sweat glands. A unique feature of the dermis is the arrangement of its upper portion into parallel rows of peglike structures called *papillae*. Papillae serve to lock the two layers of skin together and form the characteristic ripples, or fingerprints, in the epidermis at the ends of the fingers and toes. The wrinkles of old age are caused by a decrease in elastic fibers and subcutaneous fat.

Subcutaneous tissue. Subcutaneous tissue anchors the skin to the muscles and bones below. The upper portion of the subcutaneous tissue, called superficial fascia, is made of connective tissue interlaced with fat, vessels, nerves, receptors, and glands. The superficial fascia nourishes, supports, and cushions the skin. Its fat serves as reserve food for the body. The deep fascia lies beneath the superficial layer. It contains no fat and is a thin layer of dense connective tissue that covers the muscles and passes inward to form intramuscular septa. In certain areas the deep fascia thickens to produce ligaments, tendons, and aponeuroses (see Chapter 17).

Accessory organs. The accessory organs of the skin are the nails, glands, and nervous receptors.

The nails are modifications of horny epidermal cells. They grow from cells that lie at the base of each nail under the white crescent.

Hair is distributed over the entire body except the palms of the hands and soles of the feet. It is formed just as epidermis is, from a layer of stratum germinativum cells that line tiny connective tissue pockets (follicles) embedded in the dermis and subcutaneous tissue. These cells are nourished by a loop of capillary enclosed in connective tissue, called a *papilla*, found at the base of each follicle. As these cells multiply, they are pushed up, become horny in character, and form a hair. Curliness is determined by how flat or ribbonlike the shape of the hair is. Color is produced by pigment (melanin) in the cells. The visible part of a hair is called the *shaft*; the embedded part is the root. Even though the shaft may be cut off or plucked out by the root, as long as the germinating cells at the base of the follicle remain alive, hair will regenerate. In some areas of the body hair is more dense and grows at a more rapid rate than others. Hair on the head grows at about ½ inch per month. Attached to each hair follicle is a small bundle of involuntary muscle known as *arrector pili muscle*. When these muscles contract, the hairs stand on end. This contraction occurs involuntarily when an individual is cold or frightened.

There are three types of skin glands—sweat (sudoriferous), wax (ceruminous), and oil (sebaceous). All three types perform important functions for the body.

Sweat glands open onto the skin surface through their own tiny ducts, or pores. They are distributed over the entire body, especially on the palms, soles, forehead, and axillary regions. These glands play an important part in regulating body heat and, in conjunction with the kidneys, in eliminating wastes from the blood. Sweat is made up of water (99%), dissolved salts, and traces of urea. The glands are governed by the autonomic nerves. When the temperature of the blood rises in response to exercise or external heat, a nerve center in the brain triggers the glands to produce sweat. In addition to this specially triggered sweating, the body loses water through sweating every second of the day. This process is called *insensible perspiration*. It must be replaced by water intake to maintain fluid balance, just as *sensible* (recognized) *perspiration*.

Ceruminous glands are modified sweat glands

located in the external ear canal. Instead of watery sweat, they secrete cerumen, a waxy, pigmented substance that aids the hairs in trapping dust, insects, and other foreign matter that might enter the ear and cause injury.

There are at least two *sebaceous glands* for each hair. These glands secrete their oily substance called sebum about the hair shaft where it seeps up to the surface of the skin. The oil makes the hair soft and pliable and protects the skin from excess evaporation or absorption of water or heat. At the base of the eyelashes are modified sebaceous glands called *meibomian glands* whose secretions protect the delicate skin of the eyelids.

Within the skin are five different types of nervous receptors that permit the body to be in constant "touch" with the outside world. Although these microscopic receivers are scattered over the entire body, they are more concentrated in some areas than in others. They are as follows: *pain*, the most numerous of all; *Meissner's corpuscles*, especially sensitive to touch; *Krause's corpuscles*, receptors of cold; *Ruffini's corpuscles*, receptors of warmth; and *Pacini's corpuscles*, the largest of all, receptors of pressure.

DISORDERS OF THE INTEGUMENTARY SYSTEM

Characteristics of skin lesions. Disorders of the skin and many communicable and generalized diseases produce a number of typical lesions. The nurse is expected to recognize these lesions and report them accurately. Some of the most common ones are as follows:

macule discolored area on the skin that may be of various colors and shapes and is neither raised nor depressed

papule small, solid elevation varying from the size of pinhead to a pea

petechia small, purplish, hemorrhagic spot, resembling a flea bite

ecchymosis a bruise; a macule caused by hemorrhage into surface tissues

vesicle blisterlike elevation on the skin containing serous fluid

pustule small elevation filled with pus that may be flat, rounded, or depressed

bleb or **bulla** irregular elevation of the epidermis filled with fluid

wheal elevation of varying size and irregular shape that may run together, if severe, as occurs in hives (urticaria)

scale small, thin flake of dry epidermis

crust collection of dry exudate, also called a scab

excoriation an abrasion or denuded area

fissure groove, crack, or slit down into the skin

ulcer open lesions on the skin with tissue loss

gumma tumor-like lesion varying from the size of a tiny speck to the size of a pea, and from one to many; may be encapsulated

scar mark left on the skin after tissue heals

eschar depression or slough, may follow a burn

urticaria nettle rash of wheals; hives

angioneurotic edema or **angioedema** swelling of the submucous and subcutaneous tissue

comedo (plural: **comedones**) blackhead(s); discolored, dried sebum plugged the sebaceous duct(s)

keloid dense growth of connective scar tissue

Nevi. Nevi are abnormal markings of the skin that may be present at birth or later in life. They are of two general types—pigmented and vascular. Both types are caused by defects in cell growth, probably associated with heredity.

Pigmented nevi (birthmarks or moles) vary in size and color from harmless freckles to dark hairy patches. They are composed of specialized epithelial cells containing melanin, called *melanocytes*. Nevi are of medical significance because they may be quite disfiguring and may change into malignant melanomas, although this seldom happens before puberty. Treatment is surgical excision. If a nevus is in a place where it is constantly irritated or appears to be growing at a disproportional rate, it is removed because of the danger of malignancy. Disfiguring nevi are removed early in life to reduce both physical and emotional scarring.

Vascular nevi (angiomas) are localized lesions of the skin caused by an overgrowth of blood or lymph vessels. Those composed of blood vessels are called *hemangiomas*; those composed of lymph vessels are called *lymphangiomas*. Angiomas occur in about one third of all infants, but most disappear spontaneously. Some persist and create cosmetic problems.

Hemangiomas are classified as infantile (those that disappear with age) and adult (those that remain throughout life). The three most common types are nevus flammeus, nevus vasculosus, and cavernous.

Nevus flammeus (port-wine stain) are flat, purplish lesions present at birth. They usually do not fade and there is no effective treatment except hiding them with cosmetic creams.

Nevus vasculosus (strawberry mark) are raised, red lesions that are present at birth or develop soon after (Fig. 19-2). They consist of dilated capillaries, venules, and arterioles and tend to enlarge for a time and then gradually regress, leaving some degree of scarring and pigmentation. If the lesion ulcerates or is near the eye,

anus, or urethra, various treatments may be attempted to reduce the size, such as irradiation, electrocoagulation, and a tissue-hardening injection of sclerosing solutions. Surgical excisions may also be performed.

Cavernous hemangiomas are raised, red and purple lesions composed of large vascular spaces, sometimes containing lymphangiomas, connective tissue, and fat. They seldom regress by themselves, but those that do are classified as infantile. If they are life threatening and when there is no evidence of regression, surgical excision with skin grafting may be performed.

Lymphangiomas are elevated lesions composed chiefly of lymphatic vessels. They are usually yellowish tan. Treatment is by electrocoagulation or surgical excision.

A child is hospitalized when scheduled to undergo extensive surgical excision and skin grafting for a nevus. Nursing care for skin grafting is discussed later in this chapter.

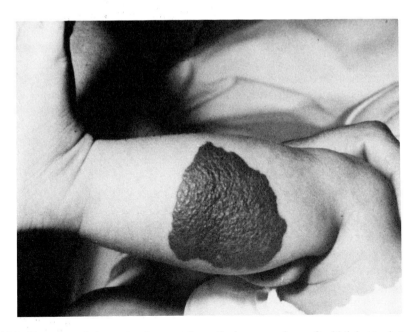

Fig. 19-2. Nevus vascularis, or strawberry mark, on the leg may enlarge after birth but tends to regress with the passage of time.

Irritations. Even with good care infants often develop such common skin irritations as miliaria, intertrigo, and diaper rash.

Miliaria, or prickly heat, is caused by an obstruction of the sweat ducts. Small vesicles develop, followed by severe itching (pruritus). The condition improves rapidly if the child is placed in a cool environment with loose clothing. A colloidal bath of starch or oatmeal and lotions may provide some relief.

Intertrigo, or chafing, occurs when two skin surfaces are in contact as occurs at the groin, axilla, and neck. Prevention and treatment involve keeping the skin clean and dry.

Diaper rash is caused by irritation from urine and stool, and is a type of contact dermatitis. It occurs more often when the infant has diarrhea, although in some infants diaper rash occurs without seeming provocation. Treatment consists of changing wet or soiled diapers promptly, washing the buttocks carefully, applying antiammonia ointment, and exposing the buttocks to warm dry air. Diapers sometimes harbor ammonia-producing bacteria or chemicals from washing products and should be washed and rinsed thoroughly.

Dermatitis. Dermatitis is a general term given to any acute or chronic inflammation of the skin. By custom, chronic dermatitis is also called *eczema*. Both infants and children are affected.

Causes. There are four general causes for dermatitis: allergy, chemical irritants, defective sebaceous glands, and infection. More than one of them may be present in any given case.

Allergic, or *atopic, dermatitis* is caused by the typical antigen-antibody mechanism discussed in the topic of allergic reactions on p. 527. There is often a family history of allergies. The condition occurs in children of all ages, but when symptoms develop in children under 2 years of age, foods are the most common antigens. An allergic child on growing older usually becomes less sensitive to foods and more sensitive to pollen. Children of all ages may be allergic to air pollutants. Often skin tests demonstrate a sensitivity to more than one allergen. Many children outgrow their sensitivities or develop immunity to them. Some, however, continue to have allergic eczema into adult life. About one half experience allergic reactions in the form of hay fever and asthma.

Symptoms of allergic dermatitis begin with redness of the cheeks that spreads to involve the entire face. Papules and vesicles form and then rupture and exude yellow sticky matter that dries and forms crusts. The infant scratches the lesions and often secondary infection results. Itching is severe. The child is irritable and sleeps poorly. Care for the child is exhausting to the parents and often discouraging because improvement (remissions) and worsening (exacerbations) are characteristic of allergic dermatitis. Until all skin eruptions are healed, the child should be kept away from anyone with skin infections because of the danger of a generalized inflammation.

Whenever possible, these children are cared for at home to avoid the many resistant organisms found in a hospital. Parents should be instructed in the expected course of the eczema, its treatment, and nursing care. If hospitalization is necessary, the child is isolated for protection. Nursing care and treatment are discussed later.

Contact dermatitis is an acute or chronic inflammation produced by substances that come in contact with the skin or mucous membrane. Such substances are numerous and include plants such as poison oak, foods such as nuts and shellfish, household items such as insect sprays and feathers, and clothing such as wool. Hot or cold weather and strong emotions may produce similar skin reactions. The most common sites of contact dermatitis eruptions are exposed portions of skin and the mucous membrane. Symptoms range from transient redness to severe pruritus, vesicle formation, hives, massive wheals, localized swelling of the lips, eyelids, face, and hands, and angioedema (Fig. 19-3). The reaction may remain localized or become generalized with widespread eruptions and angioedema of the lungs. After the offending agent is removed, inflammation gradually subsides. In severe cases symptoms may last 2 or more weeks. Treatment for allergic reactions includes giving antihistamine drugs to prevent further eruptions, epinephrine for urticaria and angioedema, and steroids for persistent symptoms. Antipruritic lotions and baths may help relieve itching. Nursing care is discussed below.

Seborrheic dermatitis is a chronic, red scaling inflammation thought to result from a defect in the amount and makeup of sebum produced by the sebaceous glands. About 50% of all infants have a mild seborrhea of the scalp called "cradle cap." In some infants the greasy crusts spread out from the scalp to behind the ears and eventually involve large areas of skin. In some places the patches are moist and produce considerable

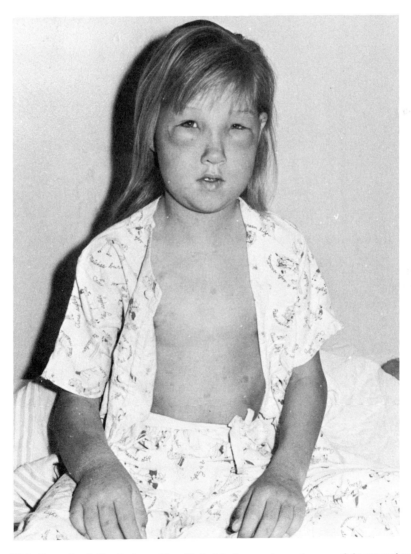

Fig. 19-3. Generalized allergic dermatitis with facial edema and macules over abdomen and arms.

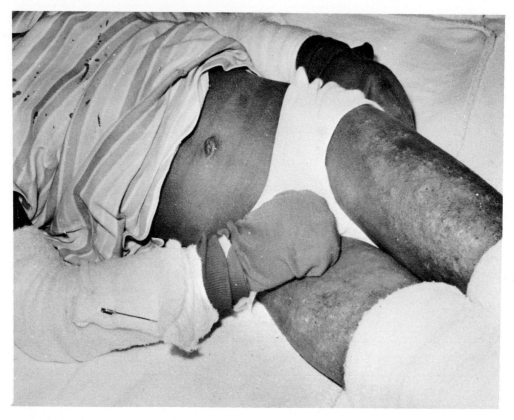

Fig. 19-4. Severe allergic dermatitis with secondary infection. Mittens on hands and bandaged extremities help prevent scratching.

exudate. In others the patches are scaly, red, and dry. Even with extensive seborrhea, there is little or no pruritus and the child's disposition is not affected.

Infectious dermatitis is an invasion of various organisms, usually secondary to some other skin condition, in which the child scratches because of pruritus. Antiseptic and antibiotic soaks may be prescribed in conjunction with treatment of the primary inflammation.

Treatment and nursing care. The treatment and nursing care of children with dermatitis from any cause are directed toward overcoming inflammation and relieving discomfort. Because allergic and infectious factors so often are re-

sponsible for childhood dermatitis, they are important considerations in the treatment.

In allergic dermatitis the causal antigens are seldom known during the initial episode. For a cure to be effective, they must be identified and removed. If they are believed to be foods, yet the skin is too inflamed for sensitivity tests, a hypoallergic diet may be prescribed for a 10-day trial. A hypoallergic diet consists of the following foods:

Milk substitute
Rice cereal
Apples and apricots
Carrots and string beans
Beef
Aqueous vitamins

At the end of the trial period the child's condition is evaluated. If there is no improvement, a second 10-day trial period is ordered during which one group of foods (such as carrots and string beans) is eliminated. A trial period is repeated for each of the food groups until the offending foods are identified. During these trial periods the nurse's responsibility is to observe and report the child's condition carefully. The importance of permitting only the foods ordered cannot be overstressed.

Dermatitis is extremely painful. Itching may keep a child from rest. Sedating drugs such as phenobarbital and chloral hydrate are usually prescribed. Antiinflammatory steroids such as prednisone and antihistamine drugs, especially diphenhydramine (Benadryl), may be ordered to reduce itching.

When a child scratches the inflamed skin, they introduce bacteria into the tissue. Serious damage also may be done to a healing area. To prevent such scratching, restraints must be applied, such as mittens and wrist, elbow, and ankle restraints (Fig. 19-4). Sometimes an extremity is bandaged to protect it from being scratched. The bandage is usually changed every 24 hours.

Colloid baths of cornstarch or oatmeal relieve itching for short periods and are especially helpful just before bedtime. Regular soap should never be used on inflamed skin. In its place a soap substitute called sodium lauryl sulfate has proved to be quite useful. When there is no infection, as in acute allergic dermatitis, Burrow's solution and potassium permanganate soaks or compresses are helpful in relieving itching and reducing inflammation. When there is an infection, antiseptic soaks may be prescribed.

In general, wet, oozing, areas of skin should not be covered with ointment. After the skin becomes dry and crusty, however, various ointments may be used to promote healing and prevent scarring. In allergic dermatitis, steroid ointment is sometimes ordered. Systemic steroids may be prescribed for brief periods.

When allergic conditions are caused by seasonal pollens, hyposensitization injections sometimes produce relief by reducing the child's sensitivity.

Acne. Acne is an inflammation of the sebaceous glands and hair follicles. It is characterized by blackheads (comedones), pustules, inflamed nodules, infected cysts, and, in severe cases infected canals and sacs. Acne, with varying degrees of severity, occurs in more than 80% of all teenagers. The effect of sex hormones on the oil-secreting glands causes them to produce an excessive amount of oil. Hereditary, vitamin deficiency, gastrointestinal disturbances, menses in girls, and psychogenic factors seem to affect the disease. Acne usually begins just before puberty and usually continues for a year or more.

Treatment for mild cases consists of (1) keeping the face clean but not scrubbed too harshly, (2) removing blackheads without traumatizing the surrounding skin (apply warm compresses and use a Schamberg loop extractor), (3) eating a balanced diet with adequate vitamins, and (4) applying topical drying agents. When crusts are removed before the underlying skin has healed, pitted scars may result. Serious cases require more extensive treatment, such as broad-spectrum antibiotics for infection, estrogen for girls, and psychological counseling. Radiation may be ordered in selected cases to reduce sebaceous gland activity.

When acute acne has finally subsided, scars may remain. To reduce these scars, a surgical procedure called *dermabrasion* or face planing may be employed, whereby the epidermis is ground down to the dermal papillae by means of a machine-powered abrasive disk. The epidermal cells between the papillary ridges then regenerate an epidermal layer that is smoother than before. The procedure may be repeated at 3-month intervals until the desired results are produced. Following dermabrasion, scabs form that drop off in about 14 days, exposing pink, tender flesh. The new skin must be protected from sun and wind. Infection and keloid formation sometimes complicate healing. Improvement in appearance after the procedure varies widely, up to 70%. A return to babysmooth cheeks cannot be expected.

Preoperatively the skin and head hair are thoroughly cleansed and the patient sedated. Postoperatively, for about 24 hours, the patient experiences intense pain until the exposed nerve endings are covered over by a crust. Then the outer bandages are removed and only the single gauze layer that has become part of the crust is left on the face until it drops off by itself. A liquid to soft diet is ordered. The patient appreciates the use of a hand mirror to help "find" the mouth with a drinking straw. Air fresheners may help overcome the putrid odor. Nurses must guard against making overly optimistic statements about the eventual outcome of the surgery because cosmetic results are not predictable.

Furuncles and carbuncles. A furuncle or boil is an acute staphylococcal infection of a hair follicle and the surrounding area with a central core of dead cells. Furuncles occur most often after puberty in males on the neck, axillae, face, and buttocks. When located in and about the nose, they may be especially painful and also more dangerous because the veins of that area lead to the brain. Treatment consists of bringing individual furuncles to a head with warm compresses and incising and removing the central core. The spread of infection to other follicles is controlled by local and systemic antibiotics and by teaching habits of personal cleanliness.

A carbuncle is a group of furuncles with extension of the infection into the subcutaneous tissue. Treatment is by antibiotics and in some cases surgical removal of the diseased tissue.

Impetigo. Impetigo is a superficial infection caused by staphylococci and streptococci that arises on apparently normal skin or complicates other skin diseases. It is highly contagious in infants and children. When impetigo affects only limited skin areas, treatment consists of soaking off the crusts and applying antibiotic ointment locally. When the infection is widespread, systemic antibiotics are also ordered. Strict isolation

technique must be used to prevent spread of the disease to other children.

Herpes simplex. Herpes simplex types I and II are recurrent virus infections characterized by the appearance on the skin or mucous membranes of single or multiple clusters of small vesicles filled with clear fluid that are painful and may spread rapidly. Type I usually infects the lips, mouth, throat, eyes, stomach, and brain. Type II usually infects the urogenital organs. Specific antiviral agents are being tested but are not widely available. Healing of both types occurs in 10 to 20 days.

When the infection involves the genital region it may spread up into the urethra and bladder or into the rectum. Such infections are extremely painful and produce serious complications resulting from urine retention. The risk of overwhelming infection to infants born through an infected vagina is so great that if the mother has a vaginal infection, cesarean section is the recommended delivery route. Cervical cancer may later occur in the infected mother. In infants and young children the mucous membrane of the mouth and gums may become inflamed, and the inflammation may lead to a generalized viral infection with a serious, even fatal, outcome. Because a specific virucidal medication has not yet been approved for systemic herpes simplex, good supportive care is essential. Regular Papanicolaou smears to detect early cervical cancer are recommended.

Warts. Warts are benign epithelial tumors caused by a virus. Although they may appear at any age, they are most common in children. Their course is not predictable. They may remain a single lesion or may spread by autoinoculation, a process called "seeding." They are named variously; the common ones found on fingers, hands, knees, and elbows are called *verrucae vulgares*. *Moist*, or *venereal*, *warts* are found in the anogenital region. *Plantar warts* are those that grow on the sole of the foot. Warts may go away completely with or without treatment. This may account for the success of various magical "cures." Treatment consists of electrosurgery, surgical excision, freezing, and certain caustics.

Dermatomycoses (ringworm). Ringworm is a superficial fungous infection of the skin. The fungus usually lives only in the dead upper cells of the epidermis but may invade living cells of persons with systemic diseases such as diabetes mellitus. Sometimes a person becomes sensitized to the fungus and develops local or generalized allergic lesions, called *dermatophytids*, which do not contain the fungus but appear when a fungous infection is anywhere in the body. The types of ringworm often seen in children are athlete's foot (*tinea pedis*), scalp ringworm (*tinea capitis*), and body ringworm (*tinea corporis*).

Diagnosis is made on the basis of the history, appearance of the lesions, and microscopic examination of skin scrapings or culture. Ringworm of the scalp produces a typical fluorescent glow when the room is darkened and a Wood's lamp is shown on the head.

Treatment of athlete's foot involves good foot hygiene. After bathing, the old dead skin should be rubbed away and the spaces between the toes dried carefully. A drying powder and the use of lightweight footwear may be helpful. During acute flare-ups, foot soaks of hot potassium permanganate solution followed by steroid lotion or various other preparations may be ordered. A systemic (oral) antibiotic called griseofulvin is used to treat ringworm of the scalp when local treatment is ineffective. Treatment of body ringworm involves the systemic administration of griseofulvin and in some cases application of a local medication, depending on the type of fungus causing the ringworm.

Pediculosis. Pediculosis is an infection of the skin and hair by lice. It is often seen among children who live in crowded unhygienic conditions. Lice are passed along by personal contact with clothing, combs, and bed linens. Once entrenched, lice are very difficult to exterminate. A single female louse can begin a whole colony.

She lays her eggs (nits) on the shaft of the hair or in the clothing. In about 3 to 14 days the nits hatch, feed off their host, and mate, and the females lay more eggs. Because lice actually bite the skin of the host, they cause severe itching. The child scratches and secondary infection is common.

Diagnosis is made on finding either the mature louse or the nits. Treatment involves killing the lice with insecticidal drugs as they hatch, before they can mate and lay more eggs. To be effective, the whole family must be treated at the same time, including clothing, combs, and bed linen. The hair and entire body of each family member must be treated several successive weeks because nits are not affected by the drug. Secondary infections are treated with antibiotic ointments.

Burns. A burn is any destruction of tissue caused by heat, chemicals, electricity, or overexposure to ultraviolet rays (sun), x-rays, or radioactive substances. Burns are classified according to the depth of tissue involved (degree) and the extent of body surface burned (percentage).

Classification. A *first-degree burn* is one in which tissue damage is limited to the outer layers of epidermis. There is redness and pain, healing is rapid with no residual scarring.

A *second-degree burn* is one in which tissue damage extends through the epidermis and involves the dermis, including superficial and deep dermal damage. There is severe pain and redness with vesicle and bleb formation. Healing is slow and scarring may result.

A *third-degree burn* is one in which the full thickness (both epidermis and dermis) of the skin is damaged. Severe pain is unusual after the acute initial pain because the nerve endings are destroyed. The skin surface may be charred, or white and lifeless, as in scalds. Sweat glands, sebaceous glands, and hair follicles are destroyed. Eschars, contractures, and keloids may result.

A *fourth-degree burn* is one in which not only

the full thickness of skin is involved, but also the subcutaneous tissue, muscle, and bone. The tissue is deeply charred and permanently damaged.

The "rule of nines" is one of the methods used to calculate the percentage of body surface burned. All degrees of burn may be present in various areas of an accident victim's body. The presence of any degree of burn is included when the percentage of body surface is calculated. Because of the change in body proportion with growth as illustrated in Fig. 2-1, the rule of nines is modified for children below 10 years of age (Table 19-1) and in other systems of calculating total body surface area (BSA) burned.

Principles of treatment. The principles of treatment for burned patients apply from the time of the accident through the initial convalescence and on to rehabilitation. They are relief of pain, prevention of shock, prevention of respiratory impairment, maintenance of fluid balance, correction of anemia, provision of adequate nutrition, control of infection, and reduction of residual handicaps. For adequate treatment, hospitalization is recommended for children under 10 years of age with 10% of the body surface burned and for those over 10 years of age with 15% of the body surface burned.

Immediate care. Emergency action calls for extinguishing flames, separating the child from the hot agent, neutralizing chemicals, or breaking the electrical circuit, depending on the cause of the burns. An assessment of the child's condition must then be made. If there is a respiratory or cardiac failure, resuscitation is of prime importance. Following resuscitation, burns from any cause are treated in a similar way.

Immediate care of *first-degree burns* consists of applying ice packs or immersing the burned part in ice water until pain stops. This treatment reduces pain and blister formation. A soothing ointment may then be applied if the skin is not broken.

Immediate care of *second-, third-,* and *fourth-degree burns* consists of leaving the area exposed, or lightly covering it with a clean cloth, and bringing the child to the emergency room at once. No medicine of any kind should be put on the wounds. On admission the child is placed on a sterile sheet and burned areas covered by sterile towels. The child's general condition receives first attention because the first 72 hours are the most critical.

In second-, third-, and fourth-degree burns shock is a serious threat. The child may be in advanced shock on admission, with cold clammy extremities, pallor, rapid respirations, thready pulse, and low blood pressure. In other cases *incipient shock* may develop gradually over several hours. In either case the nurse must be alert

Table 19-1. The rule of nines used to calculate the percentage of body surface burned

Body part burned	Over 10 years of age	10 years of age and under*
Head	9	19
Right arm	9	9
Left arm	9	9
Front of body	18	18
Back of body	18	18
Genitals	1	1
Right leg	18	13
Left leg	18	13
TOTAL PERCENTAGE OF BODY SURFACE	100	100

*For each year under 10, subtract ½ from each limb and add to head.

for shock symptoms and report them promptly. Severe pain deepens shock. Morphine, meperidine, or codeine may be ordered immediately on a continuing p.r.n. basis. These medications should not be withheld arbitrarily, but because they are respiratory depressants they should not be given if the respiratory rate is below 12 per minute. Oxygen is administered for hypoxia, and tracheostomy may be necessary to open an airway. Soon after admission an intravenous avenue for fluids is established, either by way of a cutdown operation or by a needle through which a plastic cannula is passed. Plasma and intravenous fluids are administered to combat hypovolemic shock, maintain electrolyte balance, and support kidney function because extensive burns place a great burden on the kidneys. A retention catheter may be inserted in the bladder to facilitate nursing care and maintain an accurate record of urinary output. Tetanus antitoxin is given if the patient has not had tetanus toxoid. Systemic antibiotics are given to control infection and protective isolation is instituted because burns are particularly susceptible to Pseudomonas infections.

Continuing treatment and care. After the child's general condition has stabilized, local treatment of the burned areas can proceed. If removal of devitalized and contaminated tissue (débridement) is necessary, it is carried out in surgery using general anesthesia.

There are two methods of treating burns—open and closed. In the *open method* the burned area is left exposed to the air and protective isolation technique is used. The patient is placed on sterile sheets in a room of proper temperature and humidity with a cradle over the bed. Protective isolation is maintained (Fig. 19-5). In 2 or 3 days the protein-rich exudate that oozes from the exposed areas forms a covering crust. Tub

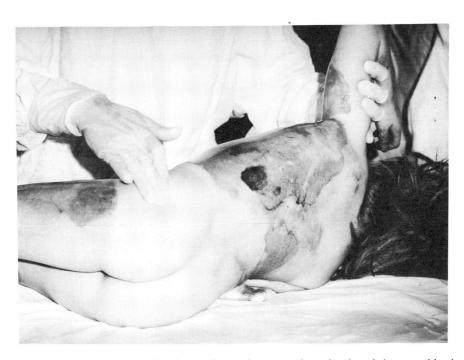

Fig. 19-5. Reverse isolation technique is used for nursing care to burned patients being treated by the open method. The nurse dons cap, mask, sterile gown, and gloves.

soaks in sterile saline solution may be ordered several times a day. In some cases cytotoxins such as tannic acid, silver nitrate, and gentian violet are applied to the tissue to reduce pain. These dyes stain the linens, furniture, and the skin of both patient and nurse. In the *closed*, or *pressure bandage, method* sterile dressings are applied over the newly cleansed burned area and bandaged tightly to produce pressure (Fig. 19-6). Bandages are removed in 4 to 14 days for inspection. If there is no infection by this time, areas of second-degree burns have begun to regenerate. Areas of third-degree burns are then evaluated for skin grafting. The area may be rebandaged or left exposed, depending on the condition of the burns. Both open and closed methods of treatment may be employed in different areas of the child's body (Fig. 19-7). If

the child is allowed to ambulate, bandaged arms and hands should be supported by slings. Bedridden patients should be maintained with the body in good alignment and joints in positions of usefulness. Passive exercises may be ordered to prevent contracture deformities.

Pain is controlled by hypnotic and analgesic drugs made more effective when given together with tranquilizing drugs. Hypnosis with posthypnotic suggestion may also be attempted.

A high-protein, high-vitamin, high-iron diet is needed for repair of body tissue. The child who is unable to eat is fed by gavage until foods can be managed. The child needs considerable encouragement and assistance at mealtime. Accurate records of intake and output are maintained with daily weight.

Progressive and severe anemia develops rap-

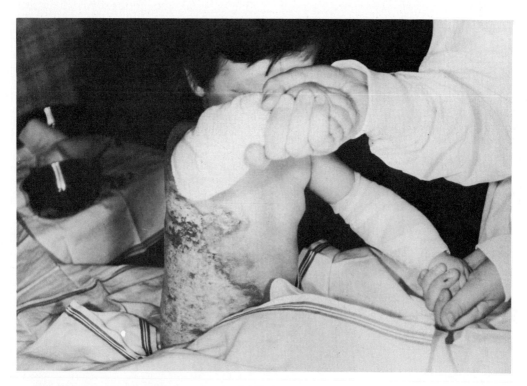

Fig. 19-6. Closed method of burn treatment. Sterile dressings are applied with strict aseptic technique. (Courtesy Children's Hospital of the East Bay, Oakland, Calif.)

idly in burned patients. Such anemia is treated with whole blood transfusions. Hemoglobin is measured frequently and when transfusions are ordered, typing and cross matching of blood is necessary.

During the long hours and days of convalescence the burned child needs diversion. An occupational therapist can be of great help to the nursing staff in planning appropriate activities for the child.

The goal in rehabilitation is to help the burned child develop and live to maximum capacity within the limits of the disabilities. This goal involves helping both the child and the parents accept disfiguring scars, sometimes repeated skin grafting procedures, and various type of handicaps.

Prevention of accidents that cause such painful and tragic aftereffects is a matter of serious public health concern. Parents should be reminded of fire hazards such as unsafe electrical appliances, open heaters, flammable materials, and hot liquids. Children should be taught not to play with matches and the dangers of other fire hazards. Constant vigilance is necessary on the part of all adults to prevent burns of all types.

Plastic surgery and skin grafting. The repair of congenital or acquired defects is accom-

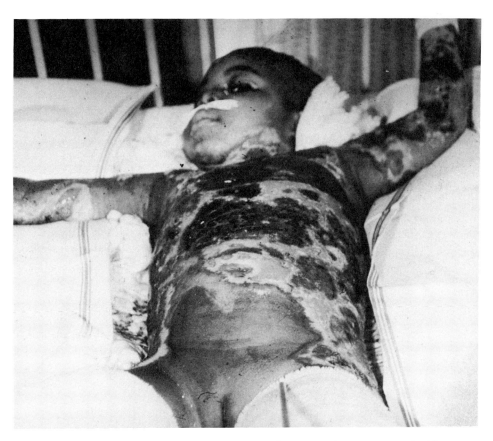

Fig. 19-7. Combined use of closed and open methods of burn care. Legs are wrapped with pressure bandages while the body, arms, and neck are left exposed.

plished by plastic surgery. Many special techniques are employed, and a variety of tissue may be grafted, such as bone, muscle, fat, skin, tendon, fascia, and nerve. Skin grafting is of particular importance in the treatment of third-degree burns because, as a result of the healing process, deforming eschars, keloids, and contractures occur.

Whenever tissue is damaged, the healthy body immediately seeks to repair itself. Wound healing takes place in the following fashion: (1) Serum, fibrin, white blood cells, and red blood cells fill in the spaces within the wound surface. (2) Epithelial and connective tissue cells multiply and capillaries penetrate the area, forming what is called *granulation tissue*. (3) Eventually the wound is filled with new cells and cell growth ceases. When there is an overgrowth of granulation tissue, keloids form; and when the connective tissue fibers contract, scars form. If, however, skin grafts are placed over granulation tissue, shrinkage and scar formation are reduced.

Skin grafts are of two general types—free and flap grafts. In *free grafts* skin is completely severed from its original position and transferred to another area of the body. Free grafts may be the full thickness of the skin or of various split thicknesses. The instrument used to slice the skin in various thicknesses is called a *dermatome*. Patch and pinch grafts are types of free grafts. *Flap grafts* are portions of skin and subcutaneous tissue that are left attached to the body at some place about the edge, permitting the flap to receive a continuous blood supply. Flap grafts may be simple, lined, tubular, or formed into a pedicle. Z-plasty is an adaptation of a flap graft. Skin grafts from one part of a person's body to another part of the same person's body or from an identical twin to the other are called *autografts*. Only autografts can be expected to grow and remain (take). Skin grafts taken from other persons are called *homografts* or *isografts*. They do not "take," but they may be used as a temporary covering for a large denuded area. Skin grafts

taken from animals are called *heterografts* and are seldom used.

For a skin graft to grow, it must be placed on a noninfected, granulating area and the patient must have a hemoglobin measurement of at least 85% of normal. The donor site is carefully selected and cleansed. The plastic surgeon calculates the depth and size of skin to be removed and then cuts out the exact size and shape of the skin to be grafted. The plastic surgeon may simply place it on denuded area or may suture it in place with delicate stitches. When the graft is in place, a pressure dressing is applied and the part immobilized by means of a cast or sling. The donor site is covered by sterile Vaseline gauze and bandages to protect it while it regenerates.

Nursing care for the casted or immobilized part includes elevating it and watching for signs of circulatory disturbances. Adequate fluids and nutrients must be maintained to support tissue rebuilding. Hemoglobin is measured frequently to check for anemia. Dressings are removed by the surgeon under aseptic conditions when it is believed that sufficient time has elapsed for the grafted skin to have begun to grow in its new position. In cases of severe deformity, many graftings, revisions, and special plastic techniques may be necessary before maximum use and cosmetic effects can be achieved.

GENERALIZED CONDITIONS
Mesenchymal (collagen) diseases

The *mesoderm* is the embryonic layer of cells that gives rise to all the connective tissues, the linings of all body cavities, and the circulatory, urogenital, and musculoskeletal systems. *Collagen* is a protein present in all mesenchymal tissues. The mesenchymal or collagen diseases are a group of conditions involving destructive change in the collagen fibrils. This change causes damage to the blood vessels and connective tissues throughout the body. The following are collagen diseases: lupus erythematosus, rheumatic fever, dermatomyositis, periarteritis, scleroderma, juvenile rheumatoid arthritis (discussed in Chapter 17), and Schönlein-Henoch purpura (discussed in Chapter 13).

Systemic lupus erythematosus. Systemic or disseminated lupus erythematosus is a disease that affects many body systems, and although the cause is unknown, it seems to run in families, appearing in girls more often than in boys. The symptoms develop slowly and diagnosis may be missed for some time because the disease tends to have periods of worsening (exacerbations) and improvement (remission). Symptoms include low-grade fever, poor appetite, weight loss, joint pains, and typical redness of the upper cheeks and bridge of the nose called a butterfly rash. The rash becomes more noticeable when exposed to sunlight and may spread to other portions of the body. Petechiae and purpura may appear, especially on the lower extremities. The spleen, liver, and lymph nodes enlarge and the heart muscle and kidneys become involved. Convulsions and psychosis may develop as a result of central nervous system involvement. Death comes as a result of kidney failure.

An interesting phenomenon of this disease (and also sometimes rheumatoid arthritis and dermatomyositis) is the alteration it produces in the nuclei of polymorphonuclear leukocytes (see Fig. 13-3). The nucleus swells, is extruded from the cell, and is engulfed by another leukocyte. This process continues until one leukocyte may contain several extruded nuclei. The greedy leukocyte is called LE cell. Identification of LE cells in a blood sample is a very useful diagnostic finding.

The prognosis of children found to have lupus erythematosus has been greatly improved since corticosteroids have become available. These drugs reduce the severity of the symptoms, return the blood to normal, and reverse some of the kidney damage. On admission to the hospital, nursing care is adjusted to the needs of the child. If acutely ill, the child feels miserable and does not want to eat or even move. The skin may be very tender and may bruise easily. Because of the inherent danger of kidney failure, intake and output records are especially important. The nurse must encourage the child to eat, give special mouth and skin care, turn tenderly, and exercise unusual patience. If there is a history of convulsions, crib and bed sides should be padded. When the child is ready for dismissal, the parents should understand the importance of continued medical supervision, whether the child is taking a maintenance dosage of corticosteroid drugs or not. Continuous medical management, low stress, and protection from unnecessary exposure to sunlight are recommended for these patients.

Rheumatic fever. Rheumatic fever is a systemic inflammatory disease that affects mesenchymal tissues throughout the body. Although the exact mechanism is unknown, the disease and its recurrences are initiated by an infection of beta-hemolytic streptococci. Frequently the child has a "strep throat" or scarlet fever and recovers; in about 3 weeks, symptoms of rheumatic fever appear. If a throat culture or blood test is taken it is positive for beta-hemolytic streptococci.

Rheumatic fever is one of the leading causes of illness and death in children, occurring most often between the ages of 7 and 10 years, with most first attacks between the ages of 6 and 8 years. The highest incidence is among poor families living in crowded, unsanitary conditions in temperate zones.

Although there are individual differences among affected children the major manifestations of rheumatic fever, called "Jones criteria," are as follows:

1. Carditis with heart enlargement, often leaving permanent damage
2. Infection and vegetation on the heart valves causing permanent malfunction
3. Pericarditis with pericardial effusion and permanent adhesions
4. Congestive heart failure

5. Migratory polyarthritis (joint inflammation that moves about and affects many different joints); it does not leave permanent joint damage
6. Sydenham's chorea in which there is involuntary muscle movement and twitching, weakness, slurred speech, and a typical awkward gait
7. Cutaneous nodules in which nontender masses appear at the back of the head, along the spine, or at the elbows, lasting for weeks or months
8. Erythema marginatum, a red raised rash that appears as a wavy red line surrounding normal skin areas
9. Fever that rises and falls periodically during each day

Less spectacular than the acute form, but of equal importance, is the smoldering type of rheumatic fever in which definite symptoms are few. The child is easily fatigued, has a persistent rapid pulse rate, a low-grade fever, and mild muscle and joint pains, often called "growing pains." Without treatment permanent heart damage may result from this type of rheumatic fever just as it may result from the more obvious type.

Diagnosis is made on the basis of the history, presenting symptoms, throat culture, various blood tests, electrocardiogram, and x-ray examination of the heart. Treatment is directed toward eradicating any remaining streptococci, preventing future reinfections with streptococci, relieving symptoms, and treating the carditis to prevent permanent heart and valve damage. For accomplishment of these treatment goals, the child is given large doses of penicillin to eliminate the infection and then a prophylactic dose of sulfadiazine or penicillin to be taken regularly for several years to prevent reinfection. Salicylates and steroids are given for joint pains. Oxygen, digitalis, diuretics, and bed rest are ordered according to cardiac needs. Tranquilizers may be prescribed to reduce the involuntary muscle movements of chorea.

Nursing care during the acute phase is planned to reduce the work of the heart while meeting the total physical and emotional needs of the child. Absolute bed rest may be necessary for several weeks or even months. During this period correct body alignment, support of the joints, and good skin care are vital. Small, frequent feedings are easier for the child to manage than are large, heavy meals. Intake and output records are important. The temperature is taken at regular intervals, and the nature and rate of the pulse should be noted and recorded. When the heart begins to recover, the child is permitted limited activity, but must be closely supervised to avoid overactivity. As soon as possible the child should assume responsibility for personal care. During the long hours and days of convalescence, the child needs diversion, recreation, and education, according to physical ability. These needs can be met in consultation with an occupational or recreational therapist and by a visiting teacher. When the child is at home, the family may need to meet the many needs. The community health nurse can provide valuable assistance both directly and by referral of the child to various community agencies. Sometimes a child cannot be returned home for limited activity convalescent care. For these children pediatric convalescent hospitals may provide that needed bridge between intensive hospital care and a return to a relatively unsupervised situation in the home.

Dermatomyositis. Dermatomyositis is a rather common collagen disease occurring most often in children 5 to 12 years of age who live in rural areas. The disease primarily affects the skin and muscles. Onset is gradual, with increasing muscle weakness, pain, and swelling, especially of the shoulder girdle. Without treatment death occurs in 40% of those afflicted as a result of paralysis of the palate and respiratory muscles. A rash appears on the upper eyelids, with edema around the eyes and sometimes a butterfly rash on the cheeks. After a time the muscles atrophy from disuse and fibrous contractures result. The rash becomes a brownish pigmentation.

Treatment is aimed at maintaining muscle action in spite of pain and swelling, thus preventing atrophy and contractures. Corticosteroids provide the symptomatic relief necessary to carry out a program of vigorous physical therapy. If this is done, muscle function returns and recovery occurs.

Nursing care during the acute phase involves close supervision for possible obstruction of the airway and suctioning to remove secretions. Although nurses must be constantly aware of the danger of respiratory failure, they must help the child overcome anxiety and fear to be able to proceed with physical therapy. The nurse and family of the child may be instructed in some of the passive exercises and may assist in giving these exercises.

Periarteritis. Periarteritis is a disease in which small- and medium-sized arteries throughout the body become inflamed, leading to an inadequate blood supply to the tissues normally supplied by those vessels. Many systems of the body are affected. There is fever, weight loss, weakness, and vague pains. The fingers and toes may become gangrenous. The kidneys gradually fail and there may be coronary involvement. There is no known cause or treatment. Prognosis is poor.

Scleroderma. The rarest of collagen diseases in children, scleroderma produces disfiguring contractures of the skin as a result of chronic inflammation of the tissue surrounding blood vessels in the skin and subcutaneous tissue. There is no specific treatment, but physical therapy may prevent contractures. Complete recovery sometimes occurs.

Allergic reactions

An allergy is a reaction of the body to certain substances called *allergens* or *antigens*. They may come from various sources, including foods, inhalants such as pollens, dust, and animal dander; infectious agents such as fungi and bacteria; contactants such as wool and metal; drugs; and physical agents such as sunlight. These allergens cause the body to manufacture *antibodies* and the body reacts by various al-

lergic responses. The mechanism that causes these responses is still obscure but seems to be related to a metabolic phenomenon. When antibodies react with antigens, histamine and other active substances are released into the body tissue. They cause such allergic conditions as hay fever, asthma, diarrhea, eczema, urticaria (hives), serum sickness, and organ transplant rejection.

Although all individuals are believed to be potentially allergic, some seem to have a special inherited proneness that, together with the degree and duration of exposure and the nature of the allergen, affects the development of an allergic state. For this reason, persons with familial tendency to allergies must be careful to avoid overexposure to known allergens. Pregnant women with known allergies to certain foods are advised to avoid those foods during the sixth to ninth months of pregnancy. Breast feeding is recommended for their newborn infants to avoid the possibility of development of an allergy to cow's milk. Highly allergenic foods such as eggs are best avoided, and solid foods of all kinds are best cooked well to reduce their allergenic properties until the baby is 3 months of age when the digestive tract is more mature.

In infants, eczema and diarrhea are more common allergic manifestations. In later years, asthma and hay fever are more common.

agnosis of the allergic origin of these conditions is made by the physician on the basis of the medical and family history, a physical examination, laboratory tests of mucus and blood to determine the percentage of eosinophils (above normal in allergies), and skin sensitivity tests such as patch, scratch, and intracutaneous to identify the responsible allergens.

Treatment of allergic conditions consists of removing the offending allergen or hyposensitizing the child (reducing the response) if the offending allergen cannot be removed. The specific symptoms are then treated according to the child's need, such as antihistamine drugs for hay fever and steroids for severe asthma.

Hyposensitization is a process whereby the

Table 19-2. Common communicable diseases

Disease	Causal agent	Mode of transmission	Incubation period	Symptoms
Chicken-pox (vari-cella)	Virus	Direct or indirect contact with secretions from mouth or moist skin lesions	10 to 21 days	Slight fever, malaise, skin lesions appear in crops, progress from papule to vesicle to pustule, which ruptures and then to crusts
Diphtheria	Klebs-Löffler bacillus (*Corynebacterium diptheriae*)	Direct or indirect contact with secretions from respiratory tract or skin lesions of patient or carrier	2 to 5 days	Sore throat, moderate fever, rapid pulse, formation of grayish white membrane on back and side of throat
Infectious hepatitis (epidemic, catarrhal)	IH virus or A virus	Direct or indirect contact with infected feces, carriers, and infected food and water	25 days	Abrupt fever, nausea, malaise, tender liver; followed in 5 days by jaundice lasting 2 to 6 weeks; severe pruritus and diarrhea
Serum hepatitis (homologous serum hepatitis)	SH virus or B virus	Transmitted by injection of infected serum (blood transfusions, needle pricks); can never donate blood	2 to 6 months	Loss of appetite, jaundice, abdominal pain, general malaise, rarely fever
Influenza	Virus, various types	Direct or indirect contact with secretions from the respiratory tract	1 to 3 days (highly contagious); epidemic every 4 years; pandemic every 40 years	Fever, prostration, aches, pains, inflammation of respiratory mucous membrane
Infectious mononucleosis	Unknown	Probably airborne	5 to 15 days	Fever and enlarged lymph gland, malaise, fatigue, headaches, sore throat, eyelid edema; lasting 1 to 12 weeks

Communicable period	Treatment and nursing care	Complications	Prevention
1 day before rash to 6 days after its onset; dry crusts are not contagious	Prevent scratching by relieving itching with lotions; bed rest during eruptive period	Skin lesions may become infected and leave scars	No vaccine; so highly contagious 7 of 10 children catch it early in life
2 weeks after onset or until organisms are no longer present in discharges; carriers may be symptomless	Antibiotics, antitoxin, and analgesics; absolute bed rest, throat irrigations, humidification, bland diet; possible emergency tracheostomy; watch for muscle weakness	Paralysis of heart and throat muscles; toxins may affect nervous system	Immunization toxoid (DPT, DT); Schick test determines immunity
From onset to 6 weeks after; carriers may be symptomless	Bed rest until jaundice, abdominal pain, and liver tenderness subside—about 3 weeks; high amount of protein, carbohydrate, and vitamin B complex for diet	Relapses occur in 5% to 15%; acute yellow atrophy of liver causes death in 0.2%	Strict isolation; passive immunity for 6 weeks with gamma globulin
Lifelong; never should donate blood for transfusions	Bed rest until liver inflammation has subsided (3 to 4 months) with gradual return to activities; enriched diet	Acute liver necrosis with cirrhosis of liver and death	Use of disposable syringes and needles; careful screening of blood donors, excluding all who have had SH
Undetermined; probably from onset of fever until mucous secretions stop	Bed rest until 2 days after temperature is normal; analgesics; light diet with high fluid intake	Secondary bacterial pneumonia	Immunization against virulent strains; good for 1 year
Undetermined	Symptomatic; bed rest during febrile period; analgesics, gargle, and lozenges; high fluid intake	Secondary infection of throat, liver inflammation, spleen inflammation with rupture, meningitis, acute myocarditis, pneumonia with pleural effusion	No vaccine

Continued.

Table 19-2. Common communicable diseases—cont'd

Disease	Causal agent	Mode of transmission	Incubation period	Symptoms
Mumps (parotitis)	Virus	Direct or indirect contact with droplets from infected person	12 to 26 days	Swelling of glands of neck, headache, moderate fever, pain on swallowing, earache
Poliomyelitis	Virus of three types—asymptomatic, nonparalytic, and paralytic	Direct or indirect contact with nose and mouth secretions and feces of infected person (most infected persons show no symptoms)	3 to 35 days	Digestive upset, headache, fever, stiffness in neck, drowsy or irritable for 3 days, then paralysis or muscle weakness Depending on affected nerves: 1. Bulbar: cranial nerves 2. Spinal: skeletal muscles, diaphragm 3. Mixed: both spinal and cranial
Pertussis (whooping cough)	Bacteria—*Bordetella pertussis*	Direct or indirect contact with nose and throat secretions of infected persons	7 to 21 days	Begins as ordinary cold with a cough; cough worsens; frequent vomiting; whoop begins in 1 to 2 weeks
Rabies	Virus with an affinity for nervous tissue	Bite of rabid dog whose saliva contains rabies virus, or through previous break in skin	10 to 365 days (usually 30 to 50 days)	Mental depression, restlessness, and fever; progresses to painful spasms of throat muscles; excessive salivation, dehydration, coma, and death
Rubella (German measles, 3-day measles)	Virus	Direct contact with nose and mouth secretions; occasionally, via placenta to fetus	14 to 21 days	Mild symptoms of cold, followed by rash on face and body about third day
Rubeola (red measles)	Virus	Direct contact with nose and mouth secretions; occasionally via placenta to fetus	10 days	Moderate fever, watery eyes, photophobia, Koplik's spots, followed by rash appearing first on head, then on body

Communicable period	Treatment and nursing care	Complications	Prevention
Undetermined, probably during early stage until swelling disappears	Bed rest; analgesics; bland, soft diet; application of heat or cold to swollen glands	Meningoencephalitis, pancreatitis, other gland inflammation (orchiditis in post-pubertal males)	Mumps vaccine or passive immunity with gamma globulin
Unknown; usually isolated for 7 days	No specific treatment, symptomatic and supportive care, bed rest, hot packs for muscle spasm, tracheostomy and respiratory aid as needed; physical therapy and rehabilitation with orthopedic surgery and devices as needed	Paralysis of affected muscles	Salk vaccine injections (three) or trivalent Sabin oral vaccine
From 7 days after exposure until 3 weeks of typical cough	Hyperimmune gamma globulin, antibiotics for secondary infections, high fluid intake, cough medication, observation for respiratory distress	Bronchitis and bronchopneumonia	Pertussis vaccine given during first year (included in DPT)
From 5 days before symptoms appear until death	No treatment once symptoms develop; immediately after bite various types of vaccine may be given with daily injections for 14 to 21 days	Certain death once symptoms develop	Vaccination of all dogs; if any animal bites, it should be confined for a 10-day observation period
From 5 days before symptoms until 5 days after they disappear	No specific treatment, symptomatic care only	Rare for victim, but may cause serious fetal defects if mother has disease during first trimester	Rubella vaccine given after 1 year and before puberty
From 4 days before rash to 5 days after rash appears	Aspirin, soothing lotions, and rest; antibiotics for secondary infections	Otitis media, pneumonia, encephalitis	Measles vaccine given at 1 year

Continued.

Table 19-2. Common communicable diseases—cont'd

Disease	Causal agent	Mode of transmission	Incubation period	Symptoms
Smallpox	Virus	Direct or indirect contact with secretions from the skin lesions or mouth	7 to 16 days	Sudden fever with flu symptoms; 1 to 5 days later skin lesions appear; may be mild or severe type
Tetanus (lockjaw)	Exotoxin of the bacterium *Clostridium tetani*; spores live for years in animal feces, soil	Contaminated wounds; burns, newborn umbilicus, and postpartum uterus predisposed	5 to 21 days after infection	Stiffness of jaw, restlessness, irritability, neck stiffness, painful convulsions, respiratory muscle paralysis, coma, death
Typhoid fever	Bacterium *Salmonella typhosa*	Direct or indirect contact with urine or feces of infected person or carrier	1 to 3 weeks	In children atypical symptoms of respiratory infection may appear at first, intestinal irritation then occurs—diarrhea, pain, ulceration of intestine with bleeding and perforation; mild "walking" cases may also occur

sensitive child is given gradually increasing doses of the offending allergen once or twice a week until an amount is reached that protects the child from the allergen but does not produce side effects. Administered by injection, there is always danger of anaphylactic shock (see below). For this reason, whenever allergens are administered, epinephrine 1:1,000 and a syringe and needle are kept on hand ready for emergency use. As a further precaution, the child should wait in the physician's office for 20 minutes after each injection. Hyposensitization may need to be repeated annually for seasonal allergies.

Various allergic manifestations are discussed in the chapters dealing with the body systems affected; they are allergic rhinitis and asthma in Chapter 13, diarrhea in Chapter 14, and allergic dermatitis in Chapter 19. A discussion of serum sickness and anaphylactic shock as generalized allergic conditions follows.

Serum sickness. Serum sickness is an allergic reaction to the animal serums (especially horse) of immunization vaccines and to penicillin and other antibiotics. In children previously sensitized to sera or antibiotics, symptoms occur soon after injection, but in those not previously sensitized, symptoms may be delayed for 1 to 2 weeks. Skin lesions are the most striking manifestation, appearing either as hives or as various types of rashes. Itching is intense. There may be a low-grade fever, enlarged lymph nodes, and stiff, swollen, painful joints. Treatment is symptomatic and includes antipruritic lotions, steroids, antihistamines, analgesics, and sedatives.

Communicable period	Treatment and nursing care	Complications	Prevention
From earliest symptoms until all crusts fall off	No specific treatment; antibiotics for secondary infection; measures to reduce fever and itching	Secondary infection of skin lesions; scars may be disfiguring	Vaccination if traveling to endemic areas—World Health Organization declared disease eradicated in 1981
Not truly communicable except through draining wound	Tetanus antitoxin or hyperimmune human antitoxin, sedation, antibiotics for wound, tracheostomy and oxygen as needed, fluid balance, and nutrition	None, if treated promptly; death, if no treatment; horse serum of vaccine may cause serum sickness	Tetanus toxoid immunization in first year of life (included in DPT); antitoxin for passive immunity
As long as typhoid bacteria appear in urine or feces; carriers are symptomless	Chloramphenicol is specific drug, other antibiotics may be ordered; isolation of stool and urine; bed rest, supportive care, adequate fluids and nutrition; blood transfusions as needed	Intestinal hemorrhage, perforation, pneumonia, thrombophlebitis, myocarditis, nephritis, meningitis	Typhoid vaccination for those traveling to endemic areas; treatment of public water; testing of food handlers

Prognosis is usually good. Death is caused by fluid in the pericardial sac or edema of the pharynx closing the airway.

As a precaution against serum sickness, preinjection skin testing should be done whenever possible. When there is a history of previous reaction to one type of serum or antibiotic, an alternate type should be used. The parents and child should be informed of the importance of reporting past reactions because of the danger of a more serious reaction once the child has been sensitized.

Anaphylactic shock. Anaphylaxis is an immediate allergic reaction that in children is almost always precipitated by an injection of serum, an antibiotic, or an insect's venom. There is a prompt antigen-antibody reaction, with release of histamine into the bloodstream. The generalized reaction that follows is characterized by dilation of the blood vessels and smooth muscle spasm, causing respiratory impairment, shock, coma, and death. Symptoms may develop immediately after the injection or may be delayed as long as 30 minutes. Only immediate action can save the child's life. If the injection site or insect bite is on an extremity, a tourniquet should be placed around it on the near side of the injection. Epinephrine is given intramuscularly at the site of the injection and an equal amount is given on the opposite side. If circulatory collapse occurs, nikethamide (Coramine) is given. Dyspnea is treated with oxygen. Tracheostomy is done in cases of laryngeal edema.

When anaphylactic shock is caused by insect

bites, prevention is difficult. The physician may recommend hyposensitization. When it is caused by a serum or antibiotic, prevention involves a medical history, caution whenever these agents are injected, and emergency epinephrine on hand in case of reactions.

Communicable diseases

A *communicable disease* is an illness caused by an infectious organism or its toxins that can be passed from one person to another by direct contact or by indirect contact with infected objects, dust particles, water insects, animals, or foods. These diseases may be caused by bacteria, viruses, molds, yeast, protozoa, and rickettsiae. The *virulence* of an organism is its ability to overcome the defenses of the host, or infected person. A *carrier* is a person or animal harboring the infectious agent without showing symptoms of the disease. A *contact* is a person or animal exposed to the infectious agent. An *incubation period* is the time between exposure to the disease and the appearance of the first symptoms. The *communicable period* is the time during which an infected person can transmit the disease directly or indirectly to another person. *Immunity* is the ability of the body to resist infectious agents. A discussion of the mechanism of immunity and current pediatric practice in protecting children against some of the communicable diseases is provided in Chapter 3. A description of some of the most common communicable diseases of concern in pediatrics is included in Table 19-2. One should remember that these diseases occasionally occur in some communities (they are *endemic*), that sudden outbursts of many cases could occur (they might become *epidemic*), or that many more cases might occur over a wide geographic area (they might become *pandemic*) if it were not for the conscientious and continuous maintenance of immunization programs. The study of the incidence of disease is called *epidemiology*.

SUMMARY OUTLINE

I. **Integumentary system**
  A. Function
  B. Structure
    1. Epidermis
    2. Dermis
    3. Subcutaneous tissue
    4. Accessory organs
II. **Disorders of the integumentary system**
  A. Characteristics of skin lesions
  B. Nevi
  C. Irritations
  D. Dermatitis
    1. Causes
    2. Treatment and nursing care
  E. Acne
  F. Furuncles and carbuncles
  G. Impetigo
  H. Herpes simplex
  I. Warts
  J. Dermatomycoses (ringworm)
  K. Pediculosis
  L. Burns
    1. Classification
    2. Principles of treatment
    3. Immediate care
    4. Continuing treatment and care
    5. Plastic surgery and skin grafting
III. **Generalized conditions**
  A. Mesenchymal (collagen) diseases
    1. Systemic lupus erythematosus
    2. Rheumatic fever
    3. Dermatomyositis
    4. Periarteritis
    5. Scleroderma
  B. Allergic reactions
    1. Serum sickness
    2. Anaphylactic shock
  C. Communicable diseases

STUDY QUESTIONS

1. What are the functions of the skin? Which parts of the skin carry out each of the functions?
2. Define macule, papule, vesicle, pustule, fissure, wheal.
3. Discuss the nursing care of children with dermatitis including baths, methods of reducing scratching, and emotional support. What is a hypoallergic diet?
4. What are the principles of treatment for all burned patients? Discuss the immediate care of a child with first-, second-, and third-degree burns over 30% of the body. Describe the open and closed methods of treating burns, including the nursing care.

5. What is a collagen disease? Describe the usual course of rheumatic fever and list the major manifestations in children.
6. Describe the symptoms of anaphylactic shock. What immediate care may save the child's life?
7. Define epidemiology, pandemic, immunity, virulence, incubation period.

REFERENCES

American Hospital Association Committee on Infections Within Hospitals: Infection control in the hospital, rev. ed., Chicago, 1976, American Hospital Association.

Anthony, C.P., and Thibodeau, G.A.: Textbook of anatomy and physiology, ed. 10, St. Louis, 1979, The C.V. Mosby Co.

Benenson, A.S., editor: Control of communicable diseases in man, ed. 12, New York, 1975, American Public Health Association.

Brooks, S.M.: Basic science and the human body; anatomy and physiology, St. Louis, 1975, The C.V. Mosby Co.

Conway, B.L.: Carini and Owens' neurological and neurosurgical nursing, ed. 7, St. Louis, 1978, The C.V. Mosby Co.

Egan, D.F.: Fundamentals of respiratory therapy, ed. 3, St. Louis, 1977, The C.V. Mosby Co.

Jacoby, F.G.: Nursing care of the patient with burns, ed. 2, St. Louis, 1976, The C.V. Mosby Co.

Larson, C.B., and Gould, M.: Orthopedic nursing, ed. 9, St. Louis, 1978, The C.V. Mosby Co.

Lyght, C.E., ed.: Merck manual of diagnosis and therapy, ed. 15, New York, 1980, The Merck Co.

Milbauer, B.: Drug abuse and addiction: a fact book for parents, teenagers, and young adults, New York, 1972, New American Library.

Netter, F.H.: The Ciba collection of medical illustrations, vols I to V, New York, 1962, Ciba Corporation.

Traisman, H.S.: Management of juvenile diabetes mellitus, ed. 3, St. Louis, 1980, The C.V. Mosby Co.

Whaley, L.F., and Wong, D.L.: Nursing care of infants and children, St. Louis, 1979, The C.V. Mosby Co.

Children in society

20
Community resources for children and parents

PHILOSOPHY, DEVELOPMENT, AND PROBLEMS OF HEALTH SERVICES

Article V of the *Declaration of the Rights of the Child*, adopted by the United Nations on November 20, 1959, states: "The child who is physically, mentally, or socially handicapped shall be given the special treatment, education, and care required by his particular condition."

The philosophy of the innate value of children and their rights to special treatment, education, and care despite physical, mental, or social handicaps has profoundly affected medical research and health services to children. No longer are defective and diseased children isolated as "hopeless" and their conditions ignored as unimportant. Tremendous intellectual and physical energy is now expended on programs of research, training of personnel, special treatment facilities, public education, and direct services to children with the goal of giving each child an opportunity to realize the maximum potential.

These programs are extremely expensive. They require leadership, planning, and coordination. No ordinary family could afford treatment for a seriously handicapped child, much less the research and development of medical programs supporting that treatment. As social and medical needs have been recognized, however, various groups within society have organized both gift- and tax-supported agencies to meet special needs. Although this support is most commendable, it has led to a multiplicity of organizations and government agencies on local, state, national, and international levels. And this very profusion of agencies has made it difficult for the needy child to receive the help originally intended.

The pediatric nurse is often the one to whom the family first indicates its needs for social services, yet the nurse may not know where to turn for help. The medical social worker, other sources of information and referral, and some of the official and voluntary agencies available to provide social service are described in the following sections.

HEALTH SERVICE COUNSELING

Medical social workers. Medical social workers are professionally prepared individuals who specialize in meeting human needs in a social setting. They are best suited to assist a family with the special problems associated with a seriously ill or handicapped child. Many large hospitals employ medical social workers as staff members to whom both inpatients and outpatients may go for help. The pediatric worker in these hospitals should learn what channels are customarily used for referral to the social service department.

Because individuals, especially children, do not live alone but in families, social workers speak of "cases." Medical casework consists of *assessment* of the social situation, *identification* of social forces and factors, *determination* of intervention measures that are needed, *participation* of the clinical team of medical and social specialists in planning, and *evaluation* of the outcome.

Other sources of information and referral. When no hospital medical social worker is available, the child and the family may be referred to the local public health department or county welfare department. In 1967, federal legislation made it mandatory that county welfare departments using federal funds provide information and referral services to every citizen of the United States regardless of financial status.

Some communities have gift-supported family service agencies in which staff social workers provide casework as just described on a free or sliding-scale fee basis. In some localities a council of social agencies office provides referral information to anyone on request.

OFFICIAL HEALTH SERVICE AGENCIES IN THE UNITED STATES

Official, or tax-supported, health service agencies are found at the federal, state, and local levels of government. Various legislative acts at each level provide the funds, name the administrative agency, and identify the uses for which funds may be spent.

Federal Social Security Act

The Social Security Act was first enacted in 1935 and has served as the framework for many of the major health and welfare programs within the United States. It has been revised from time to time as changes and expansion have been needed. The act is divided into sections called "titles," including such well-known ones as: "Title IV Grants to States for Aid and Services to Needy families with Children and for Child Welfare Services, Title V Maternal and Child Health and Crippled Children's Services, Title XVI Grants to States for Aid to the Aged, Blind, or Disabled, Title XVII Grants for Planning Comprehensive Action to Combat Mental Retardation, and Title XIX Grants to States for Medical Assistance Programs (Medicaid). These titles provide funds for a variety of services that affect the welfare of children in the United States. The monies are made available to the states through federal grants-in-aid. Regional consultants work with the state agencies to ensure the most effective use of the funds.

Federal health services

Health services at the federal level are administered by the Department of Health and Human Services (HHS). Health services are administered under the divisions of Public Health Service, Social and Rehabilitation Service, and Human Development.

Public Health Service (PHS). The Public Health Service was originally formed by act of Congress in 1798 to care for merchant seamen. Since that time its functions have been vastly expanded. At the present the three major functions of the service are (1) identification of health hazards in the environment and in the products and services that enter a person's life, and development and assurance of standards for control of such hazards; (2) support and improvement of the delivery of comprehensive and coordinated physical and mental health services for all U.S. citizens; and (3) administration and support of research in medical and related sciences and health education. Its regional consultants work with state authorities in federal-state cooperative health programs.

Social and Rehabilitation Service (SRS). The Social and Rehabilitation Service was formed in 1967 to administer federal programs providing support to states, local communities, voluntary agencies, and individuals in the provision of social, rehabilitation, income maintenance, medical, maternal, and child welfare, and other necessary services to the aged, aging, children, youth, disabled, and needy families. The division of SRS maintains regional offices throughout the nation.

Human development. The Office of Human Development (OHD) was established in 1969, and under it is the Office of Child Development (OCD). The two major bureaus in OCD are the Children's Bureau and the Bureau of Child Development Services.

The Children's Bureau, first founded in 1912, has the following important functions: (1) it develops standards and provides technical assistance to states and public and private agencies for programs related to children and parents; (2) it supports a child welfare research and demonstration grant programs and evaluates programs serving children; and (3) it informs the public through a Division of Public Education using all

communications media and publishes a wide range of publications, including the magazine *Children Today*.

The Bureau of Child Development Services grew out of Head Start and was established in 1969 to carry out many additional functions, including (1) administering Project Head Start, a nationwide comprehensive program for disadvantaged children, designed to meet their health, education, and nutritional needs; (2) directing parent and child center programs for families with children under age 3; (3) conducting such innovative programs as Home Start, Health Start, and Child Development Association, a program to develop a new profession of accredited child care workers; (4) directing programs for Indian and migrant children; and (5) planning welfare reform day care programs and preparing manuals, licensing codes, and other materials related to day care.

State health services

Within the organization of each state are departments concerned with maternal and child health, crippled children's services, child welfare, and education. Although the functions of each of these departments vary from state to state, a composite picture of their functions and activities is as follows:

Maternal and child health
1. Administration of Children's Bureau funds for maternal and child health
2. Program planning, administration, and evaluation
3. Consultation to local areas
4. Direct services such as well-child conferences and prenatal clinics
5. Standard setting
6. Education and information for lay and professional workers
7. Research and demonstration projects
8. Coordination and cooperation with other health organizations
9. Direct payment for special services such as care of premature infants

Crippled children's services

1. Administration of Children's Bureau funds for crippled children
2. Program planning, administration, and evaluation
3. Consultation to local areas
4. Direct services such as diagnostic clinics
5. Standard setting
6. Education and information for lay and professional workers
7. Research and demonstration projects
8. Coordination and cooperation with other health organizations
9. Direct payment for hospital and medical care of crippled children

Child welfare

1. Administration of Children's Bureau funds for child welfare
2. Direct services for all needy families such as counseling of children and parents, protective services, homemaker services, day care, foster care, adoption, and services to single mothers and their babies
3. Additional services to families receiving Aid to Families with Dependent Children (AFDC), such as help with training, employment, household management, and medical care
4. Standard setting
5. Cooperation and coordination with other agencies
6. Referral services and emergency assistance to any family regardless of AFDC status

Education

1. Administration of the National School Lunch Program
2. Administration of the State Vocational Rehabilitation Program
3. Administration of the education of handicapped school-aged children
4. In many states, administration of the School Health Program

Local health services

The real test of the effectiveness of health services is whether they are actually reaching mothers and children where they live. This effectiveness depends in large measure on the quality and quantity of services offered by the city and county health departments across the nation. Such services vary considerably. In some large metropolitan areas a high quality and wide variety of services are offered. In some poor rural areas health and welfare services are extremely limited. This situation is gradually being changed under the pressure of public opinion and increased federal and state funding.

VOLUNTARY HEALTH SERVICE AGENCIES

Voluntary, gift-supported organizations provide a great variety of health and welfare services to mothers and children. Their activities consists of: (1) research and experimental projects; (2) public information and professional education; (3) legislative action; (4) payment for, or delivery of, direct services; and (5) fund raising. A large part of the work of each organization is done by professional and lay volunteers. To decrease duplication and increase coordination of effort, representatives of official agencies are often members of advisory committees of voluntary agencies, and representatives of voluntary agencies are often members of advisory committees of official agencies.

Historically, voluntary agencies have grown out of a local need. For this reason the largest number and widest variety of organizations are found at the local level. Some organizations have become statewide, some nationwide with state and local branches, and some worldwide with national branches. Although some local committees have compiled their own directory of social service agencies, there are no state, national, or international directories of social services agencies to which a pediatric worker or family may turn for information. To provide a beginning, and at the risk of serious omissions, a listing of a few of the nationwide health service agencies of particular interest to pediatrics follows. Many of these agencies are prepared to offer referral information to other state and local organizations.

Alcoholics Anonymous
c/o General Service Board of A.A., Inc.
P.O. Box 459, Grand Central Station
New York, N.Y. 10017
Publications; service to alcoholics and their families through local chapters.

American Academy of Pediatrics
P.O. Box 1034
Evanston, Ill. 60204
Research, education, publication of standards for child care.

American Cancer Society, Inc.
219 E. 42nd St.
New York, N.Y. 10017
Research, education, direct services through local chapters.

American College of Nurse-Midwives
50 E. 92nd St.
New York, N.Y. 10028
Research, education, publication.

American Dental Association, Inc.
222 E. Superior St.
Chicago, Ill. 60611
Research, education, legislation.

American Diabetes Association, Inc.
1 E. 45th St.
New York, N.Y. 10017
Research, education

American Foundation for the Blind, Inc.
15 W. 16th St.
New York, N.Y. 10011
Research, consultation, legislation, scholarships, local chapters; publishes directory of agencies serving blind persons in the United States and Canada.

American Heart Association, Inc.
7320 Greenville Ave.
Dallas, Texas 75231
Research, education, publication of bulletins and newsletters; direct services through local chapters; programs for rehabilitation of children and adults.

American Hearing Society, Inc.
919 18th St., N.W.
Washington, D.C. 20006
Education; encouragement of nationwide audiometric testing; publications; direct services—hearing testing; instruction in lip reading, auditory training, hearing aid consultation, speech correction, preschool classes, vocational guidance, recreational programs.

American Hospital Association
841 N. Lakeshore Dr.
Chicago, Ill. 60611
Research, education, publication of hospital standards.

American Medical Association
535 N. Dearborn St.
Chicago, Ill. 60610
Research, education, publications, legislation.

American National Red Cross
17th and D St.
Washington, D.C. 20006
Education, training of volunteers, cooperation with the Red Cross agencies of other nations, publications, educational material, disaster relief service, service for armed forces personnel and their families.

American Nurses Association
10 Columbus Circle
New York, N.Y. 10019
Education, publications, legislation.

Arthritis and Rheumatism Foundation
10 Columbus Circle
New York, N.Y. 10019
Research, education.

Child Welfare League of America
44 E. 23rd St.
New York, N.Y. 10010
Organization of child welfare agencies offering consultation, coordination, and development of standards for child care; publications.

Cooperative for American Relief Everywhere, Inc. (CARE)
660 First Ave.
New York, N.Y. 10016
Assembles needed relief supplies and delivers them to foreign countries, including self-help gifts, medicines, and food.

La Leche League, International
9616 Minneapolis Ave.
Franklin Park, Ill. 60131
Education, publication, services to mothers through local chapters to encourage breast feeding.

Medic Alert Foundation
1000 N. Palm
Turlock, Calif. 95380
Serialized medical identification emblems provided for any person with a medical problem; information available on 24-hour basis to authorized person giving first aid in an emergency; publications and professional education.

Muscular Dystrophy Association of America, Inc.
1790 Broadway
New York, N.Y. 10019

Research, education, conferences, publications; direct services—medical supplies, clinics, physical therapy, transportation.

National Association for Mental Health, Inc.
10 Columbus Circle
New York, N.Y. 10019

Research, public information, and education; consultation for governmental agencies; direct services—clinics and child guidance centers.

National Association for Retarded Children, Inc.
386 Park Ave., South
New York, N.Y. 1O016

Research, consultation, education.

National Cystic Fibrosis Research Foundation
521 5th Ave.
New York, N.Y. 10017

Research, education, public information; direct services through local chapters—treatment and diagnostic clinics.

National Federation of Licensed Practical Nurses
250 W. 57th St.
New York, N.Y. 10019

Professional organization of practical-vocational nurses throughout United States; education, publication, legislation.

National League for Nursing
10 Columbus Circle
New York, N.Y. 10019

Research, publications, educational testing, and standards.

The National Foundation—March of Dimes
880 Second Ave.
New York, N.Y. 10017

Research on birth defects and arthritis; education on central nervous system diseases, poliomyelitis, arthritis, birth defects, virus diseases; publishes Original Article Series and Reprint Series and other informational materials; direct services—payment of medical care for children under 10 years of age.

National Hemophilia Foundation
175 Fifth Ave.
New York, N.Y. 10003

Research; through state chapters services to hemophiliacs—clinics for emergency, diagnostic, dental, and orthopedic care.

National Multiple Sclerosis Foundation, Inc.
257 Park Ave., South
New York, N.Y. 10010

Research, education; direct service through local chapters—clinics and centers for diagnosis and medical care.

National Society for Autistic Children
621 Central Ave.
Albany, N.Y. 12206

Services to families, research, publications.

National Society for Crippled Children and Adults, Inc.
2023 W. Odgen Ave.
Chicago, Ill. 60612

Research, education through publications and films, direct services through local and state societies.

National Tuberculosis Association, Inc.
1790 Broadway
New York, N.Y. 10019

Research, public information, education, publications.

Parents Anonymous
Redondo Beach, Calif. 90277

Services to parents who wish to avoid child abuse; local chapters.

The People to People Health Foundation, Inc.
2233 Wisconsin Ave., N.W.
Washington, D.C. 20007

Fund raising, information on behalf of Project Hope.

Salvation Army
120 W. 14th St.
New York, N.Y. 10011

Direct services through local corps and outposts—summer camps, children's homes, girls' and boys' clubs, family welfare, nurseries and foster homes, homes and hospitals for unwed mothers, emergency disaster relief.

United Cerebral Palsy Association, Inc.
321 W. 44th St.
New York, N.Y. 10036

Research, public and professional education; direct services—support for facilities offering care, treatment, and special education of individuals having cerebral palsy.

United States Committee for UNICEF
331 E. 38th St.
New York, N.Y. 10016

Fund raising, information on behalf of UNICEF.

U.S. Department of Health and Human Services
Washington, D.C. 20013

INTERNATIONAL HEALTH SERVICE AGENCIES
United Nations Children's Fund (UNICEF)

In 1946 the United Nations established the United Nations International Children's Emergency Fund (UNICEF) primarily to provide emergency food and clothing to war-ravaged countries. In 1950 the official title was changed to the United Nations Children's Fund. Still known by the former initials, UNICEF, the organization has expanded its work in the fields of health, nutrition, and welfare, with an emphasis on training native personnel. The primary long-term goal is to help countries establish networks of basic health services for mothers and children. To this end it works with the national govern-

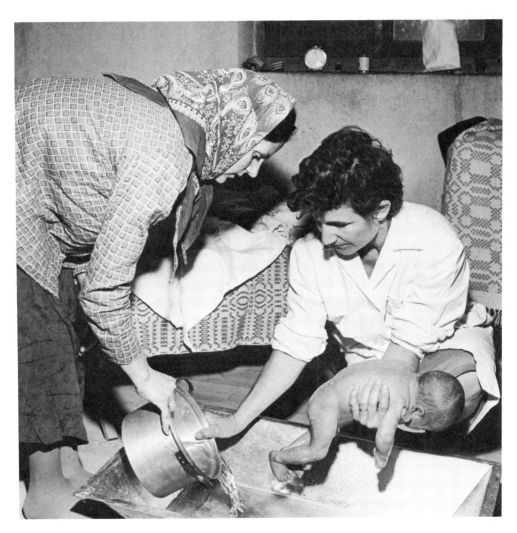

Fig. 20-1. Midwife gives a 10-day-old baby, just home from an Athens hospital, his first bath at home. Such rural health services are part of a project set up by the Greek government, assisted by UNICEF and WHO. (Courtesy UNICEF; photograph by Ilsa Kraus.)

ments and cooperates with other international agencies such as the Food and Agriculture Organization, the World Health Organization, the United Nations Bureau of Social Affairs, and the United Nations Educational, Scientific, and Cultural Organization (Fig. 20-1).

Among its specific programs are control of diseases that have a high incidence among children, such as trachoma, leprosy, and tuberculosis; maternal and child health programs, particularly prenatal, delivery, and infant care; distribution of powdered skim milk and development of safe milk production; and development of other food resources to provide better nutrition for mothers and children.

The United States Committee for UNICEF is a voluntary organization set up to work on behalf of the United Nations Children's Fund.

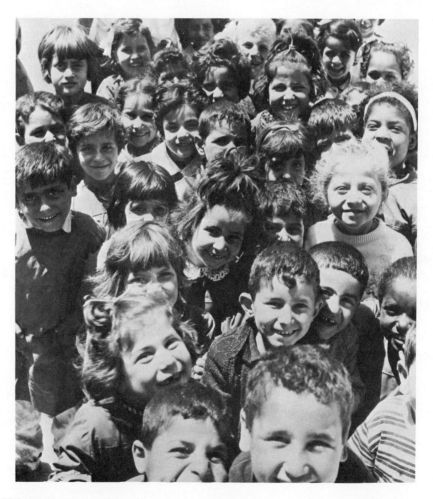

Fig. 20-2. Healthy, happy children—a national and world goal. (Courtesy UNICEF; photograph by Peter Larsen.)

World Health Organization (WHO)

The World Health Organization was established in 1948 and has become the chief international organization for health. It is composed of member nations, with each member contributing to its budget annually. The central headquarters are in Geneva, Switzerland, with regional offices in the Republic of Congo, Washington, D.C., India, Denmark, Egypt, and the Philippines.

Many programs of WHO are of direct importance to mothers and children. The organization actively fights such major infectious diseases as malaria, tuberculosis, and parasitism; provides for training of many types of health personnel, including midwives; promotes demonstration programs on the care of premature infants and the treatment of deficiency and diarrheal diseases; works with the United Nations Food and Agriculture Organization to improve the diet of people using locally available foods; assists in programs of environmental sanitation; warns of epidemics and makes available information concerning outbreaks of communicable diseases; has established a uniform set of International Sanitary Regulations; and publishes the *International Pharmacopoeia*.

In all history there has never been such effort to improve the health and welfare of children, nor have humans had the knowledge that may someday conquer the diseases that plague them. The time may indeed be near when the hope of people everywhere is realized—that of healthy, happy children (Fig. 20-2).

SUMMARY OUTLINE

  I. Philosophy, development, and problems of health services
  II. Health service counseling
    A. Medical social workers
    B. Other sources of information and referral
  III. Official health service agencies in the United States
    A. Federal Social Security Act
    B. Federal health services
      1. Public Health Service (PHS)
      2. Social and Rehabilitation Service (SRS)
      3. Human development
    C. State health services
    D. Local health services
  IV. Voluntary health service agencies
  V. International health service agencies
    A. United Nations Children's Fund (UNICEF)
    B. World Health Organization (WHO)

STUDY QUESTIONS

1. In the hospital where you work, what channel is available to you to obtain social services for one of your patients? What is a medical social worker?
2. Describe the functions of the Children's Bureau and the Bureau of Child Development Services. Which of these functions might you encounter in your work?
3. What is the difference between "official" and "voluntary" organizations? Describe the services of at least three voluntary agencies known to you.
4. Describe the services of UNICEF and WHO.

REFERENCES

King, M.H., ed.: Medical care in developing countries, New York, 1966, Oxford University Press, Inc.

U.S. Government organization manual, Washington, D.C., 1980-81, U.S. Government Printing Office.

Index